SECOND EDITION

Handbook of
Chronic Kidney
Disease
Management

SECOND EDITION

Handbook of Chronic Kidney Disease Management

Edited by

John T. Daugirdas, MD

Clinical Professor of Medicine
Division of Nephrology
University of Illinois at Chicago
Chicago, Illinois

Wolters Kluwer

Philadelphia • Baltimore • New York • London
Buenos Aires • Hong Kong • Sydney • Tokyo

Acquisitions Editor: Kate Heaney
Editorial Coordinator: Lindsay Ries
Production Project Manager: David Saltzberg
Manufacturing Coordinator: Beth Welsh
Marketing Manager: Rachel Mante-Leung
Production Service: Aptara, Inc.

Second Edition

9 8 7 6 5 4 3 2 1

Printed in China

Library of Congress Cataloging-in-Publication Data

Names: Daugirdas, John T., editor.
Title: Handbook of chronic kidney disease management / [edited by] John T.
    Daugirdas.
Description: 2. | Philadelphia : Wolters Kluwer, 2019. | Includes
    bibliographical references and index.
Identifiers: LCCN 2018026863 | ISBN 9781496343413 (pbk.)
Subjects: | MESH: Renal Insufficiency, Chronic–therapy | Guideline
Classification: LCC RC903 | NLM WJ 342 | DDC 616.6/1–dc23
LC record available at https://lccn.loc.gov/2018026863

Aseel Alsouqi, MD
Postdoctoral Fellow
Division of Nephrology and
    Hypertension
Vanderbilt University School of
    Medicine
Nashville, Tennessee

Deepa Amberker, MD
Fellow
Division of Nephrology
Washington University School of
    Medicine
St. Louis, Missouri

Cheryl A.M. Anderson, PhD, MPH, MS
Associate Professor of Preventive
    Medicine
Department of Family Medicine and
    Public Health
University of California San Diego
San Diego, California

George L. Bakris, MD
Professor of Medicine
Section of Endocrinology, Diabetes,
    and Metabolism
Pritzker School of Medicine
University of Chicago
Chicago, Illinois

David A. Calhoun, MD
Professor of Medicine
Vascular Biology and Hypertension
    Program
University of Alabama at
    Birmingham
Birmingham, Alabama

Doris T. Chan, MBBS, PhD, FRACP
Consultant Nephrologist
Department of Renal Medicine
Sir Charles Gairdner Hospital
Nedlands, Western Australia

Steven C. Cheng, MD
Associate Professor of Medicine
Division of Nephrology
Washington University in St. Louis
St. Louis, Missouri

Kai Ming Chow, MBChB, MRCP(UK)
Consultant and Chief of Service
Department of Medicine and
    Therapeutics
Prince of Wales Hospital
Sha Tin, Hong Kong, China

Jonathan C. Craig, MD, PhD
Professor of Clinical Epidemiology
School of Public Health
University of Sydney
Centre for Kidney Research
Children's Hospital at Westmead
Sydney, Australia

John T. Daugirdas, MD, FACP, FASN
Clinical Professor of Medicine
Division of Nephrology
University of Illinois at Chicago
Chicago, Illinois

Jeroen K.J. Deegens, MD, PhD
Assistant Professor of Medicine
Department of Nephrology
Radboud University Medical Center
Nijmegen, Netherlands

Christopher R. deFilippi, MD
Cardiologist
Vice-Chairman of Academic Affairs
Inova Heart and Vascular Institute
Falls Church, Virginia

Tsering Dhondup, MBBS
Fellow
Division of Nephrology and
  Hypertension
Mayo Clinic School of Medicine
Rochester, Minnnesota

Ruth F. Dubin, MD
Assistant Professor of Medicine
Division of Nephrology
University of California, San
  Francisco
San Francisco, California

Denis Fouque, MD, PhD
Professor of Nephrology
Department of Nephrology, Dialysis,
  and Nutrition
Université de Lyon
Lyon, France

Allon Friedman, MD
Associate Professor of Medicine
Division of Nephrology
Indiana University School of
  Medicine
Indianapolis, Indiana

**Jane H. Greene, RD, CSR,
LDN (retired)**
Renal Dietitian and CKD Education
  Coordinator
Vanderbilt University Medical
  Center
Nashville, Tennessee

**Lisa Gutekunst, MSEd, RD,
CSR, CDN**
Renal Dietitian
DaVita, Inc.
Buffalo, New York

Allison J. Hahr, MD
Associate Professor of Medicine
Division of Endocrinology,
  Metabolism, and Molecular
  Medicine
Northwestern University Feinberg
  School of Medicine
Chicago, Illinois

**Brenda R. Hemmelgarn,
MD, PhD**
Professor of Medicine and
  Community Health Sciences
University of Calgary
Calgary, Alberta

Michael Heung, MD, MS
Associate Professor of Medicine
Division of Nephrology
University of Michigan
Ann Arbor, Michigan

Susan Hou, MD
Professor of Medicine
Division of Nephrology and
  Hypertension
Loyola University School of
  Medicine
Maywood, Illinois

T. Alp Ikizler, MD
Professor of Medicine
Division of Nephrology and
  Hypertension
Vanderbilt University School of
  Medicine
Nashville, Tennessee

Ashley B. Irish, MBBS, FRACP
Consultant Nephrologist
Division of Nephrology and Renal
  Transplantation
Fiona Stanley Hospital
Murdoch, Western Australia

Tanya Johns, MD, MPH
Assistant Professor of Medicine
Division of Nephrology
Albert Einstein College of Medicine
Bronx, New York

David W. Johnson, MBBS (Hons), DMed(Res), PhD, FRACP
Professor of Medicine and
    Population Health
University of Queensland
City of Brisbane, Queensland

Hillary Johnston-Cox, MD, PhD
Fellow
Division of Cardiology
Hospital of the University of
    Pennsylvania
Philadelphia, Pennsylvania

Eric K. Judd, MD, MS
Assistant Professor of Medicine
Division of Nephrology
University of Alabama at
    Birmingham
Birmingham, Alabama

Rigas G. Kalaitzidis, MD
Hypertension Excellence Center
Department of Nephrology
University Hospital of Ioannina
Ioannina, Greece

Laetitia Koppe, MD, PhD
Assistant Professor of Nephrology
Deparament of Nephrology, Dialysis,
    and Nutrition
Université de Lyon
Lyon, France

Warren L. Kupin, MD
Professor of Clinical Medicine
Miami Transplant Institute
Katz Family Division of Nephrology
    and Hypertension
University of Miami Leonard M.
    Miller School of Medicine
Miami, Florida

Philip Kam-Tao Li, MBBS, MD
Chief of Nephrology and Honorary
    Professor of Medicine
Prince of Wales Hospital, Chinese
    University of Hong Kong
Sha Tin, Hong Kong, China

Joseph B. Lockridge, MD
Assistant Professor of Medicine
Division of Nephrology
Oregon Health and Sciences
    University and Portland VA
Portland, Oregon

Iain C. Macdougall, BSc, MD, FRCP
Consultant Nephrologist and
    Professor of Clinical Nephrology
Renal Unit
King's College Hospital
London, United Kingdom

Mark S. MacGregor, MSc, MBChB, FRCP(Glas)
Consultant Nephrologist
John Stevenson Lynch Renal Unit
University Hospital Crosshouse,
    NHS Ayrshire and Arran
Kilmarnock, Scotland

Timothy Mathew, MD
Emeritus Consultant Nephrologist
Renal Unit
Royal Adelaide Hospital
Adelaide, South Australia

Shona Methven, MD, MBChB, BSc
Consultant Nephrologist
Honorary Lecturer
Aberdeen Royal Infirmary, NHS
    Grampian
Aberdeen, Scotland

Edgar R. Miller, III, MD, PhD
Professor of Medicine
Division of Cardiovascular and
    Clinical Epidemiology
Johns Hopkins School of Medicine
Baltimore, Maryland

Emile R. Mohler, III, MD[†]
Associate Professor of Medicine
Division of Vascular Medicine
University of Pennsylvania School of
    Medicine
Philadelphia, Pennsylvania

[†]Deceased.

Mark E. Molitch, MD
Professor of Medicine
Division of Endocrinology,
    Metabolism, and Molecular
    Medicine
Northwestern University Feinberg
    School of Medicine
Chicago, Illinois

**Saw Yu Mon, MBBS, MMed,
MRCP, FRACP**
Nephrologist
Department of Nephrology
Princess Alexandra Hospital
Brisbane, Queensland

Keith C. Norris, MD, PhD
Professor of Medicine
David Geffen School of Medicine
University of California, Los Angeles
Los Angeles, California

Ann M. O'Hare, MD
Professor of Medicine
Division of Nephrology
University of Washington
Seattle, Washington

Ali J. Olyaei, PharmD
Professor of Medicine and
    Pharmacotherapy
Division of Nephrology and
    Hypertension
Oregon Health and Science University
Portland, Oregon

Qi Qian, MD
Professor of Medicine and
    Physiology
Division of Nephrology and
    Hypertension
Mayo Clinic School of Medicine
Rochester, Minnesota

Gregory J. Roberti, PharmD
Clinical Pharmacist
Department of Pharmacy Services
Oregon Health and Science University
Portland, Oregon

Franz Schaefer, MD
Professor of Pediatrics
Department of Pediatric Nephrology
Center for Pediatric and Adolescent
    Medicine
Heidelberg University
Heidelberg, Germany

Jenny I. Shen, MD, MS
Assistant Professor of Medicine
Division of Nephrology
David Geffen School of Medicine
Harbor-UCLA Medical Center
Los Angeles, California

Sandeep S. Soman, MD
Nephrologist
Division of Nephrology and
    Hypertension
Henry Ford Health System
Detroit, Michigan

James E. Tattersall, MD, MRCP
Specialty Doctor
Department of Renal Medicine
Leeds Teaching Hospitals NHS Trust
Leeds, United Kingdom

Allison Tong, MPH, MM, PhD
Associate Professor
Sydney School of Public Health
The University of Sydney
Sydney, New South Wales

Henry An Tran, MD
Assistant Professor of Medicine
Virginia Commonwealth University
Cardiologist
Inova Health System
Falls Church, Virginia

Agnes Trautmann, MD
Pediatric Nephrologist
Center for Pediatric and Adolescent
    Medicine
Heidelberg University
Heidelberg, Germany

Sharon I. Turban, MD, MHS
Assistant Professor of Medicine
Division of Nephrology
Johns Hopkins University School of
    Medicine
Baltimore, Maryland

Kavitha Vellanki, MD
Assistant Professor of Medicine
Division of Nephrology and
    Hypertension
Loyola University Medical Center
Maywood, Illinois

**Gerald F. Watts, DSc, MD, PhD,
FRACP, FRCP**
Professor of Medicine
University of Western Australia
    School of Medicine
Perth, Western Australia

Jack F.M. Wetzels, MD, PhD
Professor of Medicine
Department of Nephrology
Radboud University Medical Center
Nijmegen, Netherlands

Sandra F. Williams, MD
Assistant Professor of Medicine
Division of Endocrinology and
    Metabolism
Florida Atlantic University
Boca Raton, Florida

Timothy T. Yau, MD
Assistant Professor of Medicine
Division of Nephrology
Washington University School of
    Medicine
St. Louis, Missouri

Jerry Yee, MD
Professor of Medicine
Division of Nephrology and
    Hypertension
Henry Ford Hospital
Detroit, Michigan

Lenar Yessayan, MD, MS
Associate Professor of Medicine
Division of Nephrology
University of Michigan
Ann Arbor, Michigan

PREFACE

In the past 8 years since the First Edition of the *Handbook of Chronic Kidney Disease Management* was published, the basics of preventing and slowing progression of chronic kidney disease (CKD) have not changed, but incremental improvements have been realized. In this Second Edition, we decided to follow the modernist ethic of "less is more," as coined by the Chicago architect Mies van der Rohe. Thus, 44 chapters have been reduced to 31, excluding discussion of several disease-specific causes of CKD and some relatively avant-garde, but not yet clinically actionable, pathogenetic mechanisms. The goal remains the same: to increase survivability of our patients with CKD by mitigating cardiovascular risk and to slow the rate of CKD progression to the greatest extent possible.

Most of the authors who contributed to the First Edition continue to share their wisdom in this Second Edition. An important, new chapter was added about acute kidney injury and the impact this has on the causation of CKD. New chapter authors have taken on the topics of acid–base balance and heart failure.

This *Handbook* is intended not only for nephrologists, but also for the broad range of health care practitioners—internists, generalists including nurse practitioners and physician assistants, cardiologists, and endocrinologists—who care for early-stage CKD patients. I would like to express my deep and heartfelt thanks to the many chapter authors who worked so hard to make this book possible. Many thanks also to Aleksandra Godlevska for her modern art–inspired cover painting.

John T. Daugirdas, MD
Chicago, Illinois

CONTENTS

1

Assessing Kidney Function

Mark S. MacGregor and Shona Methven

WHAT THE KIDNEY DOES

Excretion of Waste Products

The kidneys are the major site for excretion of water-soluble waste products. In this task they are helped by the liver, which first converts many potentially toxic substances absorbed from the environment or produced via metabolism to water-soluble compounds, which the kidneys can then excrete into the urine.

Control of Water, Salt, Other Electrolytes, and Acid–Base (Homeostasis)

The kidneys respond continually to changes in blood volume as well as osmolality, and adjust the levels of water, sodium, potassium, calcium, magnesium, phosphorus, and many other compounds in the body by selectively excreting or reabsorbing them. The kidneys also maintain acid–base balance by excreting acid produced by metabolism of certain foods and can excrete excess alkali if necessary.

Endocrine and Metabolic Functions

The kidneys are the main site of production for a number of hormones, chiefly renin and erythropoietin. Vitamin D is activated in the kidneys by 1α-hydroxylation of 25-hydroxycholecalciferol. The kidneys affect the level of certain amino acids in the body by metabolizing or synthesizing them and also participate to a substantial degree in glucose control by gluconeogenesis.

ANATOMY

The Nephron: A Glomerulus and a Set of Renal Tubules

The kidney is set up anatomically as a filter and reabsorber connected in series. The basic unit is called the **nephron**. The nephron comprises a vascular portion, made up of a **glomerulus** and **renal venous plexus**, as well as a tubular portion, made up of a long, winding, **renal tubule**. The renal artery (Fig. 1.1, top) divides into smaller and smaller blood vessels, finally forming a very permeable meshwork of capillaries called a **glomerulus** (Figs. 1.1 and 1.2). The tuft of glomerular capillaries is supported by **mesangial cells** (a type of interstitial cell) and extracellular matrix. When blood passes through this capillary network, the hydrostatic pressure transmitted from the **afferent (upstream) arteriole** pushes a **filtrate** composed of fluid and solutes out through pores in the capillary wall into a space created by the glomerular capsule, which surrounds the glomerulus and opens into a renal tubule (Fig. 1.2).

1

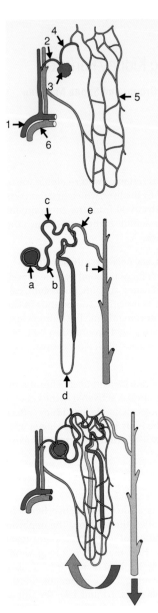

Vascular portion

1 arteriole

2 afferent arteriole

3 glomerulus

4 efferent arteriole

5 peritubular venous plexus

6 branch vein

Tubular portion

a glomerular capsule

b tubule

c proximal tubule

d hairpin turn in tubule
   (loop of Henle)

e distal tubule

f collecting duct
   (to renal pelvis)

FIGURE 1.1 Structure of the nephron, showing the vascular portion (**top**), the tubular portion (**middle**), and the two portions together (**bottom**).

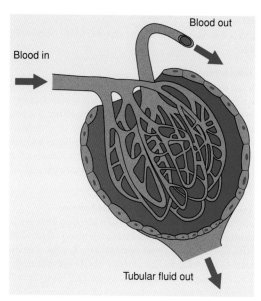

Blood out

Blood in

Tubular fluid out

FIGURE 1.2 Detail of glomerulus, showing the afferent and efferent arteriole and the glomerular capsule.

The glomerular filtrate is substantially modified as it flows through the **renal tubule**, which is lined by several distinct populations of specialized cells. The renal tubule, after taking a series of twists and turns and one hairpin loop, ultimately empties into the **renal pelvis**, from where its contents are routed to the bladder and then excreted as urine. The capillaries of the glomerulus reassemble into a single **efferent (downstream) arteriole** (see #4 in Fig. 1.1, top and Fig. 1.2), which then redivides into a very fine network of veins that form a mesh around the renal tubules (Fig. 1.1). This anatomy allows transfer of substances back and forth from the blood to different portions of the renal tubules. Some substances can be **secreted** via this network of veins into the renal tubules, effecting their excretion from the body. Also, some of the substances initially transferred from blood to the tubular fluid at the glomerulus by filtration, including water, can be **reabsorbed** from the tubules back into the blood via these tubular veins. Various hormones act along the length of the renal tubules, helping to fine-tune the absorption or secretion of a number of compounds and electrolytes.

PATHOLOGIC CHANGES WITH KIDNEY DISEASE

Functional Loss of Glomeruli

Disease affects the delicate lattices of glomeruli, tubules, and tubular veins that make up the kidney in various ways. Ultimately portions of glomeruli or entire glomeruli can become fibrosed along with their accompanying tubules, and their function is proportionately diminished or lost.

Proteinuria
Proteinuria is discussed later in this chapter in the section beginning on page 14.

Impaired Tubular Function
Many disease processes affect not only the glomeruli but also the cells lining the renal tubules and their surrounding network of veins. Tubular disease or fibrosis of the interstitium supporting the tubules can affect the transport of solutes between tubules and their surrounding veins. Kidney tubular disease usually manifests as problems in maintaining acid–base balance, resulting in acidosis or alkalosis, or as difficulties in properly adjusting potassium excretion, causing hypokalemia or hyperkalemia.

Impaired Endocrine and Sympathetic Nervous Function
With kidney disease, increased levels of renin may be secreted locally as well as into the systemic circulation. Hypoxia of renal tissue can increase the activation of renal sympathetic nerves and may cause an undesirable increase in the activity of the sympathetic nervous system. Erythropoietin production, as well as 1α-hydroxylation of vitamin D, can be impaired in diseased kidney tissue, and as a result, the amounts of circulating erythropoietin and active vitamin D can be reduced.

Measuring Renal Function
Normally each kidney contains from 500,000 to 1,000,000 glomeruli. As disease affecting the kidneys progresses, the number of functioning glomeruli is reduced, and the efficiency of remaining glomeruli may be impaired. Less blood is filtered to make tubular fluid, and the blood levels of compounds normally excreted by the kidneys increase. For this reason, one way to assess the overall health of the kidneys is to measure the blood levels of creatinine or similar substances that are normally filtered by the glomerulus.

Concept of Clearance
Glomerular Filtration Rate
One method of measuring kidney function is to determine what volume of blood the kidneys "clear" in a given unit of time. Because this clearance occurs in the glomeruli, it is called the glomerular filtration rate or GFR. The overall GFR is the sum total of the filtration by all of the individual glomeruli in the kidney. If one kidney is surgically removed, the GFR will be reduced by about 50%, because the surgeon will have removed half of the existing glomeruli (compensatory changes soon occur in the remaining nephrons to partially make up for this loss); GFR is approximately proportional to the number of **nephrons** in the two kidneys. GFR is also lower in smaller adults than in larger adults. Infants are born with the adult number of glomeruli, but GFR in children is much lower than in adults. This is because GFR is also proportional to the size of the glomeruli. For this reason, when

considering a GFR value in a given patient, one cannot decide if that value for GFR is too low, too high, or just right, unless one takes into account the size and age of the subject in which GFR was measured. In healthy individuals, GFR can increase beyond its basal level in response to certain stimuli (e.g., a protein load or pregnancy). Some believe loss of this renal functional reserve may be an early marker of renal disease.

Normalizing Glomerular Filtration Rate to Body Surface Area. The proper denominator to use when adjusting GFR to body size is a matter of debate, but traditionally, GFR is normalized in adults to body surface area (BSA)—usually per 1.73 m^2 of BSA (the average BSA in early 20th-century adults). BSA may be calculated by various formulae, including that of Gehan and George (1970) that depends on height and weight only: BSA $= 0.0235 \times W^{0.51456} \times H^{0.422446}$ where W = weight in kg and H = height in cm. When GFR is normalized to BSA, GFR/1.73 m^2 in young adult men and women is similar and is in the range of 110 to 120 mL/min. In children as young as 2 years, GFR/1.73 m^2 also remains close to 110 to 120 mL/min.

> **Example: How to normalize GFR to 1.73 m^2 BSA:**
> *Assume raw GFR is 100 mL/min*
> *If BSA = 1.5 m^2;* multiply 100 by 1.73/1.50
>   GFR/1.73 m^2 = **115 mL/min**
> *If BSA = 2.0 m^2;* multiply 100 by 1.73/2.0
>   GFR/1.73 m^2 = **86 mL/min**

The example shows two subjects with a GFR of 100 mL/min. One has a BSA of 1.5 m^2 and the other of 2.0 m^2. The BSA-normalized GFR is 115 mL/min per 1.73 m^2 in the smaller person and 86 mL/min per 1.73 m^2 in the larger person.

Decrease in Normalized Glomerular Filtration Rate With Age
As we age, a number of changes take place in the body composition, and the size as well as function of many body organs, including liver and kidneys, decrease. GFR declines with age from the third or fourth decade onward (Table 1.1). Estimates of the rate of decline vary from 0.4 to 1.2 mL/min per year. The median estimated GFR (eGFR) of 80-year-old U.S. subjects is 70 to 80 mL/min per 1.73 m^2 (see Chapter 26).

Measuring Glomerular Filtration Rate With Exogenous Markers
GFR cannot be measured directly. It can be measured indirectly using the clearance of an exogenous marker substance. Inulin is an exogenous marker that approaches the criteria for an ideal marker and is the recognized gold standard for measuring GFR. It is not widely used because of cost and inconvenience. Other exogenous markers are used occasionally in clinical practice (e.g., radioisotopes such as ^{51}Cr-EDTA, ^{125}I-iothalamate, ^{99m}Tc-DTPA, or iodinated contrast agents such as iohexol), but are limited by cost, inconvenience and exposure

TABLE 1.1	Estimated GFR/1.73 m² as a Function of Age
Age Range	**Average eGFR/1.73 m²**
20–29	116
30–39	107
40–49	99
50–59	93
60–69	85
70+	75

GFR, glomerular filtration rate; eGFR, estimated glomerular filtration rate.
From Coresh J, Astor B, Greene T, et al. Prevalence of chronic kidney disease and decreased kidney function in the adult U.S. population: Third National Health and Nutrition Examination Survey. *Am J Kidney Dis.* 2003;41:1–12, with permission.

to radioactivity, or iodinated contrast. These methods are used when it is essential to know the patient's GFR accurately (Soveri, 2014).

Estimating Glomerular Filtration Rate by Creatinine Clearance and Serum Creatinine

Creatinine is a widely used endogenous marker of GFR. It is a 113-Da molecule, which is produced at a relatively constant rate in each individual by breakdown of creatine in muscle.

Problem of Tubular Secretion of Creatinine

Creatinine is freely filtered by the glomerulus, but is also actively transferred from blood in the peritubular venous plexus to the tubular fluid by tubular secretion. For this reason, total creatinine clearance (CrCl) is the sum of GFR and tubular secretion, and so overestimates GFR. The percentage of creatinine removal by tubular secretion varies with kidney function. When GFR is high, this percentage is relatively small, but when GFR is low, the contribution of tubular secretion to CrCl becomes more important. Some drugs (e.g., trimethoprim, cimetidine) competitively inhibit creatinine secretion by the kidney tubules, and their use can result in an increase in serum creatinine that does not reflect a change in renal function or GFR.

Measurement Issues With Creatinine and Calibration to Isotope Dilution Mass Spectrometry

Most creatinine assays are based on the Jaffe colorimetric reaction with alkaline picrate. Various endogenous and exogenous substances (e.g., ketones, glucose, bilirubin) interfere with these colorimetric reactions, giving a falsely high or, less commonly, low creatinine. The degree of interference relates to the assay used and has the largest impact when serum creatinine is <1.6 mg/dL (<140 mcmol/L). Increasingly, laboratories are using enzymatic creatinine assays which are less affected by interferents. Efforts are being made to adjust all creatinine assays closer to a true creatinine level, using reference creatinine preparations and reference methods of measurement (iso-tope dilution mass spectrometry [IDMS]). IDMS-calibrated creatinine values are lower (by about 5% to 6%) than creatinine measured using the older alkaline picrate assays.

Creatinine Clearance by Urine Collection

GFR can be estimated by calculation of CrCl: a 24-hour urine speci-men is collected and its creatinine concentration is measured. A serum creatinine level is measured sometime during the collection period. It is assumed that the serum creatinine level is constant throughout the 24-hour collection period.

In adults, usually 500 to 2,000 mg/24 h of creatinine is recovered from the urine. Assume that 1,440 mg (12,730 mcmol) is recovered. Next, one calculates the serum concentration in mg/mL or mcmol/mL. Serum creatinine is usually measured per deciliter (which is 100 mL) or as mcmol/L. Assume that serum creatinine is 1 mg/dL (88.4 mcmol/L). This is equivalent to 0.01 mg/mL (0.0884 mcmol/mL). First, the creatinine excretion rate is calculated by dividing the recov-ered creatinine by the number of minutes comprising the collection period (1 day = 24 hours = $60 \times 24 = 1,440$ minutes). So if 1,440 mg (12,730 mcmol) was recovered from urine, and this was collected over 1,440 minutes, 1 mg/min (8.84 mcmol/min) is being excreted into the urine. To find out how much serum must be "cleared" per minute to get this 1 mg/min of removal, one simply divides the minute removal rate by the serum concentration:

Creatinine clearance = minute excretion rate/serum creatinine

Example (mg/dL):
minute excretion rate = 1.0 mg/min, serum creatinine = 1.0 mg/dL or 0.01 mg/mL, creatinine clearance = 1.0/0.01 = 100 mL/min

So, because each mL of serum contains 0.01 mg of creatinine, 100 mL/min would need to be cleared to account for the actual removal rate of 1 mg/min.

Example (mcmol/L):
minute excretion rate = 8.84 mcmol/min, serum creatinine = 88.4 mcmol/L or 0.0884 mcmol/mL, creatinine clearance = 8.84/0.0884 = 100 mL/min

The main pitfall with measuring CrCl is that patients often forget to urinate into the collection bottle every time. One needs to instruct the patient carefully to urinate into the toilet on rising, then note the time. Subsequently the patient needs to urinate into the collection bottle for 24 hours, and, very importantly, to urinate into the collec-tion bottle one final time on rising the next day. The exact start and end times of the collection period should be noted, with the start time being the initial urination into the toilet and the end time being the early-morning urination into the collection bottle on the following day.

TABLE 1.2	Expected Daily Creatinine Excretion Rates for Various Patients	

| | **Expected 24-hour Creatinine Excretion** | |
Patient Characteristics	mg/24 h	mmol/24 h
80 kg; man; age 20	**1,760**	15.5
80 kg; man; age 80	**1,385**	12.3
80 kg; woman; age 20	**1,380**	12.2
80 kg; woman; age 80	**1,005**	8.9
50 kg; woman; age 80	**630**	5.6

Calculations based on an equation for creatinine excretion rate by Ix et al. (2011).

The 24-hour creatinine excretion rate from the urine collection (calculated as urine concentration × volume, adjusted for 1,440 minutes) should always be compared with the expected excretion rate (Table 1.2). The expected creatinine excretion rate depends on how much muscle mass a person has, because creatinine is made from creatine, which is mostly made in muscle. Muscle mass depends on body weight, and for any given weight is higher in men than in women; and comparing African Americans to Caucasians, it is higher in the former group. Muscle mass decreases markedly as we age: creatinine excretion rate in an 80 year old is approximately 75% of that in a 20 year old with the same body weight. Patients with cachexia will also have a very low creatinine excretion rate, for example, patients with cirrhosis. Because CrCl is the minute creatinine excretion rate divided by the serum level, a person who is not generating much creatinine (because of a low muscle mass) will have a relatively low CrCl for a given level of serum creatinine. For example, Table 1.3 shows the same patients as in Table 1.2, each with a serum creatinine value of 1.3 mg/dL, along with what the calculated value of CrCl would be. Table 1.3 illustrates that a serum creatinine of 1.3 mg/dL (115 mcmol/L) can be consistent with relatively good kidney function in a muscular young man (CrCl = 94), but the same serum creatinine value in a small, elderly woman suggests a markedly reduced level of renal function (CrCl = 28). Table 1.4 shows the same calculations repeated in SI units.

TABLE 1.3	Expected Creatinine Clearances for Various Patients When Serum Creatinine Is 1.3 mg/dL (0.013 mg/mL)	

Patient Characteristics	**Clearance Calculation**	**Creatinine Clearance**
80 kg; man; age 20	**1,760**/(1,440 × 0.013) =	**94**
80 kg; man; age 80	**1,385**/(1,440 × 0.013) =	**74**
80 kg; woman; age 20	**1,380**/(1,440 × 0.013) =	**80**
80 kg; woman; age 80	**1,006**/(1,440 × 0.013) =	**54**
50 kg; woman; age 80	**630**/(1,440 × 0.013) =	**28**

Calculations based on an equation for creatinine excretion rate by Ix et al. (2011).

TABLE 1.4	Expected Creatinine Clearances for Various Patients When Serum Creatinine Is 115 mcmol/L (0.115 mcmol/mL)	
Patient Characteristics	**Clearance Calculation**	**Creatinine Clearance**
80 kg; man; age 20	**15,531**/(1,440 × 0.115) =	**94**
80 kg; man; age 80	**12,247**/(1,440 × 0.115) =	**74**
80 kg; woman; age 20	**12,176**/(1,440 × 0.115) =	**80**
80 kg; woman; age 80	**8,893**/(1,440 × 0.115) =	**54**
50 kg; woman; age 80	**5,576**/(1,440 × 0.115) =	**28**

Calculations based on an equation for creatinine excretion rate by Ix et al. (2011).

Estimating Creatinine Clearance From Serum Creatinine
A number of authors have developed equations that—using body size, sex, age, and sometimes race—attempt to predict the creatinine daily excretion rate. If this can be estimated, then the minute excretion rate can be calculated simply by dividing the estimated daily creatinine excretion rate by 1,440, the number of minutes in a day; and then the estimated CrCl can be obtained by dividing the estimated per-minute excretion rate by the serum creatinine level. Use of such equations obviates the need for 24-hour urine collection.

Cockcroft and Gault Equation. The most popular equation for estimated creatinine clearance (eCrCl) was proposed by Cockcroft and Gault (1976):

$$eCrCl = (140 - age) \times (wt\ in\ kg) \times (0.85\ if\ female) / (72 \times serum\ creatinine\ [SCr]\ in\ mg/dL)$$

or when SCr is measured in mcmol/L:
$$eCrCl = (140 - age) \times (wt\ in\ kg) \times (0.85\ if\ female) / (0.814 \times serum\ creatinine\ [SCr]\ in\ mcmol/L)$$

A new equation to predict 24-hour creatinine excretion rate was developed by Ix et al. (2011) which was validated in a number of large databases and is based on creatinine measured using an IDMS-calibrated assay. The Ix equation is used as follows:

When creatinine excretion rate is in mg/24 h and SCr is in mg/dL:
$$eCrCl = ([24\text{-hour excretion rate in mg}]/1,440)/(0.01 \times SCr)$$
24-hour excretion rate in mg = $880 - 6.2 \times age + 12.5 \times (wt\ in\ kg) + (35\ if\ black) - (380\ if\ female)$
or when SCr is measured in mcmol/L:

$$eCrCl = ([24\text{-hour excretion rate in mcmol}]/1,440)/(0.001 \times SCr)$$
24-hour excretion rate in mcmol = $8.84 \times (880 - 6.2 \times age + 12.5 \times [wt\ in\ kg] + [35\ if\ black] - [380\ if\ female])$

Note that the equation by Ix et al. (2011) has a much less steep age correction than Cockcroft and Gault, and the correction for female sex is more severe than the 0.85 term commonly used by

Cockcroft and Gault. Weight is included in both the Ix and the Cock-croft and Gault prediction equations for CrCl, because the result of these equations is the "raw" CrCl, uncorrected for BSA.

Modification of Diet in Renal Disease Equation. The Modification of Diet in Renal Disease (MDRD) equation (Levey, 1999) was developed in the course of the MDRD study, which studied patients primarily with a GFR <60 mL/min (per 1.73 m^2). GFR was measured using isotopically tagged iothalamate; iothalamate is a substance that is filtered by the glomerulus but, unlike creatinine, is not secreted by the tubules. The relationship between iothalamate-based GFR and SCr in the MDRD participants is shown in Figure 1.3. For a given value of SCr, the GFR was found to be about 26% lower in women than in men and about 18% lower in Caucasians (men or women) than in African Americans. Muscle mass in African Americans tends to be higher, so their cre-atinine excretion rate is relatively increased. There are several forms of the MDRD equation. Where the SCr measurement technique has been calibrated to IDMS standards and SCr is in mg/dL, the MDRD equation for eGFR is:

$$eGFR/1.73\ m^2 = 175 \times SCr^{-1.154} \times age^{-0.203} \times (1.21\ \text{if black}) \times (0.742\ \text{if female})$$

If the serum creatinine measurement was not calibrated to IDMS, the 175 term should be replaced with 186. When SCr is available in mcmol/L, one needs to first convert the SCr value from mcmol/L to mg/dL; this is done by dividing by 88.4.

Normalization to 1.73 m^2 Body Surface Area. The MDRD equation does not have any body-size terms, such as weight. This is because the GFR that it calculates is normalized to 1.73 m^2 of BSA, so the body-size terms cancel out. If one knows a patient's estimated BSA, one can easily normalize the Ix CrCl to 1.73 m^2, or "denormalize" the MDRD eGFR/1.73 m^2 to a non-normalized or "raw" eGFR (Table 1.5).

MDRD Equation When GFR >60. Few patients with GFR values >60 mL/min per 1.73 m^2 were included in the sample from which the MDRD equation was derived, and the MDRD equation is increasingly un-reliable if GFR is ≥60 mL/min per 1.73 m^2. Above 60, the MDRD equation underestimates GFR and has decreased precision. For this reason, some recommend that eGFR values >60 estimated using the MDRD equation be reported simply as being >60 without giving a number.

Chronic Kidney Disease Epidemiology Collaboration 2009 Equations. The Chronic Kidney Disease Epidemiology Collaboration (CKD-EPI) equations are a set of eight equations to estimate GFR from serum creatinine, and were based on a large patient sample that did include many patients with GFR >60 mL/min per 1.73 m^2 (Levey, 2009). The choice of which equation to use depends on whether the patient is

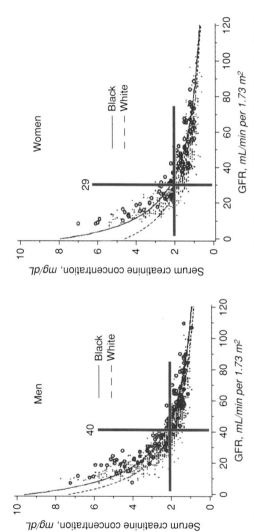

FIGURE 1.3 Relation of serum creatinine to GFR in men versus women in African Americans (*solid lines*) and in Caucasians (*dotted lines*). GFR was measured by renal clearance of iothalamate. Data from the MDRD study. The heavy lines show that (for a Caucasian aged 39), a SCr of 2.0 mg/dL corresponds to a GFR of 40 mL/min per 1.73 m² in men versus only 29 in women. (Levey AS, Bosch JP, Lewis JB, et al. A more accurate method to estimate glomerular filtration rate from serum creatinine: a new prediction equation. Modification of Diet in Renal Disease Study Group. *Ann Intern Med.* 1999;130:461–470.)

T A B L E 1.5	Effect of Normalization of Creatinine Clearance or Estimated Glomerular Filtration Rate to 1.73 m² Body Surface Area

60-Year-Old White Man, SCr = 1.0 mg/dL (IDMS)

Patient Characteristics	Body Surface Area	Ix et al. CrCl		MDRD	
		CrCl	CrCl/1.73 m²	eGFR	eGFR/1.73 m²
80 kg; height 180 cm	2.0	105	91	88	76
50 kg; height 160 cm	1.5	79	91	65	76

SCr, serum creatinine; IDMS, isotope dilution mass spectrometry; CrCl, creatinine clearance; MDRD, Modification of Diet in Renal Disease; eGFR, estimated glomerular filtration rate.

male or female, African American or Caucasian, and if the SCr is in a lower or higher range (see Appendix 1 for the equations). When eGFR is <50 mL/min per 1.73 m², the MDRD and CKD-EPI equations give similar results. Above this level, CKD-EPI gives more reliable results for eGFR. The CKD-EPI 2009 equations are now the preferred GFR estimating equations recommended by international guidelines (Kidney Disease: Improving Global Outcomes [KDIGO], 2012).

Cystatin C: CKD-EPI 2012 Equations. Cystatin C is a 13-kDa protein that is produced at a constant rate by all nucleated cells. It is freely filtered at the glomerulus and is not secreted but is reabsorbed within the tubules, where it is completely metabolized. Cystatin C shows promise as an endogenous marker of GFR, because it does not vary with muscle mass, sex, or age (although this has been challenged). The CKD-EPI collaboration developed a further set of equations to estimate GFR using creatinine, cystatin C, or both together (Inker, 2012) with the combination of creatinine and cystatin C giving the best precision and accuracy. International guidelines recommend using these cystatin C–based equations when there is concern about the accuracy of the creatinine-based equations (KDIGO, 2012). Specifically, they suggest using them if confirmation of the diagnosis of CKD is required, when creatinine-based eGFR is 45 to 59 and there are no other markers of kidney damage. The cystatin C assay is more costly, the assays have not been standardized to the same extent as creatinine, and the serum cystatin C level may be affected by inflammation or thyroid disease. These issues have limited the popularity of cystatin C–based estimates of GFR. In some populations, cystatin C–based eGFR predicts cardiovascular outcomes better than creatinine-based eGFR. Whether this means that cystatin C is a better marker of GFR or detects additional cardiovascular risk mediated by another pathway is unclear.

Web Calculators. A number of web-based calculators are available to help calculate CrCl (Ix or Cockcroft and Gault) or eGFR (MDRD or CKD-EPI) using these various equations, as detailed in Chapter 30.

Impact of Race. The MDRD and CKD-EPI formulae include terms for race (African American or Caucasian) to improve the accuracy of GFR estimate in each racial group. Factors have also been derived for other races, including Chinese and Japanese (see Chapter 27).

PROBLEMS WITH GLOMERULAR FILTRATION RATE ESTIMATES

Acute Kidney Injury

Whether based on serum creatinine or cystatin C, the eGFR prediction equations assume that kidney function is stable at the time it is measured. For example, if a patient has an SCr of 1.0 mg/dL (88 mcmol/L) and then undergoes removal of both kidneys, the next day the SCr may only have risen to 1.6 mg/dL (140 mcmol/L), and an eGFR equation may estimate that GFR is about 40 mL/min per 1.73 m^2, when the true GFR will be 0. The only way to estimate kidney function using creatinine in a changing situation is to perform a urine collection for creatinine, and then to divide the minute excretion rate by the average SCr value during the collection period.

Very Lean or Very Obese Patients

In very lean or cachectic patients with body mass index (BMI) <18.5 kg/m^2, both MDRD and Cockcroft and Gault tend to overestimate eGFR/1.73 m^2 and CrCl, respectively. Formal GFR measurement or a 24-hour collection to determine CrCl, is best done in cachectic patients, patients with cirrhosis and ascites, or patients with significant amputations. Cystatin C–based estimates of GFR may also have a role to play in these patients.

Obese patients (BMI >30 kg/m^2) present a particular problem for creatinine-based estimates of GFR. The creatinine prediction equations that incorporate weight (e.g., those by Cockcroft and Gault or Ix et al.) will overestimate CrCl, because they assume that creatinine generation rate increases as a linear function of body weight (W). In fact, creatinine generation is proportional to lean body mass (LBM; for equations to calculate, see Appendix 2), and the ratio of LBM/W decreases as BMI increases. LBM should not be directly substituted for weight into the Cockcroft and Gault or Ix equations, because LBM/W is markedly less than 1.0. Also, the ratio of LBM/W is lower in women than in men and decreases for both sexes with age. Currently there is no extensively validated equation to predict creatinine excretion in obese patients. The Salazar–Corcoran equation (1988) can be thought of as a modified Cockcroft and Gault equation that was derived from an obese population and takes into account serum creatinine, sex, actual weight, age, and height (see Appendix 1 for equations). As another complicating factor, in obese individuals, a 24% increase in CrCl has been reported that may relate to glomerular hyperfiltration because of increased kidney size, increased blood volume to kidneys, and other factors (Levey and Kramer, 2010). In obese patients, the MDRD equation gives more accurate results for GFR than Cockcroft and Gault (Froissart, 2005), but with extreme obesity, the MDRD and presumably the CKD-EPI equations, still may overestimate CrCl considerably (Pai, 2010). Thus, for very

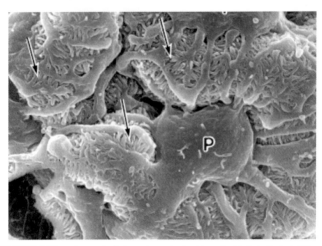

FIGURE 1.4 Photomicrograph of glomerular podocytes (visceral epithelial cells that sit like amoebas on top of the glomerular capillaries, wrapping each capillary in their foot processes [*arrows*]). P, podocyte cell body. (Modified with permission from Takahashi-Iwanaga H. Comparative anatomy of the podocyte: a scanning electron microscopic study. *Microscopy Res Tech.* 2002;57:196–202.)

obese patients in whom an accurate CrCl is required, it may be best to simply collect a 24-hour urine, or use a cystatin C–based estimate.

PROTEINURIA

Anatomy

The glomerular capillary network is surrounded by epithelial cells called **podocytes** (Fig. 1.4). These cells have foot processes that wrap around each capillary, supporting it structurally. The podocytes also secrete a **basement membrane** around the outside of each capillary wall (Figs. 1.4 and 1.5). The podocytes wrap numerous foot processes around each capillary in such a way as to form a number of **slit pores** between adjacent foot processes (Fig. 1.5). These slit pores open into the glomerular capsule, which collects the fluid filtered from the glomerular capillaries and which routes this filtrate into the kidney tubule. There is also a carbohydrate-rich layer lining the luminal aspect of endothelial cells called the glycocalyx. The endothelial glycocalyx, the pores in the endothelial cells of the capillary, the basement membrane, and the slit pores together form a **filtration barrier** between the blood in the capillary and the tubular fluid in the glomerular capsule.

Urine Proteins in Health

Large proteins in the glomerular capillary are almost completely held back from entering the filtrate in the glomerular capsule by the filtration barrier shown in Figure 1.5. Small proteins (typically molecules <4-nm diameter), however, are freely filtered. Between those extremes, the proportion filtered is determined by molecular size, conformation, and charge. For example, because the basement

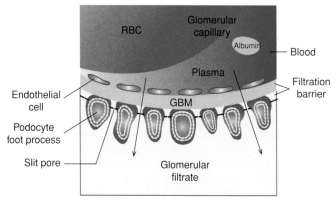

FIGURE 1.5 Detail of the filtration barrier between the blood in the glomerular capillary and the glomerular filtrate. The barrier is composed of endothelial glycocalyx (not shown), fenestrated endothelial cells, the endothelial glycocalyx (not shown), the glomerular basement membrane (GBM), and the filtration slits between adjacent podocytes.

membrane is negatively charged, negatively charged molecules such as albumin (molecular weight 55,000 Da) have an especially difficult time getting through this filtration barrier. Whatever protein is filtered is almost completely reabsorbed in the proximal tubule, where it is catabolized by tubular cells. A small quantity of protein in the tubular fluid comes from another source: It is actively secreted into the tubular fluid by the cells lining the tubules.

The upper limit of normal for the total amount of protein excreted into the urine over a day is 150 to 200 mg. For albuminuria, 30 mg/day is typically taken as the upper limit of normal, although most healthy adults excrete substantially less.

Proteinuria in Renal Disease
Pathology: Destruction of the Podocytes and the Filtration Barrier
Some pathologic processes in the kidney affect the function of the filtration barrier made up of the podocytes, the glomerular basement membrane, the glomerular capillaries, and the endothelial glycocalyx (see Fig. 1.5). As this barrier is compromised, increasing amounts of protein leak out into the glomerular filtrate, overwhelming the capacity of the tubules to absorb and metabolize the leaked protein. For this reason, one important sign of kidney disease is **proteinuria**.

Urine Proteins in Disease
In disease, the amount of proteinuria may increase dramatically and can exceed 10 g/day. Total proteinuria >3.5 g/day is described as *nephrotic-range* proteinuria. Proteinuria >1 g/day is typically due to glomerular damage. Lower levels can also be caused by tubular damage, leading to failure of reabsorption of filtered small proteins. Excess circulating protein can overwhelm tubular reabsorption (e.g., free light chains in myeloma), and is referred to as "overflow proteinuria."

The quantity of proteinuria correlates with the risk of progressive decline in kidney function, although this relationship varies in specific diseases. Whether this simply reflects severity of the glomerular injury, or whether this is because proteins are directly toxic to the tubule remains controversial. Proteinuria is also associated with an increased risk of cardiovascular events and death (Chronic Kidney Disease Prognosis Consortium, 2010).

In renal disease, albumin is usually the predominant protein in urine. Monitoring of albuminuria is useful to detect kidney disease in gradually evolving conditions, such as diabetic nephropathy. Low-level albuminuria can identify early onset of kidney disease in diabetic patients, and in both diabetic and nondiabetic patients is a marker for increased cardiovascular risk. Various other proteins also are present in urine in renal disease, and their concentrations vary independently of albumin. Their significance as predictors of outcomes remains uncertain.

In recognition of the central importance of albuminuria in renal disease, international guidelines (KDIGO, 2012) advocate a schema for quantification of albuminuria to be included in any description of chronic kidney disease (CKD). They suggest the suffix A1 (normal or mildly increased albuminuria), A2 (moderately increased, previously referred to microalbuminuria), and A3 (severely increased). Please see section entitled "Staging Chronic Kidney Disease" for further details.

Measurement
Total Proteinuria and Albuminuria
Total proteinuria is measured by various physicochemical techniques. Each assay has differing sensitivities for different proteins, making comparison between assays difficult. Total protein assays have a lower precision than albumin assays and are difficult to standardize. Urinary albumin is usually measured by immunoassays that measure albumin specifically. High-performance liquid chromatography measures consistently higher values for albumin, as it also measures some albumin fragments, and perhaps allows for earlier detection of low levels of albuminuria. Currently there is no international reference method in use or reference material for urine albumin assays, and interlaboratory variation for albuminuria is not substantially better than for total proteinuria. However, a reference method for albuminuria based on liquid chromatography mass spectrometry has been developed by the U.S.-based National Kidney Disease Education Project and other groups and is being validated.

Dipstick Urinalysis
Urine dipstick tests for total protein or albumin are cheap and easy to use. They utilize chemical or immune reactions to generate color changes in reagent pads. Machine reading improves reliability but raises cost. Dipsticks measure concentration rather than quantity, which is their main disadvantage. Urine volume varies widely according to hydration status and osmotic load. Significant proteinuria may be missed in dilute urine and may be overdiagnosed in concentrated

urine. Total protein dipsticks typically detect a protein concentration of >0.15 g/L but are less sensitive to some nonalbumin proteins, such as immunoglobulin light chains (Bence Jones protein). Albumin-specific dipsticks are sensitive to low concentrations of urine albumin (>20 mg/L) but do not address the issue of urine concentration.

Traditionally, dipstick urinalysis was used as a screening test to identify patients requiring more formal analysis. Patients with one plus or more on a dipstick would have a urine sample sent for laboratory analysis. However, given the poor positive and negative predictive value of dipsticks, guidelines increasingly recommend a formal laboratory spot urine sample for screening, diagnosis, and monitoring. There is still a role for identification of proteinuria using dipstick urinalysis in resource-poor settings (and to identify nonvisible hematuria).

Spot Urine Samples

Spot urine samples are simple to obtain and can be analyzed for total protein or albumin. Although more accurate than dipsticks, this still generates a concentration rather than a quantity.

Creatinine is excreted in urine at a relatively constant rate. Thus, if creatinine concentration is also measured, a total protein–creatinine ratio (TPCR) or albumin–creatinine ratio (ACR) can be calculated to adjust for the degree of urinary concentration. ACR correlates well with 24-hour urinary albumin excretion, and TPCR correlates well with 24-hour urinary protein excretion (Table 1.6). Spot samples from the first micturition after rising are recommended as they correlate well with 24-hour excretion and exclude orthostatic proteinuria. However, a random daytime sample will usually give acceptable accuracy.

TABLE 1.6	Measures of Albumin and Protein Excretion in the Urine			
KDIGO Classification of Albuminuria	**Albumin/ Creatinine Ratio: mg/g (mg/mmol)[a]**	**Albumin Excretion Rate: mg/ day**	**Protein/ Creatinine Ratio: mg/g (mg/mmol)[a]**	**Protein Excretion Rate: mg/ day**
A1 (normal or mildly increased)	<30 (<2.5 men, <3.5 women)	<30	<150 (<15)	<150
A2 (moderately increased)	30–300 (2.5–30 men, 3.5–30 women)	30–300	—	—
A3 (severely increased)	>300 (>30)	>300	>450 (>45)	>450
Nephrotic Range (included in A3)	—	—	>3,000 (>300)	>3,500

The albumin and total protein columns are only approximate equivalents as there is a nonlinear relationship between albuminuria and total proteinuria.
[a]Note that the TPCR values calculated using U.S. units vs. International units are only approximately 10 times higher. To accurately convert mg/g of creatinine to mg/mmol of creatinine, multiply by 0.113.

Problem With Normalizing to Creatinine

As discussed above, creatinine excretion rate varies markedly with muscle mass. In particular, women and the elderly have a lower creatinine generation rate, and this artificially inflates the ratio of protein or albumin to creatinine. Some have used a higher diagnostic threshold for ACR in women to partially address this, but this is not advocated by KDIGO (2012). A similar issue is likely to occur with different races, but there is less evidence available (Mattix, 2002).

Orthostatic Proteinuria. Protein excretion varies diurnally and with posture, with lowest values overnight and when supine. In patients with a benign condition called orthostatic proteinuria, 1 to 2 g/day of urinary protein are excreted when erect, but levels normalize when the patient is supine.

Transient Benign Proteinuria. Transient proteinuria may develop in response to stress (e.g., fever, exercise, cardiac failure). If proteinuria is detected, the sample should be repeated. It is not necessary to exclude urinary infection in asymptomatic patients.

Clinical Uses of Spot Urine Samples for Albumin–Creatinine Ratio or Total Protein–Creatinine Ratio. Proteinuria is measured for various reasons. It gives information about renal or cardiovascular risk. The level of proteinuria may be used as a threshold for investigation (e.g., renal biopsy) and/or treatment and also may be useful in monitoring disease progression and response to therapy.

Albumin–Creatinine Ratio Versus Total Protein–Creatinine Ratio. In diabetic kidney disease, albuminuria is used for screening, diagnosis, and monitoring. A spot sample for ACR is most convenient, but albumin concentration or 24-hour urine excretion is still used by some. The ACR appears to be a better predictor of renal outcomes in diabetic patients than urinary albumin concentration or 24-hour urinary albumin excretion (Lambers Heerspink, 2010). First-morning voids are more reliable than random spot urines to monitor albuminuria (Witte, 2009).

In nondiabetic kidney disease, it is more controversial as to whether total proteinuria or albuminuria is the more appropriate test to screen for kidney disease. Historically, most research studies measured 24-hour urinary total protein excretion, and thresholds for risk, investigation, and intervention arise from those studies. Albuminuria has theoretical, technical, and clinical advantages outlined above. It is also not known what level of risk is carried by proteinuric patients with low levels of albuminuria but high levels of nonalbumin proteinuria.

Low-level albuminuria in the nondiabetic population is associated with increased cardiovascular risk. This low level of urinary albumin excretion may not be reliably detected by total protein assays. But there is relatively limited evidence about which nondiabetic patients should be screened for low-level albuminuria and what treatments should be used.

Once ACR exceeds 300 mg/g, it adds no additional information to TPCR (which is cheaper). One strategy is to measure TPCR in all patients, and if TPCR is <450 mg/g, then measure ACR as well. Another is to measure ACR in all patients and then switch to TPCR if ACR exceeds 500 to 1,000 mg/g (Kidney Disease Outcomes Quality Initiative [KDOQI], 2002). However, some argue that ACR should be recommended for all, for simplicity in order to encourage the quantification of proteinuria by clinicians.

Timed Urine Collections. A timed urine collection (usually 24 hours) is traditionally the accepted gold standard for measuring proteinuria. As discussed in the section above pertaining to 24-hour urine collections for CrCl, urine collections are often poorly performed, leading to substantial inaccuracy. Collections of <24-hour duration are affected by diurnal variation in protein excretion and are less useful. Split day and night collections can be used to formally diagnose orthostatic proteinuria.

Clinical Applications. In patients with abnormal muscle mass, ACR or TPCR may give misleading results, due to uncommonly low or high urine creatinine concentrations and a 24-hour urine should be considered, particularly if results are close to thresholds for clinical decisions. If monitoring the response of proteinuria to therapy is important, ACR or TPCR may not be sufficiently reliable, and some still advocate 24-hour urines (e.g., to monitor adequacy of immunosuppression when treating lupus nephritis). Proteinuria is an indication for kidney biopsy, and commonly total proteinuria >1 g/day is used as a threshold. This threshold will be affected by the overall clinical picture—for example, if associated with hematuria, a lower threshold of 450 mg/day may be used. Proteinuria thresholds (>0.5 to 1 g/day) may also be used as indications for treatment with angiotensin-converting enzyme inhibitors.

STAGING CHRONIC KIDNEY DISEASE

The U.S. National Kidney Foundation's Kidney Disease Outcomes Quality Initiative (KDOQI) established a new classification of CKD in 2002, which has been rapidly accepted worldwide (Table 1.7).

The classification staged CKD based on eGFR/1.73 m^2 as estimated by the MDRD equation, where the levels of eGFR are multiples of 15 and 30, with stage 5 being <15 mL/min per 1.73 m^2, stage 4 being 15 to 30, stage 3 being 30 to 60, and stages 1 and 2 being >60. In this classification system, having an eGFR <60 mL/min per 1.73 m^2 is enough to have CKD, regardless of other evidence of kidney disease. To have CKD when eGFR >60 mL/min per 1.73 m^2, some other signs of kidney disease must be present. For more details about the KDOQI staging system, please see Chapters 2 and 31.

Many elderly patients with eGFR in the range of 45 to 60 mL/min per 1.73 m^2 are classified as having CKD (stage 3) by the KDOQI classification, despite the fact that in the absence of other markers of kidney

Stage	Definition	eGFR (mL/min per 1.73 m²)
1	Presence of kidney damage, with normal or raised GFR	≥90
2	Presence of kidney damage, with mildly reduced GFR	60–89
3a	Moderately reduced GFR	45–59
3b		30–44
4	Severely reduced GFR	15–29
5	End-stage kidney disease	<15

eGFR, estimated glomerular filtration rate; GFR, glomerular filtration rate.
Source: Kidney Disease: Improving Global Outcomes.

disease, their level of renal function is usually relatively stable. It may not be appropriate to label such subjects as having a disease when they are asymptomatic. The use of the term *stage* also implies that patients will progress through the stages, which for the large majority is not true. The KDOQI classification does not address the underlying cause of CKD. It is important to pursue a diagnosis in appropriate patients. However, in the majority of elderly asymptomatic patients with stable stage 3 CKD and without proteinuria or hematuria, a firm diagnosis is unlikely to be achieved despite thorough investigation. See Chapter 26 for a further discussion of CKD in the elderly.

THE KDIGO CHRONIC KIDNEY DISEASE CLASSIFICATION

KDIGO is an international collaboration which revised the KDOQI classification based on meta-analysis of CKD cohorts with ~1.5 million subjects (KDIGO, 2012). KDIGO defines CKD as abnormalities of kidney structure or function, present for at least 90 days and with implications for health. KDIGO requires CKD to be classified based on the cause of the **C**KD, the **G**FR, and the level of **A**lbuminuria (the CGA classification).

- KDIGO requires the cause of CKD to be stated, addressing previous criticisms that CKD was being treated as a diagnosis, with insufficient thought being given to the cause.
- The KDIGO GFR classification is similar to the KDOQI classification, but divides stage 3 into stage 3a and 3b (3a when 45 ≤ GFR ≤ 59, and 3b when 30 ≤ GFR ≤ 44). Stage 3a is more common than 3b (70% to 75% of stage 3) and less clearly associated with risk, particularly in the elderly.
- KDIGO also requires classification based on albuminuria: A1 ACR <30 mg/g; A2 ACR 30 to 299 mg/g (i.e., low-level albuminuria); and A3 ACR ≥300 mg/g (i.e., macroalbuminuria). This is in recognition that proteinuria is at least important as GFR for prognosis.

So for example, patients might be classified as:

- CKD G3a A1: ischemic nephropathy
- CKD G4 A3: membranous nephropathy

References and Suggested Readings

Chronic Kidney Disease Prognosis Consortium;Matsushita K, van der Velde M, Astor BC, et al. Association of estimated glomerular filtration rate and albuminuria with all-cause and cardiovascular mortality in general population cohorts: a collaborative meta-analysis. *Lancet*. 2010;375:2053–2054.

Cockcroft DW, Gault MH. Prediction of creatinine clearance from serum creatinine. *Nephron*. 1976;16:31–41.

Coresh J, Astor BC, Greene T, et al. Prevalence of chronic kidney disease and decreased kidney function in the adult U.S. population: third national health and nutrition examination survey. *Am J Kidney Dis*. 2003;41:1–12.

Coresh J, Selvin E, Stevens LA, et al. Prevalence of chronic kidney disease in the United States. *JAMA*. 2007;298:2038–2047.

Earley A, Miskulin D, Lamb EJ, et al. Estimating equations for glomerular filtration rate in the era of creatinine standardization: a systematic review. *Ann Int Med*. 2012;156:785–795.

Eckardt KU, Berns JS, Rocco MV, et al. Definition and classification of CKD: the debate should be about patient prognosis—a position statement from KDOQI and KDIGO. *Am J Kidney Dis*. 2009;53:915–920.

Fine DM, Ziegenbein M, Petri M, et al. A prospective study of protein excretion using short-interval timed urine collections in patients with lupus nephritis. *Kidney Int*. 2009;76:1284–1288.

Froissart M, Rossert J, Jacquot C, et al. Predictive performance of the modification of diet in renal disease and Cockcroft-Gault equations for estimating renal function. *J Am Soc Nephrol*. 2005;16:763–773.

Gehan E, George SL. Estimation of human body surface area from height and weight. *Cancer Chemother Rep*. 1970;54:225–235.

Graziani MS, Gambaro G, Mantovani L, et al. Diagnostic accuracy of a reagent strip for assessing urinary albumin excretion in the general population. *Nephrol Dial Transplant*. 2009;24:1490–1494.

Inker LA, Levey AS, Tighiouart H, et al. Performance of glomerular filtration rate estimating equations in a community-based sample of Blacks and Whites: the multiethnic study of atherosclerosis. *Nephrol Dial Transplant*. 2018;33:417–425.

Inker LA, Schmid CH, Tighiouart H, et al. Estimating glomerular filtration rate from serum creatinine and cystatin C. *N Engl J Med*. 2012;367:20–29.

Ix JH, Wassel CL, Stevens LA, et al. Equations to estimate creatinine excretion rate: the CKD epidemiology collaboration. *Clin J Am Soc Nephrol*. 2011;6:184–191.

Kidney Disease: Improving Global Outcomes. KDIGO 2012 clinical practice guideline for the evaluation and management of chronic kidney disease. *Kidney Int*. 2012; 1–150.

Kidney Disease Outcomes Quality Initiative. Clinical practice guidelines for chronic kidney disease: evaluation, classification and stratification. *Am J Kidney Dis*. 2002;39:S46–S75. Available from www.kidney.org/Professionals/kdoqi. Accessed May 31, 2018.

Lambers Heerspink HJ, Gansevoort RT, Brenner BM, et al. Comparison of different measures of urinary protein excretion for prediction of renal events. *J Am Soc Nephrol*. 2010;21:1355–1360.

Levey AS, Bosch JP, Lewis JB, et al. A more accurate method to estimate glomerular filtration rate from serum creatinine: a new prediction equation. Modification of Diet in Renal Disease Study Group. *Ann Intern Med*. 1999;130:461–470.

Levey AS, Kramer H. Obesity, glomerular hyperfiltration, and the surface area correction. *Am J Kidney Dis*. 2010;56:255–258.

Levey AS, Stevens LA, Schmid CH, et al; CKD-EPI (Chronic Kidney Disease Epidemiology Collaboration). A new equation to estimate glomerular filtration rate. *Ann Intern Med*. 2009;150:604–612.

Mattix HJ, Hsu CY, Shaykevich S, et al. Use of the albumin/creatinine ratio to detect microalbuminuria: implications of sex and race. *J Am Soc Nephrol*. 2002;13:1034–1039.

Pai MP. Estimating the glomerular filtration rate in obese adult patients for drug dosing. *Adv Chronic Kidney Dis*. 2010;17:e53–e62.

Salazar DE, Corcoran GB. Predicting creatinine clearance and renal drug clearance in obese patients from estimated fat-free body mass. *Am J Med.* 1988;84:1053–1060.

Seegmiller JC, Eckfeldt JH, Lieske JC. Challenges in measuring glomerular filtration rate: A clinical laboratory perspective. *Adv Chronic Kidney Dis.* 2018;25:84–92.

Soveri I, Berg UB, Björk J, et al; SBU GFR Review Group. Measuring GFR: a systematic review. *Am J Kidney Dis.* 2014;64:411–424.

Stevens LA, Coresh J, Feldman HI, et al. Evaluation of the modification of diet in renal disease study equation in a large diverse population. *J Am Soc Nephrol.* 2007;18:2749–2757.

Stevens LA, Nolin TD, Richardson MM, et al; Chronic Kidney Disease Epidemiology Collaboration. Comparison of drug dosing recommendations based on measured GFR and kidney function estimating equations. *Am J Kidney Dis.* 2009;54:33–42.

Stevens LA, Schmid CH, Zhang YL, et al. Development and validation of GFR-estimating equations using diabetes, transplant and weight. *Nephrol Dial Transplant.* 2010;25:449–457.

Vickery S, Stevens PE, Dalton RN, et al. Does the ID-MS traceable MDRD equation work and is it suitable for use with compensated Jaffe and enzymatic creatinine assays? *Nephrol Dial Transplant.* 2006;21:2439–2445.

Witte EC, Lambers Heerspink HJ, de Zeeuw D, et al. First morning voids are more reliable than spot urine samples to assess microalbuminuria. *J Am Soc Nephrol.* 2009;20:436–443.

Screening and Management Overview

Saw Yu Mon and David W. Johnson

The scope of the problem presented by chronic kidney disease world-wide is both large and growing (Bello, 2017a; Bello, 2017b). To reca-pitulate what was discussed in Chapter 1, CKD is defined on the basis of a measured or estimated glomerular filtration rate (eGFR) <60 mL/min per 1.73 m^2 and/or evidence of kidney damage for at least 3 months (Table 2.1). CKD is classified according to five GFR stages (Table 2.2) and degree of albuminuria (Table 2.3). Recent evidence has demonstrated that the degree of albuminuria provides prognostic information that is at least as important as GFR staging, such that information about both parameters should be considered for optimal staging and risk stratification (Johnson, 2015).

SCREENING

Early identification and management of CKD is highly cost effective and can reduce the risk of kidney failure progression and cardiovascu-lar disease by up to 50% (Johnson, 2015). General practitioners, other primary health care clinicians and nonrenal specialists play a crucial role in CKD early detection and management. Although the case for widespread population screening has been argued (de Jong and Brenner, 2004), the available evidence suggests that the optimal cost-effective strategy is targeted, opportunistic screening of patients with 1 or more risk factors for CKD (Collins, 2009). All people attending their doctor should be assessed for CKD risk factors as part of routine primary health encounters. Key risk factors include diabetes mellitus, obesity, hypertension, smoking, family history of kidney failure, older age (>60 years old), established cardiovascular disease, and a previ-ous history of acute kidney injury (Johnson, 2015). If a patient has any one of the key risk factors for CKD, they should undergo a Kidney Health Check as per the algorithm depicted in Figure 2.1. Guideline-based approaches to screening adult patients with CKD are described in Chapter 31. Screening programs for detection of CKD in children exist in a number of Asian countries but data on the cost effectiveness of such programs are limited (Hogg, 2009). Current American Acad-emy of Pediatrics guidelines do not recommend routine screening of children for CKD and are supported by a recent analysis that reported that screening dipstick urinalysis is not cost effective (Sekhar, 2010).

Urine testing is also very sensitive for detecting hematuria and can identify all significant bleeding. Since hematuria is often related to menstruation or urinary tract infection, a positive urinary dipstick

TABLE 2.1 Definition of Chronic Kidney Disease

1. GFR <60 mL/min per 1.73 m^2 for ≥3 mo with or without evidence of kidney damage[a]; OR
2. Evidence of kidney damage (with or without decreased GFR) for ≥3 mo, as evidenced by any of the following:
   - Albuminuria (micro or macro)
   - Proteinuria
   - Persistent hematuria (where other causes, such as urologic conditions, have been excluded)
   - Pathologic abnormalities (e.g., abnormal renal biopsy)
   - Radiologic abnormalities (e.g., scarring or polycystic kidneys seen on renal imaging)

[a]Methods for measuring or calculating GFR are discussed in Chapter 1.

TABLE 2.2 Stages of CKD According to Measured or Estimated GFR

Kidney Function Stage	GFR (mL/min per 1.73 m^2)	Description
1	≥90	Normal or increased GFR
2	60–89	Normal or slightly decreased GFR
3a	45–59	Mild–moderate decrease in GFR
3b	30–44	Moderate–severe decrease in GFR
4	15–29	Severe decrease in GFR
5	<15 or on dialysis	End-stage kidney failure

TABLE 2.3 Stages of CKD According to Albuminuria

Albuminuria Stage[a]	Urine Albumin: Creatinine Ratio (mg/mmol)	24-hr Urine Albumin (mg/day)	Urine Protein: Creatinine Ratio (mg/mmol)	24-hr Urine Protein (mg/day)
Normalbuminuria (A1)	<3 (<30 mg/g)	<30	<5	<50 (<500 mg/g)
Microalbuminuria (A2)	3–30 (30–300 mg/g)	30–300	5–50	50–500 (500–5,000 mg/g)
Macroalbuminuria (A3)	>30 (>300 mg/g)	>300	>50	>500 (>5,000 mg/g)

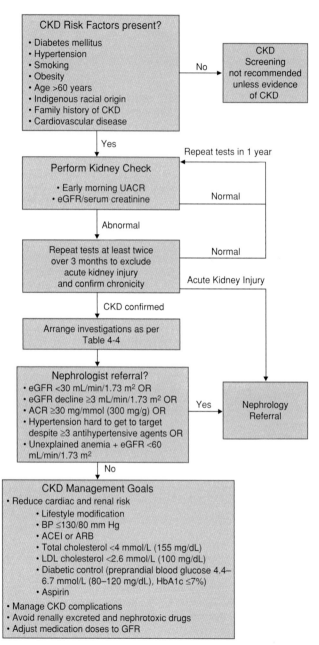

FIGURE 2.1 Algorithm for screening and management of CKD in adult patients.

for blood should be repeated and then confirmed with urine micros-copy and culture. Urine phase contrast microscopy often can help differentiate between glomerular and nonglomerular hematuria. The approach to management of persistent microscopic hematuria is detailed in Chapter 19.

ONCE CKD HAS BEEN DIAGNOSED, WHAT ADDITIONAL INVESTIGATIONS SHOULD BE ORDERED?

When CKD is initially diagnosed, it is important to be sure that acute kidney disease is not missed by assuming that the first abnormal eGFR represents a long-standing condition. An early repeat of the test is appropriate if there is any suspicion of an acute condition. Furthermore, it is also important to exclude treatable pathology, such as urinary tract obstruction, vasculitis, nephrotic syndrome, and rapidly progressive glomerulonephritis. Particular attention should be paid to symptoms (e.g., urinary symptoms, rash, arthritis, or other features of a connective tissue disorder), known medical problems, previous urinary tract infec-tions, cardiovascular risk factors, use of potentially nephrotoxic drugs (e.g., NSAIDs, intravenous drugs, previous compound analgesic use, Chinese herbal therapies), and family history of kidney disorders (e.g., polycystic kidneys). Physical examination should concentrate particu-larly on the skin, joints, cardiovascular system, and abdomen (palpable kidneys or bladder, audible renal bruits). Digital rectal examination of the prostate should be considered in older men. Recommended labora-tory investigations are listed in Table 2.4.

TABLE 2.4	Diagnostic Evaluation in Patients With Confirmed CKD

1. Generally indicated
   - Full blood count
   - Serial serum urea/electrolytes/creatinine/eGFR/albumin
   - Fasting lipids and glucose
   - Urine microscopy and culture
   - Renal ultrasound scan
2. Sometimes indicated
   - HbA1c (if diabetic)
   - Serum calcium, phosphate, parathyroid hormone and iron studies (if eGFR <60 mL/min per 1.73 m²)
   - Serum and urine electrophoresis (>40 yrs old), serum-free light chains
   - Antinuclear antibodies, extractable nuclear antigens, complement studies (if rash, arthritis, or features of connective tissue disease)
   - Antiglomerular basement membrane antibody (if pulmonary symptoms or acutely deteriorating kidney function)
   - Antineutrophil cytoplasmic antibodies, cryoglobulins (if constitutional symptoms, rash or respiratory symptoms or acutely deteriorating kidney function)
   - Hepatitis B, hepatitis C, human immunodeficiency virus serology (if risk factors)
   - Renal biopsy (especially if persistent UACR >60 mg/mmol or proteinuria >1,000 mg/day)

T A B L E 2.5	CKD Management Plan	
CKD Stage	**Review**	**Clinical Action Plan**
1–2 (eGFR >60)	Every 3–6 mo ▪ Blood pressure ▪ Weight ▪ UACR (quarterly) ▪ Urea, creatinine, electrolytes ▪ eGFR ▪ Fasting glucose ▪ Fasting lipids	▪ Initial investigations to exclude treatable CKD (Table 2) ▪ Reduce cardiovascular risk ▪ Reduce CKD progression
3a and 3b (eGFR 30–59)	Every 1–3 mo ▪ Blood pressure ▪ Weight ▪ UACR (quarterly) ▪ Urea, creatinine, electrolytes ▪ eGFR ▪ Fasting glucose ▪ Fasting lipids ▪ Full blood count ▪ Iron stores (3–6 mo) ▪ Calcium and phosphate ▪ Parathyroid hormone (quarterly)	As above plus ▪ Early detection and management of CKD complications ▪ Avoidance of renally excreted and nephrotoxic medications ▪ Adjustment of medications to levels appropriate for kidney function ▪ Appropriate specialist referral when indicated (Fig. 2.1)

MANAGEMENT OF PATIENTS WITH CKD

The review and management of patients with CKD in the primary care setting depends on the CKD stage and individual circumstances (Table 2.5, Fig. 2.1), and is described throughout this handbook.

Smoking and Drug Abuse

Smoking is associated with more severe proteinuria and kidney failure progression in patients with CKD. The clinical evidence for this association is stronger for diabetic patients. Stopping smoking has been associated with retardation of CKD progression. If required, nicotine replacement therapy or other medication should be considered to promote abstinence. Use of cocaine and injection drugs (see Chapter 3) is responsible for a substantial amount of CKD and acute kidney injury as well.

Obesity

Caloric restriction leading to weight loss has been shown to result in amelioration of CKD in overweight/obese individuals (Chapter 4), as evidenced by diminished proteinuria and improved kidney function. Ideally, body mass index (BMI) should be less than 25 kg/m^2 and waist circumference should be less than 80 cm in women and less than 94 cm in men (less than 90 cm in Asian men). Bariatric surgery may also ameliorate CKD.

Sodium and Potassium

Restriction of dietary sodium to 100 mmol/day (2.3 g sodium or 6 g salt per day) or less has been shown to reduce blood pressure and albuminuria in patients with CKD (McMahon, 2013) and is recommended. However, there are no long-term studies evaluating the impact of dietary sodium restriction on CKD progression or cardiovascular end points. Salt substitutes that contain high amounts of potassium salts should not be used in patients with CKD. A high potassium intake is associated with health benefits, as are foods high in potassium, notably fruits and vegetables (Kelly, 2017). For this reason, potassium-rich foods should not be restricted in CKD patients unless this becomes necessary based on serum potassium values nearly at, or exceeding the upper end of the normal range (Chapters 5 and 6).

Protein Restriction

A mildly restricted protein diet, consisting of 0.8 g/kg/day, with adequate energy is generally recommended for adults with CKD as discussed in Chapter 7. If prescription of a lower protein diet (≤0.6 g/kg/day) to slow CKD progression is attempted, such a diet must be closely monitored, and the potential modest benefits of such a diet on GFR decline must be weighed carefully against the concomitant risks of worsening clinical and biochemical parameters of nutrition. For children, reduction of dietary protein intake to the lowest safe amounts recommended by the World Health Organization (0.8 to 1.1 g/kg/day depending on age) has not been shown to decrease the progression of CKD.

Phosphate

It is becoming appreciated that even mildly increased levels of serum phosphate are associated with increased cardiovascular risk. However, the effect of dietary phosphate restriction has not been evaluated in patients with CKD; therefore, restriction of phosphate intake generally is not recommended in patients with early (stages 1 to 3) CKD (Johnson, 2013). Nevertheless, as described in Chapters 8 and 9, a very considerable portion of phosphate in the Western diet comes from phosphate-containing food additives. Avoiding such food additives to the greatest extent possible should be a relatively risk-free method of reducing exposure to dietary phosphate. As CKD advances, most guidelines do recommend restricting phosphate intake and even ingestion of phosphate binders as required to keep serum phosphate within the normal range (Palmer, 2016a).

Uric Acid

There is limited evidence suggesting that treating asymptomatic hyperuricemia in CKD patients with allopurinol or rasburicase may be beneficial in terms of both blood pressure control and progression of kidney disease (Bose, 2014). However, safety concerns with allopurinol and the high cost of alternative agents may limit their routine use in day-to-day clinical practice.

Advanced Glycosylation End Products

These are ubiquitous in foods, but are much higher in fatty meats and in all foods subjected to very high temperatures during preparation (e.g., food that has been grilled or fried). Serum levels of advanced glycosylation end products increase acutely after ingestion of foods containing advanced glycosylation end products (AGEs), and in the short term there is impaired flow-induced endothelial vasodilatation. In observational studies, high serum levels of AGEs are associated with increased mortality risk. One can reduce exposure to dietary AGEs by eating more boiled or steamed food and more vegetables than meats. However, the effects of dietary AGE avoidance on clinically relevant outcomes have not been systematically evaluated.

Vitamins and Supplements

The primary vitamin that may need to be supplied to patients with CKD is vitamin D, in the form of either a not-yet-activated prohormone (cholecalciferol or ergocalciferol), or as dihydroxylated, fully activated hormone or analog (calcitriol, doxercalciferol, paricalcitol). CKD patients have low 25-vitamin D levels even during early-stage disease. There may be mild deficiency of several water-soluble B vitamins in CKD patients who are following a protein-restricted diet which should be preventable with supplementation. Apart from these instances, vitamin supplementation is not required and may cause adverse effects (Chapters 8 and 10).

Fruit and Vegetables

Although current international guidelines recommend patients receive individualized, single nutrient–based dietary interventions (e.g., salt, phosphate, potassium, protein, and calories) by a qualified dietitian (Johnson, 2013), alternative approaches promoting healthy eating patterns (e.g., by increasing dietary intakes of fruit, vegetables, plant-based protein, and fiber) may have beneficial impacts on metabolic acidosis, blood pressure, CKD progression, and cardiovascular disease without appreciably increased risks of hyperkalemia (Kelly, 2017). Examples of this approach include the Mediterranean diet, Dietary Approaches to Stop Hypertension (DASH) diet, and vegetarian diets. Some CKD guidelines currently recommend that patients with early CKD consume a balanced diet rich in fruits and vegetables (Johnson, 2013).

Acidosis

As discussed in Chapter 11, CKD patients tend to have a mild to moderate degree of acidosis. The acidosis comes from the proteins in the foods we eat, and it can be neutralized by balanced dietary fruit and vegetable intake (guided by an accredited dietitian) or by ingestion of sodium (or uncommonly potassium) bicarbonate or citrate. Some studies have suggested that alkali supplementation may help maintain bone health and there is even evidence that it may slow progression of CKD. However, the risk to benefit ratio of this approach has not been evaluated. Excessive alkalinization combined with a high ingestion of calcium and vitamin D can lead to the so-called "calcium-alkali" syndrome, with hypercalcemia and rapid impairment of renal function. Alkali supplementation may also be complicated by sodium and fluid retention.

Alcohol
No specific recommendations can be made about alcohol consumption in patients with CKD due to conflicting epidemiologic evidence.

Cola Beverages
Soft drink (especially cola) consumption has been associated with diabetes, hypertension, and kidney stones. There is limited evidence to suggest that drinking two or more colas per day is associated with a significantly increased risk of CKD (Saldana, 2007). Patients with CKD should therefore minimize their intake of cola.

Fluid Intake
Drinking large amounts of water has commonly been advocated in the popular press to enhance kidney health. However, there is insufficient evidence to recommend augmenting fluid intake in most patients with CKD. Such patients should obviously avoid dehydration and overhydration. For most patients, a fluid intake of 2 to 2.5 L per day is generally sufficient, although such advice needs to be tailored to individual patient circumstances.

REDUCING RISK OF PROGRESSION OF CKD AND CARDIOVASCULAR DISEASE

Patients with CKD are at greatly increased risk of both cardiovascular disease and end-stage kidney disease. Irrespective of the underlying cause of CKD, the treatments outlined below, and described in detail in Chapters 12 to 18, will slow the decline in kidney function and decrease cardiovascular risk. Regular monitoring (at least every 3 months) is essential.

Lifestyle Modification and Exercise
Lifestyle modification can substantially reduce the risks of hypertension, as well as obesity, diabetes mellitus, cardiovascular disease, and kidney failure progression. Patients with CKD should be encouraged to undertake regular physical exercise that is appropriate for their physical ability and medical history. There is limited evidence that exercise may have beneficial effects on kidney function in patients with CKD (Johnson, 2013).

Lipid Lowering
Statins are safe and significantly reduce the risks of all-cause and cardiovascular mortality, as well as cardiovascular events, in CKD patients who are not receiving renal replacement therapy (Palmer, 2014). The effects of statins on CKD progression remain uncertain (Palmer, 2014). Based largely on the results of the SHARP trial (Baigent, 2011), the Kidney Disease Improving Global Outcomes

(KDIGO) Guidelines recommended lipid lowering medications to a broad range of patients with CKD and did not advocate ongoing monitoring of lipid levels or titrating lipid lowering medications to achieve particular lipid targets (KDIGO, 2013). Specifically, a statin or statin/ezetimibe combination is indicated in patients with nondialysis CKD, irrespective of lipid levels, if they are at least 50 years old or if they are younger and have one or more cardiovascular risk factors (e.g., coronary artery disease, previous ischaemic stroke, diabetes, or estimated 10-year incidence of fatal or nonfatal myocardial infarction above 10%). Initiation of lipid lowering therapy is not recommended after patients have commenced dialysis (KDIGO, 2013).

Glycemic Control

There is strong evidence that intensive glycemic control reduces cardiovascular and CKD progression risk in both type 1 and 2 diabetes mellitus (Chapter 13). Lifestyle modification should be first-line treatment. Metformin remains as first choice of monotherapy agent for type 2 diabetes, but dose adjustment should be applied in patients with CKD (Palmer, 2016b). Addition of newer agents such as glucagon-like peptide 1 (GLP-1) analog (liraglutide) and sodium–glucose cotransporter 2 inhibitors (e.g., empagliflozin) to standard therapy has been demonstrated to lower cardiovascular outcomes and death (Palmer, 2016b). The benefit needs to be balanced against the risk of complications (severe hypoglycemia, weight gain, and perhaps also increased mortality) that may be associated with lowering of glucose to near-normal levels. The currently recommended targets for diabetic patients with CKD are a preprandial blood glucose level of <6.1 mmol/L (110 mg/dL) and a random HbA1c of <7% (53 mmol/mol) for most (Gunton, 2014). In patients with significant comorbidities (such as established cardiovascular disease), a less intensive target (<8% or 61 mmol/mol) is recommended (American Diabetes Association, 2017).

Blood Pressure Control

Reducing blood pressure to target levels is the most important treatment step in managing cardiovascular and renal risks in CKD. The optimum BP target is a matter of current investigation and debate. Currently, the KDIGO guidelines recommend a target blood pressure of <140/90 mm Hg in patients with nondialysis CKD and normalbuminuria (with or without diabetes mellitus) (KDIGO Blood Pressure Work Group, 2012). In patients with micro- or macroalbuminuria, the BP target should be reduced to <130/80 mm Hg (KDIGO Blood Pressure Work Group, 2012). Although this lower target had also been previously suggested for all patients with diabetes and CKD, a higher BP target was suggested by KDIGO based on the findings of the ACCORD-BP (Control Cardiovascular Risk in Diabetes–Blood Pressure) trial (Cushman, 2010).

More recently, the Systolic Blood Pressure Intervention Trial (SPRINT) (Wright, 2015) demonstrated that lowering systolic blood pressure to <120 mm Hg resulted in a 25% reduction in a composite cardiovascular endpoint in older (>50 years) nondiabetic patients with a systolic blood pressure between 130 and 180 mm Hg and at least one cardiovascular risk factor. However, blood pressure was measured by automated oscillometric sphygmomanometer in the absence of a health care professional (and therefore may have yielded lower blood pressure readings than standard clinic measurements), and the intensive blood pressure group did experience a greater frequency of serious adverse events due to hypotension, syncope, serum electrolyte abnormalities (hyponatremia and hypokalemia), and acute kidney injury. Hence, the lower BP target needs to be applied judiciously, especially to elderly patients, where excessively low blood pressure may put them at increased risk. In younger patients with moderate to high cardiovascular risk, it may be reasonable to consider a lower systolic blood pressure target than is currently routinely recommended. Recently, the American Heart Association and American College of Cardiology released updated guidelines on the prevention, detection, evaluation, and management of high blood pressure in adults, which defined hypertension as a blood pressure measurement ≥130/80 mm Hg (rather than ≥140/90) and advocated a blood pressure target of <130/80 mm Hg, particularly in individuals with a high absolute cardiovascular risk (Cifu and Davis, 2017; Whelton, 2017; Wyatt, 2018).

As described in Chapters 14 and 15, multiple (often 3 to 4) antihypertensive medications are frequently required in CKD patients to reach blood pressure targets. Angiotensin-converting enzyme inhibitors (ACEIs) or angiotensin receptor blockers (ARBs) are the preferred initial blood pressure–lowering strategy, since these agents have been shown to be renoprotective, independent of blood pressure lowering. The exact role for the so-called "dual blockade" using combined ACEI + ARB therapy, or combined treatment with an ACEI or ARB plus an aldosterone antagonist, is not clear, and at least one recent study has suggested unfavorable risk:benefit with dual (ACEI + ARB) blockade.

It is prudent to measure serum creatinine and eGFR 1 and 4 weeks after initiating ACEI or ARB therapy. An acute rise in plasma creatinine concentration of less than 25% that stabilizes within the first month is expected and is associated with a beneficial long-term response compared with patients who experience no change in serum creatinine or eGFR (Johnson, 2013; Johnson, 2015). If the initial rise in creatinine level exceeds 25% above the baseline value, ACEI/ARBs should be discontinued. ACEI/ARBs should also be withdrawn if the serum potassium concentration exceeds 6 mmol/L, despite dose reduction, dietary potassium restriction, and concomitant diuretic therapy. The treatment response to ACEI or ARBs can also be monitored by quantitating albuminuria. For each 50% reduction in urinary albumin excretion, the risks of end-stage renal disease, cardiovascular events, and heart failure are reduced by 45%, 18%, and 27%, respectively (Palmer, 2007). Diuretics and dietary sodium restriction can also synergistically enhance the blood pressure and albuminuria lowering effects of ACEIs and ARBs.

In resistant hypertension or with stepwise decline in renal function with other signs of atherosclerosis, renovascular hypertension needs to be considered, although recent evidence suggests that medical management may be the best way to manage such patients (Chapters 14 and 15). Resistant hypertension often responds to attention to sodium restriction as well as to addition of drugs blocking aldosterone action or sodium channels in the distal nephron.

PERIPHERAL VASCULAR DISEASE AND STROKE RISK

CKD patients are at increased risk of both stroke and peripheral vascular disease (Chapter 16), and some of the trials studying optimal blood pressure targets find that if lower BP targets do show any additional benefit, it is in terms of enhanced protection against stroke. Aspirin has been shown to reduce cardiovascular risk in patients with CKD (Kaisar, 2008), although this potential benefit must be weighed against the significant risk of gastrointestinal bleeding. Recent trends have been to use aspirin with increased caution in terms of primary prevention due to bleeding risk.

CARDIOPROTECTION

CKD patients are at markedly increased risk of cardiovascular death, and left ventricular hypertrophy, coronary artery disease, and congestive heart failure all are quite common. As discussed in Chapters 17 and 18, the usual cardioprotective strategies used in patients with normal renal function apply, with an important caveat being slightly increased bleeding risk with anticoagulant treatment. Mineral bone disorder (Chapter 8) may impact on cardiac disease in this patient group, and adequate provision of vitamin D, and prevention of hyperphosphatemia and hyperparathyroidism may be important measures to limit both cardiac dysfunction and vascular calcification, although prospectively controlled trials focusing on the cardiovascular benefits of maintaining optimal calcium-related homeostasis have yet to be carried out.

NEPHROTIC RANGE PROTEINURIA

An important subset of CKD patients will have a high degree of proteinuria, most commonly owing to advanced diabetic nephropathy, but others will have this either due to idiopathic disease affecting the renal filtration barrier in the glomerulus, such as membranous nephropathy or focal glomerulosclerosis, and still others will have nephrotic range proteinuria as a manifestation of a systemic disease that affects multiple organs in the body, not only the kidneys. These problems are discussed in detail in Chapter 20.

ANEMIA

As CKD progresses, anemia worsens, and it was originally thought that prevention of even mild anemia might prevent the development of left ventricular hypertrophy that has been observed to occur as GFR falls. However, randomized trials using erythropoietin-stimulating agents have shown that correction of mild anemia, Hb >100 g/L (10 g/dL) to near-normal levels does not have a beneficial effect on cardiac outcomes; correction of mild anemia may increase quality of life measures slightly, but this may occur at the expense of an increased risk of strokes and overall mortality. Thus, current trends are to be cautious in terms of anemia correction, although keeping Hb >100 g/L (>10 g/dL) using iron and/or erythropoiesis-stimulating agents remains the standard of care. The controversy and recommended treatment strategies are discussed in Chapter 22.

AVOIDING CONTRAST-INDUCED COMPLICATIONS

The use of iodinated contrast for diagnostic studies is an important precipitating or aggravating cause for CKD, although the incidence is low. In patients with advanced CKD, use of magnetic resonance imaging contrast agents containing gadolinium has been associated with a fibrosing dermopathy that can be debilitating and difficult to treat although this risk has been lessened substantially with the availability of newer imaging agents.

MEDICATION REVIEW AND DRUG DOSING IN CKD

Dosage reduction or cessation of renally excreted medications is generally required once the GFR falls below 60 mL/min per 1.73 m². Optimal use of drugs is complicated by the fact that many CKD patients are also elderly, and in the elderly both renal and hepatic excretion of drugs may be diminished, and body composition is different from that of young patients. These issues, along with drug tables listing dosage recommendations are presented in Chapter 23.

CKD IN SPECIAL POPULATIONS

Children
The causes of CKD in children are different from those in adults. The measurement and estimation of GFR as well as optimal levels of blood pressure have their own special difficulties, and management of CKD in the very young is highly specialized (see Chapter 24).

Pregnant Patients
Pregnancy generally does not affect the course of renal disease in women who have normal or near-normal renal function at conception provided blood pressure is well controlled. Such individuals should not be discouraged from conceiving purely on the basis of their renal disease. CKD progression is accelerated by pregnancy in patients with poorly controlled hypertension or especially in women with pregravid plasma creatinine concentrations >200 micromol/L (2.25 mg/dL), equivalent to an eGFR <25 mL/min per 1.73 m² in a 30-year-old woman. This is discussed in more detail in Chapter 25.

Elderly
Do all elderly patients defined to have CKD really have CKD? One of the current controversies with respect to using GFR to diagnose CKD is how to take account of age-related decline in renal function in the elderly. After the age of 30 years, GFR progressively declines at an average rate of 8 mL/min per 1.73 m² per decade. It is estimated that up to 50% of adults

over the age of 70 years will have an eGFR below 60 mL/min per 1.73 m^2, although only a minority will progress to end-stage kidney disease due to the competing risk of death. There is ongoing debate as to whether this age-related GFR decline is normal or pathologic. However, an eGFR <45 mL/min per 1.73 m^2 predicts significantly increased risks of cardiovascular disease and CKD progression in all age groups and should therefore generally be considered pathologic (i.e., CKD) rather than physiologic or age appropriate. An eGFR between 45 and 60 mL/min per 1.73 m^2 (stage 3A CKD, Table 2.1) is predictive of significantly increased risks of adverse clinical outcomes in younger patients (<65 to 70 years), although the benefits of identifying older people with an eGFR between 45 and 60 mL/min per 1.73 m^2 have yet to be definitively proven. The European Renal Best Practice Group (ERBP) has recommended a clinical risk prediction model for patients aged >65 years and GFR 15 to 45 mL/min per 1.73 m^2 based on the Bansal score, Kidney Failure Risk Equation (KFRE) score, Renal Epidemiology and Information Network (REIN) score, and frailty assessment, to assist with risk stratification and clinical decision making in elderly patients with CKD (Farrington, 2017).

Other Special Groups

CKD diagnosis and management have specific nuances in different patient groups. With regard to ethnicity, a propensity to diabetes and to accelerated progression is found in patients of Hispanic and African American descent. In Asians, as discussed in Chapter 27, norms for BMI as well as prediction equations for eGFR may need to be adjusted slightly, and the strategy to optimize diet will be different in those following a non-Western pattern of food intake. Patients with kidney stones have their own particular set of management issues, as do patients with polycystic kidney disease or those suffering from HIV infection.

DETECTION AND MANAGEMENT OF CKD COMPLICATIONS

Many of the known complications of CKD, such as hypertension, secondary hyperparathyroidism, renal osteodystrophy, anemia, sleep apnea, restless legs, cardiovascular disease, and malnutrition, are often already evident by stage 3 (GFR 30 to 59 mL/min per 1.73 m^2). Other complications, such as hyperkalemia, acidosis, and hyperphosphatemia, usually become apparent in stage 4 CKD (GFR 15 to 29 mL/min per 1.73 m^2). Uremia and pulmonary edema often become manifest in stage 5 CKD (GFR <15 mL/min per 1.73 m^2). Regular monitoring for all of these complications (at least 3 monthly in stage 3 and monthly in stage 4) is essential.

WHEN SHOULD CKD PATIENTS BE REFERRED TO A NEPHROLOGIST?

The current indications for referral to a nephrologist are listed in Figure 2.1. These indications seek to identify patients who are at significant risk of progressing to end-stage kidney disease and/or who potentially have an underlying specifically treatable renal condition (e.g., primary glomerulonephritis, connective tissue disease, plasma cell dyscrasia, etc.). The decision to refer or not must always be individualized. When referring to a nephrologist, it is important to ensure that the patient has had a recent kidney ultrasound, current blood chemistry, and quantitation of albuminuria.

PREEMPTIVE TRANSPLANTATION, DIALYSIS, OR CONSERVATIVE TREATMENT?

In patients in whom CKD is expected to progress, the discussion of how best to replace lost renal function can begin at a relatively early stage of CKD, but consideration of preemptive transplantation including initiation of a pretransplant workup, must begin in earnest once eGFR has decreased to 20 to 25 mL/min per 1.73 m^2 (Chapter 28). For those contemplating dialysis, all locally available options, including home hemodialysis, peritoneal dialysis, and incenter hemodialysis need to be presented fairly and the advantages and disadvantages of each carefully debated. For those opting for hemodialysis, a reasonable lag time for creation of a well-functioning arteriovenous fistula is required, as discussed in Chapter 29.

PRACTICE-RELATED ISSUES, GUIDELINES, AND PATIENT MANAGEMENT AND EDUCATION TOOLS

The optimum method of structuring care for CKD patients depends on the health care infrastructure present in a given country. Whatever health care system is in place, the increasing use of multidisciplinary teams and a disease management approach appears to offer great potential advantages. A variety of practice guidelines are available that deal both very specifically with care for CKD patients, as well as care of those with heart disease, diabetes, or hypertension. In addition, a number of organizations throughout the world have developed toolkits and websites that offer patient- and provider-focused educational material and treatment algorithms. These are detailed in Chapter 30.

References and Suggested Readings

American Diabetes Association. Standards of medical care in diabetes—2017. *Diabetes Care*. 2017;40:S1–S132.

Baigent C, Landray MJ, Reith C, et al. The effects of lowering LDL cholesterol with simvastatin plus ezetimibe in patients with chronic kidney disease (Study of Heart and Renal Protection): a randomised placebo-controlled trial. *Lancet*. 2011;377:2181–2192.

Bello AK, Levin A, Tonelli M, et al. Assessment of global kidney health care status. *JAMA*. 2017a;317:1864–1881.

Bello AK, Levin A, Tonelli M, et al. Global Kidney Health Atlas: A Report by the International Society of Nephrology on the Current State of Organization and Structures for Kidney Care Across the Globe. Brussels, Belgium: International Society of Nephrology; 2017b.

Bose B, Badve SV, Hiremath SS, et al. Effects of uric acid-lowering therapy on renal outcomes: a systematic review and meta-analysis. *Nephrol Dial Transplant*. 2014;29:406–413.

Cifu AS, Davis AM. Prevention, detection, evaluation, and management of high blood pressure in adults. *JAMA*. 2017;318:2132–2134.

Collins AJ, Vassalotti JA, Wang C, et al. Who should be targeted for CKD screening? Impact of diabetes, hypertension, and cardiovascular disease. *Am J Kidney Dis*. 2009;53:S71–S77.

Cushman WC, Evans GW, Byington RP, et al; ACCORD Study Group. Effects of intensive blood-pressure control in type 2 diabetes mellitus. *N Engl J Med*. 2010;362:1575–1585.

de Jong PE, Brenner BM. From secondary to primary prevention of progressive renal disease: the case for screening for albuminuria. *Kidney Int.* 2004;66:2109–2118.

Farrington K, Covic A, Nistor I, et al. Clinical practice guideline on management of older patients with chronic kidney disease stage 3b or higher (eGFR<45 mL/min/1.73 m²): a summary document from the European Renal Best Practice Group. *Nephrol Dial Transplant.* 2017;32:9–16.

Gunton JE, Cheung NW, Davis TM, et al. A new blood glucose management algorithm for type 2 diabetes: a position statement of the Australian diabetes society. *Med J Aust.* 2014;201:650–653.

Hogg RJ. Screening for CKD in children: a global controversy. *Clin J Am Soc Nephrol.* 2009;4:509–515.

Johnson DW, Atai E, Chan M, et al. KHA-CARI guideline: early chronic kidney disease: detection, prevention and management. *Nephrology (Carlton).* 2013;18:340–350.

Johnson DW, Fawcett K, Harvie B, et al. Chronic Kidney Disease Management in General Practice. Adelaide, South Australia: Kidney Health Australia; 2015.

Kaisar MO, Isbel NM, Johnson DW. Recent clinical trials of pharmacologic cardiovascular interventions in patients with chronic kidney disease. *Rev Recent ClinTrials.* 2008;3:79–88.

Kelly JT, Rossi M, Johnson DW, et al. Beyond sodium, phosphate and potassium: potential dietary interventions in kidney disease. *Semin Dial.* 2017;30:197–202.

Kidney Disease: Improving Global Outcomes. KDIGO clinical practice guideline for lipid management in chronic kidney disease. *Kidney Int Suppl.* 2013;3:1–303.

Kidney Disease: Improving Global Outcomes (KDIGO) Blood Pressure Work Group. KDIGO clinical practice guideline for the management of blood pressure in chronic kidney disease. *Kidney Int.* 2012;2:337–414.

McMahon E, Bauer J, Hawley C, et al. Effect of sodium restriction on blood pressure, fluid status and proteinuria in CKD patients: results of a randomised crossover trial and 6-month follow-up. *Nephrology.* 2013;18:15–16.

Palmer BF. Proteinuria as a therapeutic target in patients with chronic kidney disease. *Am J Nephrol.* 2007;27:287–293.

Palmer SC, Gardner S, Tonelli M, et al. Phosphate-binding agents in adults with CKD: a network meta-analysis of randomized trials. *Am J Kidney Dis.* 2016a;68:691–702.

Palmer SC, Mavridis D, Nicolucci A, et al. Comparison of clinical outcomes and adverse events associated with glucose-lowering drugs in patients with type 2 diabetes: a meta-analysis. *JAMA.* 2016b;316:313–324.

Palmer SC, Navaneethan SD, Craig JC, et al. HMG CoA reductase inhibitors (statins) for people with chronic kidney disease not requiring dialysis. *Cochrane Database Syst Rev.* 2014:CD007784.

Saldana TM, Basso O, Darden R, et al. Carbonated beverages and chronic kidney disease. *Epidemiology.* 2007;18:501–506.

Sekhar DL, Wang L, Hollenbeak CS, et al. A cost-effectiveness analysis of screening urine dipsticks in well-child care. *Pediatrics.* 2010;125:660–663.

Stanifer JW, Von Isenburg M, Chertow GM, et al. Chronic kidney disease care models in low- and middle-income countries: a systematic review. *BMJ Glob Health.* 2018;3:e000728.

Umeukeje EM, Wild MG, Maripuri S, et al. Black Americans' perspectives of barriers and facilitators of community screening for kidney disease. *Clin J Am Soc Nephrol.* 2018;13:551–559.

Whelton PK, Carey RM, Aronow WS, et al. 2017 ACC/AHA/AAPA/ABC/ACPM/AGS/APhA/ASH/ASPC/NMA/PCNA guideline for the prevention, detection, evaluation, and management of high blood pressure in adults: a report of the American college of cardiology/American heart association task force on clinical practice guidelines [Epub ahead of print November 7, 2017]. *J Am Coll Cardiol.* doi: 10.1016/j.jacc.2017.11.006.

Wright JT Jr., Williamson JD, Whelton PK, et al;SPRINT Research Group. A Randomized trial of intensive versus standard blood-pressure control. *N Engl J Med.* 2015;373:2103–2116.

Wyatt CM, Chertow GM. Updated guidelines for the diagnosis and management of high blood pressure: implications for clinical practice in nephrology. *Kidney Int.* 2018;93:768–770.

3 Smoking, Substance Abuse, and Environmental Hazards

Jenny I. Shen, Sandra F. Williams, and Keith C. Norris

Environmental exposure to toxins may play an important role in triggering the onset of chronic kidney disease (CKD), modifying its progression, and impacting the adverse outcomes associated with its advanced stages. These exposures may be geographically nonspecific, such as in the near-ubiquitous presence of smoking and the high incidence of substance abuse. Other exposure risks to a particular toxin may be linked to certain working or living environments, such as occupational exposure to lead, cadmium, or mercury; exposure to lead-based paint in the home; exposure to community-related airborne levels of organic pollutants (such as polycyclic aromatic hydrocarbons, dioxins, or nitrogen oxides) or small particulate matter from vehicular exhausts and smokestack industries (Table 3.1) (Chen, 2018; Kim, 2018; Lunyera and Smith, 2017; Tsai, 2017; Wu, 2017).

TABLE 3.1	Environmental Toxins That May Affect Chronic Kidney Disease
Not Related to Geographic Location	**Geographically Specific**
Cigarette smoking	Occupational ■ Metals: lead, cadmium, mercury, boron, antimony ■ Organic compounds ■ Silica ■ Industrial and organic solvents
Substance abuse ■ Cocaine ■ Heroin ■ Methamphetamines ■ Ecstasy	Airborne pollutants ■ Toxic waste/trash dumps ■ Diesel particles (heavy industrial transportation routes) ■ Fine particulate matter ■ Persistent organic pollutants: polycyclic aromatic hydrocarbons (PAH), dioxins, nitrogen dioxides

An understanding of the risk of possible exposure to environmental toxins is an important aspect in the assessment of patients with CKD, particularly when the etiology of disease is unclear or when disease progresses despite evidence-based therapy. Such insights may aid in elucidating kidney disease diagnosis, modifying patient management, and informing local industry and public health authorities to institute appropriate prevention messages and action plans.

SMOKING

In the United States, cigarette smoking is the leading cause of preventable disease and death, and cigarettes are the most commonly used tobacco product among adults (Jamal, 2016). While current smoking has declined from nearly 21 of every 100 adults (21%) in 2005 to about 15 of every 100 adults (15%) in 2015 (Jamal, 2016), every day, nearly 400 individuals under age 18 become daily smokers. There exists a strong body of evidence associating tobacco smoking with adverse renal outcomes, particularly progression of CKD. Some of the evidence implicates smoking as a trigger for the onset of kidney disease. A meta-analysis by Xia and colleagues found an increased relative risk of incident CKD of 1.27 (95% CI 1.19–1.35) for ever-smokers, 1.34 (95% CI 1.23–1.47) for current smokers, and 1.15 (95% CI 1.08–1.23) for former smokers (Xia, 2017). A study of more than 7,000 participants enrolled in the Prevention of Renal and Vascular Endstage Disease (PREVEND) trial, plus more than 28,000 participants from the general population, found a significant correlation between urine albumin excretion rate and the number of cigarettes smoked (Pinto-Sietsma, 2000). This data points to tobacco's potential role in contributing to initiation of CKD.

Smoking and Progression of Chronic Kidney Disease

In addition to initiation of CKD, many observational analyses have found a strong link between smoking and CKD progression (Orth and Hallan, 2008). A cross-sectional study that prospectively evaluated 84 patients with type 2 diabetes taking angiotensin-converting enzyme (ACE) inhibitors noted that both cigarette smoking and increased proteinuria were interrelated predictors of nephropathy progression (Chuahirun, 2003). Similarly, a study that prospectively followed 53 patients with essential hypertension for 36 months reported that in addition to the baseline creatinine level and black race, only cigarette smoking was associated with increased progression of kidney disease (Regalado, 2000). Several large studies have also noted powerful links between smoking and progressive decline in renal function. An analysis of more than 300,000 men screened for entry into The Multiple Risk Factor Intervention Trial (MRFIT) found that in addition to elevated blood pressure, smoking was significantly associated with an increased risk for end-stage kidney disease (ESKD), although the magnitude of the effect was not reported (Klag, 1996). The relationship between smoking and the findings of progressively reduced renal function appears to be more pronounced in men (Orth and Hallan, 2008), possibly because of differences in smoking patterns, since men typically smoke more frequently and inhale more deeply.

Not all of the data have been consistent however. In the Study of Heart and Renal Protection (SHARP) which enrolled over 9,000 participants with CKD, smoking was not associated with kidney disease progression although there was a significant association with vascular and nonvascular morbidity and mortality (Staplin, 2016).

Smoking in Advanced Stages of Chronic Kidney Disease

Smoking is associated with an increased risk of developing ESKD, and also with poor outcome once ESKD has become established. For example, the above noted meta-analysis by Xia et al. found 1.51-, 1.44-, and 1.99-fold increases in relative risk for developing ESKD for ever-smokers, former smokers, and current smokers (Xia, 2017).

In nearly 2,000 patients who underwent kidney transplantation from 1981 to 2004, the rate of cardiovascular events was nearly twice as high for smokers as compared with nonsmokers (Valdés-Cañedo, 2007). Other studies have also reported an increased risk of death among smokers after renal transplantation or dialysis (Shah, 2008a). The effects of smoking on adverse cardiovascular outcomes in patients with ESKD appear to dissipate after 5 years or more of smoking cessation.

As yet not well defined is the effect of secondhand smoke on all of the above aspects of renal disease. Secondhand smoke could conceptually represent an underrecognized contributing factor to renal damage, particularly in patients who may already be afflicted with the early stages of CKD and are therefore at risk for progression. Studies are available related to fetal exposure to maternal smoking. Continued maternal smoking during pregnancy was associated with smaller kidney volume and lower estimated glomerular filtration rate (eGFR) in offspring based on later measurements when the children had reached school age (Kooijman, 2015). Prenatal exposure also has been associated with nephrotic range proteinuria in both children (Omoloja, 2013) and adolescents (Garcia-Esquinas, 2013).

Among high school students, electronic cigarette use has increased from 1.5% in the year 2011 to 16% in 2015, with similar relative increases, from 0.6% to 5.3% in middle school students. The cardiovascular effects of electronic cigarette use are consistent with the known effects of nicotine, but the potential adverse effects of electronic cigarette–related oxidants, aldehydes, particulates, and "flavorants" remain to be determined (Benowitz and Fraiman, 2017). At the time of this writing, there are no large studies reporting an association between electronic cigarette use and CKD.

Pathophysiology of Smoking and Chronic Kidney Disease

The renal lesion most strongly associated with smoking is nephrosclerosis, and significant positive associations have also been reported for glomerulonephritis. Multiple, varied, and possibly inter-related physiologic mechanisms might account for these lesions (Fig. 3.1). Chronic smoking could lead to microvascular atherosclerotic disease, which could potentially initiate nephrosclerosis, and also accelerate progression of pre-existing CKD. Microvascular disease could lead to hypertension, which could further hasten CKD progression. More than 4,000 chemicals are found in cigarette smoke, and it is yet unclear, which of these might be responsible for smoking's deleterious effects on the kidneys.

Treatment

Treatment should focus on smoking cessation as well as removal from smoke-filled environments to the greatest extent possible. A number

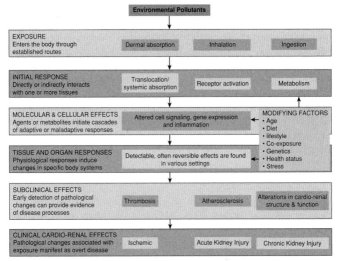

FIGURE 3.1 A framework for the characterization of the effects of environmental pollutants in cardiorenal disease. Agents enter the body through established routes, interact with one or more organs and tissues, initiating signaling cascades and physiologic responses, leading to subclinical and ultimately clinical pathologic changes. (Adapted from Cosselman KE, Navas-Acien A, Kaufman JD. Environmental factors in cardiovascular disease. *Nat Rev Cardiol.* 2015;12:627–642.)

of pharmacologic and nonpharmacologic interventions for smoking cessation have been shown to be effective (Smith, 2009). Monitoring urinary cotinine levels may be a useful tool to assess compliance (Jones-Burton, 2007). Stack and Murthy have stressed the importance of addressing the barriers and challenges that exist in achieving smoking cessation in patients with CKD (Stack and Murthy, 2010). For difficult cases electronic cigarettes have shown promise as a tool for reducing the risks of traditional smoking (McRobbie, 2014).

Nonpharmacologic Interventions
Physician counseling remains an important and effective evidence-based strategy. Other modalities that may be useful include individual psychological and behavioral therapy, group therapy, support groups such as Nicotine Anonymous, and the use of resources provided by local health departments and nonprofit organizations like the American Cancer Society. The use of mobile technology/smartphone apps and social media (e.g., via Facebook or Twitter) are recent novel interventions to reduce smoking (McCabe, 2017; Naslund, 2017) and include the use of smartphone apps such as "Clickotine" (Iacoviello, 2017). Likewise social media platforms that use Facebook and other social media platforms that create social engagement and support to promote smoking reduction show similar promise (Kim, 2017). Although potentially promising, long-term, large-scale studies documenting efficacy for these novel approaches have not been reported (Haskins, 2017), and there are no data related to their use in patients with CKD.

Pharmacologic Interventions

Nicotine replacement therapy (NRT) remains the hallmark of pharmacologic intervention for tobacco cessation. Methods include the use of nicotine patches, gum, inhalers, lozenges, and nasal spray. In patients with normal renal function, additional available pharmacologic agents include the combination therapy of atropine and scopolamine, bupropion, or varenicline (a drug that attenuates nicotine-induced dopamine stimulation) (Benowitz, 2009). The use of a nicotine replacement patch combined with a second medication has been reported to be more effective than monotherapy, without any reported differences in adverse effects or adherence (Shah, 2008b).

*Dosage Adjustments for Stop-Smoking Treatments
in Chronic Kidney Disease*

There exists the potential of accumulation of nicotine and bupropion metabolites from the use of these pharmacologic agents in patients with severely compromised renal function; accordingly appropriate dose adjustments are recommended. In dialysis patients a reduced dosage of bupropion should be given, for example, 150 mg orally every 3 days, and traditionally given doses of nicotine should be lowered by 50% to 75%. In patients with moderate or advanced CKD, the use of nortriptyline, varenicline, rimonabant, monoamine oxidase inhibitors, or selective serotonin reuptake inhibitors should be approached with substantial caution to avoid possible unexpected increases in the serum levels of these drugs (Formanek, 2018).

Public Health Implications

Collectively, public health efforts to reduce smoking have proven to be beneficial. Health care providers can and should play an active role in encouraging policies and education programs that focus on the adverse health implications of smoking in patients with CKD.

ILLICIT DRUGS AND CHRONIC KIDNEY DISEASE

A 2016 report indicated that over 10% of persons 12 years of age and over in the United States reported illicit drug use in the past month. (National Center for Health Statistics, 2017). Among frequently abused illicit substances, cocaine and heroin have been most commonly associated with CKD. More recently, synthetic cannabinoids (SCs), methamphetamines, and even Ecstasy have been increasingly recognized to have nephrotoxic effects (Pendergraft, 2014) (Tables 3.1 and 3.2). Because of the illicit nature of the use of these compounds, the identification of a distinct linkage between substance use and CKD remains difficult. Many people who use recreational drugs often do so in combination. For example, many cocaine users frequently also use alcohol, heroin, or methamphetamines. Alcohol, whether used alone or concurrently with illicit drugs, is associated with a wide range of problems, including blood chemistry abnormalities (e.g., hypokalemia, hypomagnesemia) and dehydration. These alcohol-induced abnormalities can predispose to hypoperfusion and possibly ischemia of the kidneys with not only acute kidney injury (AKI), but also, potentially, irreversible CKD.

TABLE 3.2	Relative Risk for Decline in Kidney Function Associated With Substance Abuse		
	Relative Risk for Decline in Kidney Function	**Confidence Limits**	**P**
Any drug	2.3	1.0–5.1	<0.05
Heroin	3.0	0.83–11	NS
Cocaine or crack	3.0	1.1–8.0	<0.05
Amphetamines	1.9	0.4–8.7	NS
Marijuana	2.0	0.87–4.4	NS
Psychedelics	3.9	1.1–14	<0.05
Other drugs	4.6	0.54–39	NS

NS, not significant.
Source: Vupputuri S, Batuman V, Muntner P, et al. The risk for mild kidney function decline associated with illicit drug use among hypertensive men. *Am J Kidney Dis.* 2004;43:629–635.

A recent prospective cohort study of more than two thousand community-dwelling adults residing in Baltimore, MD, found that opiate or cocaine use was associated with prevalent CKD (Novick, 2016). Taken together, the data suggest that when illicit substances are used alone or in combination, kidney damage may be initiated and/or potentiated.

Heroin
Drug overdose deaths nearly tripled in the United States during the period from 1999 to 2014, and this increase in mortality was driven by heroin and synthetic opioids other than methadone (Rudd, 2016). Heroin has been strongly associated with CKD. This agent was originally described as being the most conclusively linked illicit drug to CKD and commonly associated with a pathologic finding of focal glomerular sclerosis. However, despite early suggestive data, it remains unclear whether the identified renal lesion(s) were due to the direct use of heroin or to contaminants and/or diluents (e.g., talc, cornstarch) or even to transmittable diseases (e.g., hepatitis, human immunodeficiency virus [HIV]) associated with intravenous injection of street drugs and the sharing of needles.

Cocaine
By contrast, emerging evidence has demonstrated a strong association between the use of cocaine and CKD (Jaffe and Kimmel, 2006; Norris, 2001a,b). Cocaine use has been linked with acute rises in blood pressure and acute renal failure secondary to malignant hypertension. There have been several reports linking cocaine use to CKD progression and ESKD. Proposed mechanisms include progressive microvascular disease and/or microinfarction as a result of accelerated atherogenesis, vasospasm, and/or intermittent undocumented episodes of acute hypertension. One clinical clue to cocaine abuse is the detection of eosinophilia.

Synthetic Cannabinoids
SCs are designer drugs that bind to cannabinoid receptors. They are typically dissolved in a solvent, applied to dried plant material, and

smoked as an alternative to marijuana or sold as liquids to be vaporized and inhaled in e-cigarettes and other devices (liquid incense). These synthetic compounds with marijuana-like effects have become popular as recreational drugs and have been associated with a type of AKI (Pendergraft, 2014) characterized by acute tubular necrosis or acute interstitial nephritis; occasionally, the effects on the kidneys are severe enough to require dialysis. Some affected patients progressed from AKI to CKD. The symptoms are not highly specific and include nausea and vomiting, abdominal, flank, and/or back pain.

Methamphetamines

According to the 2012 National Survey on Drug Use and Health, approximately 440,000 people had reported using methamphetamine in the past month. Methamphetamines are strong central nervous system stimulant drugs. The drug is illicitly trafficked and sold as a white, bitter-tasting powder or pill. Crystal methamphetamine resembles glass fragments or bluish-white rocks and is chemically similar to amphetamine. Common names for methamphetamine include *chalk, crank, crystal, ice, meth,* and *speed.*

Methamphetamine-associated kidney problems manifest as AKI, most commonly through accelerated hypertension. In severe cases this can lead to irreversible renal damage and can accelerate progression of underlying CKD. Clinically, patients who chronically use methamphetamines present with symptoms such as mood swings, anxiety and confusion, problems sleeping, violent outbreaks, and weight loss.

Ecstasy

Ecstasy or Molly is *3,4-methylenedioxymethamphetamine* (MDMA), a synthetic methamphetamine analog that alters mood and perception. Initially popular in the nightclub scene and at dance parties ("raves"), the drug now is abused by a broader segment of the population.

Ecstasy has received heightened public attention recently and is commonly used by college-aged individuals. Similar to ingestion of other stimulants, Ecstasy use leads to feelings of euphoria, emotional empathy, and increased energy. There is a substantial risk for complications, including drug-induced vasculitis, hypotonic hyponatremia due to the arginine vasopressin secretagogue-like effects of the drug, hyperthermia, rhabdomyolysis, and cardiovascular collapse (Pendergraft, 2014). Recurrent episodes of rhabdomyolysis-related or other forms of AKI can lead to CKD. Rhabdomyolysis is thought to be secondary to ecstasy-induced seizures, repetitive muscular activity, or perhaps to a direct toxic effect of the drug.

Prescription Opioid Use

Chronic prescription opioid use has become a major public health epidemic in the United States (Mallappallil, 2017), and is increasingly prevalent. Up to 35% of hemodialysis patients use opioids to manage pain (Olivo, 2015). Many patients with advanced CKD are afflicted with chronic pain and the appropriate and safe use of opioids in these patients is an important component of their management. However, the inappropriate use of prescription opioids, specifically opioid overdose, can result in AKI due to dehydration, hypotension, rhabdomyolysis, and urinary retention (Mallappallil, 2017). Additionally, chronic opioid use, even if appropriate, has been associated with an increased risk of hospitalization in patients post kidney transplant, although there has been no associated increase in graft rejection rates (Kulshrestha, 2014). The data on chronic opioid use and posttransplant mortality have been conflicting, with some studies finding no differences (Kulshrestha, 2014) while others report increased mortality rates (Barrantes, 2013).

Treatment

It is essential to consider illicit drug use in the differential diagnosis of patients who present with kidney disease without a clearly evident etiology. Treatment of substance abuse issues is fraught with challenges. Because individuals with substance abuse disorders frequently have numerous complicating factors, a single nonpharmacologic or pharmacologic approach most often will not suffice. Correction of metabolic abnormalities and acute episodes of hypo/hypertension, when identified, can help to attenuate the severity of AKI events and reduce the likelihood of progression to CKD.

Nonpharmacologic Approaches

Nonpharmacologic options to address substance abuse include residential treatment programs, psychological and behavioral counseling/therapy, group therapy, family therapy, support groups, community-based support systems, and resources provided by government agencies such as the National Institute on Drug Abuse, local health departments, and not-for-profit organizations.

Pharmacologic Approaches

Pharmacologic therapy available to treat substance abuse is most effective when used in combination with psychotherapy and counseling. In many instances, pharmacologic therapy is needed in the early stages of addiction, particularly to eliminate or reduce any existing physical dependence while initiating long-term interventions aimed at the psychological dependence on illicit substances. Methadone and buprenorphine have proven to be effective medications for the treatment of opiate addiction. Other medications used to reduce withdrawal symptoms and treat mood disorders, such as antidepressants and mood stabilizers, also have proven efficacy. Management of Ecstasy (or other stimulant)-induced kidney disease includes the identification of and treatment of rhabdomyolysis with vigorous hydration and/or the identification of and treatment of hyperpyrexia utilizing dantrolene sodium. Although no specific therapies have been demonstrated to be effective in illicit opioid-related kidney disease, general interventions such as optimal control of coexisting hypertension, particularly with the use of drugs targeting inhibition of the renin–angiotensin system are among the strategies endorsed by expert opinion.

Public Health Implications

The National Institute of Drug Abuse estimates the abuse of tobacco, alcohol, illicit drugs, and prescription opioids costs nearly $750 billion annually related to entry into the criminal justice system, lost work productivity, and the need for additional health care (Office of National Drug Control Policy, 2004). Treatment and prevention of drug abuse can positively impact the costs associated with drug-related crime, as well as the spread of infectious diseases, including hepatitis and HIV/AIDS. Health care providers should, in addition to instituting indicated treatment modalities, actively engage in advocating for policies and patient education programs which focus on the adverse health implications of illicit drugs. Despite a variety of nonpharmacologic and pharmacologic interventions, there is no evidence that these measures have been successful in containing this epidemic.

ENVIRONMENTAL HAZARDS AND CHRONIC KIDNEY DISEASE

Lead

Lead, one of the heavy metals, is associated with a well-defined entity termed lead nephropathy, characterized by chronic tubulointerstitial nephritis. This presents as hypertension, often associated with gout, and evidence of renal tubular damage, the latter sometimes manifesting as glycosuria in the setting of normal serum glucose. Acute lead toxicity can occasionally be detected by the finding of elevated serum lead levels, but in the more common cases of chronic lead toxicity, serum lead levels are often normal. Chronic lead toxicity is associated with an increase in the total body lead burden, where lead is stored in soft tissue and bone. Demonstration of an elevated body lead burden may require the use of a 24-hour urine collection following the administration of chelating agents, such as ethylenediaminetetraacetic acid (EDTA) or meso-2,3-dimercaptosuccinic acid (DMSA) to mobilize soft tissue lead stores. Another diagnostic approach is the use of x-ray fluorescence to measure bone lead concentration.

Epidemiologic research indicates that lead may contribute to nephrotoxicity even at blood lead levels below 5 mcg/dL, the newly proposed threshold level of acceptability per the Centers for Disease Control and Prevention (CDC). This appears to be particularly true in susceptible populations, such as those with hypertension, diabetes, and/or pre-existing CKD. On the other hand, in one paper from Sweden, an occupational history of lead exposure (not confirmed by blood levels) was not associated with an increased risk of lead-related kidney damage (Evans, 2010). More recently, lead along with silica has been suggested to be among the toxins responsible for chronic kidney disease of unknown origin (CKDu) reported in lower-resource countries like Sri Lanka, India, and Central America (Mascarenhas, 2017). Atypical sources of excess lead exposure include the pica syndrome, especially in affected pregnant women, the use of lead-glazed pottery as food containers, retained lead bullet fragments from prior gunshot wounds, and lead bullet remnants contaminating tissues of game animals (Hamilton, 2001; McQuirter, 2003; Pain, 2010). In Asia, Africa, and South America, herbal remedies or food additives may include lead or other heavy metals (Lin, 2010).

Cadmium and Mercury

Cadmium and mercury are recognized nephrotoxic agents (Johri, 2010; Thomas, 2009). Cadmium-associated renal damage most frequently presents as CKD after prolonged exposure in an occupational setting. Mercury may cause either acute or chronic kidney disease. When mercury vapor is emitted from volcanoes, coal-burning power plants, or municipal incinerators, it returns to the earth through rainfall contaminated with metallic mercury. This metallic mercury is then converted to methyl mercury in oceans and lakes and subsequently enters the food chain via fish and other seafood.

Besides airborne and food sources, mercury levels above the FDA limit and high enough to potentially cause CKD were found in 5 of 60 skin-lightening creams, as reported in one study (Gabler and Roe, 2010). The potential of significant mercury absorption from dental amalgams remains a matter of controversy (Jarosińska, 2008) with one study reporting that the surface area of mercury-containing amalgams in the mouth was the main determinant of renal mercury concentration (Barregard, 2010); however, the clinical importance of these small amalgam-related increments in renal mercury levels remains uncertain.

Despite ongoing efforts to remove mercury from various sources, continued exposure to mercury remains an important risk factor for kidney disease (Hodgson, 2007). Minority and disadvantaged populations may be at a disproportionally increased risk of developing lead-, cadmium-, and mercury-related kidney disease since they more frequently reside in communities with higher rates of environmental and occupational exposures (Said and Hernandez, 2015).

Arsenic

Arsenic toxicity is most commonly associated with neurologic abnormalities but may lead to kidney disease in the form of tubular damage (Huang, 2009). Renal damage related to arsenic is more likely precipitated in those who ingest arsenic-contaminated well or groundwater which is a major problem in certain countries such as Bangladesh. Additionally, arsenic may be found in groundwater in many areas of the United States. Arsenic-contaminated drinking water has been linked to the development of tubulointerstitial nephritis and acute tubular necrosis which may progress to CKD (Orr and Bridges, 2017). Arsenic-induced kidney injury is characterized by hypercalciuria, albuminuria, nephrocalcinosis, and necrosis of the renal papillae (Orr and Bridges, 2017).

Chelation Therapy for Lead and Other Heavy Metals
One therapeutic option utilized to treat heavy metal exposure is chelation. Chelation has been advocated primarily in instances where exposure has resulted in unequivocally elevated serum levels of the

toxin in question. One report has suggested that 2 or 3 months of chelation therapy can improve kidney function in patients with CKD secondary to lead exposure (Lin-Tan, 2007). The efficacy of long-term chelation for prevention and/or treatment of renal damage due to lead needs confirmation, and benefits of efficacy of chelation therapy for heavy metals other than lead have yet to be defined.

Organic Solvents

Exposure to industrial and organic solvents derived from hydrocarbons also poses a risk for the development of kidney disease. These solvents include trichloroethylene, which is often found in paint thinners and degreasers (Jacob, 2007). Numerous occupations involve exposure to such solvents, but painters and various types of factory workers may be at higher risk. Widespread use of these solvents over the past decades has resulted in large amounts of trichloroethylene deposits accumulated in toxic waste sites from industrial plants, as well as contaminating groundwater sites, leading to the possibility of nonoccupational community exposure.

Airborne Small Particulate Matter and Organic Pollutants

Another important environmental exposure is to small particulate matter that is commonly expelled in exhaust fumes from large industrial plants and motor vehicles. Such pollutants have been linked to vascular damage with consequent cardiovascular disease (Cosselman, 2015) and possibly CKD (Fig. 3.1).

According to the World Health Organization, air pollution caused the deaths of approximately 7 million people worldwide in 2012. These exposures occur disproportionately in people from lower socioeconomic communities, as industrial plants and their toxic waste sites are commonly found adjacent to where people live (Hendryx, 2009). Long-term exposure to air pollution and small particulate matter, especially to PM2.5 (atmospheric particulates with a diameter less than 2.5 microns), has been associated with an increased risk of cardiovascular disease. These microparticles may mediate vascular damage via their pro-oxidant and pro-inflammatory effects, which they exert in the circulation after having been absorbed through the lungs (Bai and Sun, 2016).

The association of these pollutants with CKD is less well defined; however, several studies suggest that such a relationship may exist. Xu et al. reported long-term exposure to PM2.5 was associated with an increased risk of membranous nephropathy in China (Xu, 2016). The Veterans Administration Normative Aging Study also demonstrated that long-term PM2.5 exposure negatively affected renal function and was associated with progressive renal function decline (Mehta, 2016). Additionally, Yang and colleagues examined 21,656 Taiwanese adults and found that exposure to PM10, a somewhat larger microparticle pollutant, was associated with decreases in estimated glomerular filtration rate (Yang, 2017). A study by Bowe and colleagues, of nearly 2.5 million U.S. veterans, found that elevated levels of fine particulate matter (PM2.5) was associated with a greater than 25% increased risk of prevalent CKD and ESKD, as well as with increases in the risks of developing incident CKD, ESKD, and a 30% decline in eGFR (Bowe, 2018).

Mitigation and Treatment

The mainstay of treatment is removal of the patient from the environment contaminated by the inciting toxin(s). Separation from further environmental exposure may be more feasible in the case of occupational contaminants but may be more challenging when the toxin is present in the broader community and living space. Economic factors may preclude the ability to relocate. Compounding these challenges with some potential toxins is the lack of compelling evidence demonstrating improvement in kidney function or mitigation of risk on removal of the affected person from the offending environment. Additionally, the problem of reducing pollution of fine particulate matter is intertwined with issues relating to energy production and economic development. Health scientists can make a valuable contribution here by informing communities and governmental leaders of the risks and potential tradeoffs associated with different policy recommendations in this area (Davidson, 2005).

Public Health Implications

Globalization has led to expansion of multiple industries, which have generated an array of toxins that can adversely impact the kidney. If industrial expansion is allowed to occur unchecked and with limited environmental controls, then the risk of toxin exposure is increased, particularly in lesser developed countries as well as in low-resource communities in developed countries. The wealth and assets of one's community often influence the risk of environmental exposure to heavy metals, excess ambient air particulate matter, and other potential nephrotoxins. Perhaps partly for this reason, community-level poverty is strongly associated with a higher incidence rate for ESKD.

The problem of reducing pollution of fine particulate matter is intertwined with issues relating to energy production and economic development. Health scientists can make a valuable contribution by informing communities and governmental leaders of the risks and potential tradeoffs associated with different policy recommendations in this area (Davidson, 2005).

Chronic Kidney Disease of Unknown Origin

During the last two decades, an unexplained and highly lethal epidemic of CKD of unknown etiology has progressively emerged among farmworkers in the Pacific coastal lowlands of the Mesoamerican region, particularly in El Salvador, Nicaragua, Costa Rica, Guatemala, possibly some areas of Southeastern Mexico (Correa-Rotter, 2014), and in parts of Sri Lanka, Egypt, and India (Almaguer, 2014; Wijkstrom, 2018). This epidemic has increased in both incidence and prevalence over the last 15 years, yet there is a suspicion that it may have gone undetected for decades and that the observed upsurge in incidence is partly due to heightened awareness due to better case finding, improved general life expectancy, and growing social and political concern (Orantes-Navarro, 2017). This entity has been named Mesoamerican nephropathy or chronic kidney disease of unknown origin, and is attracting the attention of many local and regional health authorities as well as global organizations (Laux, 2016; Laux, 2012; Peraza, 2012; Torres, 2010; Wesseling, 2014). Susceptibility to this syndrome has been attributed to antecedent dehydration and heat stress leading to subclinical episodes of AKI which appears to be the trigger in many cases, and subsequently potentiated by toxic agents including possibly agrochemicals, heavy metals, and other toxins (Edirisinghe, 2018; Glaser, 2016).

What role pesticides play in this entity has been difficult to know, due to challenges in data collection and analysis (Valcke, 2017). One review of pesticides used historically by a sugarcane company in affected areas found strong or good evidence of associations between AKI and six commonly used pesticides (2,4-D, paraquat dichloride, captan, cypermethrin, glyphosate, and 1,2-dibromo-3-chloropropane [DBCP]). An analysis of 21 studies to elucidate the link between pesticide use and mesoamerican nephropathy suggested a potential causative role, but acknowledged that multiple factors may be in play (Valcke, 2017).

Public Health Implications

In settings where workers engage in heavy field labor with superimposed repetitive heat stress and dehydration, frequent episodes of undetected AKI may occur (Madero, 2017). Effective policies are needed to address working conditions and community safety standards in such agricultural communities.

References and Suggested Readings

Almaguer M, Herrera R, Orantes CM. Chronic kidney disease of unknown etiology in agricultural communities. *MEDICC Rev.* 2014;16:9–15.

Bai Y, Sun Q. Fine particulate matter air pollution and atherosclerosis: Mechanistic insights. *Biochim Biophys Acta.* 2016;1860:2863–2868.

Barrantes F, Luan FL, Kommareddi M, et al. A history of chronic opioid usage prior to kidney transplantation may be associated with increased mortality risk. *Kidney Int.* 2013;84:390–396.

Barregard L, Fabricius-Lagging E, Lundh T, et al. Cadmium, mercury, and lead in kidney cortex of living kidney donors: impact of different exposure sources. *Environ Res.* 2010;110:47–54.

Benowitz NL. Pharmacology of nicotine: addiction, smoking-induced disease, and therapeutics. *Annu Rev Pharmacol Toxicol.* 2009;49:57–71.

Benowitz NL, Fraiman JB. Cardiovascular effects of electronic cigarettes. *Nat Rev Cardiol.* 2017;14:447–456.

Bowe B, Xie Y, Li T, et al. Particulate matter air pollution and the risk of incident CKD and progression to ESRD. *J Am Soc Nephrol.* 2018;29:218–230.

Chen SY, Chu DC, Lee JH, et al. Traffic-related air pollution associated with chronic kidney disease among elderly residents in Taipei City. *Environ Pollut.* 2018;234: 838–845. doi:10.1016/j.envpol.2017.11.084.

Chuahirun T, Khanna A, Kimball K, et al. Cigarette smoking and increased urine albumin excretion are interrelated predictors of nephropathy progression in type 2 diabetes. *Am J Kidney Dis.* 2003;41:13–21.

Correa-Rotter R, Wesseling C, Johnson RJ. CKD of unknown origin in Central America: the case for a Mesoamerican nephropathy. *Am J Kidney Dis.* 2014;63:506–520.

Cosselman KE, Navas-Acien A, Kaufman JD. Environmental factors in cardiovascular disease. *Nat Rev Cardiol.* 2015;12:627–642.

Davidson CI, Phalen RF, Solomon PA. Airborne particulate matter and human health: A review. *Aerosol Sci Technol.* 2005;39:737–749.

Edirisinghe E, Manthrithilake H, Pitawala H, et al. Geochemical and isotopic evidences from groundwater and surface water for understanding of natural contamination in chronic kidney disease of unknown etiology (CKDu) endemic zones in Sri Lanka. *Isotopes Environ Health Stud.* 2018;54:244–261. doi:10.1080/10256016.2017.1377704.

Evans M, Fored CM, Nise G, et al. Occupational lead exposure and severe CKD: a population-based case-control and prospective observational cohort study in Sweden. *Am J Kidney Dis.* 2010;55:497–506.

Fischer RSB, Vangala C, Truong L, et al. Early detection of acute tubulointerstitial nephritis in the genesis of Mesoamerican nephropathy. *Kidney Int.* 2018;93:681–690.

Formanek P, Salisbury-Afshar E, Afshar M. Helping patients with ESRD and earlier stages of CKD to quit smoking. *Am J Kidney Dis.* 2018. doi:10.1053/j.ajkd.2018.01.057.

Gabler E, Roe S. FDA widens mercury-skin lightening cream investigation. Chicago Tribune. May 28, 2010. Available from www.chicagotribune.com/news/watchdog/chi-skin-creams-mercury,0,2495405.story?track = rss. Accessed July 18, 2010.

Garcia-Esquinas E, Loeffler LF, Weaver VM, et al. Kidney function and tobacco smoke exposure in US adolescents. *Pediatrics.* 2013;131:e1415–e1423.

Glaser J, Lemery J, Rajagopalan B, et al. Climate change and the emergent epidemic of CKD from heat stress in rural communities: The case for heat stress nephropathy. *Clin J Am Soc Nephrol.* 2016;11:1472–1483.

Hamilton S, Rothenberg SJ, Khan FA, et al. Neonatal lead poisoning from maternal pica behavior during pregnancy. *J Natl Med Assoc.* 2001;93:317–319.

Haskins BL, Lesperance D, Gibbons P, et al. A systematic review of smartphone applications for smoking cessation. *Transl Behav Med.* 2017;7:292–299.

Hendryx M. Mortality from heart, respiratory, and kidney disease in coal mining areas of Appalachia. *Int Arch Occup Environ Health.* 2009;82:243–249.

Hodgson S, Nieuwenhuijsen MJ, Elliott P, et al. Kidney disease mortality and environmental exposure to mercury. *Am J Epidemiol.* 2007;165:72–77.

Huang M, Choi SJ, Kim DW, et al. Risk assessment of low-level cadmium and arsenic on the kidney. *J Toxicol Environ Health A.* 2009;72:1493–1498.

Iacoviello BM, Steinerman JR, Klein DB, et al. Clickotine, a personalized smartphone app for smoking cessation: Initial evaluation. *JMIR Mhealth Uhealth.* 2017;5:e56.

Jacob S, Héry M, Protois JC, et al. Effect of organic solvent exposure on chronic kidney disease progression: the GN-PROGRESS cohort study. *J Am Soc Nephrol.* 2007;18:274–281.

Jaffe JA, Kimmel PL. Chronic nephropathies of cocaine and heroin abuse: a critical review. *Clin J Am Soc Nephrol.* 2006;1:655–667.

Jamal A, King BA, Neff LJ, et al. Current cigarette smoking among adults – United States, 2005–2015. *MMWR Morb Mortal Wkly Rep.* 2016;65:1205–1211.

Jarosińska D, Horvat M, Sällsten G, et al. Urinary mercury and biomarkers of early renal dysfunction in environmentally and occupationally exposed adults: a three-country study. *Environ Res.* 2008;108:224–232.

Johri N, Jacquillet G, Unwin R. Heavy metal poisoning: the effects of cadmium on the kidney. *Biometals.* 2010;23:783–792.

Jones-Burton C, Vessal G, Brown J, et al. Urinary cotinine as an objective measure of cigarette smoking in chronic kidney disease. *Nephrol Dial Transplant.* 2007;22: 1950–1954.

Kim SJ, Marsch LA, Brunette MF, Dallery J. Harnessing facebook for smoking reduction and cessation interventions: Facebook user engagement and social support predict smoking reduction. *J Med Internet Res.* 2017;19:e168.

Kim HJ, Min JY, Seo YS, et al. Association between exposure to ambient air pollution and renal function in Korean adults. *Ann Occup Environ Med.* 2018;30:14. doi:10.1186/s40557-018-0226-z.

Klag MJ, Whelton PK, Randall BL, et al. Blood pressure and endstage renal disease in men. *N Engl J Med.* 1996;334:13–18.

Kooijman MN, Bakker H, Franco OH, et al. Fetal smoke exposure and kidney outcomes in school-aged children. *Am J Kidney Dis*. 2015;66:412–420.

Kulshrestha S, Barrantes F, Samaniego M, et al. Chronic opioid analgesic usage post-kidney transplantation and clinical outcomes. *Clin Transplant*. 2014;28:1041–1046.

Laux TS, Barnoya J, Cipriano E, et al. Prevalence of chronic kidney disease of non-traditional causes in patients on hemodialysis in southwest Guatemala. *Rev Panam Salud Publica*. 2016;39:186–193.

Laux TS, Bert PJ, Ruiz B, et al. Nicaragua revisited: evidence of lower prevalence of chronic kidney disease in a high-altitude, coffee-growing village. *J Nephrol*. 2012; 25:533–540.

Lin CG, Schaider LA, Brabander DJ, et al. Pediatric lead exposure from imported Indian spices and cultural powders. *Pediatrics*. 2010;125:e828–e835.

Lin-Tan DT, Lin JL, Yen TH, et al. Long-term outcome of repeated lead chelation therapy in progressive non-diabetic chronic kidney diseases. *Nephrol Dial Transplant*. 2007;22:2924–2931.

Lunyera J, Smith SR. Heavy metal nephropathy: considerations for exposure analysis. *Kidney Int*. 2017;92:548–550. doi:10.1016/j.kint.2017.04.043.

Madero M, Garcia-Arroyo FE, Sanchez-Lozada LG. Pathophysiologic insight into Mesoamerican nephropathy. *Curr Opin Nephrol Hypertens*. 2017;26:296–302.

Mallappallil M, Sabu J, Friedman EA, et al. What do we know about opioids and the kidney? *Int J Mol Sci*. 2017;18. pii: E223.

Mascarenhas S, Mutnuri S, Ganguly A. Deleterious role of trace elements – Silica and lead in the development of chronic kidney disease. *Chemosphere*. 2017;177:239–249.

McCabe C, McCann M, Brady AM. Computer and mobile technology interventions for self-management in chronic obstructive pulmonary disease. *Cochrane Database Syst Rev*. 2017;5:Cd011425.

McQuirter JL, Rothenberg SJ, Dinkins GA, et al. Elevated blood lead resulting from maxillofacial gunshot injuries with lead ingestion. *J Oral Maxillofac Surg*. 2003; 61:593–603.

McRobbie H, Bullen C, Hartmann-Boyce J, et al. Electronic cigarettes for smoking cessation and reduction. *Cochrane Database Syst Rev*. 2014;Cd010216.

Mehta AJ, Zanobetti A, Bind MA, et al. Long-term exposure to ambient fine particulate matter and renal function in older men: The veterans administration normative aging study. *Environ Health Perspect*. 2016;124:1353–1360.

Naslund JA, Kim SJ, Aschbrenner KA, et al. Systematic review of social media interventions for smoking cessation. *Addict Behav*. 2017;73:81–93.

National Center for Health Statistics. Health, United States, 2016: With chartbook on long-term trends in health. 2017; Report No: 2017-1232.

Norris KC, Thornhill-Joynes M, Robinson C, et al. Cocaine use, hypertension, and end-stage renal disease. *Am J Kidney Dis*. 2001a;38:523–528.

Norris KC, Thornhill-Joynes M, Tareen N. Cocaine use and chronic renal failure. *Semin Nephrol*. 2001b;21:362–366.

Novick T, Liu Y, Alvanzo A, et al. Lifetime cocaine and opiate use and chronic kidney disease. *Am J Nephrol*. 2016;44:447–453.

Office of National Drug Control Policy. The Economic Costs of Drug Abuse in the United States: 1992–2002. Washington, DC: Executive Office of the President (Publication No. 207303); 2004.

Olivo RE, Hensley RL, Lewis JB, et al. Opioid use in hemodialysis patients. *Am J Kidney Dis*. 2015;66:1103–1105.

Omoloja A, Jerry-Fluker J, Ng DK, et al. Secondhand smoke exposure is associated with proteinuria in children with chronic kidney disease. *Pediatr Nephrol*. 2013; 1243–1251.

Orantes-Navarro CM, Herrera-Valdes R, Almaguer-Lopez M, et al. Toward a comprehensive hypothesis of chronic interstitial nephritis in agricultural communities. *Adv Chronic Kidney Dis*. 2017;24:101–106.

Orr SE, Bridges CC. Chronic kidney disease and exposure to nephrotoxic metals. *Int J Mol Sci*. 2017;18. pii: E1039.

Orth SR, Hallan SI. Smoking: a risk factor for progression of chronic kidney disease and for cardiovascular morbidity and mortality in renal patients—absence of evidence or evidence of absence? *Clin J Am Soc Nephrol*. 2008;3:226–236.

Pain DJ, Cromie RL, Newth J, et al. Potential hazard to human health from exposure to fragments of lead bullets and shot in the tissues of game animals. *PLoS One.* 2010;5:e10315.

Pendergraft WF 3rd, Herlitz LC, Thornley-Brown D, et al. Nephrotoxic effects of common and emerging drugs of abuse. *Clin J Am Soc Nephrol.* 2014;9:1996–2005.

Peraza S, Wesseling C, Aragon A, et al. Decreased kidney function among agricultural workers in El Salvador. *Am J Kidney Dis.* 2012;59:531–540.

Pinto-Sietsma SJ, Mulder J, Janssen WM, et al. Smoking is related to albuminuria and abnormal renal function in nondiabetic persons. *Ann Intern Med.* 2000;133:585–591.

Regalado M, Yang S, Wesson DE. Cigarette smoking is associated with augmented progression of renal insufficiency in severe essential hypertension. *Am J Kidney Dis.* 2000;35:687–694.

Rudd RA, Seth P, David F, et al. Increases in drug and opioid-involved overdose deaths – United States, 2010–2015. *MMWR Morb Mortal Wkly Rep.* 2016;65:1445–1452.

Said S, Hernandez GT. Environmental exposures, socioeconomics, disparities, and the kidneys. *Adv Chronic Kidney Dis.* 2015;22:39–45.

Shah DS, Polkinhorne KR, Pellicano R, et al. Are traditional risk factors valid for assessing cardiovascular risk in end-stage renal failure patients? *Nephrology (Carlton).* 2008a;13:667–671.

Shah SD, Wilken LA, Winkler SR, et al. Systematic review and meta-analysis of combination therapy for smoking cessation. *J Am Pharm Assoc.* 2008b;48:659–665.

Smith SS, McCarthy DE, Japuntich SJ, et al. Comparative effectiveness of 5 smoking cessation pharmacotherapies in primary care clinics. *Arch Intern Med.* 2009; 169:2148–2155.

Stack AG, Murthy BV. Cigarette use and cardiovascular risk in chronic kidney disease: an unappreciated modifiable lifestyle risk factor. *Semin Dial.* 2010;23:298–305.

Staplin N, Haynes R, Herrington WG, et al. Smoking and adverse outcomes in patients with CKD: the Study of Heart and Renal Protection (SHARP). *Am J Kidney Dis.* 2016;68:371–380.

Thomas LD, Hodgson S, Nieuwenhuijsen M, et al. Early kidney damage in a population exposed to cadmium and other heavy metals. *Environ Health Perspect.* 2009;117:181–184.

Torres C, Aragon A, Gonzalez M, et al. Decreased kidney function of unknown cause in Nicaragua: a community-based survey. *Am J Kidney Dis.* 2010;55:485–496.

Tsai TL, Kuo CC, Pan WH, et al. The decline in kidney function with chromium exposure is exacerbated with co-exposure to lead and cadmium. *Kidney Int.* 2017;92:710–720. doi:10.1016/j.kint.2017.03.013.

Valcke M, Levasseur ME, Soares da Silva A, et al. Pesticide exposures and chronic kidney disease of unknown etiology: an epidemiologic review. *Environ Health.* 2017;16:49.

Valdés-Cañedo F, Pita-Fernández S, Seijo-Bestilleiro R, et al. Incidence of cardiovascular events in renal transplant recipients and clinical relevance of modifiable variables. *Transplant Proc.* 2007;39:2239–2241.

Wesseling C, Crowe J, Hogstedt C, et al. Resolving the enigma of the mesoamerican nephropathy: a research workshop summary. *Am J Kidney Dis.* 2014;63:396–404.

Wijkstrom J, Jayasumana C, Dassanayake R, et al. Morphological and clinical findings in Sri Lankan patients with chronic kidney disease of unknown cause (CKDu): Similarities and differences with Mesoamerican Nephropathy. *PLoS One.* 2018;13:e0193056. doi:10.1371/journal.pone.0193056.

Wu W, Zhang K, Jiang S, et al. Association of co-exposure to heavy metals with renal function in a hypertensive population. *Environ Int.* 2018;112:198–206. doi:10.1016/j.envint.2017.12.023.

Xia J, Wang L, Ma Z, et al. Cigarette smoking and chronic kidney disease in the general population: a systematic review and meta-analysis of prospective cohort studies. *Nephrol Dial Transplant.* 2017;32:475–487.

Xu X, Wang G, Chen N, et al. Long-term exposure to air pollution and increased risk of membranous nephropathy in China. *J Am Soc Nephrol.* 2016;27:3739–3746.

Yang YR, Chen YM, Chen SY, et al. Associations between Long-term particulate matter exposure and adult renal function in the Taipei Metropolis. *Environ Health Perspect.* 2017;125:602–607.

4

Visceral Adiposity and Controlling Body Weight Through Diet and Exercise

Cheryl A.M. Anderson and Tanya Johns

Overweight and obesity are risk factors for cardiovascular disease as well as for micro- and macroalbuminuria and progression of chronic kidney disease (CKD). Waist-to-hip ratio may be a more specific measure of obesity-associated risk than body mass index (BMI), because adiposity of the abdominal viscera, including the liver, seems to be related most directly to adverse outcomes. Weight loss by dieting may be useful, especially when combined with an exercise program, and pharmaceutical drugs may help individuals achieve and maintain a healthier level of body weight and abdominal fat. Bariatric surgery may be needed to treat severe degrees of obesity.

CASE STUDY

MEASURING ADIPOSITY

Mr. G is a 53-year-old man with an extensive past medical history significant for coronary artery disease, hypertension, CKD, gout, and congestive heart failure. He presented to the nephrology clinic for an acute rise in serum creatinine that was determined to be a result of his use of indomethacin for gout. Mr. G's blood pressure is 150/90, pulse 56, weight 312 pounds (142 kg), and height 6 feet 4 inches (193 cm). His blood urea nitrogen (BUN) is 60 mg/dL (21 mmol/L) and serum creatinine is 4.2 mg/dL (370 μmol/L). Three months before this visit, his creatinine was 3.5 mg/dL (310 μmol/L). You are concerned about Mr. G's weight and visceral adiposity. What methods would you consider to assess Mr. G's level of obesity and visceral adiposity? What considerations should you give to his risk of cardiovascular and renal complications?

Body Mass Index

BMI is a practical method for assessing adiposity and is routinely used to classify obesity. The importance of BMI lies in its curvilinear relationship with all-cause mortality (Flegal, 2005). In patients <65 years of age, as BMI increases throughout the range of moderate and severe overweight, so does the increased risk of cardiovascular complications, disability, and mortality (Kuk, 2009). BMI is calculated by dividing weight by height squared when weight is in kilograms and height is in meters. Convenient equations for BMI are:

$$BMI\ (kg/m^2) = 10{,}000 \times kg/cm^2 = 703 \times lbs/in^2$$

In this particular case, Mr. G's weight was 314 pounds and height was 76 inches, so:

$$BMI = 703 \times 314/76^2 = 38.2\ kg/m^2$$

A BMI between 18.5 and 24.9 is considered normal, 25.0 to 29.9 is considered overweight, and ≥30.0 is considered to be obese. Mr. G is classified as obese by BMI criteria.

High Body Mass Index as a Paradoxical Survival Marker
Epidemiologic studies have shown that overweight and obesity are associated with improved survival in patients with endstage renal disease (ESRD), whereas a normal or low BMI increases risk of all-cause and cardiovascular death (Hsu, 2006; Johansenn, 2006). This is in contrast to findings in the general population in which both over-weight and underweight are associated with poorer survival. Based on findings of improved survival, some have suggested that obese patients with ESRD should not be counseled to lose weight, or those with normal weight should be counseled to gain weight. In contrast, other evidence suggests that physical functioning may be impaired by obesity in patients with ESRD (Salahudeen, 2003). This "reverse epidemiology" (Kalantar-Zadeh, 2003) may be due to the fact that chronically ill patients with high values for BMI may be a group that is particularly resistant to their illness, and this selection bias may overcome the normal adverse effects of adiposity. It might also be a result of intrinsic limitations of BMI in differentiating adipose tissue from lean mass in intermediate BMI ranges.

Body Mass Index in the Elderly
The optimum BMI for survival is a contentious issue, and this depends on age, culture, ethnicity, and also to what extent sick, cachectic patients are excluded from the subgroup with low BMI. Healthy elderly patients with a BMI in the "overweight" category have been reported to live longer (Flicker, 2010) and have better bone density than their counterparts with "normal" values for BMI (Doğan, 2010).

Body Mass Index in Non-Europid Ethnic Groups
The BMI norms were developed mostly in people of European (Europid) ancestry. Studies have shown that for a given value of BMI, there will be systematic differences by race/ethnicity in the average amount of body fat versus lean tissue (Hoffman, 2005). For example, at the same level of BMI, Africans and African Americans have less visceral fat than whites. In Asians, the normal range for BMI values is lower, and a BMI in the "normal" range of 18.5 to 24.9 for Asians will include a substantial number of persons who have elevated adiposity as measured by the more specific methods described below.

Visceral Adiposity
Visceral adiposity is the accumulation of adipose tissue in the abdomen and thorax, and it appears to have a particularly significant role in the determination of the renal health consequences of obesity (Elsayed, 2008a; Elsayed, 2008b). Abdominal adipose tissue comprises subcutaneous and intra-abdominal portions; the latter can be subdivided into intraperitoneal and retroperitoneal depots. The intraperitoneal fat depot is also known as visceral fat, which may contribute to insulin

resistance, glucose intolerance, dyslipidemia, hypertension, and coronary artery disease, and is associated with accumulation of fat in the liver (Björntorp, 1990; Canoy, 2007; Frayn, 2000). Evidence suggests that visceral adiposity is a key player in the development and progression of CKD (Elsayed, 2008a; Pinto-Sietsma, 2003). Therefore, assessing visceral adiposity is important when evaluating kidney disease risk. Measures of obesity that consider body fat distribution and the body's proportional components have been reported to more accurately predict adverse outcomes than BMI, but the extent of this increase in predictive value depends on which particular outcome is being examined (Vazquez, 2007).

Waist Circumference

There is some controversy as to whether waist circumference *per se* is a more useful predictor of cardiovascular risk than the BMI. Cutoff values for waist circumference depend on ethnicity, and the International Diabetes Federation has suggested "central obesity" cutoff values for different ethnic groups that are sex-specific (Table 4.1). The

TABLE 4.1	Central Obesity Defined by Waist Circumference		
Country/Ethnic Group	**Waist Circumference[a] (As Measure of Central Obesity)**		
USA ATPIII[b]	Male	≥102 cm	≥40.0 inches
	Female	≥88 cm	≥34.5 inches
Europids[b]	Male	≥94 cm	≥37.0 inches
	Female	≥80 cm	≥31.5 inches
South Asians[c]	Male	≥90 cm	≥35.5 inches
	Female	≥80 cm	≥31.5 inches
Chinese	Male	≥90 cm	≥35.5 inches
	Female	≥80 cm	≥31.5 inches
Japanese[d]	Male	≥85 cm	≥33.5 inches
	Female	≥90 cm	≥35.5 inches
Ethnic South and Central Americans	Use South Asian recommendations until more specific data are available		
Sub-Saharan Africans	Use European data until more specific data are available		
Eastern Mediterranean and Middle East (Arab) populations	Use European data until more specific data are available		

[a]See also He et al., (2010) for an understanding of the controversy around some of the ethnicity-specific waist circumference measurements.
[b]Europids are Caucasians; in the United States, the Adult Treatment Panel III (ATPIII) values (102 cm for men, 88 cm for women), which are mostly for Europids, are likely to continue to be used for clinical purposes.
[c]Based on a Chinese, Malay, and Asian Indian population.
[d]Subsequent data analyses suggest that Asian values (male 90 cm, female 80 cm) should be used for Japanese populations until more data are available.
Source: Modified from International Diabetes Federation consensus worldwide definition of the metabolic syndrome.

International Diabetes Federation cutoff values for abnormal waist circumference in Europeans are lower than the intervention values recommended by the National Cholesterol Education Project Adult Treatment Panel III, which are 102 cm (40 inches) for men and 88 cm (34.6 inches) for women. Waist circumference is obtained using a measuring tape with an individual standing comfortably, with feet 25 to 30 cm apart. The measurement is made midway between the lower margin of the last rib and the crest of the ileum, in the horizontal plane. The tape should fit snugly but not so tightly as to compress soft tissues.

Waist-to-Hip Ratio

Waist-to-hip ratio is a better index of cardiovascular and renal risk than BMI in some studies (Elsayed, 2008a; De Koning, 2007). The idea is that people with "apple-shaped" bodies are more at risk of adverse obesity-related outcomes than those with "pear-shaped" bodies, in whom excess weight is largely distributed in the buttocks and thighs (Fig. 4.1). For hip circumference, an individual should stand erect with arms at the sides and feet together. The measurement should be taken at the point yielding the maximum circumference over the buttocks, with the tape held in a horizontal plane, touching the skin, but not indenting the soft tissues. Divide the waist measurement by the hip measurement to get the ratio, which can range from 0.80 or less to above 1.0. For waist-to-hip ratio, the normal ranges are different in men and women (Table 4.2). Waist-to-hip ratios associated with risk may vary by ethnicity, but specific cutoff values by race have not been determined. Caution should be used when approaching the concept of waist-to-hip ratio in terms of cutoff values, because data suggest a continuous increase in both renal and cardiovascular risk as this ratio ranges from 0.65 to 1.3 (Elsayed, 2008a; Elsayed, 2008b).

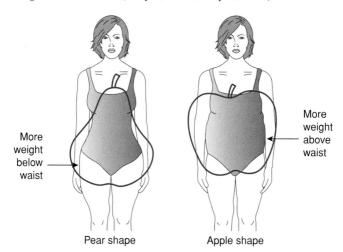

More weight below waist

More weight above waist

Pear shape

Apple shape

FIGURE 4.1 Weight gain in the area of the waist and above (apple type) is more dangerous than weight gained around the hips and flank area (pear type).

		Cardiovascular Risk
Men	**Women**	
0.78–0.95	0.65–0.87	Low
0.95–1.02	0.87–0.96	Moderate
1.02–1.28	0.96–1.20	Moderately high

Note: Initial recommendations that the waist-to-hip ratio should be kept <0.80 in women for optimum risk reduction were updated by Perry et al., 1998 which suggested 0.90 may be a more appropriate cutoff.
Source: From Elsayed EF, Tighiouart H, Weiner DE, et al. Waist-to-hip ratio and body mass index as risk factors for cardiovascular events in CKD. *Am J Kidney Dis.* 2008b;52:49–57.

Case Illustration. In this particular case, Mr. G's waist circumference was measured to be 44 inches (112 cm), and hip circumference measurement was 38 inches (96.5 cm), with a waist-to-hip ratio of 1.16. Both his waist circumference and waist-to-hip ratio are predictive of high cardiovascular risk.

Technology-Based Methods for Measuring Body Fat and Visceral Adiposity

A number of imaging methods (Kullberg, 2009) as well as bioimpedance have been used to assess both total body fat mass and visceral adiposity. Dual energy x-ray absorptiometry (DEXA), computed tomography (CT), and magnetic resonance imaging (MRI) are rarely used clinically because of their expense. Furthermore, in the clinical setting, whether a patient is obese is for the most part obvious, and response to treatment can be documented with simpler tests, such as the decrease in body weight, waist circumference, and waist-to-hip ratio.

Portable Ultrasound

Ultrasound has been used to measure both total and intra-abdominal fat. An evaluation of one method by its originator suggests a very high correlation with DEXA measurements in obese adolescents (Pineau, 2010).

Bioimpedance

Bioimpedance has been used to estimate fat mass, and results correlate reasonably well with DEXA. Foot-to-foot stand-on impedance devices, which resemble a scale and measure current and impedance from one foot to the other, are common in many health clubs. Reasonable correlations with fat mass as assessed by DEXA have been reported (Jaffrin, 2009). Norms for body fat percentage in middle-aged adults depend on the measurement method but in the non-obese typically range from 10% to 17% for men and from 15% to 23% in women. Data correlating cardiovascular or renal outcomes with body fat percentage are not available, and guideline-based targets for body fat percentage have not been proposed.

Waist Circumference or Waist–Hip Ratio and Outcomes

In a cross-sectional study of CKD patients Fabiana, (2008), found a strong association of waist circumference with visceral fat as measured by CT. In a prospective study which pooled individual patient data from two large cohort studies (the Atherosclerosis Risk in Communities Study and the Cardiovascular Health Study), waist–hip ratio, but not waist circumference or BMI, was associated with incident CKD, cardiovascular risk, and mortality (Elsayed, 2008a; Elsayed, 2008b). These data suggest that waist circumference and waist–hip ratio rather than BMI should be used as preferred anthropometric measures of obesity. When risk of CKD progression is assessed in terms of body composition, it may be better to estimate the glomerular filtration rate (GFR) using cystatin as opposed to creatinine, because serum creatinine is tied to both renal function and the amount of body muscle mass. For example Young, (2008), reported on the association between visceral adiposity and CKD in 1,300 participants from the Framingham Offspring Study. A relationship was found when the estimated glomerular filtration rate (eGFR) was measured using cystatin but not when using serum creatinine.

Obesity Microalbuminuria, Albuminuria, and Proteinuria

Obesity and Microalbuminuria or Albuminuria

Epidemiologic investigations suggest that obesity is a significant risk factor for the appearance of microalbuminuria across various populations. A population-based study of Italians (Cirillo, 1998) reported that BMI was related to albuminuria. Similar findings were seen in the PREVEND study, which investigated the relationship between body weight, fat distribution, microalbuminuria, and glomerular filtration in a European population without diabetes (Pinto-Sietsma, 2003). Those with visceral adiposity measured as waist-to-hip ratio were at increased risk for microalbuminuria. Multivariable analyses show that body mass is independently associated with albuminuria and the risk is greater in men than in women (Verhave, 2003). The occurrence of microalbuminuria or chronic renal insufficiency (GFR <60 mL/min per 1.73 m^2) is related to the number of components of the metabolic syndrome present, including central obesity, elevated fasting blood glucose level, hypertriglyceridemia, reduced high-density lipoprotein (HDL) cholesterol level, and hypertension (Gerstein, 2001).

Obesity and Proteinuria

Markedly obese patients can develop a slowly progressive proteinuria, which can reach the nephrotic range (Kambham, 2001). The appearance of proteinuria usually precedes the onset of GFR decline by several years. Weight loss in markedly obese patients often results in a reduction in proteinuria and there are multiple potential mechanisms by which this might happen (Praga, 2001), including improved blood-pressure control, improvement of serum lipid profile, improvement of insulin sensitivity, better glycemic control in diabetic patients, decrease of circulating leptin levels, reversal of glomerular hyperfiltration, and decrease of activation of the renin–angiotensin system.

Visceral Adiposity, Inflammation, and the Metabolic Syndrome

Visceral adiposity is characterized by dysfunctional adipose tissue which is a known source of proinflammatory adipokines. Proinflammatory adipokines, such as tumor necrosis factor-α, interleukin-1 and interleukin-6, leptin, and resistin, have been implicated in the development of insulin resistance (Wisse, 2004). Animal models suggest that the combination of decreased insulin sensitivity and hyperinsulinemia results in glomerular changes that include expansion and thickening of the glomerular basement membranes, as well as glomerulosclerosis (Cusumamo, 2002). The metabolic outcome of obesity is characterized by a collection of cardiovascular risk factors that includes hypertension, hyperinsulinemia, type 2 diabetes, and persistent inflammation. These clinical comorbidities are common findings in CKD, even in the absence of obesity, and suggest a synergistic relationship of these factors with cardiovascular outcomes.

WEIGHT-LOSS STRATEGIES IN CHRONIC KIDNEY DISEASE PATIENTS

Weight loss is a sensible therapeutic strategy for Mr. G, although the amount of weight loss required to achieve maximal benefit is unknown. Among the documented benefits of losing weight are reduction in proteinuria, as well as lower blood pressure and improved insulin sensitivity (Praga, 1995; Schneider, 2005). The cornerstone of therapy for management of obesity includes nonpharmacologic strategies focused on weight reduction through healthy eating and increased regular physical activity. Prevention and treatment of obesity should be a first-line objective in the therapeutic approach of patients with diabetic and nondiabetic CKD. A high BMI value is the second leading preventable cause of death after cigarette smoking (Mokdad, 2004). Although studies of intentional weight loss to slow progression of CKD have not been performed, the health benefits and recommendations for weight loss for the general population likely apply to this group. In healthy individuals, weight loss of 5% to 10% of body weight lowers blood pressure and cholesterol levels. The means by which patients lose weight is important, and healthy eating patterns and increased physical activity should be emphasized (Table 4.3).

CASE STUDY Mr. G returns to the clinic after 1 month. His blood pressure is now 168/90, his pulse is 56, and his weight has increased to 318 pounds (144.2 kg). His physical exam is within normal limits except for mild lower-extremity edema. His BUN is 28 mg/dL (10 mmol/L), creatinine is 2.4 mg/dL (212 μmol/L), and a 24-hour urine creatinine clearance is 80 mL/min (not corrected for body surface area). His 24-hour urinary protein excretion is 190 mg. **What recommendations would you make for Mr. G regarding weight loss and why?**

Dietary Approaches

Successful management requires careful planning, periodic assessment of nutritional status, and monitoring of dietary compliance. The Kidney Disease Outcomes Quality Initiative (KDOQI) clinical practice

TABLE 4.3	Lifestyle Modifications Recommended by the Seventh Report of the Joint National Committee on Prevention, Detection, Evaluation, and Treatment of High Blood Pressure

Lifestyle Component	Recommendation
Weight maintenance if BMI <25 kg/m²	Balanced diet to maintain desirable body weight
Weight loss if overweight or obese (BMI ≥25 kg/m²)	Calorie-restricted, balanced diet
Exercise and physical activity	Moderate intensity for 30 minutes/day, most days of the week
Moderation of alcohol intake	≤2 drinks/day (men) ≤1 drink/day (women)
Smoking cessation	Counseling, nicotine supplementation

BMI, body mass index.
Source: From National Kidney Foundation. KDOQI clinical practice guidelines for chronic kidney disease: evaluation, classification, and stratification. *Am J Kidney Dis.* 2002;39:S1–S266, Table 84, with permission.

guidelines are not specific to the obese patient, because data are lacking regarding optimal nutrient requirements in obese patients with CKD. Nutritional directives offered here are extrapolated from recommendations for individuals with CKD who are at normal weight.

Individualization and Monitoring
KDOQI recommends that routine care for patients include dietary advice from a registered dietitian who is experienced in counseling patients with CKD. The input of a dietitian is particularly important when managing the obese patient, as additional considerations must be made regarding energy balance and the dietary management of comorbid conditions such as diabetes and hypertension. As part of dietary management, patients should receive a comprehensive, individualized diet plan, including dietary assessment and measurement of nutrition-related laboratory parameters and anthropometrics. Dietary assessment can be completed using standardized methods such as dietary recalls, food diaries, or food frequency questionnaires. Important laboratory parameters include serum levels of albumin, prealbumin, creatinine, cholesterol, phosphorus, calcium, and blood lipid profile (i.e., cholesterol and triglycerides).

Energy Intake
In CKD stages 1 to 3, the KDOQI recommends that energy intake levels support a balanced diet and maintain desirable body weight but does not recommend specific energy intake amounts. In CKD stages 4 through 5 (GFR <30 mL/min), specific energy intake amounts are recommended: 35 kcal/kg per day for those younger than 60 years and 30 to 35 kcal/kg per day for those older than 60 years. A 30-kcal/kg diet equates to 2,400 to 2,900 kcal/day for a 150- to 180-pound patient. Obese patients should be advised to target lower energy intake levels.

Fat Intake With Hypocaloric Diets

Reducing fat as part of a low-calorie diet is a practical way to reduce energy intake. Clinical trials of diet therapy to reduce lipids and slow progression of CKD have not been conducted. Dietary fat recommendations for the obese patient with CKD should be in accordance with National Cholesterol Education Program/Adult Treatment Panel III (NCEP/ATPIII) guidelines (Expert Panel on Detection, Evaluation, and Treatment of High Blood Pressure in Adults, 2001) developed for cardiovascular risk reduction.

In stages 1 through 4 of CKD, KDOQI recommends that 25% to 35% of total energy intake come from fat with <10% of the total from saturated fat. Recommended cholesterol intake is <200 mg/day. The objective of these guidelines is to control blood lipid levels, minimizing elevated blood glucose and triglycerides. Because diets for patients with CKD sometimes are mildly restricted in protein, it may be difficult to provide sufficient energy without resorting to large intake of high-glycemic index carbohydrates that may increase triglyceride production. Another challenge when addressing fat intake is maintaining recommended macronutrient balance when lowering saturated fat in the diet. When saturated fat is reduced in the diet, it can be replaced with unsaturated fat, protein, or carbohydrate. The optimal means of replacement of saturated fat is not known. Data from dietary intervention trials suggest that a diet low in saturated fat that uses either protein or unsaturated fats to replace carbohydrates can have favorable effects on lipids.

Protein Intake in Weight Loss

The extent to which dietary protein should be restricted in various stages of CKD is controversial. It is important to maintain a minimum of high-quality biologic protein intake during any weight-loss program to avoid the development of malnutrition. Please see Chapter 9 for a detailed discussion of protein intake in CKD.

Carbohydrate Intake in Weight Loss

High dietary carbohydrate intake has been implicated as a contributor to the increased prevalence of obesity in the United States. National dietary recommendations have promoted high-carbohydrate, low-fat diets in efforts to reduce cardiovascular disease risk. These recommendations were based on observational studies in which low fat intake was associated with low risk for cardiovascular disease, presumably by lowering low-density lipoprotein (LDL) cholesterol (Grundy, 1982). However, some carbohydrates, namely fiber, have been shown to have beneficial effects on health and weight loss. In a meta-analysis of 35 studies, psyllium fiber taken before meals over multi-week spans was shown to significantly lower fasting blood glucose and glycated hemoglobin (Gibb, 2015). Another meta-analysis of 12 studies lasting 2 to 17 weeks in duration showed that fiber had a significant effect in lowering BMI, body weight, and body fat, among other makers of metabolic health (Thompson, 2017).

Macronutrient Distribution of Diets Relating to
Disease Risk and Weight Loss

There has been an ongoing debate over the last several decades as to what macronutrient distribution in diets has the most beneficial effect on health. The answer to this debate will almost certainly lie within the particular goals of the individual. To attain significant weight loss, studies have repeatedly shown that significant energy restriction over time is efficacious, regardless of the macronutrient distribution of the diet. A study with 424 adults on four different weight-loss diets with varying amounts of macronutrient distribution showed that subjects across all diet types lost significant amounts of fat and lean body mass when compared to baseline values, but no significant differences among the diet types were found at either 6 months or 2 years (de Souza, 2012). While weight loss will almost certainly improve health, more specific outcomes of disease risk do favor certain macronutrient profiles. One study of a high-protein (HP) versus high-carbohydrate (HC) diet in obese women showed that after 6 months of the dietary intervention, both groups lost significant amounts of weight from baseline, with no differences between diet types. However, there were significant differences between diets on markers of β-cell function, oxidative stress, proinflammatory cytokines, and adipokines, all favoring the HP diet. Similarly, a study between a very–low-carbohydrate (LC)/high unsaturated fat diet and a high unrefined carbohydrate (HC)/low-fat diet in obese adults showed that both groups lost similar amounts of weight over a 24-week period with no diet effect. However, the LC diet showed a significant difference over the HC diet in greater reductions of triglycerides, greater HbA1c reductions, and HDL cholesterol increases (Tay, 2014).

Very–High-Protein (Atkins-Type) Diets in Chronic Kidney Disease

Some popular weight-loss diets contain excessive amounts of nutrients that may be detrimental (e.g., protein or potassium) to patients who are in the later stages of CKD. Diets with very low-carbohydrate and HP content should be avoided as a weight-loss strategy (e.g., the Atkins diet). Atkins-type diets have been found to deliver a marked acid load to the kidney, increase the risk of stone formation, promote negative calcium balance and increase bone loss, and increase GFR (Reddy, 2002). Chronic intake of an HP diet (1.5 g/kg per day) as a strategy for weight control in obese individuals may aggravate preexisting glomerular hypertension (Friedman, 2004), the latter being a risk factor for progression of CKD. HP diets also tend to be high in phosphorus, and very high phosphorus intake may have an adverse impact on CKD progression (Chang and Anderson, 2017). Nevertheless, one 2-year trial found no adverse effect of a low-carbohydrate diet on measures of renal health (Tirosh, 2013).

Dietary Sodium Intake

Sodium retention occurs with CKD, and associated extracellular volume expansion plays a major role in the development of hypertension, peripheral edema, and congestive heart failure. In a study of 488 subjects, central obesity was significantly associated with dietary salt intake compared to nonobese subjects (Perry, 2010).

Potential Issues Related to High Water Intake

One should avoid promoting the concept of "eight glasses of water a day" or a high fluid intake in general as an aid to weight loss. A study using the Modification of Diet in Renal Disease (MDRD) database to retrospectively examine the relationship between fluid intake and renal disease progression found that sustained high urine volume and low urine osmolality were independent risk factors for faster GFR decline (Hebert, 2003). The authors concluded that high fluid intake does not slow renal disease progression and that patients should let "thirst be their guide" for how much water/fluids to drink. The controversy about the potential benefits versus harms of high water intake in various kidney conditions, including autosomal dominant polycystic kidney disease, presumably by suppressing the release of antidiuretic hormone, remains unresolved (Visconti, 2018).

Dietary Potassium Intake in Weight Loss

Even at typical levels of potassium intake, renal excretion of potassium can be affected in later stages of CKD and predispose individuals to hyperkalemia. For weight-control purposes, one usually counsels avoiding high-calorie foods such as high-glycemic index carbohydrates, fats, and oils, all of which contain little or no potassium. Highly refined foods such as white breads, pasta, rice, and certain cereals contain little potassium. A typical strategy for weight loss is to increase consumption of fruits and vegetables and high-fiber grains, all of which contain substantial amounts of potassium. Although fruits and vegetables are a major source of potassium, they can be incorporated into the diet of patients with CKD if they are carefully selected, the portion size is controlled, and the method of preparation is considered. In later stages of CKD, rich sources of potassium should be avoided (see Chapters 5 and 6 for a more complete discussion of this topic).

Dietary Phosphorus and Calcium Intake in Weight Loss

Some restriction of dietary phosphorus often is recommended in the later stages of CKD. A high calcium intake may be associated with vascular calcification. A general list of "healthy" food choices for obese patients with CKD is given in Table 4.4. Such lists always must be individualized, depending on the stage of CKD and patient preferences.

CASE STUDY 4.3   STRUCTURED WEIGHT-LOSS PROGRAMS, EXERCISE

Mr. G visited the dietitian to develop an eating plan. He experiences some highs and lows with his use of diets for weight loss. Six weeks later, Mr. G's weight is down to 309 pounds (140 kg), and his blood pressure is 170/90 mm Hg. You congratulate him on his weight loss and ask him to follow-up 2 months later. At this subsequent visit, Mr. G's weight is still 309 pounds (140 kg) but his blood pressure is now controlled at 122/50 mm Hg. **Mr. G would like additional help in meeting his weight-loss goals. He asks you about the use of a structured program. What should you tell him?**

TABLE 4.4		Food Choices to Help Obese Patients With Chronic Kidney Disease Meet Recommendations for Selected Nutrients

Nutrient	Good Food Choices for Obese Patients With CKD	Foods That Should Be Limited for Obese Patients With CKD
Sodium	Fresh, unprocessed foods Foods containing 5–10% of the recommended intake per serving (115–230 mg)	Prepackaged and processed foods, such as regular breads, cereals, cured meats, cheeses, and canned products
Saturated fat	Poultry, fish, and leaner cuts of meat Non- or low-fat dairy products Substitute unsaturated oils (e.g., olive, canola, corn) for butter or lard	Animal products, such as meats and regular-fat dairy products Butter, lard
Carbohydrate	Fruits Vegetables and legumes Complex carbohydrates, such as whole grain breads and cereals, brown rice, barley	Refined products, such as white sugar, white bread, white rice, processed honey
Phosphorus	Non- or low-fat milk and milk products Legumes Bran cereal	Regular-fat dairy products Processed meats and cheese Processed cereals
Protein	Low-protein breads and baking products Egg whites or low-cholesterol egg substitute Non- or low-fat milk Legumes Poultry and fish Low-fat meats	Animal products, such as meats and regular-fat dairy products
Potassium	*In early stages of CKD:* Fruits and vegetables *In later stages of CKD:* Potassium is widely distributed in all foods, and dietary recommendations can be met by eating fresh, unprocessed foods with low potassium content	*In later stages of CKD:* Fruits, such as tomatoes, apricots, cantaloupes, citrus, bananas Tuberous vegetables, such as potatoes (unless double boiled), soybeans, buckwheat

CKD, chronic kidney disease.
Source: From Anderson CA, Miller ER. Dietary recommendations for obese patients with chronic kidney disease. *Adv Chronic Kidney Dis.* 2006;13:394–402, with permission.

Characteristics of Structured Weight-Loss Programs

Mr. G is not unique in his struggles to maintain weight loss over the long term. Although sustained weight loss is difficult, randomized controlled trials have documented that weight loss can be achieved using structured programs that focus on lifestyle modification. Key characteristics of programs that work are long duration of the intervention, self-monitoring of calories and weight, use of group sessions, and promotion of diets with reduced portion size, reduced caloric density, and high intake of fiber and whole grains (Wadden, 2007).

Typical weight-loss interventions emphasize behavioral counseling rather than provision of information. Counseling is done in group settings with periodic one-on-one sessions. Group sessions foster accountability, provide social support, and are less costly than individual counseling. Counselors include a wide spectrum of allied health professionals, including registered dietitians, health educators, and clinical psychologists. Ideally, counselors are trained in behavioral techniques that motivate individuals to make and sustain lifestyle changes.

Most Weight-Loss Programs Have Two Phases

The first phase is an initial, intensive phase in which interventionist–participant contact occurs roughly weekly for up to 6 months. Well-designed intervention programs typically result in clinically significant weight loss for one-half to two-thirds of the participants over the initial 6 months. During initial weight-loss period, average weight loss in trials typically is 4 to 6 kg (Neter, 2003), but with a wide range.

A second or weight-maintenance phase then occurs in which individuals attempt to sustain weight loss. The weight-maintenance phase is typically less intensive than the initial weight-loss phase. Despite short-term initial success, weight regain is commonplace. Weight loss varies by factors such as sex, age, and race/ethnicity. Women generally lose less total weight than men, although the difference may be explained by differences in baseline body weight. Individuals older than age 60 generally lose more weight initially and more effectively maintain weight reductions than younger individuals. Members of minority populations generally lose less weight than their white counterparts.

For successful weight loss, patients must have an excellent attendance record at group sessions and maintain adherence with behavioral recommendations. It has been estimated that to achieve weight loss of 1 pound per week, a daily calorie deficit of 500 kcal is required. Such a calorie deficit is difficult to achieve through increased physical activity alone. Hence, contemporary weight-loss programs typically emphasize calorie restriction as a means to lower weight.

Importance of Exercise

Exercise has been shown to (a) modestly contribute to weight loss in overweight and obese adults, (b) decrease abdominal fat, (c) increase cardiorespiratory fitness, and (d) help with maintenance of weight loss. Exercise should be recommended for the obese patient with CKD as part of a comprehensive weight-loss therapy and weight-control program. Exercise, as well as simply avoiding physical inactivity, can be beneficial in obese patients with CKD in controlling comorbidities such as hypertension, diabetes, cardiovascular disease, and hyperlipidemia (Zelle, 2017). As such, exercise is recommended as part of the

National Kidney Foundation's KDOQI clinical practice guidelines for hypertension and antihypertensive agents in CKD (guideline 6). This particular guideline suggests moderate-intensity exercise for 30 min/day, most days of the week (see Table 4.3).

Effectiveness of Exercise in Chronic Kidney Disease

Studies of the effects of exercise training in earlier stages of CKD are infrequent, and the majority of published research has been conducted in patients with ESRD. Exercise in combination with a structured weight-loss program has been shown to be effective in one small study (MacLaughlin, 2010). Beneficial effects of exercise training have been seen in terms of improved blood-pressure control, physical function, and health-related quality of life, and notably, skeletal muscle function (Roshanravan, 2017). In patients with type-1 diabetes with or without CKD, physical activity was associated with improved survival (Tikkanen-Dolenc, 2017).

Prior Medical Screening

Before exercise is incorporated into a patient's weight-loss program, a medical screening should be completed and consideration made for coexisting diseases, including blood-pressure control and volume status. Exercise plans need to be carefully individualized and monitored for each patient. Ideally, exercise should be undertaken in combination with behavioral therapy that targets the patient's motivation levels and other factors that contribute to the success of an exercise program. Based on data from the National Weight Control Registry, high levels of physical activity, ongoing self-monitoring, restrained eating, and comparatively small amounts of television time are all factors associated with sustained weight loss (Raynor, 2006).

CASE STUDY 4.4

PHARMACOLOGIC DRUGS FOR WEIGHT LOSS IN CHRONIC KIDNEY DISEASE

Mr. G is having a difficult time trying to lose weight through lifestyle modification (diet and exercise). This is typical for patients attempting weight loss. At this visit, his blood pressure is 172/90 mm Hg, pulse is 80, and his weight is back up to 318 pounds (144 kg). **Do you think it might be appropriate to suggest pharmacologic approaches to weight loss?**

General Effectiveness Versus Risks of Weight-Loss Drugs

The use of pharmacologic approaches for weight loss may become necessary if obesity-associated renal disease cannot be prevented or retarded by using lifestyle modification. It has been estimated that current weight-loss drugs produce an additional mean weight loss of only 3 to 5 kg above that of diet and placebo over 6 months, and more effective pharmacotherapy of obesity is needed. Currently there are five drugs approved by the U.S. FDA for weight loss, and each has shown some degree of efficacy, namely weight loss exceeding 5% over a 1-year period (Khera, 2016).

Specific Weight-Loss Drugs
Orlistat (Xenical)

Orlistat (Roche Laboratories, Nutley, NJ) acts by inhibiting lipases in the gut to reduce fat absorption. Malabsorption of fat can markedly increase gut absorption of oxalate, and this can cause either oxalate stones or, acutely, oxalate-induced kidney injury. On the other hand, there was no evidence of deterioration of kidney function in 33 patients with CKD given orlistat as part of a structured weight-loss program (MacLaughlin, 2010). Cholestyramine (to bind bile salts) and calcium supplementation (to bind gut oxalate) have been used to reduce oxalate excretion in patients with fat malabsorption due to small bowel surgery. Whether such adjunctive treatments might mitigate any hyperoxaluria occurring with orlistat treatment has not been investigated. The continued episodic reports of worsening of CKD associated with orlistat, presumably because of precipitation of oxalate crystals in the kidney, remains a cause for concern (Solomon, 2017). Use in patients with hyperoxaluria or kidney stones would require additional caution.

Phentermine–Topiramate (Qsymia)

Qsymia is a combination of immediate-release phentermine hydrochloride, a noradrenergic appetite suppressant, and extended-release topiramate, a fructose derivative used as an anticonvulsant (Shin and Gadde, 2013). A 24-week phase II trial of the combination drug showed a −10.7% body weight change compared to −2.1% for placebo. A phase III trial showed similar weight loss results with additional reductions in systolic blood pressure, triglycerides, and fasting insulin. For safety, it is recommended that in patients with moderate (creatinine clearance ≥30 to <50 mL/min) and severe (<30 mL/min) kidney dysfunction, the maximum dose of PHEN/TPM should not exceed 7.5/46 mg.

Lorcaserin (Belviq)

Lorcaserin is a selective serotonin 2C receptor antagonist used for appetite suppression. In a randomized controlled trial, overweight or obese patients on lorcaserin lost an average of 5.8 kg compared to 2.2 kg in those taking a placebo, at 52 weeks. At that time, those subjects initially randomized to lorcaserin were split into two treatment groups that received either placebo or lorcaserin for an additional year. At the 2-year time point, more subjects on lorcaserin (68%) maintained their weight loss than the placebo group (50%). The most common adverse effects reported with locaserin were headache, dizziness, and nausea (Smith, 2010). Lorcaserin may be used in patients with mild renal impairment, but is not recommended for those with moderate or severe kidney dysfunction or ESRD (Gustafson, 2013).

Naltrexone–Bupropion (Contrave)

Contrave is a combination of naltrexone and bupropion, and the exact mechanism of action has not been fully described. Naltrexone and bupropion both act on regions of the brain that may influence food intake, cravings, and other aspects of eating (Billes, 2014). In a 52-week study, subjects taking Contrave lost an average of 8.1% body weight compared to 1.4% in patients taking a placebo. Interestingly, a study in which smokers received the weight-loss dose of Contrave showed a significant decrease in nicotine use, and in subjects with depression, a decrease of depressive symptoms. Treatment with Contrave has not been tested in patients with renal or hepatic impairment. Dosage recommendations for these populations are based on the data for naltrexone and bupropion individually. Contrave is not recommended for individuals with ESRD (Sherman, 2016).

Liraglutide 3.0 mg (Saxenda)

Liraglutide is a long-acting glucagon-like peptide-1 receptor agonist. As discussed in Chapter 13, liraglutide is completely metabolized in the body, and the kidney is not a major organ of elimination, so it requires no dosage adjustment in stages 2 or 3 of CKD. The label suggests caution when initiating Saxenda in patients with more advanced stages of CKD, as instances of worsening of CKD have been reported in postmarketing surveillance, perhaps linked to dehydration consequent to nausea and vomiting, which is a side effect of the drug.

BARIATRIC SURGERY AND CHRONIC KIDNEY DISEASE

For some obese patients, for whom lifestyle modifications prove ineffective for weight loss, gastric bypass surgery may be an option. This surgical intervention can result in weight loss that improves a variety of disease risk factors, and can also prove beneficial for individuals with CKD (Friedman, 2018). The Roux-en-Y gastric bypass procedure may show more favorable results than sleeve gastrectomy in patients (Imam, 2017). However, caution is warranted for individuals with CKD who are considering bariatric surgery. Studies have shown that adverse events and mortality rates are higher in individuals with CKD and identification for specific risk factors remains a high priority (MacLaughlin, 2010). Specifically, CKD stage predicts higher complication rates, though it is worth noting that the incidence of complications remains at <10% (Turgeon, 2012).

CASE STUDY 4.5

Mr. G decides not to use a pharmacologic approach for weight loss. It is now 13 months after his initial visit, and Mr. G returns to the clinic. His weight is now 331 pounds (151 kg). His blood pressure is 132/76 mm Hg. His serum creatinine is 2.3 (203 µmol/L). He tells you that his wife recently had laparoscopic gastric bypass surgery and inquires whether you think this might be a good approach for him. What do you say?

Bariatric surgery has become an important tool in the treatment of obese patients with CKD and often results in improvement or complete remission of the comorbidities of obesity.

CASE STUDY 4.6

You make a surgical referral, but the surgeon is hesitant to consider Mr. G for surgery for fear of potential complications related to his CKD. What knowledge can you share with the surgeon about the benefits of bariatric surgery in patients with CKD?

The scientific literature on bariatric surgery in patients with CKD is limited. Benefits documented in case reports must be weighed against the risk of postsurgery complications such as acute kidney injury on CKD, cardiopulmonary complications, wound infection, dehydration, kidney stones, and possibly death. The most successful bariatric surgeries reduce body weight by 35% to 40%. Significant improvements have been noted postsurgery in eGFR, urinary albumin excretion, diabetes, hypertension, and dyslipidemia, as well as improvement in the quality of life (Buchwald, 2004; Izzedine, 2005; Owen, 2018). In some patients, significant improvements in glycemia and hypertension are seen within days of bariatric surgery, allowing tapering or withdrawal of antidiabetic and/or antihypertensive medications. Inflammatory markers and leptin and angiotensin also decline after surgery. This trend continues throughout the first year after surgery. The durability of resolution rates has been shown out to 10 to 15 years. In type 2 diabetic patients, cost-effectiveness of bariatric surgery is enhanced by marked decrease in the use of diabetic medications as well as reductions in total annual health care costs (Makary, 2010).

Enteric Hyperoxaluria Risk With Bariatric Surgery
By causing some degree of fat malabsorption, some forms of bariatric surgery may increase urinary excretion of oxalate. The unabsorbed fat binds to calcium, preventing calcium binding to oxalate. This can increase the risk of kidney stones after bariatric surgery and may even cause oxalate-mediated impairment of renal function. It is prudent to measure urinary oxalate excretion after bariatric surgery and to assure an adequate intake of calcium, and to limit ingestion of high-oxalate containing foods. (Tarplin, 2015; Asplin, 2016).

CASE STUDY 4.7 The surgeon is convinced by your argument, and Mr. G has bariatric surgery. Sixteen months later, he has lost 100 pounds (45.4 kg) and now weighs 218 pounds (99 kg). His blood pressure has decreased to 102/70 mm Hg.

References and Suggested Readings

Asplin JR. The management of patients with enteric hyperoxaluria. *Urolithiasis.* 2016;44:33–43.
Billes SK, Sinnayah P, Cowley MA. Naltrexone/bupropion for obesity: An investigational combination pharmacotherapy for weight loss. *Pharm Res.* 2014;84:1–11.
Björntorp P. "Portal" adipose tissue as a generator of risk factors for cardiovascular disease and diabetes. *Arteriosclerosis.* 1990;10:493–496.
Buchwald H, Avidor Y, Braunwald E, et al. Bariatric surgery: A systematic review and meta-analysis. *JAMA.* 2004;292:1724–1737.
Canoy D, Boekholdt SM, Wareham N, et al. Body fat distribution and risk of coronary heart disease in men and women in the European Prospective Investigation Into Cancer and Nutrition in Norfolk cohort: A population-based prospective study. *Circulation.* 2007;116:2933–2943.
Chang AR, Anderson C. Dietary phosphorus intake and the kidney. *Annu Rev Nutr.* 2017;37:321–346.

Cirillo M, Senigalliesi L, Laurenzi M, et al. Microalbuminuria in nondiabetic adults. *Arch Intern Med.* 1998;158:1933–1939.

Cusumamo AM, Bodkini NL, Hansen BC, et al. Glomerular hypertrophy is associated with hyperinsulinemia and precedes overt diabetes in aging, rhesus monkeys. *Am J Kidney Dis.* 2002;40:1075–1085.

De Koning L, Merchant AT, Pogue J, Anand S S. Waist circumference and waist-to-hip ratio as predictors of cardiovascular events: Meta-regression analysis of prospective studies. *Eur Heart J.* 2007;28:850–856.

de Souza RJ, Bray GA, Carey VJ, et al. (2012). Effects of 4 weight-loss diets differing in fat, protein, and carbohydrate on fat mass, lean mass, visceral adipose tissue, and hepatic fat: results from the POUNDS LOST trial. *Am J Clin Nutr.* 2012;95:614–625.

Doğan A, Nakipoğlu-Yüzer GF, Yildizgören MT, et al. Is age or the body mass index (BMI) more determinant of the bone mineral density (BMD) in geriatric women and men? *Arch Gerontol Geriatr.* 2010;51:338–341.

Elsayed EF, Sarnak MJ, Tighiouart H, et al. Waist-to-hip ratio, body mass index, and subsequent kidney disease and death. *Am J Kidney Dis.* 2008a;52:29–38.

Elsayed EF, Tighiouart H, Weiner DE, et al. Waist-to-hip ratio and body mass index as risk factors for cardiovascular events in CKD. *Am J Kidney Dis.* 2008b;52:49–57.

Expert Panel on Detection, Evaluation, and Treatment of High Blood Pressure in Adults. Executive summary of the third report of the National Cholesterol Education Program (NCEP) Expert Panel on Detection, Evaluation, and Treatment of High Blood Cholesterol in Adults (Adult Treatment Panel III). *JAMA.* 2001;285:2486–2497.

Fabiana MR, Sanches CM, Avesani, MA, et al. Waist circumference and visceral fat in CKD: A cross-sectional study. *Am J Kidney Dis.* 2008;52:66–73.

Flegal KM, Graubard BI, Williamson DF, et al. Excess deaths associated with underweight, overweight, and obesity. *JAMA.* 2005;293:1861–1867.

Flicker L, McCaul KA, Hankey GJ, et al. Body mass index and survival in men and women aged 70 to 75. *J Am Geriatr Soc.* 2010;58:234–241.

Frayn KN. Visceral fat and insulin resistance—causative or correlative? *Br J Nutr.* 2000;83:S71–S77.

Friedman AN. High protein diets: Potential effects on the kidney in renal health and disease. *Am J Kidney Dis.* 2004;44:950–962.

Friedman AN, Wahed AS, Wang J, et al. Effect of bariatric surgery on CKD risk. *J Am Soc Nephrol.* 2018;29:1289–1300.

Gerstein HC, Mann JF, Yi Q, et al. Albuminuria and risk of cardiovascular events, death and heart failure in diabetic and nondiabetic individuals. *JAMA.* 2001;286:421–426.

Gibb RD, McRorie Jr JW, Russell DA, Hasselblad V, D'Alessio DA. Psyllium fiber improves glycemic control proportional to loss of glycemic control: a meta-analysis of data in euglycemic subjects, patients at risk of type 2 diabetes mellitus, and patients being treated for type 2 diabetes mellitus. *Am J Clin Nutr.* 2015:102;1604–1614.

Grundy SM, Bilheimer D, Blackburn H. Rationale of the diet-heart statement of the American Heart Association. *Circulation.* 1982;65:839A–854A.

Gustafson A, King C, Rey JA. Lorcaserin (Belviq): A selective serotonin 5-HT2C agonist in the treatment of obesity. *P T.* 2013;38:525–534.

He M, Li ET, Harris S, et al. Canadian global village reality: Anthropometric surrogate cutoffs and metabolic abnormalities among Canadians of East Asian, South Asian, and European descent. *Can Fam Physician.* 2010;56:e174–e182.

Hebert LA, Greene T, Levey A, et al. High urine volume and low urine osmolality are risk factors for faster progression of renal disease. *Am J Kidney Dis.* 2003;41:962–971.

Hoffman DJ, Wang Z, Gallagher D, et al. Comparison of visceral adipose tissue mass in adult African Americans and whites. *Obes Res.* 2005;13:66–74.

Hsu CY, McCulloch CE, Iribarren C, et al. Body mass index and risk for end-stage renal disease. *Ann Intern Med.* 2006;144:21–28.

Izzedine H, Coupaye M, Reach I, et al. Gastric bypass and resolution of proteinuria in an obese diabetic patient. *Diabet Med.* 2005;22:1761–1762.

Imam TH, Fischer H, Jing B, et al. Estimated GFR before and after bariatric surgery in CKD. *Am J Kidney Dis.* 2017;69:380–388.

Jaffrin MY. Body composition determination by bioimpedance: An update. *Curr Opin Clin Nutr Metab Care.* 2009;12:482–486.

Johansenn KL, Kutner NG, Young B, et al. Association of body size with health status in patients beginning dialysis. *Am J Clin Nutr*. 2006;83:543–549.

Kalantar-Zadeh K, Block G, Humphreys MH, et al. Reverse epidemiology of cardiovascular risk factors in maintenance dialysis patients. *Kidney Int*. 2003;63:793–808.

Kambham N, Markowitz G, Valeri AM, et al. Obesity-related glomerulopathy: An emerging epidemic. *Kidney Int*. 2001;59:1498–1509.

Khera R, Murad MH, Chandar AK, et al. Association of pharmacological treatments of obesity with weight loss: A systematic review and meta-analysis. *JAMA*. 2016;315:2424–2434.

Kuk JL, Ardern CI. Influence of age on the association between various measures of obesity and all-cause mortality. *J Am Geriatr Soc*. 2009;57:2077–2084.

Kullberg J, Brandberg J, Angelhed JE, et al. Whole-body adipose tissue analysis: Comparison of MRI, CT and dual energy x-ray absorptiometry. *Br J Radiol*. 2009;82:123–130.

MacLaughlin HL, Cook SA, Kariyawasam D, et al. Nonrandomized trial of weight loss with orlistat, nutrition education, diet, and exercise in obese patients with CKD: 2-year follow-up. *Am J Kidney Dis*. 2010;55:69–76.

Makary MA, Clarke JM, Shore AD, et al. Medication utilization and annual health care costs in patients with type 2 diabetes mellitus before and after bariatric surgery. *Arch Surg*. 2010;145:726–731.

Mokdad AH, Marks JS, Stroup DF, et al. Actual causes of death in the United States, 2000. *JAMA*. 2004;291:1238–1245.

Neter JE, Stam BE, Kok FJ, et al. Influence of weight reduction on blood pressure: A meta-analysis of randomized controlled trials. *Hypertension*. 2003;42:878–884.

Owen JG, Yazdi F, Reisin E. Bariatric surgery and hypertension. *Am J Hyperten*. 2018;31:11–17.

Patel DK, Stanford FC. Safety and tolerability of new-generation anti-obesity medications: a narrative review. *Postgrad Med*. 2018;130:173–182.

Perry AC, Miller PC, Allison MD, et al. Clinical predictability of the waist-to-hip ratio in assessment of cardiovascular disease risk factors in overweight, premenopausal women. *Am J Clin Nutr*. 1998;68:1022–1027.

Perry IJ, Browne G, Loughrey M, Harrington J, Lutomski J, Fitzgerald AP. Dietary salt intake and related risk factors in the Irish population. *Cork: SafeFood Ireland*. 2010.

Pineau JC, Lalys L, Bocquet M, et al. Ultrasound measurement of total body fat in obese adolescents. *Ann Nutr Metab*. 2010;56:36–44.

Pinto-Sietsma SJ, Navis G, Janssen WM, et al. A central body fat distribution is related to renal function impairment, even in lean subjects. *Am J Kidney Dis*. 2003;41:733–741.

Praga M, Hernandez E, Andres A, et al. Effects of body weight loss and captopril treatment on proteinuria associated with obesity. *Nephron*. 1995;70:35–41.

Praga M, Hernandez E, Morales E, et al. Clinical features and long-term outcome of obesity-associated focal segmental glomerulosclerosis. *Nephrol Dial Transplant*. 2001;16:1790–1798.

Raynor DA, Phelan S, Hill JO, et al. Television viewing and long-term weight maintenance: Results from the National Weight Control Registry. *Obesity (Silver Spring)*. 2006;14:1816–1824.

Reddy ST, Wang CY, Sakhaee K, et al. Effect of low-carbohydrate high protein diets on acid base balance, stone forming propensity and calcium metabolism. *Am J Kidney Dis*. 2002;40:265–274.

Roshanravan B, Gamboa J, Wilund K. Exercise and CKD: Skeletal muscle dysfunction and practical application of exercise to prevent and treat physical impairments in CKD. *Am J Kidney Dis*. 2017;69:837–852.

Salahudeen AK. Obesity and survival on dialysis. *Am J Kidney Dis*. 2003;41:925–932.

Schneider R, Golzman B, Turkot S, et al. Effect of weight loss on blood pressure, arterial compliance, and insulin resistance in normotensive obese subjects. *Am J Med Sci*. 2005;330:157–160.

Sherman MM, Ungureanu S, Rey J. Naltrexone/Bupropion ER (Contrave): Newly approved treatment option for chronic weight management in obese adults. *P T*. 2016;41:164–172.

Shin JH, Gadde KM. Clinical utility of phentermine/topiramate (QsymiaTM) combination for the treatment of obesity. *Diabetes Metab Syndr Obes.* 2013;8:131–139.

Smith SR, Weissman NJ, Anderson CM, et al. Multicenter, placebo-controlled trial of lorcaserin for weight management. *N Engl J Med.* 2010;363:245–256.

Solomon LR, Nixon AC, Ogden L, et al. Orlistat-induced oxalate nephropathy: An under-recognised cause of chronic kidney disease. *BMJ Case Rep.* 2017;pii: bcr-2016-218623.

Srivastava G, Apovian C. Future pharmacotherapy for obesity: New anti-obesity drugs on the horizon [Epub ahead of print march 5, 2018]. *Curr Obes Rep.* 2018 doi: 10.1007/s13679-018-0300-4.

Tarplin S, Ganesan V, Monga M. Stone formation and management after bariatric surgery. *Nat Rev Urol.* 2015;12:263–70.

Tay J, Luscombe-Marsh ND, Thompson CH, et al. A very low-carbohydrate, low-saturated fat diet for type 2 diabetes management: A randomized trial. *Diabet Care.* 2014;37:2909–2918.

Thompson SV, Hannon BA, An R, Holscher HD. Effects of isolated soluble fiber supplementation on body weight, glycemia, and insulinemia in adults with overweight and obesity: a systematic review and meta-analysis of randomized controlled trials. *Am J Clin Nutr.* 2017;106:1514–1528.

Tikkanen-Dolenc H, Wadén J, Forsblom C, et al. FinnDiane Study Group. Physical activity reduces risk of premature mortality in patients with type 1 diabetes with and without kidney disease. *Diabet Care.* 2017;40:1727–1732.

Tirosh A, Golan R, Harman-Boehm I, et al. Renal function following three distinct weight loss dietary strategies during 2 years of a randomized controlled trial. *Diabet Care.* 2013;36:2225–2232.

Turgeon NA, Perez S, Mondestin M, et al. The impact of renal function on outcomes of bariatric surgery. *J Am Soc Nephrol.* 2012;23:885–894.

Vazquez G, Duval S, Jacobs DR Jr, et al. Comparison of body mass index, waist circumference, and waist/hip ratio in predicting incident diabetes: A meta-analysis. *Epidemiol Rev.* 2007;29:115–128.

Verhave JC, Hillege HL, Burgerhof JG, et al. Cardiovascular risk factors are differently associated with urinary albumin excretion in men and women. *J Am Soc Nephrol.* 2003;14:1330–1335.

Visconti L, Cernaro V, Calimeri S, et al. The myth of water and salt: From aquaretics to tenapanor. *J Ren Nutr.* 2018;28:73–82.

Wadden TA, Butryn ML, Wilson C. Lifestyle modification for the management of obesity. *Gastroenterology.* 2007;132:2226–2238.

Wisse BE. The inflammatory syndrome: The role of adipose tissue cytokines in metabolic disorders linked to obesity. *J Am Soc Nephrol.* 2004;15:2792–2800.

Young JA, Hwang S, Sarnak MJ, et al. Association of visceral and subcutaneous adiposity with kidney function. *Clin J Am Soc Nephrol.* 2008;3:1786–1791.

Zelle DM, Klaassen G, van Adrichem E, et al. Physical inactivity: A risk factor and target for intervention in renal care. *Nat Rev Nephrol.* 2017;13:152–168.

5

Sodium and Potassium Intake

Sharon I. Turban and Edgar R. Miller, III

Low-sodium and high-potassium diets have important health benefits, including lowering blood pressure. In epidemiologic studies, low-sodium and high-potassium intake are associated with reduced risk of stroke and heart disease. In patients with chronic kidney disease (CKD), these effects are particularly relevant, given that hypertension and cardiovascular disease occur commonly in this population. CKD is also associated with greater "salt sensitivity": dietary sodium is excreted less efficiently and results in increased extracellular fluid volume and blood pressure.

Although increased potassium intake has been shown to be beneficial in individuals without CKD, benefits have not been well-studied in CKD patients. With more advanced CKD stages, there may be a delicate balance between the health benefits of increased potassium intake and the risk of hyperkalemia. The level of kidney dysfunction at which dietary recommendations should change from a high-potassium diet, such as the Dietary Approaches to Stop Hypertension (DASH) diet (Appel, 1997), to potassium restriction is uncertain.

CASE STUDY 5.1   RECOMMENDED SODIUM INTAKE

A 48-year-old African American man presents for a routine clinic visit. He was diagnosed with hypertension 10 years ago and has been compliant with lisinopril (angiotensin-converting enzyme inhibitor) 20 mg per day. Blood pressure is 142/90. Serum creatinine is 1.5 mg/dL (133 mcmol/L), estimated glomerular filtration rate (eGFR) using the CKD-EPI equation (as described in Chapter 1) is 63 mL/min per 1.73 m^2 (stage 2 CKD), and urine protein-to-creatinine ratio is 750 mg/g. Serum potassium is 4.0 mmol/L. In addition to increasing the dose of lisinopril, you give the patient dietary advice.

Question: What are your recommendations for sodium intake?

For the general population, several groups recommend consumption of *less than* 2.3 g (100 mmol) per day of sodium (Table 5.1). A further reduction in sodium intake to <1.5 g (65 mmol) per day has been recommended by some organizations for certain populations, including African Americans, age >50 years, and for individuals with kidney disease, diabetes mellitus, or hypertension; this sodium target has also been recommended by the American Heart Association (AHA) for all populations (Eckel, 2014). Because sodium reduction to this degree has been found to be difficult to achieve, the AHA recommends sodium reduction by at least 1 g/day even if the desired daily sodium intake has not yet been achieved (Van Horn, 2016). Therefore, while an exact target has not been agreed upon, multiple organizations agree

TABLE 5.1	Observed Versus Recommended Daily Intakes of Sodium

Sodium Intake Range

g/day	mmol/day	Comments
4.1	180	Average intake in U.S. men.
3.6	158	Average intake in 45 countries in the INTERSALT study (both sexes).
3.0	129	Average intake in U.S. women.
2.3–2.4	100–102	Maximum recommended intake by the U.S.-based Institute of Medicine, the United States Department of Agriculture (USDA), Health Canada, Australian National Health and Medical Research Council, and other authorities (for the general population). **Maximum upper limit by K/DOQI for CKD stages 1–4.**
1.5–1.6	65–70	Maximum intake recommended by the American Heart Association (2013 Guidelines).
0.46–0.92	20–40	Adequate intake according to the Australian National Health and Medical Research Council and the New Zealand Ministry of Health (all individuals).

K/DOQI, Kidney Disease Outcomes Quality Initiative.

that excess sodium intake should be reduced; they agree that this is likely to have significant public health benefits.

For adults with stage 1 or 2 CKD, the National Kidney Foundation Kidney Disease Outcomes Quality Initiative (K/DOQI) recommends less than 2.4 g (104 mmol) per day of sodium (2004).

CONTROVERSY OVER RECOMMENDATIONS FOR SODIUM REDUCTION

Although numerous studies report the negative effects of a high-sodium diet and the benefit from a low-sodium diet, there is controversy in the literature about the safety and benefits of a low-sodium diet, whether sodium reduction should be universally recommended, what the target intake should be, and if the target intake should vary among certain populations. In particular, there are concerns about the well-documented activation of the renin–angiotensin and sympathetic nervous systems and reported adverse effects on lipids and insulin resistance that may occur in response to sodium reduction. However, the clinical relevance of these potential adverse effects is speculative. Although the controversy about whether sodium intake should be restricted in individuals with normal blood pressure may continue, this controversy may not necessarily apply to patients with CKD, because this group tends to be salt sensitive.

CURRENT AVERAGE INTAKES

In the United States, typical daily sodium intake is estimated to be 4.1 g (180 mmol) for adult men and 3.0 g (129 mmol) for adult women, with an overall mean of 3.6 g (154 mmol) per day (Bailey, 2016); see Table 5.1. In an analysis of sodium intake of individuals in 45 countries in a study in which daily sodium intake was estimated from 24-hour urinary excretion, the mean was 3.6 g (158 mmol) per day (McCarron, 2013).

> **Converting sodium intake from grams to mmol:** The molecular weight of sodium is **23**. To convert sodium from grams to mmol, multiply by 1,000/**23**. So a sodium intake of 2.3 g/day = 2.3 × 1,000/23 = 100 mmol/day.

> **Salt versus sodium:** Some studies and guidelines refer to salt rather than sodium. Table salt is NaCl, with a molecular weight of 58.4, because 23 (Na) + 35.4 (Cl) = 58.4. To convert from salt to sodium, divide by 2.54. For example, 6 g/day salt = 6/2.54 = 2.36 g/day Na.

BENEFITS OF SODIUM REDUCTION

Dietary Sodium and Blood Pressure

Increased blood pressure is an important biologic mediator of risk for adverse kidney and cardiovascular events. In studies across different populations, there is a dose-dependent relationship between blood pressure and average daily sodium intake. In populations in which sodium intake is extremely low, there is an attenuation of age-related increases in blood pressure. One limitation of these ecologic studies is that it is difficult to distinguish the relative importance of diets low in sodium from diets that are high in potassium, because populations with low sodium intake tend to have high potassium intake. The best evidence for the health benefits of sodium reduction depends on results of well-conducted clinical trials that test the effects of sodium reduction in isolation.

DASH Diet

The **DASH** diet was shown to lower blood pressure and serum cholesterol in adults with prehypertension or stage 1 hypertension not on antihypertensive medications. The DASH diet is widely recommended to achieve these goals. This diet is rich in fruits, vegetables, and low-fat dairy, modestly high in protein, and has reduced saturated and total fat.

DASH-Sodium Trial

The DASH-Sodium Trial (Sacks, 2001) was a randomized controlled feeding trial that tested the effects of dietary patterns and sodium intake on blood pressure in adults with prehypertension and stage 1 hypertension, who were not on antihypertensive medications. In this trial, adoption of the DASH diet resulted in a lower blood pressure at all sodium levels compared with a control diet similar to what many Americans consume. In addition, blood pressure decreased in those participants on the DASH diet as well as in those on the control diet when daily sodium intake was lowered from the amount typically consumed by adults in the United States, 3.4 g (150 mmol) per day, to 2.3 g (100 mmol) per day. An even greater blood-pressure reduction was achieved with consumption of either diet at a lower level of sodium, 1.5 g (65 mmol) per day.

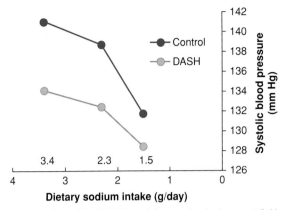

FIGURE 5.1 The effects of the DASH diet and dietary sodium intake on systolic blood pressure in African American hypertensive individuals not on antihypertensive medications. (Adapted from Bray GA, Vollmer WM, Sacks FM, et al. A further subgroup analysis of the effects of the DASH diet and three dietary sodium levels on blood pressure: Results of the DASH-Sodium Trial. *Am J Cardiol.* 2004;94:222–227, with permission.)

Larger reductions in blood pressure with sodium reduction were seen in certain subgroups. For example, for African American hypertensive participants who were consuming the control diet, changing from high-to-low sodium was associated with a 9.4-mm Hg systolic blood-pressure reduction (Fig. 5.1) (Bray, 2004). While consuming the DASH diet, the systolic blood pressure–lowering effect was 5.7 mm Hg. The blood-pressure effects observed in the DASH and DASH-Sodium Trials were achieved while participants were eating sufficient calories to maintain their initial body weight; there was no overall weight loss.

Salt Sensitivity of Blood Pressure

Within a population of healthy individuals, there is substantial variation in the blood-pressure responses to changes in sodium intake. The term "salt sensitive" has been used to refer to individuals whose blood pressure increases in response to increased sodium intake; however, this is not an all-or-none phenomenon. Changes in blood pressure in response to changes in sodium intake appear to have a continuous distribution; it is the magnitude of this response that varies. There is no agreed-upon definition of salt sensitivity and no current strategies to identify salt-sensitive people on an individual level; however, certain groups appear to be more salt sensitive, including African Americans, older individuals, those with diabetes or hypertension, and, most pertinent to the topic at hand, patients with CKD.

Other Benefits of Sodium Reduction

Although many of the effects of sodium reduction are mediated through resultant lower blood pressure, **additional benefits of sodium reduction beyond blood pressure** have been described.

Dietary Sodium and Cardiovascular Disease

High sodium intake has been linked to left ventricular hypertrophy and increased risk of cardiovascular events, especially stroke. Higher risk may be mediated by both blood pressure–dependent and blood pressure–independent mechanisms (e.g., increased oxidative stress and upregulation of mineralocorticoid receptor signals). Differentiating the relative contributions of blood pressure or alternate etiologies is difficult in epidemiologic studies. Additionally, most trials investigating the effects of sodium reduction have not been large enough or of sufficient duration to adequately assess the effects of sodium on cardiovascular outcomes. However, one provocative finding in the long-term follow-up of the Trials of Hypertension Prevention (TOHP) (Cook, 2007) was that participants originally randomized to sodium reduction showed reduced risk of cardiovascular events when assessed 10 to 15 years later.

Sodium reduction is commonly recommended for patients with congestive heart failure, in part because sodium retention drives fluid retention. This is often performed in conjunction with a diuretic. In patients with resistant hypertension, multidrug therapy including diuretics is often required, and the further addition of a low-sodium diet can sometimes markedly improve blood-pressure control (Pimenta, 2009). A low-sodium diet can augment the effects of diuretics, making it easier to control volume overload (Jessup, 2009). However, there are conflicting results in the literature regarding the association of dietary sodium intake in heart failure patients (who are typically on a diuretic) with hospitalization and mortality. Therefore, more studies are needed to further investigate the effects of dietary sodium on cardiovascular disease and to determine the optimal intake in patients at risk for, or who have, cardiovascular disease.

Dietary Sodium and Chronic Kidney Disease

Sodium intake may modify the rate of progression of kidney disease by both blood pressure–dependent and blood pressure–independent mechanisms. Individuals with CKD tend to be "salt sensitive" because of a decreased ability to excrete sodium. He (2016) and others have demonstrated that a high-sodium intake in CKD patients (based on 24-hour urinary excretion) was associated with a higher risk of CKD progression and all-cause mortality. Lower-sodium diets have been shown to decrease proteinuria (He, 2009; Swift, 2005), including in the setting of fixed-dose angiotensin-converting enzyme inhibition (Keyzer, 2017). However, there are insufficient studies in humans to determine the long-term effects of alterations in sodium intake on CKD.

RECOMMENDED POTASSIUM INTAKE

For the general population, an **"adequate intake" for potassium is set at 4.7 g (120 mmol) per day** for all adults (Institute of Medicine of the National Academies. Panel on Dietary Reference Intakes for Electrolytes and Water, Standing Committee on the Scientific Evaluation of Dietary Reference Intakes, Food and Nutrition Board, 2004). For adults with stage 1 or 2 CKD, the K/DOQI group recommends daily consumption of **at least 4 g**

TABLE 5.2 Observed Versus Recommended Daily Intakes of Potassium

Potassium Intake Range

g/day	mmol/day	Comments
4.7	120	Potassium content of the DASH diet (per 2,100 calories). Recommended level of adequate intake for both men and women (healthy individuals without kidney disease) according to the Institute of Medicine.
4.0	102	**Recommended intake by K/DOQI for patients with stages 1–2 CKD (GFR/1.73 m² ≥60 mL/min with evidence of kidney damage).**
3.1–3.3	80–85	Observed average intake in the U.S. population for men (NHANES 2011–2012).
2.0–4.0	51–102	**Recommended intake by K/DOQI for patients with stages 3–4 CKD (GFR/1.73 m² between 15 and 59 mL/min).**
2.4	60–62	Observed average intake in the U.S. population for women (NHANES 2011–2012).

DASH, Dietary Approaches to Stop Hypertension; K/DOQI, Kidney Disease Outcomes Quality Initiative; CKD, chronic kidney disease; GFR, glomerular filtration rate; NHANES, National Health and Nutrition Examination Survey.

(102 mmol) of potassium. Table 5.2 shows the typical potassium intake for the U.S. population as well as recommended intakes.

> **Converting potassium intakes from grams to mmol:** The molecular weight of potassium is **39.1 g/mol**. To convert potassium from g per day to mmol per day, multiply by 1,000/**39.1**. For example, 4.7 g/day = 4.7 × 1,000/39.1 = 120 mmol/day.

What is considered to be an "adequate intake" by the Institute of Medicine is a level of potassium thought to be high enough to reduce the adverse effects of sodium chloride intake on blood pressure, reduce the risk of kidney stones, and possibly decrease bone loss. A higher potassium intake may be especially beneficial in hypertensive persons and African American individuals. There is no upper limit set for potassium intake in individuals without significant kidney disease, because in these individuals, excess potassium is excreted in the urine, and there do not appear to be adverse effects associated with levels above the adequate intake. Although large amounts of potassium were present in the prehistoric diet, potassium in the modern era is often removed during the processing of commercially prepared foods. Most people in the United States eating modern Western diets are not consuming an "adequate" amount of potassium, as shown in Table 5.2.

Potassium Intake and Blood Pressure

In both normotensive and hypertensive individuals without kidney disease, increased potassium intake, either from potassium-rich foods or supplements, has been shown to lower blood pressure. The antihypertensive effects of potassium may be mediated via increased sodium excretion by the kidney, by vasodilation, and/or by other vasculoprotective effects. With an average supplemental potassium dose that resulted in doubling of usual intake, the amount of blood-pressure reduction reported in several meta-analyses of randomized controlled clinical trials typically has ranged from 3.5 to 8.2 mm Hg for systolic pressure and 1.0 to 4.5 mm Hg for diastolic pressure (Cappuccio and MacGregor, 1991; Geleijnse, 2003; Whelton, 1997). Greater effects were observed in African Americans and those with hypertension. Individuals with CKD were not included in these trials.

Sodium sensitivity of blood pressure is markedly affected by potassium intake. Decreased potassium intake may lead to higher blood pressure in response to sodium loading, whereas a high potassium intake may attenuate the rise in blood pressure due to a higher sodium intake. Similarly, potassium is more likely to lower blood pressure when sodium intake is high than low.

Potassium Intake and Cardiovascular Disease

As with sodium, the effects of potassium on cardiovascular and kidney disease may be mediated through blood pressure–dependent and blood pressure–independent pathways. Low potassium intake may lead to increased oxidative stress and inflammation, whereas increased potassium intake inhibits these processes. Evidence from epidemiologic studies and animal models shows that diets rich in potassium reduce risk for stroke, cardiovascular events, and mortality. Prospective studies have shown that high dietary potassium intake was associated with reduced risk of stroke mortality after adjustment for blood pressure. Reduced serum potassium levels appear to increase the risk of ventricular arrhythmias and cardiovascular disease events in patients with heart disease. One small trial showed that the use of potassium-enriched salt as compared with regular salt resulted in a reduced risk of cardiovascular events (Chang, 2006). Again, whether the effects of healthy diets are from the high potassium or low sodium, or from other ingredients in these diets, is difficult to determine.

Potassium Intake and Chronic Kidney Disease

In addition to lowering blood pressure, a major risk factor for CKD, animal studies show that increasing dietary potassium protects against kidney damage independent of blood-pressure effects. This may in part be mediated by modulation of inflammatory pathways. Chronic potassium depletion has been shown to be associated with more rapid progression of kidney disease, the onset of interstitial nephritis, and increased renal cyst formation in both animals and humans. However, as with sodium, the effects of increased potassium intake as a means to prevent or slow progression of CKD have not been well-studied.

RECOMMENDED SODIUM AND POTASSIUM INTAKES FOR CASE 5.1

Given that this patient has stage 2 CKD and a normal serum potassium, the current recommendations are to reduce dietary sodium intake to 2.3 g (100 mmol) per day (possibly lower) and to consume at least 4.0 g (102 mmol) of potassium per day; the amount of recommended dietary intake would be influenced by serum potassium and by the presence of potassium-altering medications.

CASE STUDY

5.2

DIETARY RECOMMENDATIONS FOR SODIUM AND POTASSIUM INTAKE IN STAGES 3 AND 4 CHRONIC KIDNEY DISEASE

A 62-year-old Caucasian woman presents to your clinic. She was diagnosed with hypertension 30 years ago and has slow progressive worsening of her kidney function. Her serum creatinine is 2.2 mg/dL (194 mcmol/L), with an eGFR/1.73 m^2 of 23 mL/min; stage 4 CKD. She is on a stable dose of valsartan (angiotensin receptor blocker). Her home blood pressure readings have been slightly elevated, and she has been trying to lower her sodium intake. Serum potassium level is 4.3 mmol/L.

What should dietary sodium and potassium recommendations be at this point?

Sodium Intake for Stages 3 and 4 Chronic Kidney Disease

The current recommendation for **sodium intake** for patients with stages 3 to 4 CKD is the same as for the general population and for patients with stages 1 to 2 CKD: a maximum of 2.3 g (100 mmol) per day. An upper daily limit of 1.5 g may be more optimal in these patients, but there is not enough data to make this recommendation.

Potassium Intake for Stages 3 and 4 Chronic Kidney Disease

Despite the known benefits of increased potassium intake on blood pressure and cardiovascular disease, there is uncertainty about the optimal potassium intake for individuals with stages 3 to 4 CKD because of the risk of the development of hyperkalemia, particularly for patients on potassium-sparing agents such as angiotensin-converting enzyme inhibitors, angiotensin receptor blockers, or aldosterone antagonists (Table 5.3). Although there are reports to suggest that the renal excretion of potassium does not appear to be substantially impaired until the glomerular filtration rate is markedly decreased, this has not been well studied.

The current recommendation by K/DOQI for potassium intake for individuals with stages 3 or 4 CKD is 2 to 4 g (50 to 100 mmol) per day, which is lower than the minimum 4 g (100 mmol) per day recommended for stages 1 and 2 CKD or the adequate intake of 4.7 g (120 mmol) per day recommended for the general population. However, it is not clear whether or not this recommendation is optimal for individuals with CKD and normal serum potassium levels; reducing potassium intake could lead to potential negative effects on blood pressure and avoidance of foods that may otherwise be healthy.

The DASH diet in its original form (4.7 g potassium/2,100 kcal/day) is not currently recommended for patients with stages 3 through 4 CKD, though a pilot feeding study of the DASH diet for 1 to 2 weeks in 11 participants with stage 3 CKD did not demonstrate any acute metabolic events; furthermore, nocturnal BP improved in the DASH group (Tyson, 2016). The ideal serum potassium level for CKD patients

TABLE 5.3	Medications That May Raise Serum Potassium Level	
	Drug	**Mechanism**
Antihypertensives or potassium-sparing diuretics	ACE inhibitors and ARBs	Decrease aldosterone
	Spironolactone, eplerenone	Decrease aldosterone
	Aliskiren	Direct renin inhibitor
	Triamterene	Blocks sodium channel in distal tubule
	Amiloride	Blocks sodium channel in distal tubule
	β-blockers	Decrease aldosterone synthesis and may decrease cellular uptake of potassium
Other medications	NSAIDs and COX-2 inhibitors	Decrease aldosterone
	Trimethoprim	Blocks sodium channel in distal tubule
	Heparin	Decreases aldosterone
	Calcineurin inhibitors (cyclosporine and tacrolimus)	Decrease aldosterone and decrease activity of sodium-potassium ATPase pumps in principal cells

ACE, angiotensin-converting enzyme; ARBs, angiotensin receptor blockers; COX-2, cyclooxygenase-2; NSAIDs, nonsteroidal anti-inflammatory drugs.

is also not known; there are conflicting studies. A prospective study of 820 individuals with stages 3 to 5 CKD showed that serum potassium levels between 4.1 and 5.5 mmol/L were associated with the lowest risk for mortality, and that serum potassium levels ≤4.0 mmol/L seemed to predict mortality to a greater degree compared with when levels were ≥5.5 (Korgaonkar, 2010). In patients with CKD stage 3 or 4, the mortality risk of individuals with serum potassium 5.5 to 5.9 in a study by Einhorn was increased fivefold compared to patients without hyperkalemia (2009), though the mortality risk was higher in non-CKD compared to CKD patients.

There is, therefore, a delicate balance that must be kept. It may be worthwhile to increase potassium intake in patients with moderate CKD who have good urine output and no evidence of hyperkalemia to provide them with the benefits of a higher potassium intake, but these patients should be monitored carefully given the documented mortality risks of hyperkalemia.

POTASSIUM INTAKE IN PATIENTS TAKING POTASSIUM-SPARING DRUGS

CKD patients often are treated with angiotensin-converting enzyme inhibitors, angiotensin receptor blockers, or aldosterone antagonists to treat hypertension, reduce proteinuria, or slow CKD progression. Patients receiving one or more potassium-sparing drugs are at risk of potentially life-threatening hyperkalemia; serum potassium must be monitored carefully. If serum potassium approaches upper limits of normal, then a potassium binder (see below) and/or stringent reduction of dietary potassium may be required to allow them to continue taking these medications that may raise serum potassium levels (see Table 5.3). In addition, use of medications known to increase the serum potassium level such as nonsteroidal anti-inflammatory drugs (Table 5.3), should be avoided when possible, especially when serum potassium is high, and in particular when ACE inhibitors, angiotensin receptor blockers, or aldosterone antagonists are also being prescribed.

CKD patients who become hyperkalemic are sometimes given sodium polystyrene sulfonate (SPS), an ion-exchange resin (brand name Kayexalate), though its safety and long-term efficacy have been questioned. There are potential concerns about its use leading to colonic necrosis, though most of the reported cases of serious gastrointestinal adverse events associated with SPS occurred when it was administered with the osmotic laxative sorbitol. There is also a lack of controlled trials regarding the efficacy of SPS (Sterns, 2010). A newer agent, patiromer, is available for the treatment of hyperkalemia that is not acute or life-threatening. Patiromer is a nonabsorbed, cation-exchange polymer that binds potassium in the colon in exchange for calcium. In clinical trials, patiromer significantly reduced serum potassium levels in CKD patients with mild-to-severe hyperkalemia (Weir, 2015), as well as in individuals with CKD, mild-to-moderate hyperkalemia, and type 2 diabetes mellitus who were receiving renin–angiotensin–aldosterone system inhibitors (Bakris, 2015). Patiromer can be prescribed chronically along with a medication such as an ACE inhibitor that can raise serum potassium. Patiromer should be taken at least 3 hours before or 3 hours after certain other medications because of the potential of binding of patiromer to other drugs, lowering their efficacy. In one study in healthy volunteers, there is little clinical evidence for such drug binding during coadministration of patiromer with some drugs, while with ciprofloxacin, clopidogrel, metformin, and metoprolol, a 3-hour window was required to minimize reduced absorption of the target drug (Lesko, 2017). Patiromer administration can lower the serum magnesium levels slightly; the clinical importance of this is not known.

Sodium zirconium cyclosilicate (ZS-9) is an inorganic, nonabsorbable crystalline compound that exchanges sodium and hydrogen ions for potassium throughout its transit in the intestines. ZS-9, was demonstrated in clinical trials to lower potassium more than placebo. Treatment of hyperkalemia is discussed in more detail in Chapters 11 and 29.

Some medications are associated with a lowering of the serum potassium level, either by increasing renal or gastrointestinal excretion, or by driving potassium into cells. See Table 5.4. The impact of diuretics on serum potassium is discussed in Chapters 14 and 23.

TABLE 5.4	Medications That Can Lower Serum Potassium Level	
	Drug Name	**Mechanism**
Diuretics (potassium nonsparing)	Hydrochlorothiazide Chlorthalidone Furosemide, bumetanide, torsemide Metolazone	Increase kidney excretion of potassium
Other medications	Steroids (fludrocortisone, prednisone, hydrocortisone) Aminoglycosides Amphotericin B Cisplatin Some penicillins Lithium	Increase kidney excretion of potassium
	Laxatives	Increase potassium losses into the stool
	Sodium polystyrene	Nonspecific sodium–cation-exchange resin
	Patiromer ZS-9 (not approved yet by the FDA)	Bind potassium (cation exchangers)
	β-Adrenergic agonists Insulin	Drive potassium into cells

CASE STUDY 5.3

ASSESSING AND ENSURING ADHERENCE WITH SODIUM AND POTASSIUM RECOMMENDATIONS

Each of the two patients described above returns to your clinic 3 months later, reporting adherence with medications and dietary sodium reduction. The patient described in case 5.1 reports "no problem" adhering to your recommendations, but you suspect noncompliance. The patient described in case 5.2 is having difficulty figuring out how to measure her sodium intake; she asks if there is a way to determine this. You decide that measuring sodium intake by quantifying urinary sodium excretion may have benefits in both cases by providing a method for assessing adherence and for use as a counseling tool.

How can dietary compliance be ensured and assessed?

Tools to Assess and Help Ensure Dietary Adherence

The clinician's office provides a powerful setting to advocate and promote lifestyle and dietary changes. Provider-directed dietary changes can be accomplished, but success depends on several factors, including the communication skills and knowledge of the provider, available resources, adequate time for counseling, and patient willingness to modify dietary practices. Unfortunately, patients often forget details of advice given to them. Food labels are not required to list potassium content. Although sodium content is listed on food labels, it may still be difficult for individuals to calculate the total sodium content of their foods. Patients who are successful with dietary changes typically are highly motivated and may seek outside resources. When possible, providers should refer patients to a dietitian. Most insurance programs, including Medicare, will cover dietitian counseling if the patient has documented CKD. For patients who lack insurance, referral to community-based organizations may be equally effective. Multiple visits and contacts are key ingredients for success. Detailed advice on educating patients about sodium and potassium from a dietitian's perspective is described in Chapter 6.

Evaluation of Sodium Intake

Twenty-four hour urine sodium collections can be used to help determine a patient's intake of sodium. These urine collections should always include concurrent analyses of creatinine excretion to determine the adequacy of the urine collection (see Appendix 1 for expected daily creatinine excretion rates). The 24-hour urine sodium excretion closely reflects sodium intake during the preceding day but may not accurately reflect the overall typical intake. Several formulas have been proposed to convert a spot urine sodium and creatinine result into an estimate of 24-hour urinary sodium excretion, though this is not optimal; however, it is a consideration in settings where a 24-hour urine collection is not feasible. Use of dipstick tests to measure urinary chloride-to-creatinine ratio (Mann and Gerber, 2010) is another proposed technique used to approximate sodium intake that has not been well-studied.

The urinary sodium-to-potassium ratio may be useful to measure. Higher ratios have been shown to be associated with an increased risk of hypertension and cardiovascular disease, although there are no set recommended targets for this ratio (a ratio of <1.0 has been proposed as the most ideal target).

References and Suggested Readings

Appel LJ, Anderson CA. Compelling evidence for public health action to reduce salt intake. *N Engl J Med.* 2010;362:650–652.

Appel LJ, Moore TJ, Obarzanek E, et al. A clinical trial of the effects of dietary patterns on blood pressure. DASH Collaborative Research Group. *N Engl J Med.* 1997;336:1117–1124.

Bailey RL, Parker EA, Rhodes DG, et al. Estimating sodium and potassium intakes and their ratio in the American diet: Data from the 2011–2012 NHANES. *J Nutr.* 2016;164:745–750.

Bakris GL, Pitt B, Weir MR, et al. Effect of patiromer on serum potassium level in patients with hyperkalemia and diabetic kidney disease: The AMETHYST-DN randomized clinical trial. *JAMA.* 2015;314:151–161.

Bray GA, Vollmer WM, Sacks FM, et al. A further subgroup analysis of the effects of the DASH diet and three dietary sodium levels on blood pressure: Results of the DASH-Sodium Trial. *Am J Cardiol.* 2004;94:222–227.

Cappuccio FP, MacGregor GA. Does potassium supplementation lower blood pressure? A meta-analysis of published trials. *J Hypertens.* 1991;9:465–473.

Chang HY, Hu YW, Yue CS, et al. Effect of potassium-enriched salt on cardiovascular mortality and medical expenses of elderly men. *Am J Clin Nutr.* 2006;83:1289–1296.

Cook NR, Cutler JA, Obarzanek E, et al. Long term effects of dietary sodium reduction on cardiovascular disease outcomes: Observational follow-up of the trials of hypertension prevention (TOHP). *BMJ.* 2007;334:885–888.

Eckel RH, Jakicic JM, Ard JD, et al; American College of Cardiology/American Heart Association Task Force on Practice Guidelines. 2013 AHA/ACC guidelines on lifestyle management to reduce cardiovascular risk: A report of the American College of Cardiology/American Heart Association Task Force on Practice Guidelines. *Circulation.* 2014;129:S76–S99.

Einhorn LM, Zhan M, Hsu VD, et al. The frequency of hyperkalemia and its significance in chronic kidney disease. *Arch Intern Med.* 2009;169:1156–1162.

Geleijnse JM, Kok FJ, Grobbee DE. Blood pressure response to changes in sodium and potassium intake: A metaregression analysis of randomised trials. *J Hum Hypertens.* 2003;17:471–480.

Georgianos PI, Agarwal R. Revisiting RAAS blockade in CKD with newer potassium-binding drugs. *Kidney Int.* 2018;93:325–334.

He FJ, Marciniak M, Visagie E, et al. Effect of modest salt reduction on blood pressure, urinary albumin, and pulse wave velocity in white, black, and Asian mild hypertensives. *Hypertension.* 2009;54:482–488.

He J, Mills KT, Appel LJ, et al. Urinary sodium and potassium excretion and CKD progression. *J Am Soc Nephrol.* 2016;27:1202–1212.

Institute of Medicine of the National Academies. Panel on Dietary Reference Intakes for Electrolytes and Water, Standing Committee on the Scientific Evaluation of Dietary Reference Intakes, Food and Nutrition Board. Dietary Reference Intakes for Water, Potassium, Sodium, Chloride, and Sulfate. Washington, DC: The National Academies Press; 2004:186–268.

Jessup M, Abraham WT, Casey DE, et al. 2009 focused update: ACCF/AHA Guidelines for the diagnosis and management of heart failure in adults: A report of the American College of Cardiology Foundation/American Heart Association Task Force on Practice Guidelines: Developed in collaboration with the International Society for Heart and Lung Transplantation. *Circulation.* 2009;119:1977–2016.

Keyzer CA, van Breda GF, Vervloet MG, et al. Effects of vitamin D receptor activation and dietary sodium restriction on residual albuminuria in CKD: The ViRTUE-CKD Trial. *J Am Soc Nephrol.* 2017;28:1296–1305.

Kidney Disease Outcomes Quality Initiative (K/DOQI). K/DOQI clinical practice guidelines on hypertension and antihypertensive agents in chronic kidney disease. *Am J Kidney Dis.* 2004;43:S1–S290.

Korgaonkar S, Tilea A, Gillespie BW, et al. Serum potassium and outcomes in CKD: Insights from the RRI-CKD cohort study. *Clin J Am Soc Nephrol.* 2010;5:762–769.

Lesko LJ, Offman E, Brew CT, et al. Evaluation of the potential for drug interactions with Patiromer in healthy volunteers. *J Cardiovasc Pharmacol Ther.* 2017;22:434–446.

Mann SJ, Gerber LM. Estimation of 24-h sodium excretion from a spot urine sample using chloride and creatinine dipsticks. *Am J Hypertens.* 2010;23:743–748.

McCarron DA, Kazaks AG, Geerling JC, et al. Normal range of human dietary sodium intake: A perspective based on 24-hour urinary excretion worldwide. *Am J Hypertens.* 2013;26:1218–1223.

Nerbass FB, Calice-Silva V, Pecoits-Filho R. Sodium intake and blood pressure in patients with chronic kidney disease: a salty relationship. *Blood Purif.* 2018;45:166–172.

Pimenta E, Gaddam KK, Oparil S, et al. Effects of dietary sodium reduction on blood pressure in subjects with resistant hypertension: Results from a randomized trial. *Hypertension.* 2009;54:475–481.

Sacks FM, Svetkey LP, Vollmer WM, et al. Effects on blood pressure of reduced dietary sodium and the Dietary Approaches to Stop Hypertension (DASH) diet. DASH-Sodium Collaborative Research Group. *N Engl J Med.* 2001;344:3–10.

Sterns RH, Rojas M, Bernstein P, et al. Ion-exchange resins for the treatment of hyperkalemia: Are they safe and effective? *J Am Soc Nephrol.* 2010;21:733–735.

Swift PA, Markandu ND, Sagnella GA, et al. Modest salt reduction reduces blood pressure and urine protein excretion in black hypertensives: A randomized control trial. *Hypertension.* 2005;46:308–312.

Tyson CC, Lin PH, Corsino L, et al. Short-term effects of the DASH diet in adults with moderate chronic kidney disease: A pilot feeding study. *Clin Kidney J.* 2016;9:592–598.

Van Horn L, Carson JA, Appel LJ, et al. Recommended dietary pattern to achieve adherence to the American Heart Association/American College of Cardiology (AHA/ACC) guidelines: A scientific statement from the American Heart Association. *Circulation.* 2016;132:e505–e529.

Weir MR, Bakris GL, Bushinsky DA, et al. Patiromer in patients with kidney disease and hyperkalemia receiving RAAS inhibitors. *N Engl J Med.* 2015;372:211–221.

Whelton PK, He J, Cutler JA, et al. Effects of oral potassium on blood pressure: Meta-analysis of randomized controlled clinical trials. *JAMA.* 1997;277:1624–1632.

6

Dietary Sodium and Potassium: A Dietitian's Perspective

Jane H. Greene

The previous chapter detailed the recommended sodium and potassium intakes for patients with chronic kidney disease (CKD). Here we present practical methods for achieving dietary sodium and potassium restriction.

SODIUM

As a review, the maximum sodium intake is recommended to be 2.3 g (100 mmol) per day, with possible increased benefits by lowering sodium intake to 1.5 g (65 mmol) per day. Whereas in primitive societies the sodium intake of the diet typically is low, in developed countries, it averages about 3.7 g (160 mmol) per day. This is 60% higher than the upper limit of normal recommended for CKD patients. Thus, for most patients a marked change in eating habits will be necessary to achieve suggested sodium targets. The challenge for dietitians is to help the patient understand where sources of dietary sodium are coming from so that patients can alter their diets to reduce sodium content to recommended levels while still maintaining a healthful mix of nutrients; avoiding problems of excessive protein, phosphate, and potassium; and limiting intake of foods believed to be associated with cardiovascular disease such as transsaturated and saturated fats.

Sources of Sodium in the Diet

The great majority of sodium (about 77% as shown in Fig. 6.1) in food consumed in the average Western diet has been added to the food during processing. Only 5% is added during the process of cooking after the food has been purchased, and another 6% is added by the person eating the food at the time of the meal. What this means is that it is not very effective to focus counseling on "putting away the salt shaker." Rather, patients must be taught how to understand and read food labels, and where they have the financial and discretionary ability to control food choices, patients need to be taught how to identify low-sodium varieties of the foods that they like to eat and where they can obtain such foods.

An Operational Approach to Controlling Sodium

Food intake is linked to how a patient functions within his or her social network and depends on the patient's ability to control selection of food as well as final preparation of the food that has been procured. Finances are important, given that some patients do not

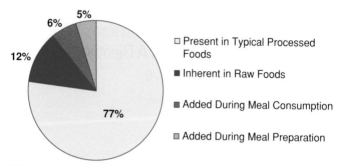

FIGURE 6.1 Approximate dietary sodium sources based on typical Western diets. (Adapted from Mattes RD, Donnelly D. Relative contributions of dietary sodium sources. *J Am Coll Nutr.* 1991;10:383–393. See also Centers for Disease Control and Prevention. Sodium intake among adults—26 States, the District of Columbia, and Puerto Rico, 2013. *MMWR Morb Mortal Wkly Rep.* 2015;64:695–698.)

have the resources to change the selection of food that they eat. Generally, patients eat in three different settings: in their home, with friends or family, and in restaurants. When counseling a patient with regard to diet, it is important to first determine what proportion of food is consumed at each venue.

Who Buys and Prepares the Food That the Patient Eats?
In cases in which the majority of food is consumed at home, the next question should be "Who buys the food?" It is of little benefit to educate a patient with regard to how to read food labels if the majority of the food purchases are being made by some other family member. In many instances, another family member is the main preparer of food, and that person is emotionally involved with assuring that the food tastes good and pleases other family members. In patients with multiple comorbid conditions, the patient's family members may already be burdened with having to assist in the patient's care, and they may not have the time or energy to change the way the household eats for the sake of the patient's health care problems. This problem becomes more acute in patients who live in large, extended families, where their dietary needs are overshadowed by a tradition of the way the family has always eaten together. Forcing an entire family to change their dietary habits for the sake of the patient may arouse resentments and arguments.

Fast Foods (Life in the Fast Lane)
As our lives have become more fast-paced, the food industry has responded by providing us with more and more options for "eating on the run." Although not always true, usually the faster a product is to prepare, the higher it is in sodium.

Patients Who Get Most of Their Food From Restaurants
A different set of problems may be encountered in patients who primarily live alone and eat in restaurants. Many restaurants provide

nutritional information, including sodium content of menu items, on their websites to aid in food selection when dining out.

Food Insecurity

According to the U.S. Department of Agriculture (USDA)'s *Current Population Surveys,* 13% of U.S. households were food insecure at some time during 2015. *Food insecure* means these households were at times uncertain of having enough food, or were unable to acquire sufficient food for all household members because they had insufficient money and other resources for food. Low socioeconomic status is associated with both development and progression of CKD, thus food insecurity plays a role in the dietary adherence of CKD patients (Shoham, 2005; Young, 1994). People who depend on community resources for food generally do not have the privilege of selecting only foods prescribed by their health care provider. The majority of foods distributed from food banks and government programs are not low-sodium foods, and some of these foods may also be high in potassium and/or phosphorus.

Dealing With Operational Issues of Food Provision

Although the list of problems detailed above appears daunting, at least partial solutions are available. When the patient is not the person purchasing and/or preparing the food in the house, then the purchaser/preparer should be counseled. For patients eating primarily fast foods, dietitians can help with meal planning and give instructions on how to prepare simple low-sodium meals.

At the Market

Sodium Food Labels

Sodium Content per Serving Size. Food labels are structured differently in countries around the world. In the United States, sodium content is listed in mg according to "serving size," which is the "reference amount customarily consumed per eating occasion" as determined by the U.S. Food and Drug Administration (FDA) based on their research (USFDA Title 21: Food and Drugs, Subpart A, General Provisions. 101.12). Criteria for allowable food claims with regard to sodium are given in Table 6.1. Although sodium content per serving size is a useful measure, individually packaged food items may contain more than one serving and total sodium content per package should be considered.

T A B L E 6.1	Sodium Content Claims on U.S. Food Labels
Claim	**Sodium Content per Serving Size**
Sodium-free	<5 mg (0.22 mmol)
Very low sodium	≤35 mg (1.5 mmol)
Low sodium	≤140 mg (6.1 mmol)
Unsalted or no added salt	Only contains the sodium that naturally occurs in the food

Sodium: Calorie Ratio. Though not standard, one way to compare sodium content of foods in a way different from serving size using the information on the food label is to look at the ratio of sodium in mg to calories per serving size. This is useful, for example, in comparing the sodium content of breads (Daugirdas, 2013), where serving sizes may have a wide range. For breads, the sodium:calorie ratio can range from less than 1 to more than 3.

Order of Ingredients. In the United States, the ingredients must be listed in order of abundance, from greatest to least amount. This is useful in looking at all sodium-containing ingredients in packaged food products.

Monosodium Glutamate and Baking Soda. Monosodium glutamate (MSG) is a flavor enhancer and can be found in meat tenderizers, soups, sauces, and gravies. Baking soda is used as a leavening agent in baked goods, cookies, and crackers. Baking soda should not be confused with baking powder. Baking soda is pure sodium bicarbonate, whereas baking powder is a mixture of sodium bicarbonate, an acidifying agent (cream of tartar), and a drying agent (usually starch). Sodium content from these ingredients will be included in the food label for sodium content.

Low-Sodium Aisle of Chain Grocery Stores, Specialty Grocery Stores
Most people in the United States buy their food from large chain grocery stores. Many of these, depending on the degree of urbanization of the region and the awareness of healthy foods, will have an aisle where low-sodium versions of many different foods will be kept. In many larger cities, grocery chains specializing in healthy foods will have outlets. Dietary counseling should include informing the person who purchases food for a patient's family about these options when they exist.

Buying Low-Sodium Food via the Internet
Depending on the country, numerous websites are usually available specializing in the sale of various low-sodium foods, including meats and sausages, soup stocks, breads, and various condiments. For patients living in areas where low-sodium food shopping is difficult, purchase of low-sodium foods via the Internet can be very helpful.

In the Kitchen
In food preparation at home, it is important to avoid the use of very–high-sodium ingredients such as broth to flavor soups and casseroles, bouillon cubes, and "flavoring packets." One should always read the ingredient list and the amount of sodium per serving for such items before use. As mentioned previously, when the patient is not preparing the meals, or when the patient is preparing meals for the entire family, family involvement in the education process regarding the benefits of sodium restriction, and how to prepare flavorful meals using less sodium, is needed. To people who are accustomed to a very–high-salt diet, lower-sodium food often will taste

bland. However, this blandness typically wears off about one week after changing to a lower sodium intake. Seasoning suggestions using herbs and spices instead of table salt are listed later in the text.

Salt Added to Water While Making Rice, Pasta, or Potatoes
This is unnecessary and should be avoided.

Salt Added to Meat, Fish, and Other Sauces
The amount of salt added should be minimized. Family members can add salt to taste using a salt shaker, whereas it is impossible for the patient to remove additional salt from the sauce.

Soy Sauce, Teriyaki Sauce, Barbecue Sauce, Flavorings, Spices, and Commercial Meat Rubs. The sodium content of these sauces, particularly soy sauce, is very high. It is worthwhile to shop for lower-sodium varieties of these sauces or to make them from scratch. Spice and rub mixtures very often contain salt as the main ingredient. Patients should read the ingredient label and choose salt-free versions or prepare spice mixtures at home. There are many Internet resources for salt-free spice mixture recipes. Additionally, patients may find no-salt spice mixtures at their local farmer's market or at a spice specialty market. Use of these low-sodium alternative seasoning agents is very helpful to prevent a lower-sodium diet from tasting bland. This increases acceptability of the diet to all members of a patient's family and reduces the need for separate food preparation for the patient.

Using Only Part of the Seasoning Packets for Processed Food. Seasoning packets, which contain mostly salt, commonly accompany vegetables and prepared dishes. If a low-sodium alternative is not available, the supplied seasoning packet can often be used, but the patient can be advised to use only ¼ of the supplied packet, limiting the sodium content of the seasoned food.

Tips for Using Herbs and Spices in Food Preparation

- Begin with no more than ¼ teaspoon of dried spice or ¾ teaspoon of fresh spice per pound of meat; adjust spice to taste preferences.
- Crush dried herbs to release their flavor before adding to foods.
- Whole spices should be added at the beginning, or 1 hour before the end, of the cooking time.
- Ground or crushed spices should be added during the last 15 minutes of the cooking period.
- Try basil, bay leaf, curry, marjoram, rosemary, thyme, tarragon, or sage with meats, poultry, and fish in place of salt.
- Fresh lemon juice or zest, garlic, and olive oil should always be available in the kitchen of the CKD patient. These three ingredients will enhance the flavor of just about any food that normally would have salt added to it.

How Much Sodium Is in One Teaspoon of Table Salt, Baking Soda, or Baking Powder?

When making cakes and cookies, as well as other baked goods, recipes often call for salt, baking soda, and/or baking powder. How much sodium does this add? One-quarter teaspoon of table salt contains 590 mg of sodium (25 mmol). One-quarter teaspoon of baking soda contains 250 to 300 mg (11 to 13 mmol) of sodium. Some baking powders contain a large amount of sodium, whereas others contain none. One should refer to the food label to determine how much sodium a given baking powder product contains.

Low-Sodium Cookbooks and Websites

A number of excellent low-sodium cookbooks are available. Some are written by patients who had severe congestive heart failure or hypertension and have markedly improved their health by following a low-sodium diet. Browsing through such books will help patients' caregivers get ideas about preparing tasty low-sodium meals. Other authors have extended the reach of their books by companion websites where further tips on buying and preparing low-sodium foods are available. Available cookbooks change over time, and their appropriateness and usefulness depend on the patient's primary language and country; therefore, they are best found using Internet search engines. One popular cookbook available in the United States is published by the American Heart Association. Not all low-sodium recipes are appropriate for CKD. For those CKD patients who need to limit potassium intake, the low-sodium recipes in cookbooks need to be evaluated to ensure that they do not contain excessively high amounts of potassium.

Various kidney societies and U.S. dialysis service providers also sponsor cookbooks and recipes for kidney patients on their websites that may be useful. Many of these target dialysis patients and are unnecessarily restrictive for patients with early-stage CKD.

At Restaurants and Social Events

Most restaurant chains have nutrition information available at the establishment or on their website. Helping patients obtain this information enables them to select the lowest-sodium option available. If nutrition information is not available, general principles for restaurants include:

- Inform the wait staff that you are limiting sodium, and ask that your food be prepared without additional salt.
- Eat only a taste of the sauces on meats and vegetables; sauces usually are highly salted.
- If meat has been ordered that has a salty surface, or with deep-fried dishes, where the breading usually contains extremely large amounts of salt, the surface rub can be deftly scraped off or the breading removed before eating the dish.
- Each dinner roll or biscuit will usually contain from 250- to 500-mg sodium, with some biscuits having as much as 800-mg sodium. These should be eaten sparingly.

- Order salad dressing "on the side." Dip your fork tips into the dressing cup before spearing the salad, to get the flavor of the dressing while consuming only a small amount. Generally low-fat or fat-free dressings have a higher sodium content than full-fat salad dressings.
- Consider sorbet, sherbet, or fruit for dessert.

At social events:

- Choose fruits and raw vegetables (without dip) instead of nuts, chips, and crackers.
- Limit intake of hard, highly salted cheese or dishes with cheese.
- Limit casseroles. These usually contain high-sodium ingredients such as canned soup.

At the Table
Use of the Salt Shaker
Whether a patient should be counseled to completely avoid the use of surface salting depends on the patient. If a patient and family are both very compliant in stopping addition of salt to food during preparation, allowing surface salting to taste of low-sodium food adds back only about 20% of the salt that would have been present if the food were prepared in the normal fashion (Shepherd, 1989). On the other hand, allowing the salting of food at the table does send a mixed message. It is better to ban the salt shaker for those patients who are struggling with the concept of sodium restriction or who, for various reasons, are not able to meaningfully eliminate salt from food eaten at mealtime.

Salt Substitutes
Most salt substitutes contain potassium (Table 6.2). This is not necessarily a problem for patients with stage 1 or 2 CKD who are not taking potassium-sparing medications and in whom the serum potassium is well within the normal range. However, for patients with more advanced CKD, those taking potassium-sparing drugs, and for any patient in whom the serum potassium level is close to the upper limit of normal, salt substitutes are best avoided.

Nutrition Databases for Food Sodium Content
United States Department of Agriculture Agricultural Research Service USDA Food Composition Databases
This database is the major authoritative source of information about food composition in the United States. The website allows you to search by food item, food group, or manufacturer's name for nutrient profiles (including all nutrients of interest for CKD patients). The database contains data on almost 9,000 food items and up to 150 food components in familiar portion sizes. The database can be found on the USDA's website https://ndb.nal.usda.gov/ndb.

▰▰▰▰▰ TABLE 6.2	Potassium Content of Salts, Salt Substitutes, and Baking Powders	
Product	**Sodium (mg per ¼ teaspoon)**	**Potassium (mg per ¼ teaspoon)**
No salt	0	650
Morton Salt Substitute	0	610
Adolph Salt Substitute	0	600
McCormick Unseasoned Salt Substitute	0	585
Diamond Crystal Salt Substitute	0	550
Co-Salt	0	495
Morton Lite Salt	245	375
Table salt	590	0
Sea salt	560	0
Salt Sense	390	0
Lessalt	310	170
Baking soda	250–300	0
Baking powder[a]	80	0
Monosodium glutamate	125	0

[a]There are many different types of baking powders, and the sodium content varies widely.

SELFNutritionData

Condé Nast Publications has developed an interface that users can employ to search the data in the USDA Nutrient Database for Standard Reference. The interface is available at no charge on the web.

One of the most useful features of the nutritiondata.com website is the "find foods by nutrient" section. The current web address for this page is www.nutritiondata.self.com/tools/nutrient-search. Using this interface, one can compare the nutrient (e.g., sodium) amounts in similar foods. This can be useful in searching for low-sodium alternatives to high-sodium foods. One potential problem: the sodium content can only be searched by either 100-g (3.5-ounce) serving or by 200-calorie serving, which may be confusing to some patients.

Specific Recommendations for Sodium Reduction by Meal
Breakfast

Typical choices for breakfast in a Western diet include bread (English muffin, a bagel, biscuit, or toast), eggs, breakfast meat (bacon, ham, or sausage), cheese, hot or dry cereal, pancakes, and juice. Fruit is also commonly taken. Alternately, sweet rolls, donuts, or muffins commonly are eaten in place of bread.

Bread Products. The salt content of bread is deceptive because bread usually does not taste salty. Often bread will contain more sodium than snack chips, on which the salt is largely on the surface of the food. Fresh bakery breads such as French breads may or may not be a lower-sodium alternative, as recipes vary. Because bread is such a large part of the Western diet, finding a source of lower-sodium bread can be of great help in achieving overall dietary sodium reduction.

Finding low-sodium bread may be challenging. Geographic availability may be limited and, because the bread is perishable, it is often not cost effective to buy it over the Internet. Low-sodium breads at grocery stores are usually found in the frozen food section rather than on the shelf with other baked goods. Other alternatives include dried low-sodium "flat breads" that can be purchased by mail order and will keep for a long time and low-sodium matzos. Those with time and an interest in cooking can make their own bread using any of a variety of bread makers.

Food That Is Spread on Bread. This includes butter, margarine, or some amalgam of butter and oil, mayonnaise, tomato ketchup, peanut butter, and fruit jellies or preserves. Unsalted butter contains no sodium. Sometimes mixtures of butter and vegetable oils are highly salted, and these should be avoided. Mayonnaise contains 100-mg sodium per tablespoon. Peanut butter usually contains a substantial amount of sodium. Tomato ketchup can be very high in sodium. Low-sodium versions of both peanut butter and ketchup are readily available in most grocery stores. Sodium is usually absent from jams and jellies, but inexplicably can be found in some, but not all, apple butters and apple sauces.

Cheese. There is tremendous variability in the sodium content of cheese. The best way to illustrate this is to use the "nutrient search" tool at nutritiondata.self.com; input "foods lowest in sodium" and search by "dairy and egg products," and then to reverse the search for "foods highest in sodium." Using this tool, you can search either by 200-calorie or 100-g portion. Searching by 100-g portion is usually more useful. One hundred grams is about 3.5 ounces, and the usual serving size for cheese is 1 ounce. One then finds that low-sodium cheeses are available containing only essentially zero sodium per 100 g (three-and-a-half 1-ounce servings), a large number of cheeses with a reasonable sodium content containing <200 mg of sodium per 100-g portion, and some processed cheeses containing a very large amount of sodium, up to 1,500 mg per 100-g portion.

Bacon, Ham, Sausage, and Other Processed Meats. If there were a single dietary recommendation that one could make to CKD patients in terms of reducing sodium content in food eaten in the home, it would be to reduce or eliminate consumption of processed meats! Such meats can contain an enormous amount of sodium. Consumption of processed meats has been associated with decreased survival (Micha, 2010). In contrast to processed meats, regular meat is low in sodium. For example, a 100-g (3.5-ounce) portion of poultry contains only about 50 mg of sodium, and this is similar for beef, pork, and lamb. Thus, if possible, having the patient or spouse cook unprocessed meat in advance and then store it for use in sandwiches and breakfast can result in a marked reduction in daily sodium intake. Low-sodium varieties of bacon and bologna are available, and this is another possible option. It should be noted that meats containing lower amounts of sodium do spoil more rapidly.

Breakfast Cereals. Hot cereals commonly eaten include oats, cream of wheat, and grits. Dry cereals, such as toasted oats, shredded wheat, and corn flakes are usually eaten with milk. Grains prepared as hot cereals contain very low amounts of sodium, but when sold in "instant" or "flavored" forms, they can contain considerable amounts of added sodium. Cold dry cereals intrinsically contain little or no sodium (for example, shredded wheat squares), but to most brands, sodium has been added, such that a typical serving of corn flakes may contain about 200 mg of sodium per 1-cup (28 g) serving.

Dairy. Milk is neither a low-sodium nor high-sodium food, as it usually contains about 120 mg per 8-ounce serving. Yogurt has a sodium content similar to milk. Cottage cheese is a high-sodium food; its sodium content is commonly three times higher than milk, and its higher sodium content is deceptive in that it does not taste salty. Low-sodium cottage cheese is available.

Eggs and Omelets. Two large eggs contain about 120 mg of sodium. The high sodium content of many omelets is mainly due to the inclusion of high-sodium cheese and/or processed meat such as "honey-cured ham."

Pancakes. Pancakes are made from various amounts of flour, eggs, and milk and sometimes contain butter or oil. The sodium content is derived from the eggs and milk as well as from added table salt and a sodium-containing baking powder. Large pancakes usually contain about 200 mg of sodium each, but some pancake mixes make pancakes with twice this amount.

Breakfast Juices. Common choices are orange, apple, and tomato juice. Orange and apple juice contain only a small amount of sodium. Tomato juice is not intrinsically high in sodium, but usually has a very large amount of sodium added to it, about 700 mg per 8-ounce glass. Low-sodium tomato or vegetable juice is available. As discussed later, most vegetable juices are quite high in potassium.

Sweet Rolls and Muffins. These are relatively high in sodium, and their salty taste is masked by their high sugar content.

Breakfast Sodium Reduction: Summary. Most of the sodium consumed during breakfast is from processed meats, ketchup, mayonnaise, high-sodium cheese, and breads. All of these are amenable to the sodium-lowering strategies outlined above.

Lunch
The type of food eaten at lunch varies widely. Soup, sandwich, and salad combinations are common.

Sandwiches. The sodium content of sandwiches can be deduced from what was described for breakfast. Each slice of bread usually contains about 140 mg of sodium; therefore, if two slices are used for a sandwich, bread will contribute 300 mg of sodium. Mayonnaise or salted butter/margarine adds another 100 mg, and then the bulk of sodium at lunch can be found in processed meat and high-sodium cheese. It is not uncommon for all of the ingredients in a sandwich to contain 1.0 to 1.5 g of sodium. Mitigation strategies include use of lower-sodium bread, substituting precooked meat for processed deli meats, using low- or lower-sodium cheese and either unsalted butter or low-sodium mayonnaise, and using either low-sodium ketchup or mustard (a tablespoon of regular mustard has 170 mg of sodium).

Soups. Most soups from cans or mixes contain an enormous amount of sodium added during processing. The amount of sodium is often underestimated. A can of soup usually contains two servings, with a sodium content of 600 to 1,000 mg per serving. It is easy to consume more than a single serving. Reduced-sodium canned soups are available in the low-sodium section of many grocery stores, which generally reduce sodium content by 30% to 50%, but many of these products contain potassium chloride in place of salt. Otherwise soups can be prepared "from scratch" using fresh ingredients or recipes from low-sodium cookbooks. Low-sodium soup stocks are available on the Internet from manufacturers such as Redi-Base (Redi-Base Soup) and others.

Salads. Salad vegetables contain essentially no sodium. All of the sodium in a salad comes from salad dressing or other toppings such as meat and cheese. Standard oil and vinegar mixtures contain no additional salt; however, large amounts of salt are added to most store-bought salad dressings such that they typically contain 200 to 260 mg per 30-mL serving. Because salad dressings stay so long in the refrigerator, it makes sense to purchase a set of low-sodium salad dressings (10 to 30 mg per 30-mL serving) from a healthy foods store or via the Internet. Croutons often add a large sodium load and should be avoided.

Dinner
The classical Western main meal of meat or fish, potatoes or other starch, vegetables, and a salad, is intrinsically low in sodium. As discussed earlier, meats are essentially low-sodium foods. The sodium content in potatoes and all fresh vegetables, as well as salad greens, is also quite low on a per-serving basis. Most of the sodium load during dinner comes from processed food. Increasingly, local supermarkets are selling food that has been partially prepared for cooking. Although convenient, this often includes some form of sodium addition, as in selling meat presoaked in marinade. Rotisserie-cooked chicken is a popular way to buy food in the grocery store. Chicken prepared in this way usually has a high sodium content. In addition, poultry,

especially, often is injected with meat tenderizers containing high amounts of both sodium and phosphate.

Otherwise, high sodium loads are coming from the condiments, including high-sodium tomato-based pasta sauces, barbecue sauce, and, common with vegetables, high-sodium seasoning packets, as mentioned above.

Snacks and Desserts. Sodium in desserts is found mainly in puddings, pastries, and pies, where it has been added as table salt and/or sodium-containing leavening agents. The sodium content of milk-based desserts, such as ice cream, is similar to that for whole milk. Puddings can contain enormous amounts of sodium. On the other hand, fruits intrinsically contain very small amounts of sodium. Potato chips taste salty, but their sodium content often is about the same as or less than that in bread.

POTASSIUM

To review the recommendations discussed in the previous chapter: For potassium intake, a relatively high amount (4.0 g [100 mmol] per day) is recommended for CKD patients in stage 1 or 2 (eGFR/ 1.73 m^2 >60 mL/min). For patients with more advanced CKD, and potentially for patients with earlier-stage CKD who are taking drugs that reduce kidney excretion of potassium, a lower potassium target of 2 to 4 g (50 to 100 mmol) per day is appropriate. Hyperkalemia is a potentially life-threatening situation as it can cause respiratory failure due to muscle weakness and sudden cardiac arrest. So in all patients in whom serum potassium level is on the high side, strict attention to potassium in the diet is required. Even a transient increase in ingestion of high-potassium foods in such patients can cause marked hyperkalemia.

Ranges of Serum Potassium
These will vary somewhat according to the individual laboratory, but in general, 4.0 to 5.0 mmol/L is a relatively safe zone, although patients at the higher end of this range should be counseled about the importance of avoiding bingeing on potassium-rich foods. Levels between 5.0 and 5.5 mmol/L can be thought of as a "caution zone" and require prompt attention to potassium restriction and close follow-up. Levels >5.5 mmol/L have been associated with a markedly increased short-term mortality risk and need urgent attention (see Chapters 5, 11, and 29 for more information on strategies to avoid and treat hyperkalemia).

Food Labeling for Potassium
In the past, food manufacturers did not have to list potassium content on the Nutrition Facts panel, but that is changing. In May 2016, the FDA announced a new Nutrition Facts label for foods to reflect new scientific information, including the link between diet and chronic diseases.

The FDA determined that potassium was a "nutrient of concern" for the general U.S. population because of the benefits of potassium intake in lowering blood pressure. The fact that mandatory labeling of potassium would help people with CKD was not a factor the FDA considered in the new labeling requirements. Renal dietitians don't care about the exact reason why the potassium labeling was added. They are just happy that all consumers, but especially CKD patients, will finally be able to find the potassium content of a food on the label.

Manufacturers had until July 26, 2018 to comply with the final rule, and manufacturers with less than $10 million in annual food sales had an additional year to make changes. In addition, the nutrient databases previously discussed can be used to provide the potassium content of foods.

Dietary Potassium Recommendations for Chronic Kidney Disease Patients With Serum Potassium in the Normal Range

In such patients there is no need to restrict potassium, and in fact, many such patients will have a potassium intake that is below the recommended target of 4.0 g (120 mmol) per day.

Dietary Potassium Restriction for Chronic Kidney Disease Patients With Serum Potassium in the Caution or Danger Zone

In such patients potassium intake must be restricted. These patients should be educated about foods containing high amounts of potassium and should be counseled to especially avoid periods of bingeing on high-potassium foods as it may result in severe hyperkalemia.

Potassium Across Various Food Categories

Potassium is found primarily in what are considered "healthy" foods. Foods that are considered high in potassium are primarily fruits and vegetables, especially potatoes, tomatoes, lentils, and beans. Potassium content is also relatively high in dairy products, nuts, and seeds. Whole grains contain more potassium than refined grains. Most high-potassium foods are generally considered to be healthful. For this reason, when restricting potassium in the diet, special care should be taken to try to substitute lower-potassium alternative foods to maintain a balanced diet. Also, it is important that the alternate choices provide the benefit of healthy nutrients found in the offending high-potassium foods that will be restricted. The potassium content of foods usually thought to be high in potassium is listed in Table 6.3.

Potassium in Fruits

When restricting potassium, the patient should be interviewed carefully about intake of fruits and fruit juices. Potassium content of fruits, although high, varies among different fruits. The amount depends not only on the particular fruit, but on how it is prepared. Canning fruits in heavy sugar can leach out potassium into the syrup, not all of which is consumed. As shown in Table 6.4, almost all fruits and berries contain large amounts of potassium, with apples and pears

Food	Typical Serving	Potassium Content	
Banana	1 small, 6–7 inches long	360 mg	9.3 mmol
Cantaloupe	1 cup diced	420 mg	11 mmol
Orange juice	½ cup from frozen, reconstituted with water	240 mg	6.1 mmol
Prunes	5, dried, uncooked	350 mg	8.9 mmol
Avocado	Raw, ½ cup sliced	350 mg	9.0 mmol
Potato	Baked, 2¼–3-inch diameter, peel eaten	920 mg	23 mmol
Potato	Baked, 2¼–3-inch diameter, peel not eaten	510 mg	13 mmol
Spinach	1 cup cooked	840 mg	21 mmol
Brussels sprouts	1 cup cooked	490 mg	13 mmol
Broccoli	1 cup cooked flowerets	290 mg	7.4 mmol
Milk	1 cup, whole milk	350 mg	8.9 mmol
Yogurt	Fruit variety, from low-fat milk, 1 cup	440 mg	11 mmol
Dried beans	1 cup cooked, most varieties	880 mg	23 mmol

being on the lower end, cherries and plums in the middle range, and oranges, grapefruit, apricots, peaches, melons, kiwi fruit, bananas, and avocados in the higher range.

Fruits and Vegetable Juices
The potassium content for various juices is given in Table 6.5. Per cup (240 mL), potassium content of juices ranges from 200 mg (5 mmol) for cranberry juice to 500 mg (13 mmol) or higher for tomato juice. In terms of potassium content, cranberry or apple juice is a better choice than orange juice. The potassium content of some tomato juices is as high as 800 mg (20 mmol) per cup. Low-sodium versions of tomato and vegetable juice have unchanged levels of potassium.

Fruit Bingeing
At times fruits are eaten in large quantities over a short period, especially in summer, when a supply of delicious fruit suddenly becomes available. Patients with hyperkalemia should be counseled to not only limit fruit intake on a continuing basis, but to refrain from fruit bingeing as well. Because potassium is found in substantial amounts in foods other than fruits, eating a large amount of food at any one time, such as family reunions or parties, should be avoided in general.

Dried Fruits
On a weight basis, dried fruits can contain greatly larger amounts of potassium than fresh fruits. This becomes a problem with the popularity of various trail mixes containing raisins, dried figs, apples, or cherries. Patients with hyperkalemia should probably avoid eating dried fruit for this reason, including dried fruit roll-ups that are now commonly sold as a "healthy" snack food.

TABLE 6.4 Fruits: Potassium Content per 250-g Serving (About 1 Cup)

mg mmol	125–249 3.2–6.39	250–374 6.4–9.59	375–499 9.6–12.79	500–624 12.8–15.99	>625 >16.0
Listed from lower to higher within each column range	Blueberries, frozen or canned	Apples, raw	Strawberries, raw	Gooseberries, raw	Melons, cantaloupe, raw
	Apples or pears, canned	Pineapple, raw	Plums, canned or raw	Pummelo, prickly pear, raw	Guavas, raw
	Tangerines, canned	Rhubarb, frozen	Mangos, raw	Melons, honeydew, raw	Rhubarb, raw
	Fruit salad	Pears, rose apples, raw	Blackberries, raw	Figs, raw	Guavas, raw
	Cranberries, raw	Cherries, frozen or canned	Litchis, raw	Papayas, raw	Kiwi fruit, raw
		Apricots or peaches, canned	Cherries, raw	Apricots, raw	Currants, raw
		Lemons, raw	Oranges, raw		Passion fruit, raw
		Grapefruit, raw	Melons, casaba, raw		Bananas, raw
			Peaches, raw		Avocados, raw
			Grapes, raw		Plantains, cooked
			Crabapples, quinces, raw		Breadfruit, raw
					Tamarinds, raw
					Persimmons, raw
					Raisins
					Dried currants, peaches, apricots

Source: From Nutritiondata.self.com, which is based on the USDA National Nutrient Database for Standard Reference, with permission.

TABLE 6.5 Potassium in Fruit and Vegetable Juices

Fruit Source	mg per Cup (~240 mL)	mmol per 240 mL
Cranberry	195	5.0
Apple	275	7.0
Grapefruit	400	10
Orange	465	12
Tomato	500	13

TABLE 6.6	Potassium Content of Vegetables

Lower Potassium Content	Higher Potassium Content
Asparagus	Artichokes
Beans (green beans or wax beans)	Bamboo shoots
Cabbage	Beans and lentils
Carrots	Beets
Cauliflower	Broccoli, Brussels sprouts
Celery	Chinese cabbage, greens
Corn	Kohlrabi
Cucumber	Mushrooms
Eggplant	Parsnips
Kale	Potatoes (white or sweet)
Lettuce	Pumpkin
Mixed vegetables	Rutabaga
Okra	Spinach
Onions	Squash (Hubbard)
Peas	Tomatoes
Peppers	
Radish	
Rhubarb	
Squash (summer)	
Watercress	
Water chestnuts	
Zucchini	

Source: Modified from the U.S. National Kidney Foundation website: https://www.kidney.org/atoz/content/potassium.

Potassium in Vegetables

Vegetables contain substantial amounts of potassium, and very high amounts of potassium in relation to the calories they provide. A list of vegetables that are lower versus higher in potassium content is given in Table 6.6. Tomatoes are high in potassium, and tomatoes are consumed not only in fresh form, but also as vegetable juice, tomato ketchup, and tomato sauce for various pasta dishes. Dried tomatoes, sometimes eaten as a snack, should be avoided. A number of other vegetables in the higher-potassium group are commonly believed to have health benefits. A low-potassium diet strategy should be to limit portion size but not necessarily avoid these vegetables completely.

Food Boiling and Soups

There can be marked differences in potassium content of the same food depending on the method of food preparation. Processing methods such as double boiling (see below) can reduce potassium. On the other hand, taking a large quantity of a particular food and cooking it down for a soup or sauce can result in a very–high-potassium dish. As an example, ½ cup fresh tomato slices contains 186-mg potassium, whereas ½ cup tomato sauce contains 387-mg potassium.

Canned Versus Fresh Vegetables
Fresh vegetables are low in sodium but high in potassium, and canned vegetables are high in sodium but may be low in potassium. There are low-sodium canned vegetables available, so patients should be encouraged to use these products when hyperkalemia is an issue.

How to Remove Some of the Potassium From Potatoes and Other Tuberous Vegetables
Potatoes, sweet potatoes, and similar tuberous vegetables have a relatively high potassium content (Table 6.3). The following double-boiling method (Burrowes and Ramer, 2006; 2008) will remove a substantial amount (about 50%) or more of potassium from such food:

- Peel (the skin contains a substantial amount of potassium)
- Slice into small pieces (about ⅛ inch thick)
- Boil for at least 10 minutes using a large pot of water
- Discard this water, refill the pot with fresh water, and boil again until done

Potassium Content of Foods Other Than Fruits or Vegetables
See Table 6.7.

Bread and Pasta Group
In general, rice, noodles, pasta, and bread do not contain large amounts of potassium, with the exception that bread and pasta made from whole grains can have a higher potassium content. High-fiber breakfast cereals containing bran are high in both potassium and phosphate content. Again, here is an example when intake of "healthy foods" must be curtailed.

Dairy Foods
These are high in both potassium and phosphorus.

Tree Nuts
Tree nuts are high in potassium. Peanuts (a legume) and peanut butter are also high in potassium.

TABLE 6.7	Potassium Content of Foods Other Than Fruits or Vegetables
Lower Potassium Content	**Higher Potassium Content**
Rice	Whole-grain pasta and breads
Noodles	Cereals containing bran
Pasta	Milk, yogurt, cheese
Refined breads	Nuts and seeds
Pies without chocolate or high-potassium fruit	Some salt-free broths and soup stocks
Cookies without nuts or chocolate	Salt substitutes

Chocolate

Chocolate has been touted as a new health food that is good for the cardiovascular system. Chocolate is moderately high in potassium and is very high in oxalate and so can exacerbate oxalate-based kidney stones. Chocolate should be eaten sparingly in hyperkalemia-prone patients.

Potassium in Salts and Salt Substitutes

There are many options in the supermarkets for seasoning foods, and many contain sodium and/or potassium in varying amounts. Seasoning labels and content lists must be reviewed closely to make sure the product is safe for CKD patients. Hyperkalemia-prone patients should avoid all salt substitutes containing potassium (Table 6.2).

Potassium in Commercially Prepared Low-Sodium Soups and Other Foods

In some low-sodium soups and other foods, potassium has been substituted by the processor for sodium to maintain a salty taste. Hyperkalemia-prone patients should use such products with caution and first inform themselves as to their potassium content.

Sources of Potassium You May Not Think About

Because most patients with CKD have other comorbidities, somewhere along the way they have been given dietary advice that had nothing to do with kidney disease. This advice may result in the patient eating foods high in potassium that the clinician may not think about. Examples include:

- The patient with years of hypertension may have been on a potassium-wasting diuretic and so has been told to "eat a banana and drink orange juice every day." The diuretics may have been changed with progression of CKD, but no one told the patient to stop eating these high-potassium fruits every morning.
- The patient with congestive heart failure who was told to avoid salt but whose cardiologist told her that she could use a potassium-containing salt substitute instead.
- The patient with diabetes for 20 years has always used orange juice to treat low blood sugar, because years ago that is what the patient was told to use. Now with advanced CKD, the patient is having more episodes of hypoglycemia and is still treating those low glucose levels with orange juice.

Also, although this source has little to do with comorbidity, occasionally it is the cause of mysterious hyperkalemia. Chewing tobacco is high in potassium, which is absorbed as the tobacco is chewed.

CONCLUSIONS

Patients become confused and frustrated when trying to limit potassium in their diet, especially if they have multiple health care providers telling them what not to eat. Even diet lists from very reputable sources may provide conflicting information, because potassium content depends so much on the amount of food eaten and how the food has been prepared. Patients need guidance from experienced nephrology dietitians to help them sort out fact from fiction. People with kidney disease face many challenges when advised to limit multiple nutrients in their diet. Balancing mineral restrictions while also trying to follow dietary guidelines for other medical conditions such as heart disease and diabetes is especially challenging. Health care providers should be food coaches, not food police, and help their patients do the best they can with the tools and resources that are available.

References and Suggested Readings

Academy of Nutrition and Dietetics. Chronic kidney disease (CKD) evidence-based nutrition practice guideline. Executive summary. 2010. Available from https://www.andeal.org/category.cfm?cid=14. Accessed April 26, 2018.

Beer-Borst S, Luta X, Hayoz S, et al. Study design and baseline characteristics of a combined educational and environmental intervention trial to lower sodium intake in Swiss employees. *BMC Public Health*. 2018;18:421.

Burrowes JD, Ramer NJ. Removal of potassium from tuberous root vegetables by leaching. *J Ren Nutr*. 2006;16:304–311.

Burrowes JD, Ramer NJ. Changes in potassium content of different potato varieties after cooking. *J Ren Nutr*. 2008;18:530–534.

Cordain L, Eaton SB, Sebastian A, et al. Origins and evolution of the Western diet: health implications for the 21st century. *Am J Clin Nutr*. 2005;81:341–354.

Cupisti A, Kovesdy CP, D'Alessandro C, et al. Dietary approach to recurrent or chronic hyperkalaemia in patients with decreased kidney function. *Nutrients*. 2018;10: E261. doi: 10.3390/nu10030261.

Daugirdas JT. Potential importance of low-sodium bread and breakfast cereal to a reduced sodium diet. *J Ren Nutr*. 2013;23:1–3.

Gazzaniga DA. The No-Salt, Lowest-Sodium Cookbook. New York: St. Martin's Press; 2002.

Karanja NM, Obarzanek E, Lin PH, et al. Descriptive characteristics of the dietary patterns used in the dietary approaches to stop hypertension trial. DASH Collaborative Research Group. *J Am Diet Assoc*. 1999;99:S19–S27.

Kidney Disease Outcomes Quality Initiative (K/DOQI). K/DOQI clinical practice guidelines on hypertension and antihypertensive agents in chronic kidney disease. *Am J Kidney Dis*. 2004;43:S1–S290.

Mattes RD, Donnelly D. Relative contributions of dietary sodium sources. *J Am Coll Nutr*. 1991;10:383–393.

Micha R, Wallace SK, Mozaffarian D. Red and processed meat consumption and risk of incident coronary heart disease, stroke, and diabetes mellitus: a systematic review and meta-analysis. *Circulation*. 2010;121:2271–2283.

Nerbass FB, Pecoits-Filho R, McIntyre NJ, et al. Demographic associations of high estimated sodium intake and frequency of consumption of high-sodium foods in people with chronic kidney disease stage 3 in England. *J Ren Nutr*. 2014;24:236–242.

Parpia AS, L'Abbé M, Goldstein M, et al. The impact of additives on the Phosphorus, Potassium, and Sodium content of commonly consumed meat, poultry, and fish products among patients with chronic kidney disease. *J Ren Nutr*. 2018;28:83–90.

Shepherd R, Farleigh CA, Wharf SG. Limited compensation by table salt for reduced salt within a meal. *Appetite*. 1989;13:193–200.

Shoham DA, Vupputurri S, Kshirsagar AV. Chronic kidney disease and life course socioeconomic status: a review. *Adv Chronic Kidney Dis*. 2005;12:56–63.

U.S. Department of Agriculture. Household food security in the United States in 2015. Available from https://www.ers.usda.gov/publications/pub-details/?pubid=79760. Accessed April 26, 2018.

U.S. Department of Agriculture. Nutrient data laboratory. National nutrient database. Available from https://ndb.nal.usda.gov/ndb. Accessed April 26, 2018.

U.S. Food and Drug Administration. Changes to the nutrition facts label. Available from https://www.fda.gov/food/guidanceregulation/guidancedocumentsregulatoryinformation/labelingnutrition/ucm385663.htm. Accessed April 26, 2018.

Young EW, Mauger EA, Jiang KH, et al. Socioeconomic status and end-stage renal disease in the United States. *Kidney Int*. 1994;45:907–911.

7

Protein Intake

Laetitia Koppe and Denis Fouque

Nutritional management in chronic kidney disease (CKD) has triple goals: protect renal function, prevent metabolic disorders and protein-energy wasting. There is evidence that eating a low amount of protein may be beneficial to patients with CKD, especially in terms of reduction of proteinuria. Whether a low-protein diet can slow the progression of CKD is still being debated. In some CKD patients, a low-protein diet may worsen nutritional status if not properly implemented, and the overall burden of multiple dietary restrictions that CKD patients face should always be kept in mind. The goal is to provide patient education, dietitian support, and regular physician follow-up so that CKD patients can maximize the benefits afforded by a modest reduction in protein intake.

WHAT ARE THE USUAL PROTEIN REQUIREMENTS AS A FUNCTION OF AGE AND BODY SIZE?

In large national surveys of protein intake in Western countries, actual protein intake depends on age, ideal body weight (IBW), and sex. In the National Health and Nutrition Examination Survey (NHANES), for example, daily protein intake averaged 91 g/day in young adults (1.35 g/kg per day) compared with 66 g/day (1.0 g/kg per day) in subjects older than age 70. Young men eat more protein (1.5 g/kg per day) than young women (1.2 g/kg per day), but the sex difference narrows as subjects get older, such that men and women older than 70 eat similar amounts, about 1.0 g/kg IBW per day. In patients with more advanced stages of CKD, daily protein intake averages 0.85 g/kg per day (Garg, 2001; Kopple, 2000).

Minimum Recommended Dietary Allowance for Protein

A number of international health bodies, including the World Health Organization, have issued minimum recommended dietary allowances (RDA) for protein intake. This is the level that would ensure that almost all individuals would be in nitrogen balance and maintain stable body weight. The minimum RDA for protein intake is generally agreed to be around 0.8 g/kg per day. This recommendation assumes that protein from mixed plant and animal origin is being ingested (Rand, 2003). Usually, the RDA for protein is the same for both sexes and does not differ for adults based on age. However, higher protein intake per day has been suggested for healthy older adults (1.0 to 1.2 g/kg per day) and at least 1.2 to 1.5 g/kg per day in patients with acute or chronic illnesses to counteract disease-induced hypercatabolism and sarcopenia (Deutz, 2014).

Adjusted Body Weight

According to the 2000 Kidney Disease Outcomes Quality Initiative (KDOQI) nutrition guidelines, the IBW (minus the weight of any edema fluid, i.e., edema-free body weight) should be used for protein and energy requirement calculations only when this weight is between 95% and 115% of the median weight for standard body weight (stdBW). StdBW is the normal weight of healthy Americans of similar sex, age, height, and skeletal frame size, obtained through the NHANES II. In the other case, adjusted body weight (adjBW) should be used. The equation is:

$$adjBW = IBW + (stdBW - IBW) \times 0.25$$

Example 1 (obese patient): Current body weight of a patient who is 60 years old and 72-inches (183-cm) tall is 300 pounds (136 kg). He has no edema. What is the adjusted body weight?

Step 1 is to look up the median standard weight for such patients. If the patient is American, the NHANES II data table can be used (Appendix 2). Assuming a medium frame size, the median weight for men aged 55 to 74 who are 183 cm tall is 81 kg.

$$adjBW = 136 + (81 - 136) \times 0.25 = 123 \text{ kg}$$

So the daily protein RDA for this patient, assuming 0.8 g/kg, would be $0.8 \times 123 = 98$ g instead of $0.8 \times 136 = 110$ g. In even heavier patients, a maximum protein intake of 100 g/day probably should not be exceeded.

Example 2 (very lean patient): Assume that this male patient of the same frame size, age, and height has an actual edema-free body weight of 155 pounds (70 kg), where the median standard weight was 81 kg. Now:

$$adjBW = 70 + (81 - 70) \times 0.25 = 73 \text{ kg}$$

So protein requirement RDA would be $0.8 \times 73 = 58$ g instead of $0.8 \times 70 = 56$ g/day.

Protein Intake Requirements as a Function of Energy Intake

Protein intake requirement cannot be looked at in the absence of energy intake, and in patients with suboptimal energy intake, which may include many CKD patients, the required minimum protein intake may be higher. Usual energy intake in CKD patients is not different from that in subjects with normal renal function and is in the range of 30 to 35 kcal/kg per day to guarantee an optimal metabolic balance. It is admitted (yet unproven) that older patients have a lower dietary energy requirement due to the loss of lean mass and lower physical activity. KDOQI guidelines state that advanced CKD patients who are <60 years of age should meet 35 kcal/kg per day, whereas for patients ≥60 years of age the recommended intake is reduced to 30 kcal/kg per day (Kopple, 2001).

Quality of Protein and Essential Amino Acids

Proteins in the human body are made up mostly of 20 amino acids. Eight of these are considered essential in adults because the body does not synthesize them: phenylalanine, valine, threonine, tryptophan, isoleucine, methionine, leucine, and lysine. An additional four—histidine, tyrosine, cysteine, and arginine—are required in food for growing children. If some essential amino acids (EAA) are not available, the qualitatively deficient ingested protein cannot be used by the body to make new protein but is then deaminated and converted to carbohydrate and fat.

Both animal- and plant-based food contain EAA, but some sources contain more complete sets of EAA than others. Particularly good sources of EAA are milk, eggs, meat, and fish. Near-complete plant-based sources of EAA are grains that are not commonly eaten, such as amaranth, buckwheat, and quinoa. Soy protein is relatively complete but slightly deficient in the sulfur-containing amino acids methionine and cysteine. Grains are deficient in lysine but beans are high in lysine, providing a rationale for combining grains and beans in a balanced vegan diet. Plant-based diets can supply a complete set of amino acids, but combinations of different plant-based foods must be eaten to ensure a supply of all EAA. The RDA of protein assumes that a mixture of animal and plant-based foods are eaten that is supplying the required amounts of all EAA.

WHAT ARE THE RISKS OF SARCOPENIA AND OSTEOPOROSIS IN THE ELDERLY, AND HOW ARE THESE RELATED TO PROTEIN INTAKE?

Sarcopenia

Ageing is accompanied by changes in the body composition with a gradual increase in the proportion of fat mass and decline in lean mass. Lean mass is the main reservoir of protein and it has an important role in movement, regulation of metabolism, and storage of energy. Sarcopenia is a loss of muscle tissue that occurs as a natural part of both aging and disease. Its mechanisms and risk factors are still poorly identified. There is strong evidence linking reduced physical activity to the occurrence of sarcopenia with age, and this appears to be the most important factor. Moderately increasing daily protein intake from 0.8 to 1.0 g/kg per day may enhance muscle anabolism during exercise training, thereby reducing the progressive loss of muscle mass with age (Campbell and Leidy, 2007; Tieland, 2012).

Osteoporosis

In some epidemiologic studies, a higher dietary protein intake is associated with a lower risk of osteoporosis and hip fracture (Misra, 2011). Similarly, in the elderly, a body mass index in the overweight range is associated with better bone density compared with a normal-range body mass index. The effect of dietary protein intake on osteoporosis and the fracture risk overall remain controversial, and in a recent meta-analysis, only the lumbar spine bone mineral density showed moderate evidence to support benefits of higher protein intake (Shams-White, 2017).

Protein, Acid Load, and Bone
When protein is metabolized, it generates an acid load as a result of breakdown of its phosphorus- and sulfur-containing amino acids. An acid load increases excretion of calcium in the urine and has a catabolic effect on bone and so is bad for bone health. The degree of acid load associated with vegetable proteins is less than with animal proteins, but vegetarian diets have been shown to contain lower amounts of calcium, vitamin D, vitamin B_{12}, and omega-3 fatty acids, all of which have important roles in maintaining bone health. The debate is unresolved at this time, whether ingestion of animal versus plant protein is better in terms of maintenance of healthy bone (Tucker, 2014).

WHAT ARE THE THEORETICAL MECHANISMS WHEREBY REDUCED PROTEIN INTAKE MIGHT SLOW PROGRESSION OF CHRONIC KIDNEY DISEASE?

The main mechanism by which a low-protein diet is thought to slow progression of CKD is by lowering the degree of proteinuria and by resulting in better control of blood pressure, the major determinants of the progression of CKD (Table 7.1). In addition, a high protein intake usually is associated with a higher intake of phosphorus, sodium, and saturated fats, each of which may, directly or indirectly, adversely affect kidney function. The higher acid load seen with high-protein diets may adversely affect kidney function as well as bone metabolism. Also, insulin resistance and oxidative stress, which may affect both cardiovascular and renal disease risk, may be improved with a lower-protein diet. Finally, there is some evidence that protein intake influences uremic toxin levels and production, as detailed below.

 TABLE 7.1 Potential Benefits Versus Risks of a Protein-Restricted Diet in Chronic Kidney Disease Patients

Benefits	Cautions
Reduction in proteinuria	Worsening of sarcopenia
Slowing of progression (nondiabetic patients)	Worsening of bone density and increased fracture risk
Reduction of phosphate load	
Reduction of sodium intake and blood pressure	
Reduction of acid load	
Reduction of intake of saturated fats	
Improved insulin sensitivity	
Reduced uremic toxin production	

Uremic Toxin Production

CKD is characterized by the accumulation of toxins that the kidney is not able to eliminate. Use of a low-protein diet was initially based on the rationale that decreased amino acid degradation and urea synthesis result in lowered urea accumulation. Long considered to be of negligible toxicity, urea is reemerging as a uremic toxin and several studies demonstrate both direct (increased oxidative stress) and indirect (by carbamylation of proteins) toxicity of urea (Lau and Vaziri, 2017). Other uremic toxins are produced from amino acid breakdown by intestinal microbiota, including p-cresyl sulfate (PCS) and indoxyl sulfate (IS)—these last two in particular have been associated with morbidity and mortality in CKD patients. Trimethylamine-N-oxide (TMAO), a degradation product of choline and L-carnitine (which come from animal proteins such as red meat and eggs), is also associated with cardiovascular complications. IS, PCS, and TMAO have deleterious effects on renal function and metabolic parameters (Koppe, 2015).

Recent data highlight that uremia is associated with the modification of the intestinal microbiota that could strongly increase transformation of amino acids into uremic toxins. Influx of urea and other toxins as well as pH alterations due to local production of ammonium exert a selection pressure in the intestinal lumen, resulting in the expansion of bacteria that express urease, uricase, and indole- and p-cresol–forming enzymes. Protein intake, intestinal microbiota, and uremic toxin production are closely linked. To demonstrate the importance of diet on intestinal uremic metabolite levels Patel (2012), showed that PCS and IS production rates were markedly lower in vegetarians than in individuals consuming an unrestricted diet. This difference could be explained by the fact that a vegetarian population has reduced protein intake. Two studies confirm that a very–low-protein diet supplemented with keto-analogs (KAs) reduced IS and PCS serum levels in CKD patients and healthy adults (Marzocco, 2013; Poesen, 2015). The influence of a low-protein diet on intestinal microbiota is still unknown. A low-protein diet minimizes the accumulation of urea and other toxins and this suggests a clinical benefit in terms of slowing the progression of CKD.

One factor modulating the rate at which gut bacteria generate uremic toxins is the gastrointestinal transit time. In patients who have frequent bowel movements, there is simply less time for bacteria to generate uremic toxins, and this may be one mechanism whereby high-fiber diets are associated with a cardiovascular benefit in the general population (Park, 2011). In patients with CKD, dietary advice limiting fiber and fluid intake coupled with a lack of physical activity conspire to markedly prolong gastrointestinal transit time. At least one study shows that a high fiber intake is associated with relatively lower blood levels of IS and PCS (Rossi, 2015). Dietary protein–fiber ratio associates with circulating levels of IS and PCS in CKD patients (Rossi, 2015). If this association proves to depend on reduced gut transit time, then this would point to the importance of maintaining regular bowel movements and avoiding constipation in CKD patients. Interestingly, hyperkalemia (but not dietary potassium intake) may be linked with constipation as suggested by St-Jules (2016).

Proteinuria Reduction and Slowing of Chronic Kidney Disease Progression

An oral protein load or infusion of amino acids rapidly and transiently increases the glomerular filtration rate (GFR). Chronic increases in the GFR over time, as observed during diabetes or with severe obesity, can lead to microalbuminuria and ultimately to impairment of kidney function. Clinically, a low-protein diet reduces proteinuria (Gansevoort, 1995; Kaysen, 1988; Walser, 1996). This decrease in proteinuria is important because proteinuria is an independent risk factor for progressive renal disease. Although proteinuria reduction is primarily targeted using angiotensin-converting enzyme inhibitors and/or angiotensin receptor blockers, addition of a low-protein diet confers further protection to the kidney and may postpone end-stage renal failure (Locatelli and Del Vecchio, 1999; Gansevoort, 1995). In many, but not all, studies in CKD patients in which proteinuria reduction is achieved, the short-term change in proteinuria (percentage of reduction and residual proteinuria) correlates with the subsequent rate of progression of kidney disease and identifies the patients who are likely to benefit from dietary prescription. The most important benefit is observed in patients with high baseline proteinuria: The greater the reduction in proteinuria, the greater the renal protection (Brantsma, 2007).

Phosphate

Although amino acids themselves contain no phosphorus, protein content and phosphorus content of commonly eaten foods are strongly associated, such that food containing 1 g of protein commonly contains approximately 11 to 15 mg of phosphorus. For this reason, reducing protein intake limits oral phosphate load. A direct and independent association between serum phosphate levels and mortality has been reported. A high phosphate intake decreases the antiproteinuric response to a low-protein diet (Cozzolino, 2017; Di Iorio, 2013). A dietary phosphate intake of 800 mg daily is the maximum recommended limit, which generally corresponds to 45 to 50 g of protein (e.g., 0.8 g/kg per day in a 60-kg adult). An increase in phosphorus intake can induce a series of physiopathologic cascades such as an increase in fibroblast growth factor 23. The latter is reported to be a cardiac toxin (Faul, 2011) and is associated with progression of CKD (Fliser, 2007). Protein intake is a significant determinant of fibroblast growth factor 23 (Di Iorio, 2012). Practical aspects of controlling phosphate and protein in the diet are discussed further in Chapter 11.

Sodium and Blood Pressure

Reducing protein intake may help to control blood pressure as a result of decreased dietary sodium ingestion. Consumption of proteins from animal origin, especially eating processed meats as well as salt-containing sauces commonly used with meats, is associated with elevated sodium intake. In one study of blood pressure in CKD patients receiving a low-protein diet supplemented with ketoanalogs blood pressure decreased from 143/84 to 128/78 mm Hg. The reduction by 30% in protein intake was associated with a 30% decrease in sodium intake (Bellizzi, 2007).

Lipid Profile

Because a reduced protein intake generally entails eating less protein of animal origin (e.g., meat and dairy products), intake of saturated fat is concomitantly decreased, and this can result in an improved serum lipid profile. In one study, reducing daily protein intake from 1.1 to 0.7 g/kg per day for 3 months effected an increase in serum lipoprotein A-I levels and in the Apo-A-I/Apo-B ratio, changes that are considered beneficial in terms of cardiovascular risk (Bernard, 1996). The origin of protein also plays a role in lipid profile as observed in a recent study in CKD patients where soy protein substitution had a beneficial lipid-lowering effect (Chen, 2005).

Insulin Resistance

Insulin resistance is frequently observed during the course of CKD. After a 3-month low-protein diet, patients improved their sensitivity to insulin, reduced their fasting serum insulin as well as daily insulin needs, and reduced both blood glucose level and endogenous glucose production (Gin, 1994). Recently, the implications of uremic toxins in glucose homeostasis have emerged. For example, studies have demonstrated the role of PCS and urea in insulin resistance and may explain the benefits of low-protein diet on glucose homeostasis by reducing these toxins (Koppe, 2013; Koppe, 2016).

Acid Load

Metabolism of proteins generates acid, and this effect is more pronounced with animal protein versus vegetarian diets. An increase in serum bicarbonate from 24.2 to 26.5 mmol/L was reported after 1 year of a very–low-protein diet (0.3 g/kg per day) supplemented with ketoanalogues (Chauveau, 1999). During the Modification of Diet in Renal Disease (MDRD) study, achieved reduction of protein intake was associated with an increase in serum bicarbonate (Mitch and Remuzzi, 2004). A post hoc analysis of the MDRD study showed that lower plasma bicarbonate levels increased the risk of outcomes such as renal death and mortality (Menon, 2010). An increase in blood pH associated with a low-protein diet may be partially responsible for the renoprotective effects of a low-protein diet (Kalantar and Fouque, 2017).

WHAT ARE THE RESULTS OF CLINICAL STUDIES OF THE EFFECTS OF A LOWER-PROTEIN DIET ON CHRONIC KIDNEY DISEASE PROGRESSION?

More than 100 studies have evaluated the effects of reducing protein intake in CKD. The most recent studies, including 10 randomized controlled trials (RCT) in nondiabetic patients and 13 RCT in patients with diabetes, are of great interest, and exhaustive analysis of each of these trials can be found in reviews and meta-analyses (Fouque and Laville,

2009; Nezu, 2013). In more than 1,400 nondiabetic patients, reducing protein intake resulted in a 40% decrease on average in the number of patients starting dialysis or who died during the trial (Fouque and Laville, 2009). In diabetic patients, a recent meta-analysis enrolling 779 patients (Nezu, 2013) highlighted that a low-protein diet was associated with a significant improvement in GFR; however, proteinuria was not different between diets. There are three other meta-analyses on this issue. The meta-analysis by Pedrini (1996) reported beneficial effects of low-protein diets; however, they combined RCTs and nonrandomized crossover trials. In addition, they used a composite outcome of GFR or albuminuria. Two other meta-analyses (Pan, 2008; Robertson, 2007) did not show significant effects on kidney function. These discrepant results may be explained by the difference in the pooled study number and population size. Satisfactory adherence to a low-protein diet was observed in approximately 50% of the patients. While the results of the studies on the effects of a low-protein diet on the rate of progression of renal failure remain inconclusive, they are highly significant when initiation of dialysis is the primary outcome.

WHAT ARE THE RECOMMENDATIONS OF CURRENT GUIDELINES REGARDING PROTEIN INTAKE IN CHRONIC KIDNEY DISEASE?

The various groups issuing CKD guidelines have come up with slightly different recommendations with regard to the extent of dietary protein restriction in CKD patients. These are summarized in Table 7.2. All guidelines are supportive of mild protein restriction in CKD patients, to the level of the RDA (0.8 g/kg per day) or lower, with KDOQI supporting a diet with more severe daily protein restriction to 0.6 g/kg per day for patients with GFR <25 mL/min per 1.73 m². The International Society of Renal Nutrition and Metabolism (ISRNM) suggests a protein intake of 1 g/kg per day in sick patients. However, all of these guideline groups are concerned about the risk of malnutrition with low-protein diets, emphasizing the need to maintain a high caloric intake and to monitor dietary intake on a regular basis. Despite several studies confirming that low-protein diets are nutritionally safe (Bellizzi, 2015; Chauveau, 2009), a few guidelines do specifically recommend against the use of a very–low-protein diet for CKD patients.

USE OF KETOANALOGS OF AMINO ACIDS

During the past 60 years, various levels of protein restriction have been studied. Indeed, the protein metabolism of a healthy or CKD adult enables adaptation to an intake as low as 0.3 g/kg per day of protein if energy and EAAs are supplied. To avoid nutritional deficits, supplements can be added as EAA pills or KAs of amino acids if levels of protein intake are below 0.6 g/kg per day (Aparicio, 2012). After transamination, KAs can recapture nitrogen from waste endogenous uremic products and then be used to synthesize the corresponding EAAs. Adding EAAs or KAs to a low-protein diet allows a greater variety of food to be selected because the patients are not restricted to only

TABLE 7.2		**Protein Restriction Recommendations in Chronic Kidney Disease Patients**		
Guideline	**Last Updated**	**Target Patient Subgroup**	**Recommended Daily Protein Intake**	**Comments**
KDOQI Nutrition	2000	GFR[a] <25, patients not yet on dialysis	0.6 g/kg or up to 0.75 g/kg for patients who cannot tolerate 0.6 g/kg	50% protein should be of high biologic value (guideline #24); guideline #25 suggests a daily energy intake of 35 kcal/kg for patients older than age 60, and 30–35 for patients younger than age 60.
International Society of Renal Nutrition and Metabolism	2013	CKD	0.6–0.8 g/kg per day If illness, then 1.0 g/kg per day (based on ideal body weight [IBW])	Greater than 50% of high biologic value protein (complete protein sources containing the full spectrum of essential amino acids).
KDOQI Diabetes and CKD	2007	Diabetes and CKD stages 1–4 (GFR >15)	0.8 g/kg	50–75% protein should be of high biologic value.
CARI Nutrition and Growth in Renal Disease	2005		Not lower than 0.75 g/kg IBW	50–66% protein should be of high biologic value; daily energy intake should be 35 kcal/kg IBW.
British Renal Association	2010	CKD	0.75 g/kg	Daily energy intake 30–35 kcal/kg IBW upon age and physical activity.
European Dialysis and Transplant Nurses Association/ European Renal Care Association	2003	CKD	0.6–1.0 g/kg, >0.75 g/kg when GFR >30	Very restricted protein diets (<0.5 g/kg) require supplements.
Canadian Society of Nephrology	2008	CKD	0.80–1.0 g/kg	Their opinion is that there is lack of convincing evidence of slowing of progression with daily intakes <0.7 g/kg.

[a]All GFR values as mL/min per 1.73 m^2.
KDOQI, Kidney Disease Outcomes Quality Initiative; GFR, glomerular filtration rate; CKD, chronic kidney disease; CARI, Caring for Australasians with Renal Impairment.
Note: See Chapter 31 for a description of the various United States and International Guidelines cited in this table.

high-quality protein foods such as meat or eggs. One caveat: if protein intake is greater than the minimum requirements, for example, 0.7 to 0.8 g/kg per day, adding KAs will not be followed by transamination, and these supplements will be oxidized rather than incorporated into new protein.

The effectiveness and safety of KA supplementation is emerging. Initially, the largest study addressing KAs, for example, the MDRD Study, provided conflicting results: the protein-restricted diet only marginally reduced the decline in GFR; the advantage was small and apparently caused by the protein restriction, not the KA supplementation. However, a large RCT published in 2016 suggested that KAs are nutritionally safe and might defer dialysis initiation by ameliorating CKD-associated metabolic disturbances in patients with CKD; KA supplementation seemed to have specific advantages (Garneata, 2016). This was confirmed in a meta-analysis that indicated that a very–low-protein diet supplemented with KAs could delay the progression of CKD, decrease hyperphosphatemia, prevent hyperparathyroidism, and benefit blood pressure control without causing malnutrition (Jiang, 2016).

HOW TO ADAPT PROTEIN INTAKE TO THE CHRONIC KIDNEY DISEASE STAGE, AND SHOULD WE FAVOR VEGETABLE PROTEIN?

Studies have assessed a number of different protein restrictions (Fouque and Laville, 2009). The nutritional status of patients following a supplemented very–low-protein diet (0.3 g/kg per day) is conserved after starting hemodialysis or receiving a kidney transplant (Aparicio, 2000; Vendrely, 2003). Survival of these patients was as good, if not better, 1 year after dialysis start as that of patients who did not receive a low-protein diet and KA supplement (Vendrely, 2003).

To date there is no optimal level of protein restriction; however, from a metabolic view, it is tempting to say that more restriction is better. A subgroup analysis based on the level of protein restriction, although defined after the trials had been completed, suggested that the more restricted diets (0.3 to 0.6 g of protein/kg per day) were associated with a greater benefit than diets that were less restrictive (Fouque and Laville, 2009). The degree of protein restriction should be chosen based on individual patient acceptance and the skills and availability of dietitians, as well as baseline nutritional status.

There is no metabolic, nutritional, or evidence-based rationale to progressively decrease protein intake based on CKD stage or rapidity of progression. In our opinion, diet optimization should be started at a relatively early stage of CKD—that is, when normalized GFR falls below 60 to 50 mL/min because at this level of renal function, many metabolic disorders are already present.

Vegan–vegetarian diets are becoming increasingly widespread, thus setting the groundwork for easier integration of moderate protein restriction. Moreover, results of small studies suggest that a vegetarian protein diet compared to an animal protein diet can delay the progression of CKD, protect vascular endothelium, help to control high blood pressure, improve phosphorus homeostasis, and can decrease proteinuria (Gluba-Brzózka, 2017; Zhang, 2014). However, these potential benefits remain to be proven by large RCTs.

DOES PRESENCE OF MARKED PROTEINURIA CHANGE THE RECOMMENDATION FOR PROTEIN RESTRICTION?

Protein intake recommendations do not need to be increased in patients with proteinuria. Indeed, in such patients, there is a clear positive relationship between protein intake and proteinuria (Kaysen, 1988), and increasing protein intake will induce an elevation in proteinuria. Even in the case of nephrotic-range proteinuria, starting a low-protein diet will lower proteinuria and increase serum albumin. If malnutrition occurs in severe nephrotic syndrome, the mechanisms are far more complex than just the renal loss of 5 to 10 g of protein per day, which could be replaced by ingestion of one or two egg whites; this is why the dietary protein intake recommendation in patients with proteinuria is 0.6 to 0.8 g/kg per day of protein plus 1 g of dietary protein intake for each 1 g of daily urinary protein excretion. The mechanisms of protein depletion during the nephrotic syndrome depends more on catabolic factors associated with the disease and urinary loss of anabolic compounds (Maroni, 1997).

HOW SHOULD ONE MONITOR NUTRITIONAL INTAKE DURING CHRONIC KIDNEY DISEASE?

In all patients with CKD, especially in those with GFR values below 20 mL/min per 1.73 m^2 and in those following an intensive program of protein restriction, nutritional status must be closely monitored because PEW can suddenly worsen as GFR falls into a range in which anorexia can be induced. The monitoring strategy is ideally implemented with the aid of a renal dietitian and includes repeated discussions with the patient about diet, use of structured food questionnaires when required, and a method called subjective global assessment. Laboratory values should include serum albumin and/or prealbumin as well as cholesterol (a drop in serum cholesterol may indicate poor nutrition) (Table 7.3).

TABLE 7.3	Nutritional Monitoring

Every Month for 4 Months, Then Quarterly:
Dietary interview
    Develop a care plan
    Tailor diet to patient's taste and economic situation
Home 3-day food record
    Record energy intake
24-hour urinary urea
    Estimate protein intake

Quarterly:
Body weight, anthropometry (optional), Subjective Global Assessment (optional)
Serum albumin, serum prealbumin, serum cholesterol

Example of Monitoring Patient Adherence With 24-Hour Collection of Urinary Nitrogen

Example: Stable noncatabolic 80-kg adult patient prescribed a dietary protein restriction of 0.6 g/kg per day.

Patient's daily urinary nitrogen appearance (UNA) from 24-hour collection: 5.2 g
Add estimate of nonurinary excretion (NUN): $0.031 \times BW = 2.48$ g per day

Total nitrogen appearance (TNA):
UNA + NUN = $5.2 + 2.48 = 7.68$ g/day

Dietary protein intake estimate (DPI):
DPI = $6.25 \times TNA$
    = 6.25×7.68
    = 48 g/day

DPI/kg = $48/80 = 0.6$ g/kg
Assessment: This patient is compliant with the prescribed diet.

For a more complete discussion of this topic, see Masud T, Manatunga A, Cotsonis G, et al. The precision of estimating protein intake of patients with chronic renal failure. *Kidney Int.* 2002;62:1750–1756.

Subjective Global Assessment

This is a rating based on six scales: weight, dietary intake, gastrointestinal symptoms, functional capacity, comorbidities related to nutritional needs, and physical examination (focusing on muscle wasting, subcutaneous fat loss, and edema) (Sacks, 2000).

URINARY NITROGEN APPEARANCE

After collecting a 24-hour urine sample and determining the daily urinary nitrogen excretion or appearance (UNA), one can use the following equation (Masud, 2002) to estimate nitrogen intake:

$$N \text{ intake (g/day)} = UNA \text{ (g/day)} + 0.031 \times BW \text{ (kg)}$$

Where BW is the actual body weight and UNA is the 24-hour urinary urea nitrogen output (see Table 7.4); then, to convert N intake into protein intake, multiply N intake by 6.25.

References and Suggested Readings

Aparicio M, Bellizzi V, Chauveau P, et al. Keto acid therapy in predialysis chronic kidney disease patients: final consensus. *J Ren Nutr.* 2012;22:S22–S24.

Aparicio M, Chauveau P, De Précigout V, et al. Nutrition and outcome on renal replacement therapy of patients with chronic renal failure treated by a supplemented very low protein diet. *J Am Soc Nephrol.* 2000;11:708–716.

Bellizzi V, Calella P, Hernández JN, et al. Safety and effectiveness of low-protein diet supplemented with ketoacids in diabetic patients with chronic kidney disease. *BMC Nephrol.* 2018;19:110.

Bellizzi V, Chiodini P, Cupisti A, et al. Very low-protein diet plus ketoacids in chronic kidney disease and risk of death during end-stage renal disease: a historical cohort controlled study. *Nephrol Dial Transplant.* 2015;30:71–77.

Bellizzi V, Di Iorio BR, De Nicola L, et al. Very low protein diet supplemented with ketoanalogs improves blood pressure control in chronic kidney disease. *Kidney Int.* 2007;71:245–251.

Bernard S, Fouque D, Laville M, et al. Effects of low-protein diet supplemented with ketoacids on plasma lipids in adult chronic renal failure. *Miner Electrolyte Metab.* 1996;22:143–146.

Brantsma AH, Atthobari J, Bakker SJ, et al. What predicts progression and regression of urinary albumin excretion in the nondiabetic population? *J Am Soc Nephrol.* 2007;18:637–645.

Campbell WW, Leidy HJ. Dietary protein and resistance training effects on muscle and body composition in older persons. *J Am Coll Nutr.* 2007;26:696S–703S.

Chauveau P, Aparicio M, Bellizzi V, et al; European Renal Nutrition Working Group of the ERA-EDTA. Mediterranean diet as the diet of choice for patients with chronic kidney disease. *Nephrol Dial Transpl.* 2018;33:725–735.

Chauveau P, Barthe N, Rigalleau V, et al. Outcome of nutritional status and body composition of uremic patients on a very low protein diet. *Am J Kidney Dis.* 1999; 34:500–507.

Chauveau P, Couzi L, Vendrely B, et al. Long-term outcome on renal replacement therapy in patients who previously received a keto acid-supplemented very-low-protein diet. *Am J Clin Nutr.* 2009;90:969–974.

Chen ST, Ferng SH, Yang CS, et al. Variable effects of soy protein on plasma lipids in hyperlipidemic and normolipidemic hemodialysis patients. *Am J Kidney Dis.* 2005;46:1099–1106.

Cozzolino M, Foque D, Ciceri P, et al. Phosphate in chronic kidney disease progression. *Contrib Nephrol.* 2017;190:71–82.

Deutz NE, Bauer JM, Barazzoni R, et al. Protein intake and exercise for optimal muscle function with aging: recommendations from the ESPEN Expert Group. *Clin Nutr.* 2014;33:929–936.

Di Iorio BR, Bellizzi V, Bellasi A, et al. Phosphate attenuates the anti-proteinuric effect of very low-protein diet in CKD patients. *Nephrol Dial Transplant.* 2013;28:632–640.

Di Iorio B, Di Micco L, Torraca S, et al. Acute effects of very-low-protein diet on FGF23 levels: a randomized study. *Clin J Am Soc Nephrol.* 2012;7:581–587.

Faul C, Amaral AP, Oskouei B, et al. FGF23 induces left ventricular hypertrophy. *J Clin Invest.* 2011;121:4393–4408.

Fliser D, Kollerits B, Neyer U, et al. Fibroblast growth factor 23 (FGF23) predicts progression of chronic kidney disease: the Mild to Moderate Kidney Disease (MMKD) Study. *J Am Soc Nephrol.* 2007;18:2600–2608.

Fouque D, Laville M. Low protein diets for chronic kidney disease in non diabetic adults. *Cochrane Database Syst Rev.* 2009;CD001892.

Gansevoort RT, de Zeeuw D, de Jong PE. Additive antiproteinuric effect of ACE inhibition and a low-protein diet in human renal disease. *Nephrol Dial Transplant.* 1995;10:497–504.

Garg AX, Blake PG, Clark WF, et al. Association between renal insufficiency and malnutrition in older adults: results from the NHANES III. *Kidney Int.* 2001;60:1867–1874.

Garneata L, Stancu A, Dragomir D, et al. Ketoanalogue-supplemented vegetarian very low-protein diet and CKD progression. *J Am Soc Nephrol.* 2016;27:2164–2176.

Gin H, Combe C, Rigalleau V, et al. Effects of a low-protein, low-phosphorus diet on metabolic insulin clearance in patients with chronic renal failure. *Am J Clin Nutr.* 1994;59:663–666.

Gluba-Brzózka A, Franczyk B, Rysz J. Vegetarian diet in chronic kidney disease—a friend or foe. *Nutrients.* 2017;9:pii: E374.

Jiang Z, Zhang X, Yang L, et al. Effect of restricted protein diet supplemented with keto analogues in chronic kidney disease: a systematic review and meta-analysis. *Int Urol Nephrol.* 2016;48:409–418.

Kalantar-Zadeh K, Fouque D. Nutritional management of chronic kidney disease. *N Engl J Med.* 2017;377:1765–1776.

Kaysen GA. Albumin metabolism in the nephrotic syndrome: the effect of dietary protein intake. *Am J Kidney Dis.* 1988;12:461–480.

Koppe L, Mafra D, Fouque D. Probiotics and chronic kidney disease. *Kidney Int.* 2015;88:958–966.

Koppe L, Nyam E, Vivot K, et al. Urea impairs β cell glycolysis and insulin secretion in chronic kidney disease. *J Clin Invest.* 2016;126:3598–3612.

Koppe L, Pillon NJ, Vella RE, et al. p-Cresyl sulfate promotes insulin resistance associated with CKD. *J Am Soc Nephrol.* 2013;24:88–99.

Kopple JD. National Kidney Foundation K/DOQI clinical practice guidelines for nutrition in chronic renal failure. *Am J Kidney Dis.* 2001;37:S66–S70.

Kopple JD, Fouque D. Pro: The rationale for dietary therapy for patients with advanced chronic kidney disease. *Nephrol Dial Transpl.* 2018;33:373–378.

Kopple JD, Greene T, Chumlea WC, et al. Relationship between nutritional status and the glomerular filtration rate: results from the MDRD study. *Kidney Int.* 2000;57:1688–1703.

Lau WL, Vaziri ND. Urea, a true uremic toxin: the empire strikes back. *Clin Sci (Lond).* 2017;131:3–12.

Locatelli F, Del Vecchio L. How long can dialysis be postponed by low protein diet and ACE inhibitors? *Nephrol Dial Transplant.* 1999;14:1360–1364.

Maroni BJ, Staffeld C, Young VR, et al. Mechanisms permitting nephrotic patients to achieve nitrogen equilibrium with a protein-restricted diet. *J Clin Invest.* 1997; 99:2479–2487.

Marzocco S, Dal Piaz F, Di Micco L, et al. Very low protein diet reduces indoxyl sulfate levels in chronic kidney disease. *Blood Purif.* 2013;35:196–201.

Masud T, Manatunga A, Cotsonis G, et al. The precision of estimating protein intake of patients with chronic renal failure. *Kidney Int.* 2002;62:1750–1756.

Menon V, Tighiouart H, Vaughn NS, et al. Serum bicarbonate and long-term outcomes in CKD. *Am J Kidney Dis.* 2010;56:907–914.

Misra D, Berry SD, Broe KE, et al. Does dietary protein reduce hip fracture risk in elders? The Framingham Osteoporosis Study. *Osteoporos Int.* 2011;22:345–349.

Mitch WE, Remuzzi G. Diets for patients with chronic kidney disease, still worth prescribing. *J Am Soc Nephrol.* 2004;15:234–237.

Nezu U, Kamiyama H, Kondo Y, et al. Effect of low-protein diet on kidney function in diabetic nephropathy: meta-analysis of randomised controlled trials. *BMJ Open.* 2013;3:pii: e002934.

Pan Y, Guo LL, Jin HM. Low-protein diet for diabetic nephropathy: a meta-analysis of randomized controlled trials. *Am J Clin Nutr.* 2008;88:660–666.

Park Y, Subar AF, Hollenbeck A, et al. Dietary fiber intake and mortality in the NIH-AARP diet and health study. *Arch Intern Med.* 2011;171:1061–1068.

Patel KP, Luo FJ, Plummer NS, et al. The production of p-cresol sulfate and indoxyl sulfate in vegetarians versus omnivores. *Clin J Am Soc Nephrol.* 2012;7:982–988.

Pedrini MT, Levey AS, Lau J, et al. The effect of dietary protein restriction on the progression of diabetic and nondiabetic renal diseases: a meta-analysis. *Ann Intern Med.* 1996;124:627–632.

Poesen R, Mutsaers HA, Windey K, et al. The influence of dietary protein intake on mammalian tryptophan and phenolic metabolites. *PLoS One.* 2015;10:e0140820.

Rand WM, Pellett PL, Young VR. Meta-analysis of nitrogen balance studies for estimating protein requirements in healthy adults. *Am J Clin Nutr.* 2003;77:109–127.

Robertson L, Waugh N, Robertson A. Protein restriction for diabetic renal disease. *Cochrane Database Syst Rev.* 2007;CD002181.

Rossi M, Johnson DW, Xu H, et al. Dietary protein-fiber ratio associates with circulating levels of indoxyl sulfate and p-cresyl sulfate in chronic kidney disease patients. *Nutr Metab Cardiovasc Dis.* 2015;25:860–865.

Sacks GS, Dearman K, Replogle WH, et al. Use of subjective global assessment to identify nutrition-associated complications and death in geriatric long-term care facility residents. *J Am Coll Nutr.* 2000;19:570–577.

Shams-White MM, Chung M, Du M, et al. Dietary protein and bone health: a systematic review and meta-analysis from the National Osteoporosis Foundation. *Am J Clin Nutr.* 2017;105:1528–1543.

St-Jules DE, Goldfarb DS, Sevick MA. Nutrient non-equivalence: does restricting high-potassium plant foods help to prevent hyperkalemia in hemodialysis patients? *J Ren Nutr.* 2016;26:282–287.

Tieland M, Dirks ML, van der Zwaluw N, et al. Protein supplementation increases muscle mass gain during prolonged resistance-type exercise training in frail elderly people: a randomized, double-blind, placebo-controlled trial. *J Am Med Dir Assoc.* 2012;13:713–719.

Tucker KL. Vegetarian diets and bone status. *Am J Clin Nutr.* 2014;100:329S–335S.

Vendrely B, Chauveau P, Barthe N, et al. Nutrition in hemodialysis patients previously on a supplemented very low protein diet. *Kidney Int.* 2003;63:1491–1498.

Walser M, Hill S, Tomalis EA. Treatment of nephrotic adults with a supplemented, very low-protein diet. *Am J Kidney Dis.* 1996;28:354–364.

Zhang J, Liu J, Su J, et al. The effects of soy protein on chronic kidney disease: a meta-analysis of randomized controlled trials. *Eur J Clin Nutr.* 2014;68:987–993.

8

Mineral and Bone Disorders

Deepa Amberker and Steven C. Cheng

The presence of chronic kidney disease (CKD) has a variety of effects on mineral metabolism. The term *mineral bone disorder of CKD* encompasses not only **bone disease** but also **vascular and soft tissue calcification**, as well as abnormalities in calcium, phosphorus, parathyroid hormone (PTH), and vitamin D metabolism.

As kidney function worsens and glomerular filtration rate (GFR) falls, the body attempts to maintain mineral homeostasis through a cascade of compensatory mechanisms. Fibroblast growth factor (FGF23), a hormone that promotes phosphate excretion, is increased. Hydroxylation of vitamin D to the active form (1,25-D) is decreased and PTH secretion rises. Unfortunately, many of these adaptive changes also have adverse effects, including high bone turnover, left ventricular hypertrophy, and vascular calcification.

The goal of therapy is to keep the bone and vasculature healthy, minimizing these adverse effects by reducing the need for compensatory hormonal changes. This is achieved through avoidance of hyperphosphatemia, control of serum calcium, maintenance of active vitamin D levels, and limiting the degree of parathyroid hyperplasia and PTH secretion.

PATHOPHYSIOLOGY

As Glomerular Filtration Rate Falls, the Kidney Needs to Increase Fractional Phosphate Excretion

As kidney function falls, the number of functioning nephrons is reduced (see Chapter 1 for a definition of *nephron*). Unless intake is reduced, the total amount of phosphate that needs to be excreted remains unchanged, so the *fractional excretion of phosphate* by the remaining nephrons needs to be increased.

Serum FGF23 Levels Rise to Increase Fractional Renal Phosphate Excretion

FGF23, which is made by bone cells, regulates phosphate excretion by the kidney. FGF23 acts on receptors in the renal tubules to block reabsorption of filtered phosphate thereby increasing phosphate excretion. FGF23 also suppresses PTH and reduces activation of vitamin D. When GFR falls even slightly, the kidney signals the bone to make more FGF23. FGF23 increases early in the course of CKD, maintaining serum levels of phosphate within the normal range. However, as kidney disease progresses to its later stages, the rise of FGF23 may be insufficient to excrete the daily phosphate load and serum phosphorus levels begin to rise. Contributing to this is the reduction in tissue expression of Klotho, a critical cofactor for FGF23, as GFR declines.

Activation of Vitamin D Is Reduced

In normal individuals, vitamin D is "activated" in the kidney by 1α-hydroxylase, an enzyme which converts 25-D (a relatively inactive precursor of activated vitamin D) to the active 1,25-D. 1,25-D then interacts with vitamin D receptors (VDRs) located in the gut to increase enteric absorption of phosphorus and calcium. This multi-step process is shown in Table 8.1. However, as GFR falls, the rising

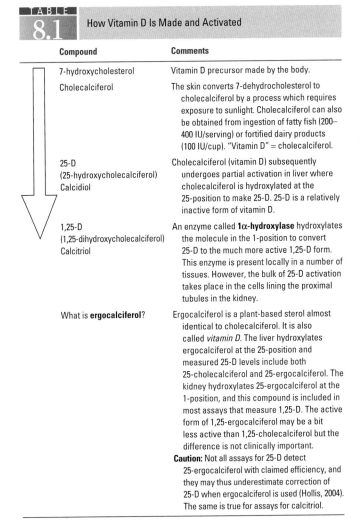

TABLE 8.1 How Vitamin D Is Made and Activated

Compound	Comments
7-hydroxycholesterol	Vitamin D precursor made by the body.
Cholecalciferol	The skin converts 7-dehydrocholesterol to cholecalciferol by a process which requires exposure to sunlight. Cholecalciferol can also be obtained from ingestion of fatty fish (200–400 IU/serving) or fortified dairy products (100 IU/cup). "Vitamin D" = cholecalciferol.
25-D (25-hydroxycholecalciferol) Calcidiol	Cholecalciferol (vitamin D) subsequently undergoes partial activation in liver where cholecalciferol is hydroxylated at the 25-position to make 25-D. 25-D is a relatively inactive form of vitamin D.
1,25-D (1,25-dihydroxycholecalciferol) Calcitriol	An enzyme called **1α-hydroxylase** hydroxylates the molecule in the 1-position to convert 25-D to the much more active 1,25-D form. This enzyme is present locally in a number of tissues. However, the bulk of 25-D activation takes place in the cells lining the proximal tubules in the kidney.
What is **ergocalciferol**?	Ergocalciferol is a plant-based sterol almost identical to cholecalciferol. It is also called *vitamin D*. The liver hydroxylates ergocalciferol at the 25-position and measured 25-D levels include both 25-cholecalciferol and 25-ergocalciferol. The kidney hydroxylates 25-ergocalciferol at the 1-position, and this compound is included in most assays that measure 1,25-D. The active form of 1,25-ergocalciferol may be a bit less active than 1,25-cholecalciferol but the difference is not clinically important. **Caution:** Not all assays for 25-D detect 25-ergocalciferol with claimed efficiency, and they may thus underestimate correction of 25-D when ergocalciferol is used (Hollis, 2004). The same is true for assays for calcitriol.

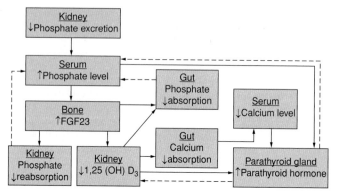

FIGURE 8.1 How phosphate loading raises fibroblast growth factor 23 levels and how this then affects 1,25-D and parathyroid hormone. *Solid arrows* signify stimulation; *dotted arrows* signify inhibition. (From Seiler S, Heine GH, Fliser D, et al. Clinical relevance of FGF-23 in chronic kidney disease. *Kidney Int Suppl.* 2009;76:S34–S42, with permission.)

levels of FGF23 inhibit activity of 1α-hydroxylase, thereby decreasing the activation of vitamin D and reducing enteric phosphorous absorption (Fig. 8.1).

Furthermore, as kidney function is lost, there are fewer healthy renal tubular cells available to carry out conversion of 25-D to 1,25-D in CKD (Fig. 8.2).

In Chronic Kidney Disease, Serum Levels of 25-D Tend to Be Low

As shown in Table 8.1, 25-D is the substrate for 1α-hydroxylase and the immediate precursor of 1,25-D. Levels of 25-D depend on sun

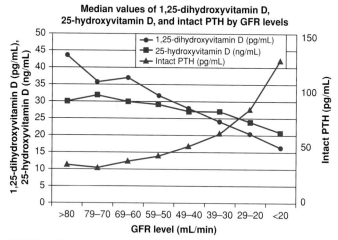

FIGURE 8.2 Changes in parathyroid hormone, 25-D, and 1,25-D as glomerular filtration rate falls. (From Levin A, Bakris GL, Molitch M, et al. Prevalence of abnormal serum vitamin D, PTH, calcium, and phosphorus in patients with chronic kidney disease: results of the study to evaluate early kidney disease. *Kidney Int.* 2007;71:31–38, with permission.)

exposure and dietary intake (cholecalciferol is found naturally in fish and is added to dairy products). Serum levels of 25-D have been measured in a number of large population studies and levels believed to be suboptimal (<30 ng/mL [75 nmol/L]) or severely low (<15 ng/mL [37 nmol/L]) are quite commonly found. In addition, 25-D levels seem to be decreasing in recent years as people spend more time indoors. 25-D levels are also substantially lower in African Americans, perhaps, because of a reduced efficiency of melanin-laden skin in converting cholesterol-based precursors to cholecalciferol. The 25-D levels in CKD patients are almost invariably low, and as shown in Figure 8.1, 25-D levels decline as CKD progresses. The reason for this has not been well studied. It may be due to diet, less sun exposure, or uremic inhibition of cholecalciferol synthesis in UV-exposed skin. There is also some evidence that uremia and hyperparathyroidism may impair 25-hydroxylation of cholecalciferol in the liver (Michaud, 2010).

Effect on Parathyroid Hormone
As CKD progresses, the serum PTH level begins to rise. This is due to the following factors:

1. *Reduced calcium absorption by the gut and relative hypocalcemia.* Low 1,25-D levels reduce calcium absorption in the gut. The resulting low serum calcium levels then directly stimulate PTH.
2. *Removal of direct inhibitory effect of 1,25-D on the parathyroid gland.* Synthesis of PTH is suppressed by VDRs in the parathyroid gland. When 1,25-D levels are low, this inhibition is lost, and the parathyroid gland cells multiply to cause hyperplasia and secondary hyperparathyroidism.
3. *High serum levels of phosphate and resistance to FGF23.* Serum phosphorus stimulates PTH secretion, although the direct mechanism of this effect remains unclear. In addition, the inhibitory effect of FGF23 on the parathyroid gland is reduced due to declining levels of the cofactor Klotho in CKD.

Parathyroid Hormone Effects on the Kidney in Chronic Kidney Disease

Phosphaturia
PTH has an effect on the kidney similar to that of FGF23 in that it acts on the tubules to block phosphate reabsorption, causing the kidney to excrete phosphorus. Functionally, this is consistent with the role of PTH in maintaining serum calcium levels, since high phosphate levels can lower the serum calcium.

Stimulation of 1α-Hydroxylase
The effects of PTH and FGF23 on 1α-hydroxylase run in opposite directions: Whereas FGF23 inhibits this enzyme, PTH stimulates it. The resulting increase in 1,25-D stimulates enteric absorption of calcium, thus raising levels of serum calcium—a net effect which reflects the role of PTH in protecting serum calcium levels. However, the stimulatory

effect of high PTH on 1α-hydroxylase generally is negated by the inhibitory effects of FGF23 and the reduced nephron mass.

Summary of Pathophysiology

The mechanism of mineral bone disorder in CKD is secondary hyperparathyroidism, in which the parathyroid glands undergo hyperplasia because of chronic stimulation. This is mediated by three mechanisms: (a) stimulation by low serum calcium levels (due to reduced gut calcium absorption from low 1,25-D), (b) removal of suppression by 1,25-D (due to low levels of 1,25-D and reduced sensitivity to 1,25-D), and (c) stimulation by increased serum phosphate levels.

BONE DISEASE

High-Turnover Bone Disease

The classical form of bone disease seen with CKD is similar to the bone disease found in primary hyperparathyroidism called *osteitis fibrosa cystica*. It is the result of sustained elevation in PTH. PTH has a number of actions in bone, all of which accelerate bone turnover. Both bone formation and reabsorption, mediated by osteoblasts and osteoclasts, respectively, are increased, and marrow fibrosis is often seen to be increased on bone marrow biopsy. In severe disease, cystic lesions can occur in areas of marked bone resorption. Bone pain can be present and fracture risk is increased.

Adynamic Bone Disease

Other forms of bone disease have been described as well. Low-turnover bone disease, or **adynamic bone disease**, is characterized by reduced bone formation and resorption. The cause of this form of renal osteodystrophy is poorly understood. It is distinguished by low PTH levels in contrast to the high PTH levels found most commonly in CKD. Bones tend to be brittle and there is a higher fracture rate than in those with high-turnover bone disease. Patients with adynamic bone also tend to become hypercalcemic easily because the bone loses its capacity to buffer extraneous calcium loads.

Osteomalacia

Osteomalacia is also a low-turnover type of bone disease, but it is characterized by an increase in unmineralized bone. This can be seen in patients with severe vitamin D deficiency.

Osteoporosis

Osteoporosis is common in the elderly CKD population. In patients with early CKD (stages 1 to 3), osteoporosis is diagnosed (e.g., by dual energy x-ray absorptiometry [DEXA] scanning) and treated (using bisphosphonates, selective or nonselective estrogens, or teriparatide if PTH is persistently low, and vitamin D) in the usual fashion. In more advanced CKD, DEXA scanning becomes unreliable to detect osteoporosis, and the optimum treatment of bone disease is uncertain.

Bone Biopsy

Bone biopsy is the gold standard method of determining the type of bone disease present in CKD. The vast majority of patients with underlying mineral bone disease can be identified and correctly treated from the laboratory values (described below) alone. Biopsy is currently used to clarify when there are conflicting laboratory data or an unusual presentation, including unexplained hypercalcemia. Biopsy also is helpful before parathyroidectomy when there is a history of aluminum exposure or concern of possible adynamic disease, because the removal of parathyroid glands and subsequent reduction of PTH may be detrimental in patients who already demonstrate low bone turnover.

Bone samples are typically obtained from the iliac crest after a time-spaced administration of two doses of tetracycline, which are deposited on the bone surface. This provides information regarding the bone's microarchitecture and kinetic properties, as indicated by the amount of formation and mineralization found between the two separate layers of bone labeled by tetracycline.

CARDIOVASCULAR RISK FACTORS ASSOCIATED WITH MINERAL BONE DISORDER OF CHRONIC KIDNEY DISEASE

The mineral bone disorder of CKD results in laboratory abnormalities and compensatory mechanisms that have effects beyond the bone. As shown in Tables 8.2 and 8.3, many of these changes, including high phosphate, high PTH, and low 25-D, are associated specifically with cardiovascular risk, including vascular calcification. PTH levels have been linked to the presence of left ventricular hypertrophy as well, possibly through its effect on raising intracellular calcium concentrations. In addition, FGF23 and deficiency of Klotho have been identified as risk factors for cardiovascular disease and vascular calcification in CKD patients (Nasrallah, 2010; Scialla, 2014).

LABORATORY TESTS

Early detection is the first step in managing the mineral bone disorder in CKD (see Tables 8.2 and 8.3).

Calcium

In CKD patients, the normal serum calcium level is 8.5 to 10.2 mg/dL (2.1 to 2.55 mmol/L). Only 1% of calcium is extracellular, so serum levels are a poor reflection of body stores. While serum-ionized calcium is usually 40% to 50% of the total serum calcium, the ionized fraction can be relatively increased in the hypoalbuminemic state.

There is a tendency for the serum calcium to decrease as the GFR falls, particularly if vitamin D is not replaced adequately. The recommendation from guideline bodies like Kidney Disease: Improving Global Outcomes (KDIGO, 2017) is to avoid hypercalcemia. Careful calcium supplementation can be given if serum calcium is low and PTH is elevated. However, KDIGO guidelines do not recommend

	TABLE 8.2	Levels of Calcium, Phosphate, and Magnesium in Chronic Kidney Disease		
Mineral	Normal Blood Level	Target Level in CKD	Risk Associations in Outcomes Studies	Comments
Calcium	8.5–10.5 mg/dL 2.12–2.65 mmol/L	8.5–9.5 (lower) 2.12–2.37 (lower)	Mortality risk in predialysis CKD patients is lowest when serum Ca is at the low end of the normal range.	When PTH levels are high and serum Ca levels are low, some recommend giving Ca supplements, but this may increase risk of vascular calcification.
Phosphate	2.7–4.6 mg/dL 0.87–1.48 mmol/L	2.7–4.6 (same) 0.87–1.48 (same)	Mortality risk keeps improving as serum P levels fall. High levels linked to left ventricular hypertrophy and vascular calcification in dialysis patients. Very-low levels may reflect malnutrition.	The effect of P restriction on FGF23 and benefits of doing this have not been established.
Magnesium	1.8–3.0 mg/dL 1.4–2.1 mmol/L	no data no data	Risk of mortality and cardiovascular disease higher at lower serum Mg levels in population studies and in dialysis patients). High Mg suppresses PTH.	CKD patients may be Mg depleted because of relative avoidance of high-Mg foods such as nuts, seeds, dairy, vegetables, and fruits. Also, diuretics, proton pump inhibitors, and possibly patiromer can lower serum Mg. **Caution:** Risk of severe hypermagnesemia from laxatives and supplements in patients with lower GFR values.

CKD, chronic kidney disease; Ca, calcium; PTH, parathyroid hormone; P, phosphate; FGF, fibroblast growth factor; Mg, magnesium; GFR, glomerular filtration rate.

TABLE
8.3

Parathyroid Hormone, Alkaline Phosphatase, and 25-Vitamin D

Hormone or Enzyme	Normal Blood Level	Target Level in CKD	Risk Associations in Outcomes Studies	Comments
Parathyroid hormone	35–70 pg/mL 3.7–7.4 pmol/L	CKD3: 35–70 CKD4: 70–110 CKD5: 150–300 CKD3: 3.7–7.4 CKD4: 7.4–11.6 CKD5: 12–36	High PTH associated with high-turnover bone disease, increased mortality, vascular calcification, and left ventricular hypertrophy	Intact PTH assays have high variability and detect 7–84 receptor-blocking fragment. Latest KDIGO guidelines admit that optimal PTH levels are NOT known, and suggest treatment should be based on persistence and magnitude of PTH elevation and also on trends in both PTH and alkaline phosphatase.
Alkaline phosphatase	45–150 IU/L	Normal range	Mortality lowest when serum levels in the 50–75 range	Useful to help detect high-turnover bone disease in conjunction with serum PTH monitoring.
25-Vitamin D	15–50 ng/mL 40–125 nmol/L	>15–30 >40–75	Mortality risk linked to low 25-D levels in both general and CKD populations	Caution should be used when treating patients with hypercalciuria, calcium stones, those receiving alkali therapy, and patients at risk for nephrocalcinosis or calciphylaxis.

CKD, chronic kidney disease; PTH, parathyroid hormone.

127

aggressive supplementation of calcium to the upper limit of the normal range in an attempt to suppress PTH.

Serum Phosphate

The normal range of serum phosphate is shown in Table 8.2, and the 2017 KDIGO recommends that decisions about phosphorus-lowering treatments be based on treating patients with progressively or persistently elevated serum phosphorus levels. The upper limit of normal for serum phosphorus is 4.6 mg/dL (1.48 mmol/L).

In predialysis CKD patients, a strong relationship has been reported between serum phosphate and mortality (Kovesdy, 2010). The risks of vascular calcification and cardiac hypertrophy are strongly related to the serum phosphate level. Elevated serum phosphate also accelerates the rate of aortic valve calcification with or without aortic stenosis (Linefsky, 2014). Interestingly, the risk of higher serum phosphate levels and mortality extends even to patients with normal or near-normal renal function for reasons that are unclear. In chronically ill populations, the risk between phosphate and mortality is U shaped, and the high mortality risk in patients with very low serum phosphate levels likely reflects poor nutritional status.

Magnesium

Two-thirds of magnesium is stored in bone, one-third is intracellular, and only 1% is extracellular. Serum magnesium measures total magnesium, of which 30% is bound to albumin, 15% to various anions, and 55% is free. Normal serum levels are 1.8 to 3.0 mg/dL (1.4 to 2.1 mmol/L). Urinary magnesium excretion is maintained until GFR falls to <30 mL/min. However, severe hypermagnesemia has been reported in elderly CKD patients taking large doses of magnesium-containing laxatives. A relative magnesium deficiency can occur in CKD when a low-potassium or low-phosphate diet is being eaten, as many magnesium-rich foods are also high in potassium or phosphate, or from urinary magnesium wasting that is due to diuretics, particularly thiazides. Low serum magnesium levels increase the propensity to vascular calcification (Bressendorff, 2017) and are associated with increased risk of all-cause mortality in CKD patients (Ferrè, 2017). Patients taking gastrointestinal proton pump inhibitors are susceptible to hypomagnesemia, and the K-binder patiromer also has been associated with low serum magnesium levels. Whether cautious supplementation of magnesium might lower the rate of progression of CKD or reduce the risk for mortality is not yet established.

Serum Parathyroid Hormone

Because uremia imparts a degree of resistance to the effects of PTH, patients with later stages of CKD require higher levels of PTH to have the same effect in mobilizing calcium and phosphorus from bone stores. Therefore, target levels of PTH may be variable and highly influenced by the degree of renal disease and the type of assay used. In the 2017 KDIGO guidelines, the workgroup acknowledged that it could not define a precise range for desirable PTH levels in each stage of CKD. Instead, they recommend lowering PTH levels when elevations are persistent, increasing over time, and were undesirable in the context of other markers of mineral and bone disorder, including serum phosphorus, serum calcium, and serum alkaline phosphatase. Previous guidelines provided by KDOQI for an appropriate intact PTH range (35 to 70 pg/mL in stage 3 CKD, 70 to 110 pg/mL in stage 4 CKD, and 150 to 300 pg/mL in stage 5 CKD) should now be interpreted in the larger context of the individual patient, their laboratory trends, the assay used, and other mineral markers. A PTH level persistently and progressively elevated indicates high bone turnover and osteitis fibrosa cystica. A persistently low PTH is consistent with low bone activity and is seen with adynamic bone disease.

Parathyroid Hormone Assays
PTH is an 84-amino-acid peptide. Each amino acid is labeled from the N-terminus (NH_4 group), starting with the number 1, to the C-terminus (carboxyl group), number 84. The first two amino acids close to the N-terminus are particularly important for receptor binding and activation. Incomplete fragments of PTH can also be found in circulation. Those without the first two amino acids on the N-terminus are functionally inactive; however, fragments including amino acids (7–84) may actually have some inhibitory properties. Currently used PTH assays measure "intact" PTH, but the detection sites of many assays do not include the key 1, 2 positions of the molecule, so they also detect other fragments including the 7–84 fragment. Some assays, referred to as the *biointact* PTH, measure specifically the entire PTH peptide (1–84), thus avoiding fragments in which the crucial 1,2 amino acids are absent. Levels of biointact PTH are approximately 55% of the corresponding "intact" PTH levels. Biointact PTH has yet to gain wide acceptance because of limited availability and technical considerations. There is also some controversy as to whether the use of biointact PTH is necessary because both intact and biointact assays correlate quite well with one another. Current guidelines for target PTH levels use intact PTH levels.

Of note, results from PTH assays may be quite variable, as preparations differ in the antibodies used to detect PTH and its fragments. Furthermore, although PTH levels are used as a surrogate marker for bone activity, the results do not always correlate with actual bone status as determined by biopsy, and several studies have reported patients with PTH at target range with adynamic bone disease. Thus, PTH results must be taken in the context of the entire clinical picture, including other laboratory data such as serum calcium which may be elevated in low-turnover disease, and serum alkaline phosphatase which is discussed below.

Serum Alkaline Phosphatase
Alkaline phosphatase, as commonly measured, is a mixture of phosphatases active in the liver, bone, and other tissues. In the absence of

liver disease, serum alkaline phosphatase reflects bone alkaline phosphatase and is a measure of the bone osteoblast activity in patients with CKD. As such, serum alkaline phosphatase is a measure of PTH-induced bone disease and secondary hyperparathyroidism. A serum alkaline phosphatase level obtained concomitantly with a PTH level may often help illuminate whether a borderline PTH level has deleterious effects on bone. High levels indicate not only bone disease but also are associated with increased levels of inflammatory markers and mortality (Kovesdy, 2010). Bone-specific alkaline phosphatase is a readily obtainable test that reflects bone formation and should be measured when the source of a high serum alkaline phosphatase is in doubt.

Serum 25-D and 1,25-D Assays and Levels

25-D Levels

The most commonly used assay to assess vitamin D stores measures 25-D. In theory, the 25-D assay should detect both 25-cholecalciferol and 25-ergocalciferol to properly assess the response to treatment in patients taking ergocalciferol-based vitamin D repletion (Table 8.1). Accurate detection of 25-D may be limited by an assay's affinity for both forms of 25-D.

What constitutes a sufficient blood level of 25-D is a matter of contention and debate. There is little debate that levels <10 to 15 ng/mL (22 to 37 nmol/L) are insufficient, but not all authorities recommend that levels be kept >30 ng/mL (75 nmol/L) (Table 8.3). There also is no consensus as to what the desirable upper limit should be. It should be kept in mind that 25-D levels do not necessarily reflect 1,25 levels, and they certainly will not reflect VDR activation in patients being treated with calcitriol or active analogs such as doxercalciferol or paricalcitol, described later.

1,25-D Levels

As with 25-D, levels of 1,25-D fall as CKD progresses (Fig. 8.2). 1,25-D levels can be extremely difficult to accurately measure as circulating concentrations can be 1,000 times lower than 25-D values. As with 25-D, low 1,25-D levels, with a cutoff of 25 ng/L in one study, were associated with increased mortality risk (Zittermann, 2009).

MONITORING

One monitoring strategy, recommended by the KDIGO mineral bone disorder guidelines (2017) for CKD, is shown in Table 8.4. Serum calcium, phosphorus, PTH, and, when indicated, alkaline phosphatase should be measured regularly, with increasing frequency as CKD progresses. A 25-D level should also be drawn at baseline and repeated if necessary based on initial value and interventions. A lateral abdominal radiograph can be done to assess aortic calcification, and an echocardiogram can be used to screen for cardiac vascular/valvular calcification.

TABLE 8.4	Monitoring Recommendations
What to Monitor	**How Often**
Serum calcium, phosphorus	CKD3: Every 6–12 months CKD4: Every 3–6 months CKD5: Every 1–3 months
PTH (and serum alkaline phosphatase as an option)	CKD3: Based on baseline level and CKD progression CKD4: Every 6–12 months CKD5: Every 3–6 months
25-D	Depends on baseline level
Lateral abdominal radiograph	Baseline
Echocardiogram for vascular/ valvular calcification	Baseline

CKD, chronic kidney disease; PTH, parathyroid hormone.

TREATMENT STRATEGY

Given the pathogenesis of CKD-associated mineral bone disorder discussed above, a logical approach would be to limit the phosphate load to the kidney early on in the course of CKD, although this strategy has not been evaluated in clinical trials. In theory, at least, phosphate restriction in early CKD might be pursued even in the absence of overt hyperphosphatemia to limit the need for a compensatory increase in FGF23. In one small study in CKD stages 3 and 4 patients, a combination of dietary phosphate restriction and use of phosphate binders (lanthanum carbonate) did lower urinary phosphate excretion as well as serum levels of FGF23 (Isakova, 2013).

Adequate levels of both 25-D and 1,25-D should be maintained in order to preserve the actions of active D on enteric calcium absorption and the parathyroid gland, thereby preventing hyperplasia and limiting the increase in serum PTH.

Restriction of Phosphate Intake

The usual recommendation for CKD patients is to restrict phosphate intake to about 0.8 to 1.0 g per day. The usual phosphate intake in the Western diet ranges from 1.0 to 1.6 g per day and is considerably higher in men than in women. A substantial portion of this is due to phosphorus in foods that also have a high protein content. It's important to realize that the phosphorus is not part of the amino acid structure of proteins per se, but is found in other compounds present in commonly eaten high-protein foods. High–biologic-value proteins, such as those found in eggs, milk products, meat, or fish, normally contain about 8 to 10 mg phosphate per g of protein. If high-protein foods were the only source of phosphorus intake, a diet providing 60 g per day of protein, which would equal the recommended daily allowance (RDA) of 0.8 g/kg for a 75-kg patient, would contain only 0.5 to 0.6 g per day of phosphorus. Phosphorus restriction is made more difficult, however, because many foods such as dairy products contain a higher amount of phosphorus per g of protein. Also, the food industry routinely adds phosphate additives to baked goods, meats, and cereals in very substantial amounts, such that 30% to 50% of the ingested phosphate may be due to food additives. Phosphate from food additives is especially important because it is more readily absorbed in the gut compared to phosphorus present naturally in foods. More information about phosphate content of various foods and how to structure a phosphate-restricted diet is provided in Chapter 9.

Control of Serum Phosphate Levels

Target Values

The 2017 KDIGO guidelines recommend treating hyperphosphatemia in those CKD patients in whom the increase is above the normal range and is persistent and/or progressive. The upper limit of normal for most phosphorus assays is 4.6 mg/dL (1.48 mmol/L).

Phosphate Binders

Phosphorus binders should be used when dietary restriction is not sufficient to control serum phosphorus levels. These agents should be dosed with meals, as they bind phosphorus in ingested food and form compounds that are not absorbed in the gut. The amount of binder taken with each meal should be proportional to the estimated phosphate content of the food being eaten. A variety of substances have been used to form these insoluble complexes with phosphorus, including calcium, magnesium, sevelamer, and lanthanum, and, in earlier times, aluminum (Table 8.5). For a review on their relative abilities to bind phosphate, see Daugirdas (2011). Not all compounds have approved indications for phosphate binding in predialysis CKD patients by local regulatory authorities (e.g., the U.S. Food and Drug Administration [FDA]); product approval varies by country.

Calcium-Containing Phosphate Binders. In patients with stages 3 and 4 CKD, calcium-based binders are commonly used as first-line agents. These binders are predominately available as either calcium carbonate (TUMS, Caltrate, and OsCal) or calcium acetate (PhosLo). Both agents are effective phosphorus binders that also provide calcium supplementation. There are slight differences between calcium carbonate and calcium acetate in regard to cost, availability, and efficacy. Calcium carbonate is available in the generic form, giving it the advantage of lower cost and wider availability. On the other hand, calcium acetate has been shown to be more effective in binding phosphorus (Delmez, 1992), and it has a lower content of elemental calcium (25% vs. 40% in calcium carbonate). Although calcium-based binders are frequently used, the exposure to additional calcium may be of concern in a population at risk for vascular calcification and cardiovascular mortality. For CKD patients

TABLE 8.5

Phosphate Binders

Binder Source	Rx Required?	Forms	Starting Dose	Elemental Ca Content	Potential Advantages	Potential Disadvantages
Calcium acetate	Yes/No	Capsule, tablet	Dose/tablet: 667 mg. Start: 1–2 tablets PO three times per day with meals	25% elemental Ca (169-mg elemental Ca/tablet)	More effective phosphate binding than $CaCO_3$; less elemental calcium.	More expensive than $CaCO_3$; GI side effects; potential for hypercalcemia.
Calcium carbonate	No	Tablet, capsule, gum	Dose/tablet: 500 mg. Start: 1–2 tablets PO three times per day with meals	40% elemental Ca^{2+} (200-mg elemental Ca^{2+}/tablet)	Effective; inexpensive; readily available.	GI side effects; potential for hypercalcemia.
Magnesium/calcium carbonate	No	Tablet	Dose/tablet: 300-mg $MgCO_3$/250-mg $CaCO_3$. Start: 1 tablet PO three times per day with meals	Approx 28% Mg^{2+} (85 mg/tablet) and 25% elemental Ca (100 mg/tablet)	Effective; reduces calcium exposure.	GI side effects (diarrhea); hypermagnesemia; not well studied.
Magnesium carbonate/calcium acetate	Yes	Tablet	Dose/tablet: 235-mg $MgCO_3$/435-mg Ca acetate. Start: 1 tablet PO three times per day with meals	Approx 50 mg of elemental Mg and 110 mg of elemental Ca/tablet	Effective; reduces calcium exposure.	Lack of availability, assumed to have similar effects of its components.
Sevelamer carbonate	Yes	Tablet	Dose/tablet: 800 mg. Start: 1 tablet PO three times per day with meals	N/A	Effective; no calcium/metal for tissue deposition; reduces plasma concentration of LDL-C.	Cost; GI side effects.
Lanthanum carbonate	Yes	Wafer, chewable	Dose/tablet: 500/750/1,000 mg. Start: 500 mg PO three times daily with meals	N/A	Effective; no calcium; chewable.	Cost; potential for lanthanum accumulation; GI side effects.
Niacinamide	Yes	Tablet	Dose/tablet: 500 mg. Start: 1 tablet once or twice per day	N/A	May also beneficially affect lipids.	Thrombocytopenia; not well studied in CKD.
Ferric citrate	Yes	Tablet	2 tablets (1 tablet = 210 mg of ferric iron) three times daily with meals	N/A	No calcium. Potential to increase iron stores.	GI side effects. Potential aluminum overload.
Sucroferric oxyhydroxide	Yes	Tablet/chewable	1 tablet (500 mg of iron) three times daily with meals	N/A	No calcium. Lower pill burden.	GI side effects.

Rx, prescription; Ca, calcium; PO, by mouth; GI, gastrointestinal; N/A, not applicable; LDL-C, low-density lipoprotein cholesterol; CKD, chronic kidney disease.
Source: Modified with permission from KDIGO 2009 CKD-MBD Guidelines, Table 19.

who demonstrate radiographic evidence of existing vascular calcification or low-turnover bone disease, we suggest limiting additional calcium exposure and using non–calcium-based binders instead, although further research is needed to investigate this issue. The 2017 KDIGO guidelines recommend restriction of calcium-based phosphorus binders for all adult CKD patients, realizing that this is often not possible for economic reasons. For all patients, total binder dose should perhaps supply no more than 1.5 g/day of elemental calcium (i.e., give no more than 3.75 g of calcium carbonate or 6.0 g of calcium acetate per day), although the maximum "safe" dose of calcium-containing phosphorus binders is not known.

Magnesium–Calcium Binders. Contain a mixture of magnesium carbonate and either calcium carbonate or calcium acetate. Because magnesium also binds phosphate, a lower amount of calcium carbonate (as present in MagneBind) or calcium acetate (as present in OsvaRen) can be used than if these calcium-containing binders were used alone. However, magnesium-based binders do not have an FDA-approved indication for this purpose in the United States, and there is a theoretical risk of hypermagnesemia. Use of magnesium/calcium–phosphorus binders has the theoretical advantage of not only limiting calcium absorption but avoiding hypomagnesemia, hypothetically offering some protection against vascular calcification.

Non-Calcium Binders. Although calcium-containing binders are widely available and inexpensive, the increased exposure to calcium may warrant concern, particularly in patients with reduced urinary excretion of calcium. Studies have suggested that the use of non-calcium binders attenuates the progression of vascular calcification in comparison with calcium-containing binders, at least in the dialysis population. Currently available non-calcium binders are described below.

Lanthanum Carbonate. Lanthanum carbonate (Fosrenol) has good phosphate-binding properties and a low level of absorption. Lanthanum is approved for predialysis CKD patients in the United Kingdom as of 2010. It is available as 250-, 500-, 750- and 1,000-mg chewable wafers. A reasonable starting dose is 500 mg three times a day with upward titration as needed, not exceeding doses of 1,250 mg three times a day. So far there has been no evidence of toxic accumulation of lanthanum or adverse effects on bone metabolism.

Sevelamer Carbonate. Sevelamer carbonate (Renvela) is a non-aluminum, non–calcium-based phosphorus binder that traps phosphorus in the bowel through ion exchange and hydrogen binding. This drug replaced sevelamer hydrochloride (Renagel) and has an advantage of not generating an acid load, which its precursor, sevelamer hydrochloride, did. It also has the advantage of lowering LDL cholesterol due to gut binding of bile acids.

Iron-Based Phosphate Binders. Ferric citrate and sucroferric oxyhydroxide are the two forms currently available. Because some of the iron in ferric citrate is absorbed, it offers the advantage of concurrent iron supplementation in CKD patients with iron deficiency. This reduces the need for other forms of iron treatments, translating into decreased treatment costs. In contrast, The iron present in the phosphate binder sucroferric oxyhydroxide is not absorbed to an appreciable extent.

Aluminum-Based Phosphate Binders. These agents are potent binders of phosphorus that were previously considered first line. However, their use has been curtailed because of toxic effects of aluminum accumulation, including anemia, neurologic changes, and impaired bone mineralization. KDIGO 2017 guidelines recommend against the long-term use of aluminum-based phosphate binders in predialysis CKD patients.

Niacinamide

Niacin and niacinamide are the two principal forms of vitamin B_3. Although they do not function as phosphorus binders, they do inhibit the sodium–phosphate transporter in the gastrointestinal system, thereby reducing the amount of absorbed phosphate. Studies in the dialysis population have shown an effective reduction of serum phosphate with once- to twice-daily dosing of these compounds (Cheng and Coyne, 2007). These agents may offer a smaller pill burden and beneficial effects on cholesterol (see Chapter 12), but long-term experience is limited thus far. In one trial where extended-release niacin was given to a broad range of subjects, the subset with CKD had a very slight lowering of serum phosphorus but no effect on serum levels of FGF23, PTH, or vitamin D metabolites (Malhotra, 2018).

Tenapanor

Tenapanor is an inhibitor of the intestinal sodium–proton exchanger NH_3 that increases stool sodium and phosphorus in healthy volunteers. In one pilot study in dialysis patients with hyperphosphatemia, tenapanor given over 4 weeks resulted in a substantial lowering of elevated serum phosphorus levels (Block, 2017). Studies of tenapanor in nondialysis CKD patients have not been reported.

Calcium Supplementation

Calcium containing salts can be administered as either a phosphorus binder or as a calcium supplement. When the intended use is phosphate binding, calcium should be dosed with meals. This results in a smaller amount of calcium absorption, as calcium forms nonabsorbable complexes with phosphorus. In contrast, when the intended use is calcium supplementation, calcium salts should be given apart from meals to maximize calcium availability and absorption. Because PTH is stimulated by low levels of serum calcium, supplementation may have an ancillary effect on controlling secondary hyperparathyroidism.

There are, however, concerns about calcium supplementation in a patient population that is already at risk for vascular calcification. In patients with normal kidney function, calcium supplementation has been associated with an increase in the rate of myocardial infarction (Bolland, 2010), a potential risk that may be even more concerning for CKD patients who frequently have pre-existing coronary artery calcification. In one small study of mineral kinetics, the use of calcium supplementation in CKD patients resulted in a net positive calcium balance which exceeded the positive balance in bone—suggesting some retention of calcium into other body tissues.

Therefore, the decision to implement calcium supplementation should be based not only on a low or low-normal serum calcium level but on other markers of mineral metabolism as well. If PTH is within the normal range, there is no compelling indication to dose supplemental calcium. If PTH is elevated, the correction of low serum calcium levels may help to suppress PTH, but correction of 25-D deficiency, if present, is a better initial approach, since this can increase enteric calcium absorption and suppress PTH, thereby reducing or eliminating the need for calcium supplementation. Calcium supplementation should be avoided in patients with high serum phosphorus, as there may be an increased risk of calcium/phosphate precipitation and tissue calcification.

Vitamin D Supplementation

As long as serum phosphate levels are reasonably well controlled, some form of vitamin D supplementation is commonly given to patients with CKD. In early (e.g., stages 1 to 3) CKD, often either cholecalciferol or ergocalciferol is given. In the later stages (4 to 5) of CKD, conversion of 25-D to 1,25-D may be impaired, and maintaining serum 25-D levels alone may not be sufficient to suppress elevated serum PTH levels. At that point, either calcitriol or one of the active vitamin D analogs can be given either in addition to, or in place of, ergocalciferol or cholecalciferol.

Usual Doses of Cholecalciferol and Ergocalciferol

The RDA for cholecalciferol for adults has traditionally been in the range of 200 to 400 international unit (IU). Health authorities are considering raising this value to 800 IU, and 800 to 2,000 IU are usually required to increase 25-D levels above 30 ng/mL in CKD patients.

In the United States, because cholecalciferol is available as an over-the-counter product only, ergocalciferol is commonly used to increase 25-D levels. Ergocalciferol is a plant-based analog of cholecalciferol with similar biologic activity (some authorities believe ergocalciferol is roughly 20% to 30% less potent than cholecalciferol, but this is controversial). Ergocalciferol typically is given monthly as a 50,000-IU capsule. The dose can be increased up to weekly × 4 in patients in whom serum 25-D levels are below 15 ng/mL (37 nmol/L). An extended-release formulation of calcifediol (25-cholecalciferol) has become available in the United States for lowering serum PTH levels in CKD patients (Sprague, 2016). The dose is 30 to 60 mcg given once daily at bedtime.

Dosing Strategy for Ergocalciferol. One dosing strategy for ergocalciferol based on 25-D levels might be as follows:

25D level <5 ng/mL (<12 nmol/L): Ergocalciferol 50,000 IU/week × 12, then monthly × 3

25D level 5 to 15 ng/mL (12–37 nmol/L): Ergocalciferol 50,000 IU weekly × 4, then monthly × 5

25D level 15 to 30 ng/mL (37–75 nmol/L): Ergocalciferol 50,000 IU monthly × 6

Cautions Regarding Cholecalciferol or Ergocalciferol Treatment. One should avoid giving very large doses of these agents unless 25-D levels are monitored. A subpopulation of CKD patients will have hypercalciuria. Patients on concomitant high doses of calcium supplementation as well as patients with diabetes or on anticoagulation, who may be at increased risk for vascular calcification, should be followed closely, and serum 25-D targets should not be higher than 30 to 40 ng/mL (75 to 100 nmol/L).

Effect of Vitamin D on Parathyroid Hormone Levels
One early sign of vitamin D insufficiency is an increase in intact PTH levels. As GFR decreases, the bone becomes less sensitive to the effects of PTH, and the desirable range of PTH values shifts upward (Table 8.3). An important goal of vitamin D therapy is to keep serum PTH within a desirable range, understanding that the ideal range of PTH at various levels of CKD is not completely known.

Use of Active Vitamin D
Active vitamin D can be considered when phosphorus restriction, calcium supplementation, and vitamin D replacement are not sufficient to reduce a persistently or progressively elevated PTH level. However, it should not be prescribed by rote. Calcitriol is 1,25-D, the product of 1α-hydroxylation in the kidney and an effective suppressor of PTH. Because calcitriol stimulates gut absorption of both calcium and phosphorus, it should be used cautiously as it can increase the load of calcium and phosphorus in the body. Although hypercalcemia and hyperphosphatemia appear to be less common in patients with residual renal function, serum levels of calcium and phosphorus should be checked monthly for 3 months and then followed at 3-month intervals after initiation. If hypercalcemia or hyperphosphatemia develops, calcitriol should be held until the mineral levels normalize. In patients who develop hypercalcemia, use of a calcimimetic might be more appropriate.

Use of Active Vitamin D Analogs
Active vitamin D analogs are compounds designed to interact with VDRs in the parathyroid gland, suppressing PTH secretion as calcitriol does, but which also have been designed to have reduced affinity for VDRs in the gut. As a result, the analogs in general cause less of an increase in serum calcium and phosphorus while still maintaining

TABLE 8.6	Active Vitamin D Analogs		
Medication	**Trade Name**	**Dosing Information**	**Comments**
Calcitriol	Rocaltrol	0.25 mcg PO daily or 0.5 mcg PO three times per week (dose range: 0.25–2 mcg daily)	Monitor calcium and phosphorus monthly for 3 months after initiation, then every 3 months thereafter. Escalate dose to attain target PTH. If hypercalcemia/ hyperphosphatemia develops with calcitriol, treatment should be held until mineral abnormalities normalize. Consider switch to doxercalciferol or paricalcitol, which suppress PTH with less effect on calcium/ phosphorus absorption in the gut.
Doxercalciferol	Hectorol	2.5–5 mcg three times per week, titrate by 2.5 mcg every 8 weeks	None.
Paricalcitol	Zemplar	1–2 mcg PO daily, titrate by 1-mcg increments *or* 2–4 mcg PO three times per week, titrate by 2-mcg increments	None.

PO, by mouth; PTH, parathyroid hormone.

effective suppression of PTH. Table 8.6 lists commonly available vitamin D analogs, their differences, and typical starting doses.

Nontraditional Actions of Vitamin D

Activation of VDRs by calcitriol or active vitamin D analogs may have effects beyond the gut and parathyroid gland. VDRs are distributed throughout the body and mediate a wide range of effects beyond mineral homeostasis. In the cardiovascular system, studies have focused on the role of VDR in regulating the formation of atherosclerotic calcified plaques and the attenuation of medial calcification in the uremic milieu. VDRs also have direct effects on the heart, especially in regulating the development of left ventricular hypertrophy. These effects are thought to be mediated by a decrease in myocardial fibrosis and by decreased activation of the renin–angiotensin system. Of particular interest in the CKD population is the reduction of proteinuria in patients treated with the active vitamin D analog paricalcitol

(Alborzi, 2008; de Zeeuw, 2010), an effect that appears to be independent of PTH suppression or improved hemodynamics.

Dual Supplementation With Cholecalciferol Plus an Active Form of Vitamin D

Because 25-D may have important biologic effects of its own resulting from local conversion to 1,25-D in tissues, there is a theoretical argument for maintaining levels of 25-D in the normal range, even in patients to whom an active form of vitamin D (e.g., calcitriol, paricalcitol, doxercalciferol) is already being given (Jones, 2010). This was supported in recent studies that demonstrated further decrease in serum PTH levels with dual therapy in hemodialysis patients, though the long-term effects of such therapy still need to be elucidated.

Calcimimetic Drugs

Calcimimetics are agents that increase the sensitivity of the calcium-sensing receptor in the parathyroid gland, potentiating the feedback inhibition of PTH. Studies evaluating the use of calcimimetic agents in CKD-5D show effective suppression of PTH to target levels, with similar efficacy to active vitamin D. In one large randomized trial in hemodialysis patients, calcimimetic treatment did not translate into improved cardiovascular morbidity or mortality (Chertow, 2012), although secondary adjusted analyses did suggest some benefit, including in older patients (KDIGO, 2017).

Patients on calcimimetics may develop significant elevations in serum phosphate level along with increased incidence of hypocalcemic episodes, but the degree of harm associated with usually mild hypocalcemia is uncertain. Nausea and vomiting are prominent side effects. Calcimimetics are currently available in an oral form, as cinacalcet, and an intravenous form, etelcalcetide. The KDIGO 2017 guidelines recommend the use of either a calcimimetic or active vitamin D derivative when treating hyperparathyroidism in CKD-5D patients, and it was the opinion of some members of the KDIGO workgroup that calcimimetics might be more appropriate (than active vitamin D compounds) as a first-line agent.

In the United States, there is no FDA-approved on-label indication for use of calcimimetic drugs in nondialysis CKD. Calcimimetics are being used outside of the United States in nondialysis CKD patients, and there are claims of reduction in cardiovascular events and even fracture risk (Evans, 2018), but this evidence is from observational data, and the benefits of calcimimetics are far from being definitively established (Sekercioglu, 2016).

Phosphorus Binders, Vitamin K, Magnesium, and Vascular Calcification

One major problem in CKD is vascular calcification. The propensity of serum to calcify is linked to adverse outcomes (Pasch, 2017). Several modifiable factors, notably vitamin K level and serum magnesium, reduce the propensity of calcification in the serum. A number of phosphorus binders can lower serum vitamin K values by binding to vitamin K, with sucroferric oxyhydroxide and sevelamer carbonate being notable exceptions (Neradova, 2017). Vitamin K and/or magnesium supplementation may potentially lower vascular calcification risk, and trials are currently underway to study this.

Calcium–Alkali Syndrome

This syndrome was initially known as milk–alkali syndrome and manifested as acute kidney injury in patients who were treating duodenal ulcers by following a diet rich in milk and antacids (Patel and Goldfarb, 2010). With the availability of acid-reducing medications and *Helicobacter pylori* treatment, the syndrome is seen in this context only rarely. However, patients concerned about osteoporosis often take large amounts of calcium supplements and relatively high doses of vitamin D, and may follow a self-imposed alkalinizing regimen with the hope of maintaining bone health. They may be taking thiazide diuretics for hypertension or kidney disease, which is also a well-known cause of hypercalcemia, thus increasing the risk of calcium–alkali syndrome. The pathogenesis of this syndrome involves a complex interplay of many factors including bone, kidney, and intestine. To minimize the occurrence of this syndrome, the dose of calcium supplements given to CKD patients who are being concomitantly treated with alkali should be limited. Also, if vitamin D is being supplemented, levels of 25-D should be monitored in high-risk individuals (e.g., those with hypercalciuria and/or alkalosis), and 25-D levels above the middle of the normal range should be avoided. If alkali therapy is being given, the serum bicarbonate target probably should be no higher than 22 mEq/L, and the serum bicarbonate should be monitored regularly to avoid overcorrection.

SPECIAL CIRCUMSTANCES

As noted previously, patients with adynamic bone disease tend to have low intact PTH. Although the cause is still uncertain, it is clear that many of the measures discussed in the management of secondary hyperparathyroidism would only worsen the poor bone turnover in these patients. One opinion is that in contrast to patients with high bone turnover, patients with low PTH should not be placed on a phosphorus restriction or given binder therapy. Phosphorus levels, perhaps, should be permitted to rise slightly in these patients to stimulate PTH secretion and restore dynamic activity in the bone. Such patients should not be given calcium, as the added calcium load would likely lead to hypercalcemia and PTH would be further suppressed. Whether they should be given vitamin D is controversial. On the one hand, vitamin D therapy would be expected to maintain or even increase the suppression of the parathyroid gland, worsening adynamic bone disease, but on the other hand, in observational studies of dialysis patients, active vitamin D treatment has been associated with improved survival, regardless of whether PTH was high or low. The latter would argue for, perhaps, treating such patients with a low dose of active vitamin D which would provide the "benefits" of VDR activation throughout the body without significant suppression of PTH.

References and Suggested Readings

Alborzi P, Patel NA, Peterson C, et al. Paricalcitol reduces albuminuria and inflammation in chronic kidney disease: a randomized double-blind pilot trial. *Hypertension*. 2008;52:249–255.

Block GA, Rosenbaum DP, Leonsson-Zachrisson M, et al. Effect of tenapanor on serum phosphate in patients receiving hemodialysis. *J Am Soc Nephrol*. 2017;28: 1933–1942.

Bolland MJ, Avenell A, Baron JA, et al. Effect of calcium supplements on risk of myocardial infarction and cardiovascular events: meta-analysis. *BMJ*. 2010;341:c3691.

Bressendorff I, Hansen D, Schou M, et al. Oral magnesium supplementation in chronic kidney disease stages 3 and 4: efficacy, safety, and effect on serum calcification propensity—a prospective randomized double-blinded placebo-controlled clinical trial. *Kidney Int Rep*. 2017;2:380–389.

Cheng SC, Coyne D. Vitamin D and outcomes in chronic kidney disease. *Curr Opin Nephrol Hypertens*. 2007;16:77–82.

Chertow GM, Block GA, Correa-Rotter R, et al; EVOLVE Trial Investigators. Effect of cinacalcet on cardiovascular disease in patients undergoing dialysis. *N Engl J Med*. 2012;367:2482–2494.

Daugirdas JT, Finn WF, Emmett M, et al. The phosphate binder equivalent dose. *Semin Dial*. 2011;24:41–49.

Delmez JA, Tindira CA, Windus DW, et al. Calcium acetate as a phosphorus binder in hemodialysis patients. *J Am Soc Nephrol*. 1992;3:96–102.

de Zeeuw D, Agarwal R, Amdahl M, et al. Selective vitamin D receptor activation with paricalcitol for reduction of albuminuria in patients with type 2 diabetes (VITAL study): a randomised controlled trial. *Lancet*. 2010;376:1543–1551.

Evans M, Methven S, Gasparini A, et al. Cinacalcet use and the risk of cardiovascular events, fractures and mortality in chronic kidney disease patients with secondary hyperparathyroidism. *Sci Rep*. 2018;8:2103.

Evenepoel P, Meijers B, Viaene L, et al. Fibroblast growth factor-23 in early chronic kidney disease: additional support in favor of a phosphate-centric paradigm for the pathogenesis of secondary hyperparathyroidism. *Clin J Am Soc Nephrol*. 2010;5:1268–1276.

Ferrè S, Li X, Adams-Huet B, et al. Association of serum magnesium with all-cause mortality in patients with and without chronic kidney disease in the Dallas Heart Study. *Nephrol Dial Transplant*. 2017. doi: 10.1093/ndt/gfx275.

Hollis BW. Editorial: The determination of circulating 25-hydroxyvitamin D: no easy task. *J Clin Endocrinol Metab*. 2004;89:3149–3151.

Isakova T, Barchi-Chung A, Enfield G, et al. Effects of dietary phosphate restriction and phosphate binders on FGF23 levels in CKD. *Clin J Am Soc Nephrol*. 2013;8: 1009–1018.

Jones G. Why dialysis patients need combination therapy with both cholecalciferol and a calcitriol analogs. *Semin Dial*. 2010;23:239–243.

Kalantar-Zadeh K, Kuwae N, Regidor DL, et al. Survival predictability of time-varying indicators of bone disease in maintenance hemodialysis patients. *Kidney Int*. 2006;70:771–780.

Kestenbaum B, Sampson JN, Rudser KD, et al. Serum phosphate levels and mortality risk among people with chronic kidney disease. *J Am Soc Nephrol*. 2005;16: 520–528.

Kidney Disease: Improving Global Outcomes. KDIGO clinical practice guideline for the diagnosis, evaluation, prevention, and treatment of chronic kidney disease–mineral and bone disorder (CKD-MBD). *Kidney Int Suppl*. 2017;7:S1–S59.

Kovesdy CP, Anderson JE, Kalantar-Zadeh K. Outcomes associated with serum phosphorus level in males with non-dialysis dependent chronic kidney disease. *Clin Nephrol*. 2010;73:268–275.

Kovesdy CP, Kalantar-Zadeh K. Bone and mineral disorders in pre-dialysis CKD. *Int Urol Nephrol.* 2008;40:427–440.

Kovesdy CP, Ureche V, Lu JL, et al. Outcome predictability of serum alkaline phosphatase in men with pre-dialysis CKD. *Nephrol Dial Transplant.* 2010;25:3003–3011.

Linefsky JP, O'Brien KD, Sachs M, et al. Serum phosphate is associated with aortic valve calcification in the Multi-ethnic Study of Atherosclerosis (MESA). *Atherosclerosis.* 2014;233:331–337.

Malhotra R, Katz R, Hoofnagle A, et al. The effect of extended release niacin on markers of mineral metabolism in CKD. *Clin J Am Soc Nephrol.* 2018;13:36–44.

Melamed ML, Eustace JA, Plantinga L, et al. Changes in serum calcium, phosphate, and PTH and the risk of death in incident dialysis patients: a longitudinal study. *Kidney Int.* 2006;70:351–357.

Menon MC, Ix JH. Dietary phosphorus, serum phosphorus, and cardiovascular disease. *Ann N Y Acad Sci.* 2013;1301:21–26.

Michaud J, Naud J, Ouimet D, et al. Reduced hepatic synthesis of calcidiol in uremia. *J Am Soc Nephrol.* 2010;21:1488–1497.

Nasrallah MM, El-Shehaby AR, Salem MM, et al. Fibroblast growth factor-23 (FGF-23) is independently correlated to aortic calcification in haemodialysis patients. *Nephrol Dial Transplant.* 2010;25:2679–2685.

Neradova A, Schumacher SP, Hubeek I, et al. Phosphate binders affect vitamin K concentration by undesired binding, an in vitro study. *BMC Nephrol.* 2017;18:149.

Nitta K, Nagano N, Tsuchiya K. Fibroblast growth factor 23/klotho axis in chronic kidney disease. *Nephron Clin Pract.* 2014;128:1–10.

Parker BD, Schurgers LJ, Brandenburg VM, et al. The associations of fibroblast growth factor 23 and uncarboxylated matrix Gla protein with mortality in coronary artery disease: the Heart and Soul Study. *Ann Intern Med.* 2010;152:640–648.

Pasch A, Block GA, Bachtler M, et al. Blood calcification propensity, cardiovascular events, and survival in patients receiving hemodialysis in the EVOLVE trial. *Clin J Am Soc Nephrol.* 2017;12:315–322.

Patel AM, Goldfarb S. Got calcium? Welcome to the calcium-alkali syndrome. *J Am Soc Nephrol.* 2010;21:1440–1443.

Schlieper G, Schurgers L, Brandenburg V, et al. Vascular calcification in chronic kidney disease: an update. *Nephrol Dial Transplant.* 2016;31:31–39.

Scialla JJ, Xie H, Rahman M, et al. Fibroblast growth factor-23 and cardiovascular events in CKD. *J Am Soc Nephrol.* 2014;25:349–360.

Sekercioglu N, Busse JW, Sekercioglu MF, et al. Cinacalcet versus standard treatment for chronic kidney disease: a systematic review and meta-analysis. *Ren Fail.* 2016;38:857–874.

Slatopolsky E, Cozzolino M, Lu Y, et al. Efficacy of 19-Nor-1,25-(OH)2D2 in the prevention and treatment of hyperparathyroid bone disease in experimental uremia. *Kidney Int.* 2003;63:2020–2027.

Sprague SM, Crawford PW, Melnick JZ, et al. Use of extended-release calcifediol to treat secondary hyperparathyroidism in stages 3 and 4 chronic kidney disease. *Am J Nephrol.* 2016;44:316–325.

Teng M, Wolf M, Ofsthun MN, et al. Activated injectable vitamin D and hemodialysis survival: a historical cohort study. *J Am Soc Nephrol.* 2005;16:1115–1125.

Westerberg PA, Sterner G, Ljunggren O, et al. High doses of cholecalciferol alleviate the progression of hyperparathyroidism in patients with CKD Stages 3-4: results of a 12- week double-blind, randomized, controlled study. *Nephrol Dial Transplant.* 2018;33:466–471.

Zittermann A, Schleithoff SS, Frisch S, et al. Circulating calcitriol concentrations and total mortality. *Clin Chem.* 2009;55:1163–1170.

9

Restricting Protein and Phosphorus: A Dietitian's Perspective

Lisa Gutekunst

The potential medical benefits of restricting protein and phosphorus have been described in Chapters 7 and 8. When restricting protein, one must always keep in mind the risk of protein malnutrition. Those with chronic kidney disease (CKD) often don't eat enough because of uremia-induced anorexia, altered taste sensation, overly restricted diets, and the inability to procure or prepare meals. Also, some comorbidities induce a catabolic response that causes proteins to be broken down even when protein and calorie intake are adequate. For this reason, CKD patients who are following a protein-restricted diet must be carefully monitored, and as detailed in Chapter 7, careful attention needs to be paid to ensure an adequate daily energy intake: at least 35 kcal/kg for younger patients and 30 kcal/kg for older patients.

Protein and phosphate go hand in hand—that is, foods that are traditionally high in phosphate are also good sources of protein. By restricting one, you automatically restrict the other. However, the ratio of phosphate to protein differs considerably among foods, and the practice of adding phosphorus-containing additives to foods is increasing.

PROTEIN

High and Low Biologic Value Proteins

Amino acids are the chemical units or building blocks that make up proteins. Amino acids that must be obtained from the diet are called *essential amino acids* (EAAs). Other amino acids that the body can manufacture internally from other food sources are called *nonessential amino acids*. Foods containing all EAAs are known as *high biologic value (HBV)* proteins, and those that are missing at least one EAA are known as *low biologic value (LBV)* proteins (Burke, 2003). HBV proteins are found in eggs, meat, fish, and dairy products. On the vegan side, soybeans as well as buckwheat and amaranth are HBV. HBV proteins are metabolized with great efficiency, thus conserving body protein. Those who consume a low-protein diet, either by choice or by medical necessity, use the amino acids found in HBV proteins more efficiently than those who consume large amounts of protein; in the latter case, the excess protein is simply converted to carbohydrate or fat and burned for fuel.

LBV proteins are found in fruits, vegetables, legumes, nuts, seeds, and whole grains. In a sense, "low biologic value" is a misnomer. It's not that the proteins in many plant-based foods are of little biologic value, but by virtue of missing one or several amino acids, they must be eaten in combination with other foods that contain these missing amino acids so that the body can use the ingested amino acid mixture to build new protein. A vegetarian diet can be of "high biologic value" as long as foods such as grains which are usually deficient in the amino acid lysine, for example, are eaten in combination with other vegetables (such as beans) that are rich in lysine (see more on vegan diets below).

Degree of Protein Restriction

As detailed in Chapter 7, Table 7.2, guideline bodies from various countries differ in the degree of protein restriction they recommend for CKD patients. The Kidney Disease Outcomes Quality Initiative (KDOQI) 2000 Nutrition Guidelines recommend a protein restriction of 0.6 to 0.75 g of protein per kg per day for those patients who have a glomerular filtration rate of <25 mL/min. The KDOQI 2007 Diabetes and CKD guidelines recommend 0.80 g/kg per day for most people; this means limiting the diet to 40 to 60 g of protein per day. KDOQI and other guideline-writing committees recommend that at least 50% of proteins in a CKD patient diet come from HBV sources, meaning that 20 to 30 g should come from eggs, meat, fish, dairy, and/or soy.

Building a Low-Protein Diet

Using nutritional values from the National Renal Diet (Knochel, 2006), 1 ounce of meat (beef, poultry, pork, lamb, game) or fish contains on average 7 g of protein, and 1 large chicken egg has 6 g of protein. Dairy products vary from 4 g to 15 g of protein per ½-cup or 1-ounce serving. Soy products vary in protein content depending on the soy product.

Sample Meal Plan

Protein portions should be spread throughout the day's meals. An example of how this can be accomplished on a 60-g protein diet (≥30 g HBV) is shown in Table 9.1. Once the HBV value is established, LBV protein sources can be added in divided servings throughout the day. Working with the starting menu developed in Table 9.1, the full 60 g of protein can be distributed throughout the day. Finally, to ensure

TABLE 9.1	Sample Menu Step 1		
Meal	**HBV Proteins**	**LBV Proteins**	**Additional Calories**
Breakfast	½-cup low-fat milk (4 g)		
Lunch	2 hard-boiled eggs (12 g)		
Dinner	3 ounces broiled pork chops (21 g)		
Total protein	**37 g**		

HBV, high biologic value; LBV, low biologic value.

TABLE 9.2	Sample Menu Step 2		
Meal	**HBV Proteins**	**LBV Proteins**	**Additional Calories**
Breakfast	½-cup low-fat milk (4 g)	1 cup cornflakes (2 g) 1 toasted bagel (4 g)	1 tablespoon cream cheese 1 tablespoon jelly 6 ounces juice
Lunch	2 hard-boiled eggs (12 g)	1½ cups green salad containing carrot slices, cucumber slices, radishes (2 g) 1 large hard roll (4 g)	3 tablespoons oil and vinegar dressing 2 tablespoons butter or margarine 1 medium apple
Snack 1		8 vanilla wafer cookies (2 g)	1 cup fresh grapes
Dinner	3 ounces broiled pork chops (21 g)	1 cup white rice (4 g) 1 cup green beans (1 g) 1 slice Italian bread (2 g)	1 teaspoon butter or margarine
Snack 2		1 slice pound cake (2 g)	½ cup fresh strawberries 2 tablespoons whipped topping
Total protein	**37 g**	**23 g**	

HBV, high biologic value; LBV, low biologic value.

adequate calories, high-calorie low-phosphorus foods are added, to result in the meal plan shown in Table 9.2, providing 2,700 calories and 60 g protein.

Additional Tips for Patients

It is important to provide the CKD patient with choices. Although the above example provides a realistic and seemingly food-laden meal plan, those just starting the diet may still feel restricted. Below are a few tips for patients to use when planning meals at home:

- Consider vegetables and grains as your entrée and your meat as your side dish.
- Prepare kebabs using small pieces of meat and lots of vegetables.
- Make fried rice with vegetables and small amounts of meat or fish.
- Start your meals off with soup or salad to help fill you up.
- Incorporate your meat, egg, and seafood portions into a salad.
- Add rice or pasta to your soups to make them more filling.
- Use thinly sliced meats for sandwiches—it looks like more.
- Add lettuce, spinach, alfalfa sprouts, sliced cucumber, chopped celery, or apple to your sandwiches.
- When making casseroles, decrease the amount of meat; increase the starch, pasta, or rice; and use low-sodium soups when the recipe calls for soup.

■ Add low-protein pastas and breads when possible.
■ Use stronger-tasting cheeses such as sharp cheddar, Parmesan, or Romano—you'll need much less to get the same amount of flavor.

PHOSPHATE

As discussed in Chapter 8, limiting daily dietary phosphate to 800 to 1,000 mg and prescribing phosphate binders reduce the risk of developing osteodystrophy and metastatic calcification. The normal phosphate intake in population studies is about 1,800 mg/day for men and 1,000 mg/day for women, so a reduction to 800 mg/day represents a much larger change in the diet for men versus women. The U.S. recommended daily allowance for phosphorus is 700 mg/day, and reductions down to this level should have few adverse consequences on nutrition. However, in some patients, apparent "adherence" with a low-phosphorus diet based on a lowering of serum phosphate level may in fact be due to a reduction of protein intake because of some intercurrent illness. Additionally, the source of phosphate should be considered as the bioavailability among sources varies from 40% to 100%.

Phosphate Sources

Organic Phosphate
Phosphate found in animal and vegetable products are bound to either protein or to phytate, reducing the amount of phosphate available for absorption. Though literature suggests the bioavailability of phosphorus varies from 40% to 60% (Kalantar-Zadeh, 2010), food preparation can increase or decrease the true bioavailability (Ando, 2015; Cupisti, 2006; Karp, 2012a; Karp, 2012b; Schlemmer, 2009).

Animal Products
All foods contain phosphate. In a standard, nonvegan diet, the main sources of phosphorus are meat, fish, eggs, and dairy products. The phosphate content of these, as mg phosphorus per g of protein, is shown in Table 9.3. The phosphate content of chicken (assuming that the bones are not eaten) is generally lower (6 mg/g) than that of beef or pork (about 8 mg/g). Phosphate content of fish can range from 6 (cod) to 9 (canned tuna) to 12 mg/g for salmon. At the higher end of the range are eggs (13 mg/g) and liver (17 mg/g). Dairy products range from 10.7 (cottage cheese) to 28.3 (reduced fat milk).

However, the bioavailability of phosphate in these foods varies from 5 (cottage cheese) to 27 (reduced fat milk) (Karp, 2012a; Karp, 2012b) as shown in Table 9.4.

Additionally, boiling meat can also alter the bioavailability of phosphate in meat with little alteration in protein content. Boiling meat for 30 minutes has been shown to decrease phosphate content by 20% to 62% (Ando, 2015; Cupisti, 2006). As an example, the mg

	Milligrams of Phosphorus per Gram Protein Content of Common Protein-Rich Foods

Protein Range (mg phosphorus per g)	Food Source and Value
<5.0	Egg white (1.4)
5.1–7.0	Cod (6.0) Chicken, dark meat (6.5) Shrimp (6.5)
7.1–10.0	Turkey (7.1) Beef, tenderloin (8.3) Rabbit, wild (7.3) Beef, bottom round (8.5) Chicken, white meat (7.4) Pork (8.9) Goat (7.4) Lobster (9.0) Lamb, leg (7.4) Venison, loin steak (9.1) Crab, Dungeness (7.8) Tuna, canned (9.2) Ground beef, 95% lean (7.8); ground beef, 80% lean (9.6) Beef, brisket (8.1) Haddock (10.0) Tuna, yellow fin (8.2)
10.1–11.9	Halibut (10.7) Cottage cheese, 2% low fat (10.9) Salmon, farm raised (11.4)
12–14.9	Catfish (13.0) Peanut butter, crunchy (13.0) Egg, whole (13.2) Crab, Alaska King (14.5) Peanut butter, smooth (14.5)
15.0–20.0	Peanuts (15.0) Salmon, canned (15.8) Pinto beans (16.3) Soy nuts (16.4) Liver, beef, and chicken (17.5) Soy milk, regular, not enriched (17.9)
>20.0	Cheddar cheese (20.6) Swiss cheese (21.3) Almonds (25.3) Milk, 2% low fat (27.6) American cheese (30.7) Cashews (32.3)

Source: Data from Pennington JAT, Douglas JS, eds. *Bowes & Church's Food Values of Portions Commonly Used.* 18th ed. Baltimore, MD: Lippincott Williams & Wilkins; 2005.

TABLE 9.4 Bioavailability of Animal and Plant Foods

Product	Total P/100 g (mg)	Digestible P/100 g (mg)	Protein/ 100 g (g)	Total P/Protein (mg/g)	Digestible P/ Protein (mg/g)	% Digestibility
Meat and Dairy Products						
Milk, 1.5% fat	108	85	3.2	33.8	26.6	78.7
Skimmed milk	122	75	3.3	36.9	22.7	61.5
Processed cheese, individually packed slice, 5% fat	574	589	23	24.9	25.6	102.6
Processed cheese, individually packed slice, 12% fat	647	720	24	27.0	30.0	111.2
Processed cheese, individually packed slice, 23% fat	584	576	21	27.8	27.4	98.6
Cheese spread, 9% fat	892	794	18	49.6	44.1	89.0
Cheese spread, 22% fat	755	772	19	39.7	40.6	102.3
Hard cheeses pool, 5–17% fat	638	484	30.3	21.1	16.0	75.9
Hard cheeses pool, 25–29% fat	529	282	26.5	20.0	10.6	53.3
Cottage cheese	146	71	13.8	10.6	5.1	48.6
Processed sausage, 18% fat	210	224	9	23.3	24.9	106.7
Processed sausage, light, 10% fat	241	242	10	24.1	24.2	100.0
Frankfurter pool, 20% fat	175	144	9.2	19.0	15.3	82.3
Frankfurter pool, light, 13% fat	186	130	10	18.6	13.0	69.9
Sausage, dry, salami type	244	171	21.5	11.4	7.9	70.0
Sausage cold cuts	184	164	10.7	17.2	15.4	89.1
Boiled ham	279	255	17.9	15.6	14.3	91.4
Raw pork steak	212	161	21	10.1	7.7	75.9
Raw chicken fillet	229	191	23	10.0	8.3	83.4
Raw beef	199	147	22	9.1	6.7	73.8
Raw rainbow trout fillet	232	207	16.8	13.8	12.3	89.2

Grain, Seed, Legume Products

Rye bread pool	208	123	8.2	25.4	15.0	59.1
Rye crisp	291	191	10.1	28.8	18.9	65.6
Mixed grain bread with seeds	189	116	9.7	19.5	12.0	61.4
Muffin pool	212	201	6.6	32.1	30.5	94.8
Sweet bun pool	116	60	7.7	15.1	7.8	51.7
Cookie pool	125	43	6.1	20.5	7.0	34.4
Sesame seed (with hull)	667	42	26.9	24.8	1.6	6.3
Tofu (firm)	164	51	16.5	9.9	3.1	31.1
Green bean	57	24	1.9	30.2	12.4	42.1
Green pea (frozen)	118	50	5.1	23.1	9.7	35.6
Chickpea (soaked)	149	53	8.4	17.7	6.3	35.6
Red lentil	432	167	23.8	18.2	7.0	38.7
Green lentil	400	120	24.4	16.4	4.9	30.0

Source: Adapted from Karp H, Ekholm P, Kemi V, et al. Differences among total and in vitro digestible phosphorus content of meat and milk products. *J Ren Nutr*. 2012;22:334–349; Karp H, Ekholm P, Kemi V, et al. Differences among total and in vitro digestible phosphorus content of plant foods and beverages. *J Ren Nutr*. 2012;22:416–422.

phosphorus per g protein for chicken breasts was reduced from 12.3 to 9.5 (Cupisti, 2006) and beef was reduced from 9.1 to 3.5 (Ando, 2015). To increase the palatability of the boiled meat, the patient can add herbs to the boiling water, add the meat to soups, or choose to brown the meat in the oven.

Plant-Based Products

Phosphates found in plant products are attached to phytic acid or phytate and though the absolute phosphate content as well as the mg phosphorus per g protein is considered high, as shown in Table 9.3, true bioavailability is quite low, as shown in Table 9.4.

In the Western diet, rich in animal-based proteins, humans have very little ability to digest phytate, releasing the phosphate (Schlemmer, 2009), thus allowing for the inclusion of more plant-based foods in patients' diets. In one preliminary clinical study in CKD patients with an estimated glomerular filtration rate in the range of 20 to 45 mL/min, serum phosphorus was about 10% lower in patients eating a plant-based diet compared with the same patients eating a diet in which protein was supplied by meat (Moe, 2011).

Preparation of plant products also affects the bioavailability of phosphate (Schlemmer, 2009). Factors that increase phosphate availability include storing plant-based products in hot and humid conditions, germinating legumes, malting grains, fermentation, and the addition of the commercial enzyme phytase. Factors that have reduced phosphate availability or have little effect on availability include storing plant-based products in cool and dry conditions, boiling legumes, soaking grains and legumes, and germinating seeds and grains. Additionally, oats are heat treated to prevent rancidity thus reducing phosphate bioavailability.

In recent years, dietitians have expanded the CKD diet to include whole grains and seeds; however, it is still too soon to know if we can add legumes. Though boiling in water has little effect on the phosphate bioavailability, it is not known how bioavailability is affected with commercial manufacturing and cooking in other liquids.

Tips Regarding Vegan/Vegetarian Diets

In cultures where life-long vegetarianism or veganism is a mainstay, the body has adapted to producing more phytase to harness the phosphate from plant products (Schlemmer, 2009). This may also be true of those who choose a vegan or vegetarian lifestyle later in life. Additional vegetarian diet support is available through the Seventh-day Adventist Dietetic Association. Attention must be paid to phosphate or sodium added to processed vegetarian foods—for example, tricalcium phosphate–fortified soy milk (see the section below on phosphate additives).

Inorganic Phosphate

Phosphate additives are inorganic phosphate salts that are added to food that perform a variety of functions in the food product. Table 9.5 lists the most common phosphate additives used.

TABLE 9.5	Most Common Phosphate Additives and Their Uses in Foods

Phosphate Additive Common Name	Uses
Dicalcium phosphate	Mineral source, dough conditioner, leavening agent
Disodium phosphate	Sequestrant, emulsifier, buffering agent, absorbent, pH control agent, protein modifier, source of alkalinity, stabilizer
Monocalcium phosphate	Acidulant, leavening acid, nutrient, dietary supplement, yeast food dough conditioner, calcium source for fortification or enrichment
Magnesium phosphate	Nutritional source of magnesium and phosphorus, pH control agent, dietary supplement
Monopotassium phosphate	PH control agent, buffering agent, acidulant, leavening agent, nutrient source
Phosphoric acid	Acidulant, pH control agent, buffering agent, flavor enhancer, sequestrant, stabilizer, thickener, synergist
Sodium hexametaphosphate	Sequestrant, neutral salt, curing agent, firming agent, dough strengthener, emulsifier, flavor enhancer, flavoring agent, humectant, nutrient supplement, processing aid, synergist
Sodium tripolyphosphate	Sequestrant, pH control agent, emulsifier, alkalinity source, buffering agent, protein modifier, antioxidant, curing agent, flavor enhancer, humectant, thickener and stabilizer, texturizer, moisture retention
Tetrasodium pyrophosphate	Buffering agent, pH control agent, alkalinity source, dispersing agent, protein modifier, coagulant, sequestrant, moisture retention, antioxidant, color stabilizer
Tricalcium phosphate	Anticaking agent, absorbent, calcium supplement
Trisodium phosphate	Buffer, emulsifier, stabilizer, protein modifier, provides "meltability" in processed cheese, quickens cooking time of cooked breakfast cereals, color agent

Source: Data from Murphy-Gutekunst L, Urribari J. Hidden phosphorus-enhanced meats: Part 3. *J Ren Nutr.* 2005;15:e1–e4.

Phosphate-Containing Calcium, Iron, or Magnesium Salts Used for Mineral Fortification

The food industry is under consumer pressure to increase the calcium and/or iron content of many foods that otherwise contain small amounts of these minerals. Some food is enriched in magnesium for the same reasons. Minerals are added to achieve fortification, restore minerals lost during processing, or standardize and compensate for natural variations in nutrient level. Common examples of calcium-fortified foods are those consumed by growing children including orange juice, breads, cereals, and even some processed cheese spreads and milk. Flour and some beverages also can be fortified with calcium, iron, and/or magnesium. Perhaps the most common form of calcium supplement added to foods for this purpose is calcium carbonate, but the use of various phosphate salts (dicalcium phosphate or tricalcium phosphate) also is quite common. Phosphate salts often are preferred because they usually have little effect on the taste or color of the fortified food.

Processed Meats

A variety of chemicals have been used by the meat industry to keep meat from drying out and to help it retain water, enhancing its succulence and helping increase its storage life. In the past, high salt concentrations were used for this purpose, but given recent pressures by the food industry to lower salt, sodium chloride–based compounds are increasingly being replaced by compounds containing phosphate for this purpose. Phosphates not only reduce the amount of sodium chloride needed but also have additional attractive properties. For example, they compensate for the oxidative effect of sodium chloride, protecting against rancidity. They also help the appearance and taste of seafood on storage. Sodium tripolyphosphate is a popular additive used for this purpose.

Leavening Acids and Dough Conditioners in Baked Goods

Various baked goods, including biscuits, muffins, and pancake mixes, contain one or more of a variety of baking powders, the purpose of which is to create CO_2 bubbles in the dough to make it lighter and fluffier. Often a combination of a bicarbonate source and an acid agent are used. Many of the acid leavening agents include phosphate, such as monocalcium phosphate monohydrate (MCP), monocalcium phosphate anhydrous (MCP-A), dicalcium phosphate dihydrate (DCP-D), calcium acid pyrophosphate (CAPP), and sodium aluminum phosphate (SALP). Sodium-containing leavening agents and baking powders can contribute substantially to the sodium content of food, which the food industry is under pressure to reduce. Hence, the food industry is experimenting with various alternative leavening agents containing cations other than sodium. However, there is no pressure to reduce the amount of phosphate; therefore, most baked goods and mixes will contain substantial amounts.

Phosphoric Acid as an Acidulant in Colas

Acidulants are used to give a sharp taste to foods. The most commonly used is citric acid. Phosphoric acid is used as the acidulant in many carbonated cola drinks because its harsh, biting taste is believed to complement the cola flavor. Not all dark cola drinks contain phosphoric acid as the acidulant as many alternative acids are available.

Phosphates as Calcium or Magnesium Salts in Multivitamins or Bone Care Supplements

A number of multivitamins and supplements targeting prevention of osteoporosis contain mineral supplements, primarily calcium and magnesium, in which the accompanying anion is phosphate. Alternative products in which nonphosphate salts are used are easily substituted.

Heightened Absorption of Phosphate From Additives

Phosphate additives are absorbed differently into the body than organic phosphate found naturally in food. Organic phosphate is attached to either a protein or a phytate limiting absorbability to about 70% (absorption may be higher in the presence of vitamin D) (Ramirez, 1986). Inorganic phosphate (i.e., phosphate additive) is almost 100% absorbed. So, although a glass of cola may contain only 25 to 60 mg of phosphate from phosphoric acid, categorizing it as a low-phosphate food, 100% of this phosphate is absorbed.

Medications Containing Phosphates

Not often considered by nephrologists is the phosphate content of medications. One study analyzed the phosphate content of medications used in one dialysis company (Sherman, 2015). Of the 200 most prescribed medications, 23 (11%) contained phosphorus. The phosphate content ranged from 1.4 mg/tablet (clonidine 0.2 mg, Blue Point Laboratories, Dublin, Ireland) to 111 mg/tablet (paroxetine 40 mg, GlaxoSmithKline, Philadelphia, PA).

Content varied among manufacturers (10 mg amlodipine made by Lupin Pharmaceuticals, Mumbai, India, contained 8.6 mg of phosphorus while Greenstone LLC, Peapack, NJ, contained 28 mg of phosphorus, and Qualitest Pharmaceuticals, Huntsville, AL, topped out at 40 mg phosphorus), and even the renal vitamins varied in their content of phosphorus (1.7 mg for Reno Caps, Nnodum Pharmaceuticals, Cincinnati, OH, to 34 mg for Rena-Vite, Cypress Pharmaceuticals, Madison, MS). The researchers also found that phosphorus content varied among the strength of certain medications. For example, Blue Points 5, 20, and 40 mg lisinopril contained 18 mg, 21 mg, and 31 mg of phosphorus, respectively.

The researchers hypothesized that this could be an added phosphorus burden to patients and provided a hypothetical example of one patient taking Greenstone's 10-mg amlodipine, Blue Point's 10-mg lisinopril, and a Rena-Vite. These medications would increase the patient's phosphorus intake by 110 mg.

Another researcher reviewed over 3,700 commonly used medications available in Italy for phosphate compounds (Cupisti, 2016). In total, 472 medications (12%) listed phosphate as part of their inactive ingredients. Researchers noted that the calcium hydrogen phosphate was included in 78% of the medications, followed by trisodium phosphate and sodium dihydrogen phosphate dihydrate included in 5% of medications.

Food Labels and Other Information Sources on Phosphate Content

Food Labels

By law, food manufacturers must list sodium content per serving, including that of any food additives, on the label, allowing easy comparison among foods to assist in making food choices. In the United States, there is no law requiring listing of phosphate content of foods in a quantitative sense on food labels. However, all ingredients must be listed and with the exception of some terms such as *baking powder* or *flavoring agent*, it is usually fairly clear whether a food additive present in the ingredient list contains phosphate, as it will most often be one of the additives listed in Table 9.5. Such additives will contain the letters *phosph,* either as *phosphate, phosphoric acid,* or the like. For example, it is fairly easy when buying soft drinks to avoid those that have phosphoric acid in the ingredient list. One problem is that one does not know if the additive in a particular food supplies a trivial or a substantial amount of phosphate.

Food and Recipe Analysis Sources

As discussed in Chapter 6, the U.S. Department of Agriculture (USDA) maintains a National Nutrient Database for Standard Reference in which data for a very large number of food items are provided, including phosphorus. The database web address can be found by searching for the appropriate link on the Agricultural Research Service's website: www.ars.usda.gov/.

Condé Nast Publications has developed an interface that users can employ to search the data in the USDA Nutrient Database for Standard Reference. The interface is available at no charge on the web. One of the most useful features of the nutritiondata.self.com website is the "Find Foods by Nutrient" section. The current web address for this page is www.nutritiondata.self.com/tools/nutrient-search. Using this interface, one can compare the nutrient (e.g., phosphate) amounts in similar foods. Phosphate content can be searched by either a 100-g serving or a 200-calorie serving.

There are reference materials that either the patient can purchase or the clinician can get from companies that sell phosphate binders. Diet analysis computer software programs can assist the motivated patient by comparing protein and phosphate content of many foods. Also, patients can analyze their diets to keep on track with their meal plan. Alternately, patients can purchase reference food lists that also have the nutrient analysis of foods; however, manual analysis of diets is tedious. Finally, free education material and food lists are readily available from the companies that make phosphate binders. The companies' representatives provide research articles regarding phosphate control, educational materials, and additional tips to help patients meet their phosphate restriction.

Limitations of Food Databases With Regard to Phosphate Additives

Manufacturers change the formulations of their products regularly depending on the cost of raw supplies. Also, under pressure to reduce the sodium content of foods, sodium additives are in the process of being replaced by additives containing phosphate for a number of foods. The phosphate content of one food may change throughout the year and the only way for consumers to know of the change is by reading the ingredient list on the nutrition facts label of the product.

Strategies for Limiting Dietary Phosphate Intake

Phosphorus is a hard nutrient to avoid in the diet. Limiting the intake of protein and high-phosphorus foods and avoiding hidden sources is the basic strategy. Teaching the patient to look for "phos" in the ingredients is the best tip for limiting phosphate in the diet. Additionally, working with your renal dietitian to identify low-phosphorus, high-protein foods is imperative as we are learning more about the bioavailability of phosphate.

Often overlooked is the phosphate load from medications. We don't yet know the true burden this presents; however, prescribing medications to be taken at meals, when phosphate binders are also administered, may reduce phosphate absorption.

Phosphate Binders

As phosphate intake increases, the need to start or increase phosphate binders becomes more of a consideration. Binders are a medication taken every time the CKD patient eats to help absorb some phosphorus found in foods. It can be a tedious task and an inconvenience for the patient, as well as an additional cost burden. Phosphate binder use is discussed in Chapter 8. It is important to titrate the amount of binder taken to the amount and type of phosphate eaten. When switching from one phosphate binder to another, utilizing the phosphate binder equivalent dose (Daugirdas, 2011) is a valuable tool.

SPECIAL-NEEDS POPULATIONS

Low and Fixed Income

Those with CKD often face serious financial hurdles. Many such patients are older, retired, and living on a fixed income. Others may be no longer able to work because of the extent of their disease and other health complications. In addition to their monthly expenses related to housing, the CKD patients also need to pay for medications. Typically, CKD patients take multiple medications, including those for high blood pressure, glycemic control (if diabetic), hyperlipidemia, cardiac disease, phosphate binding, and nutrition (supplemental vitamins and minerals). Many are left with very little money to purchase healthy kidney-friendly food. To stretch their grocery budget, low- and fixed-income patients may choose to shop at superstores and low-cost grocery stores. Shelves in such stores often are stocked primarily with processed foods that are a source of hidden phosphorus. For example, some superstores stock mostly enhanced meat products, giving the shopper few economical choices in terms of buying fresh unprocessed meat. More patients are turning to food pantries in these hard economic times. Local and governmental food assistance centers provide canned meats and vegetables and provide protein sources in the form of cheeses and legumes, both of which tend to be high in phosphorus. Asking the low-income patient to avoid such free food because it has a higher phosphate content is not a feasible strategy as such patients often rely heavily on these food sources to feed not only themselves but also their families. Instead, developing the meal plan around available food is the only way to meet nutritional needs while limiting protein and phosphorus intake to the greatest extent possible.

Pregnant Chronic Kidney Disease Patients

The nutritional goals for supporting the pregnant CKD patient are to support the growth of the fetus, maintain the nutritional status of the mother, and reduce the risk of uremic toxicity. Intake of both protein and calories needs to be increased. Nutritional issues in the pregnant CKD patient are discussed further in Chapter 25.

SUMMARY

There are many challenges faced by the clinician when developing the protein- and phosphate-restricted diet; however, the challenge can be met through careful consideration of the CKD patient's lifestyle, the patient's involvement in developing his or her meal plan, the use of tips for protein and phosphate control, the use of low-protein and low-phosphorus food products, and a positive presentation of the diet to the patient. The more choices the patient has, the more likely the patient will be successful in following his or her meal plan. Continual, ongoing support of the patient is essential, as what is being required is a lifestyle change involving one of our core values: food.

ADDITIONAL RESOURCES

1. The National Kidney Foundation, 30 East 33rd Street, New York, NY 10016. www.kidney.org
2. Academy of Nutrition and Dietetics, 120 South Riverside Plaza, Suite 2000, Chicago, IL 60606. www.eatright.org

References and Suggested Readings

The American Dietetic Association. Pre-end-stage renal disease. In: *Manual of Clinical Dietetics*. 6th ed. Chicago, IL: The American Dietetic Association; 2000:487–499.

Ando S, Sukuma M, Morimoto Y, et al. The effect of various boiling conditions on reduction of phosphorus and protein in meat. *J Re Nutr*. 2015;25:504–509.

Byham-Gray L, Wiesen K, eds. *A Clinical Guide to Nutrition Care in Kidney Disease*. 2nd ed. Chicago, IL: Academy of Nutrition and Dietetics; 2013.

Cupisti A, Comar F, Benini O, et al. Effects of boiling on dietary phosphate and nitrogen balance. *J Ren Nutr*. 2006;16:36–40.

Cupisti A, Moriconi D, D'Alessandro C, et al. The extra-phosphate intestinal load from medications: is it a real concern? *J Nephrol*. 2016;29:857–862.

Cupisti A, D'Alessandro C, Gesualdo L, et al. Non-traditional aspects of renal diets: focus on fiber, alkali and vitamin K1 intake. *Nutrients*. 2017;9:E444.

Daugirdas J, Finn W, Emmet M, et al. The phosphate binder equivalent dose. *Semin Dial*. 2011;24:41–49.

Institute of Medicine, Food and Nutrition Board. Phosphorus. In: *Dietary Reference Intakes: Calcium, Phosphorus, Magnesium, Vitamin D, and Fluoride*. Washington, DC: National Academy Press; 1997:146–189.

Kalantar-Zadeh K, Gutekunst L, Mehrotra R, et al. Understanding sources of dietary phosphorus in the treatment of patients with chronic kidney disease. *Clin J Am Soc Nephrol*. 2010;5:519–530.

Karp H, Ekholm P, Kemi V, et al. Differences among total and in vitro digestible phosphorus content of meat and milk products. *J Ren Nutr.* 2012a;22:334–349.

Karp H, Ekholm P, Kemi V, et al. Differences among total and in vitro digestible phosphorus content of plant foods and beverages. *J Ren Nutr.* 2012b;22:416–422.

Knochel PJ. Phosphorus. In: Shils ME, Shike M, Ross AC, et al., eds. *Modern Nutrition in Health and Disease.* 10th ed. Baltimore, MD: Lippincott & Wilkins; 2006:211–222.

Kuhlmann MK. Practical approaches to management of hyperphosphatemia: can we improve the current situation? *Blood Purif.* 2007;25:120–124.

Kuhlmann MK, Hoechst S, Landthaler I. Patient empowerment in the management of hyperphosphatemia (Review). *Int J Artif Organs.* 2007;30:1008–1013.

Kung CW. Milk alternatives. *J Ren Nutr.* 2010;20:e7–e15.

McCann L, ed. *Pocket Guide to Nutrition Assessment of the Patient With Chronic Kidney Disease.* 5th ed. New York: The National Kidney Foundation; 2015.

Moe SM, Zidehsarai MP, Chambers MA, et al. Vegetarian compared with meat dietary protein source and phosphorus homeostasis in chronic kidney disease. *Clin J Am Soc Nephrol.* 2011;6:257–264.

Morton RA, Hercz G. Calcium, phosphorus, and vitamin D metabolism in renal disease and chronic renal failure. In: Kopple JD, Massry SG, eds. *Nutritional Management of Renal Disease.* Baltimore, MD: Lippincott Williams & Wilkins; 1997:341–370.

National Kidney Foundation. Clinical practice guidelines for nutrition in chronic renal failure. K/DOQI, National Kidney Foundation. *Am J Kidney Dis.* 2000;35:S1–S140.

National Kidney Foundation. K/DOQI clinical practice guidelines for bone metabolism and disease in chronic kidney disease. *Am J Kidney Dis.* 2003;42:S1–S201.

Parpia AS, Abbe ML, Goldstein M, et al. The impact of additives on the phosphorus, potassium, and sodium content of commonly consumed meat, poultry, and fish products among patients with chronic kidney disease. *J Ren Nutr.* 2018;28:83–90.

Ramirez JA, Emmett M, White MG, et al. The absorption of dietary phosphorus and calcium in hemodialysis patients. *Kidney Int.* 1986;30:753–759.

Robinson P. Nutritional status and requirements in cystic fibrosis. *Clin Nutr.* 2001;20:S81–S86.

Savica V, Calò LA, Monardo P, et al. Salivary phosphate-binding chewing gum reduces hyperphosphatemia in dialysis patients. *J Am Soc Nephrol.* 2009;20:639–644.

Schiro-Harvey K, ed. *National Renal Diet: Professional Guide.* 2nd ed. Chicago, IL: The American Dietetic Association; 2002.

Schlemmer U, Frolich W, Prieto RM, et al. Phytate in foods and significance for humans: food sources, intake, processing, bioavailability, protective role and analysis. *Mol Nutr Food Res.* 2009;53:S330–S375.

Sherman RA, Mehta O. Phosphorus and potassium content of enhanced meat and poultry products: implications for patients who receive dialysis. *Clin J Am Soc Nephrol.* 2009;4:1370–1373.

Sherman RS, Ravella S, Kopoian T. A dearth of data: the problem of phosphorus in prescription medications. *Kidney Int.* 2015;87:1097–1099.

Wolfson M. Causes, manifestations, and assessment of malnutrition in chronic renal failure. In: Kopple H, Massry S, eds. *Nutritional Management of Renal Disease.* Baltimore, MD: Lippincott Williams & Wilkins; 1997:245–256.

Vitamins, Trace Minerals, and Alternative Medicine Supplements

T. Alp Ikizler, Aseel Alsouqi, and Allon Friedman

Many individuals, especially those afflicted with a chronic disease, often look to improve their health through "natural" means, resorting to ingestion of a variety of vitamins, supplements, and "superfoods" that they hope might help prevent progression of their illness, ward off complications, or increase life span. In some ethnic groups, use of herbal medicines is quite popular. Nutritional supplement stores and Internet websites afford easy access to vitamins in which doses can be much higher than recommended dietary allowances (RDAs). A number of high-dose vitamins and supplements can do more harm than good, and it is wise to query chronic kidney disease (CKD) patients carefully about vitamin, mineral, and supplement intake, as well as use of alternative medicine preparations.

VITAMINS

Guidelines Targeting Either the General Population or Non–Chronic Kidney Disease Populations

Selected recommendations regarding vitamin supplementation (excluding vitamin D) by various guideline-writing groups are shown in Table 10.1. A National Institutes of Health (NIH) consensus panel, the American Association of Clinical Endocrinologists, and the American Heart Association all found that routine use of multivitamins, whether for healthy patients or for patients with either diabetes or heart disease, could not be recommended based on available evidence. The American Academy of Ophthalmology does recommend the use of a relatively high dose (500 mg) of vitamin C, along with vitamin E, β-carotene, zinc, and copper for prevention of progression of intermediate-grade, age-related macular degeneration; this advice was based on the results of a randomized controlled Age-Related Eye Disease Study (AREDS) trial. The US Preventive Services Task force recommends daily supplementation of 0.4 to 0.8 mg of folic acid to all women who are planning or capable of pregnancy to prevent neural tube defects, starting at least one month prior to conception and continuing to 2 to 3 months of pregnancy (Bibbins-Domingo, 2017). (Grade A).

Guidelines Focusing on Chronic Kidney Disease Patients

Most patients with predialysis CKD are not much different in terms of their nutritional needs than patients with "normal" renal function,

T A B L E 10.1	Guideline Recommendations for Vitamin Intake (Excluding Vitamin D)		
Group	**Date Issued**	**Targeted Population**	**Recommendation**	**Comments**
NIH State of the Art Conference	2006	General population, for the purpose of chronic disease prevention	"… the present evidence is insufficient to recommend either for or against the use of multivitamins by the American public to prevent chronic disease."	Final panel statement can be found here: http://consensus.nih.gov/2006/multivitaminstatement.htm
American Association for Clinical Endocrinologists	2007	Patients with diabetes and nonhealing wounds	One daily multivitamin.	No recommendation for patients with diabetes, without nonhealing wounds.
American Heart Association	2010	Healthy patients, patients with heart disease	"We recommend that healthy people get adequate nutrients by eating a variety of foods in moderation, rather than by taking supplements."	"Although antioxidant supplements are not recommended, antioxidant food sources—especially plant-derived foods such as fruits, vegetables, whole-grain foods, and vegetable oils—are recommended."
American Academy of Ophthalmology	2008	Intermediate-grade age-related macular degeneration	AREDS vitamins: 500 mg C, 400 IU E, 15-mg β-carotene, 80-mg zinc oxide, 2-mg cupric oxide.	The addition of lutein and zeaxanthin plus fish oil is being evaluated.
CARI	2005	Predialysis CKD patients	CKD patients following a protein-restricted diet should receive supplementation with thiamine (>1 mg/day), B_2 (1–2 mg/day), and B_6 (1.5–2.0 mg/day).	None of the other kidney guideline bodies, including KDOQI, KDIGO, British Renal Association, and EDTNA/ERCA have issued definitive guidelines about vitamin supplementation (other than D) for predialysis CKD patients.

(continued)

Group	Date Issued	Targeted Population	Recommendation	Comments
USPSTF	2017	Women of childbearing age	"… all women who are planning or capable of pregnancy take a daily supplement containing 0.4 to 0.8 mg (400–800 µg) of folic acid."	(Grade A) recommendation for the prevention of neural tube defects in the developing fetus.

TABLE 10.1 — Guideline Recommendations for Vitamin Intake (Excluding Vitamin D) *(Continued)*

NIH, National Institutes of Health; AREDS, Age-Related Eye Disease Study; CARI, Caring for Australasians with Renal Disease; CKD, chronic kidney disease; KDOQI, Kidney Disease Outcomes Quality Initiative; KDI-GO, Kidney Disease: Improving Global Outcomes; EDTNA/ERCA, European Dialysis and Transplant Nurses Association/European Renal Care Association; USPSTF, United States Preventative Services Task Force.

and there are few studies evaluating the vitamin status or needs of predialysis CKD patients in a controlled fashion. CKD patients who are severely restricting the intake of vegetables and fruits because of hyperkalemia, those following a low-protein diet, and those with nephrotic syndrome, however, are subpopulations in which the possibility of vitamin deficiency should be considered.

Nutrition Guidelines Regarding B Vitamins in CKD Patients not on Maintenance Dialysis

For adult predialysis CKD patients, the only recommendation from any of the major guideline-writing groups has been from Caring for Australasians with Renal Insufficiency (CARI). As shown in Table 10.1, CARI "nutrition and growth" guidelines (Pollock, 2005) recommend supplemental vitamin B_1 (thiamine) (>1 mg per day), vitamin B_2 (riboflavin) (1 to 2 mg per day), and vitamin B_6 (pyridoxine) (1.5 to 2.0 mg per day) for those CKD patients following a low-protein diet. Other guideline organizations—Kidney Disease Outcomes Quality Initiative (KDOQI), the Canadian Society of Nephrology, the British Renal Association, and the European Renal Care Association—make no recommendations in this area. B vitamins normally are present in protein-rich food, and this CARI guideline is based on studies that found relatively low measured levels of B vitamins in patients eating low-protein diets. A summary of serum and/or red blood cell levels of various vitamins in predialysis CKD patients is provided in Table 10.2.

Multiple Vitamin Deficiencies in Nephrotic Syndrome

The most commonly recognized vitamin deficiency in nephrotic syndrome is that of vitamin D, in which measured 25-D levels often are low. However, because vitamin D–binding protein levels also are low, the clinical importance of lower total 25-D levels and the need for supplementation require individualization. Less well known are case reports of deficiencies of B vitamins in children with nephrotic

TABLE 10.2	Commonly Recognized Abnormalities in Vitamins in Patients With Chronic Kidney Disease Who Are Not on Any Vitamin Supplementation
Vitamin	**Serum or Plasma Concentrations in Chronic Kidney Disease**
Thiamin	Decreased or normal
Riboflavin	Decreased or normal
Pyridoxine	Decreased or normal in serum, decreased in erythrocytes
Cobalamin	Increased
Folic acid	Decreased or normal in serum and increased or normal in erythrocytes
Ascorbic acid	Decreased or normal
Vitamin A	Increased in serum
Vitamin E	Variable
Vitamin D	Decreased

Note: Serum levels of many trace elements and vitamins may be reduced in the nephrotic syndrome because of increased urinary losses and low serum levels of binding proteins.
Sources: Adapted from Chazot C, Kopple JD. Vitamin metabolism and requirements in renal disease and renal failure. In: Kopple JD, Massry SG, eds. *Nutritional Management of Renal Disease.* Baltimore, MD: Williams & Wilkins; 1997:415–478; Tucker BM, Safadi S, Friedman AN. Is routine multivitamin supplementation necessary in US chronic adult hemodialysis patients? A systematic review. *J Ren Nutr.* 2015;25:257–264.

syndrome, especially B_1 (thiamine) and B_6 (pyridoxine) (Nishida, 2009; Podda, 2007). Deficiencies of vitamin K–dependent glycoproteins also have been found (Ozkaya, 2006).

Vitamin B_{12} and Folate

Vitamin B_{12} Deficiency in the Elderly and Anemia. In elderly patients, low blood levels of vitamin B_{12} as well as folate are not uncommon (Dali-Youcef and Andrès, 2009), although the clinical importance of these deficiencies is not clear. Low folate levels are more strongly associated with degree of anemia than low levels of B_{12} (den Elzen, 2008). Because vitamin B_{12} is poorly absorbed orally, in patients with deficiency it needs to be given either parenterally or orally in doses of 0.5 to 1.0 mg per day, amounts that are far above the usual RDA. There are no published data suggesting that B_{12} or folate-related anemia is more prevalent in predialysis elderly CKD patients compared with those with near-normal renal function.

Homocysteine and B_{12}. Homocysteine, a metabolite of the essential amino acid methionine, has been implicated as an atherogenic agent and is a strong risk factor for cardiovascular disease. Plasma homocysteine levels are considerably higher in patients with stages 4 and 5 CKD than in patients with more normal levels of renal function. The metabolism of homocysteine depends on vitamins B_{12}, B_6, and folate. Supplementation with these vitamins does reduce plasma homocysteine levels. In contrast to the general population, however, CKD patients with low glomerular filtration rate (GFR) values require very high vitamin doses to lower homocysteine. Randomized interventional trials in CKD patients that employed such high doses of folic acid, B_{12}, and B_6

to reduce homocysteine levels reported no improvement in cardiovascular or all-cause mortality (Nigwekar, 2016; Pan, 2012; Bostom, 2011).

Vitamins B₁₂, B₆, and Folate and Progression of Diabetic Nephropathy. In a meta-analysis on nine trials including 1,354 patients studying the effect of supplementation of vitamin B or its derivatives on diabetic nephropathy, there was no evidence of improvement or delay in the progression of diabetic nephropathy. Only one trial showed reduction in albuminuria in one of the arms that provided thiamine supplements (Raval, 2015).

Vitamin C (Ascorbic Acid)
Observational studies show that high serum vitamin C levels are associated with a lower risk for atherosclerosis and are associated with lower blood pressures. In contrast, randomized interventional studies of vitamin C and other "antioxidant" vitamins have not conclusively shown benefit.

Few studies of vitamin C in CKD patients are available. Furosemide increases urinary excretion of ascorbate, and ascorbate excretion also is increased in diabetic nephropathy. In CKD patients, especially those in stage 5D (receiving dialysis), some studies have suggested an increased response to erythropoietin-stimulating drugs after patients are given supplemental vitamin C. However, current KDOQI anemia guidelines do not recommend the use of supplemental vitamin C for this purpose.

Potential Adverse Effects of Vitamin C That Are due to Oxalate. Oxalate is a metabolic end product of ascorbic acid. In patients with CKD, oxalosis is an important risk associated with excessive vitamin C supplementation. Patients with low GFR and those with hypercalciuria with or without calcium oxalate kidney stones should be especially careful to avoid higher doses of vitamin C.

Current Recommendations Regarding Vitamin C. In patients with CKD stages 3 to 5, current recommendation is to provide the adult RDA for vitamin C (60 mg per day) and no more. In the general population, in patients with age-related macular degeneration, guidelines based on the AREDS trial recommend supplementing with vitamin C at a dose of 500 mg per day. The safety of this moderately increased dose of vitamin C in CKD patients is unknown. A macular protective effect might still be substantial at a lower level of vitamin C, which would be safer in CKD.

Vitamin A
Vitamin A promotes normal nocturnal vision, cellular differentiation, morphogenesis, and immune response. RDA of vitamin A is 5,000 IU in healthy adults and a daily intake above 25,000 IU appears to be toxic even in normal adults. In CKD, high plasma vitamin A levels have been described. Toxicity is associated with skin and central nervous system changes, alopecia, and hypercalcemia. Even low-protein

diets prescribed to CKD patients contain normal vitamin A amounts. Accordingly, vitamin A deficiency is rare, and even small amounts of supplementation (i.e., >7,500 IU per day) can cause vitamin A toxicity in CKD patients. In nephrotic syndrome patients, a daily intake of the RDA for vitamin A appears to be adequate. Some "eye vitamins" targeting protection against macular degeneration contain daily vitamin A doses well above the RDA and these should be avoided.

Antioxidant Supplements for Chronic Kidney Disease Patients
CKD is associated with increased oxidative stress, even in the early stages of the disease. Given the robust clinical and experimental data supporting the concept that an increase in oxidative stress contributes to cardiovascular disease in CKD patients, it is logical to hypothesize that antioxidant therapy may be beneficial in reducing these complications. However, in the general population, large randomized clinical trials of antioxidant therapy either for primary or secondary cardiovascular prevention have generally failed to demonstrate any benefit. Given the weight of these large trials, a high standard of evidence for clinical efficacy should be demonstrated before antioxidants are routinely recommended for CKD patients.

Vitamin E. Vitamin E is the main antioxidant in biologic membranes, and it is considered to be an antiatherogenic agent. Supplementation with vitamin E has been shown to increase erythrocyte life span. Main dietary sources of vitamin E are vegetable oils. Even protein-restricted diets generally provide adequate amounts of vitamin E. Accordingly, supplementation of vitamin E is not generally recommended in CKD patients.

Alpha Lipoic Acid. This is an endogenous thiol antioxidant. Experimental studies demonstrated protection of renal function in animal models of kidney ischemia/reperfusion injury. In diabetic animal models, alpha lipoic acid (ALA) protects against the development of glomerulosclerosis and kidney failure. In one prospective study in patients, 600 mg of ALA given over 18 months prevented an increase of albumin excretion in patients with diabetic nephropathy (Morcos, 2001). Currently, there are no established guidelines for ALA administration to CKD patients, although the supplement is considered to be safe in general.

Vitamin K. Vitamin K has two forms. Vitamin K_1 (phylloquinone) is found in leafy green vegetables, fruits, and, to a lesser extent, vegetable oils. Vitamin K_2 (menaquinone) is made by bacteria in the colon. The main dietary source is fermented foods and dairy products such as cheese.

Vitamin K (*Koagulations-Vitamin* in the German and Scandinavian languages) is important for the normal coagulation cascade. Vitamin K_2 is important in bone metabolism and is used in Japan in an attempt to prevent osteoporosis. Vitamin K is required for the synthesis of a number of inhibitors of vascular calcification such as matrix Gla protein. Vitamin K deficiency is more common in CKD patients than in control groups, and this is thought to be contributing to the high incidence of vascular calcification in this population.

Whether vitamin K supplementation improves cardiovascular outcomes in the general population is not clear (van Ballegooijen and Beulens, 2017). Insulin sensitivity may be improved with vitamin K supplementation in patients with diabetes (Li, 2018). The kidneys play no major role in vitamin K metabolism, and even low-protein diets provide normal amounts of vitamin K. However, vitamin K indices are reduced in CKD patients, and reduction correlates with markers of poor nutrition status (Holden, 2010). It has been speculated that vitamin K supplements may be beneficial to CKD patients in terms of preventing vascular calcification (Krueger, 2009), and several prospective studies are ongoing to examine its benefits in CKD. Vitamin K is important for the carboxylation of Matrix GIa Protein (MGP) which inhibits vascular calcification. A case control study showed an association between low carboxylated MGP and calciphylaxis in ESRD patients on maintenance hemodialysis. This suggests a possible role for vitamin K in the prevention and or the treatment of calciphylaxis in this population (Nigwekar, 2017).

Summary

If vitamin supplementation is given to patients with CKD, supplements should be limited primarily to usual supplemental doses of the B and C vitamins (Table 10.3). Patients with nephrotic syndrome and those following a lower-protein diet are those most at risk for vitamin deficiency.

TABLE 10.3	Recommended Daily Supplemental Vitamins in Addition to the Patient's Daily Intake of Vitamins From Foods. For Individuals With Stages 3–5 Chronic Kidney Disease (Not On Dialysis)
Vitamin	**Stages 3–5 CKD**
Thiamine (mg/day)	1.2
Riboflavin (mg/day)	1.3
Pantothenic acid (mg/day)	5
Niacin (mg/day)	16
Pyridoxine HCl (mg/day)	5
Vitamin B_{12} (mcg/day)	2.4
Vitamin C (mg/day)	60
Folic acid (mg/day)	1
Vitamin A	No additional (avoid in CKD 3–5)
Vitamin D	See Chapter 8
Vitamin E (mg/day)	15
Vitamin K	None

Note: There is no additional supplementation recommendation for stages 1 and 2 CKD patients except in patients with nephrotic syndrome.
CKD, chronic kidney disease.
Source: Adapted Chazot C, Kopple JD. Vitamin metabolism and requirements in renal disease and renal failure. In: Kopple JD, Massry SG, eds. *Nutritional Management of Renal Disease.* Baltimore, MD: Williams & Wilkins; 1997:415–478.

FISH OIL AND OTHER OMEGA-3 FATTY ACIDS

The three major fish oil–derived omega-3 fatty acids are eicosapentaenoic (EPA), docosapentaenoic (DPA), and docosahexaenoic (DHA) acids. Plant-based sources of omega-3 fatty acids include walnuts, flaxseeds, canola oil, and soybeans. Based on evidence that omega-3 fatty acids have cardioprotective benefits, the American Heart Association, the American Diabetes Association, and other guideline bodies have recently established intake guidelines (Table 10.4) (Bantle 2008; Kris-Etherton, 2003). Not all analyses of data regarding fish oil benefits are positive, however (Kimmig and Karalis, 2013; Kwak, 2012). No guidelines regarding fish oil have been established for the CKD population, although a handful of small studies have explored, without conclusive results, whether omega-3 fatty acids reduce levels of inflammation or beneficially affect markers of sudden cardiac death in CKD patients. A randomized trial showed that daily fish oil supplements did not decrease loss of graft patency within 12 months of initiation of hemodialysis (Lok et al., 2012). Another retrospective

TABLE 10.4	American Heart Association and American Diabetes Association Guideline Recommendations Regarding Fish Oil and DHA/EPA Supplementation

American Heart Association

The AHA recommends that all adults eat fish (particularly fatty fish) at least two times a week. Fish is a good source of protein and is low in saturated fat. Fish—especially oily species like mackerel, lake trout, herring, sardines, albacore tuna, and salmon—provides significant amounts of the two kinds of omega-3 fatty acids shown to be cardioprotective, EPA and DHA. The AHA also recommends eating plant-derived omega-3 fatty acids. Tofu and other forms of soybeans, walnuts and flaxseeds and their oils, and canola oil all contain ALA.

For patients with documented CHD, the AHA recommends 1 g of EPA and DHA (combined) per day. This may be obtained from the consumption of oily fish or from omega-3 fatty acid capsules, although the decision to use the latter should be made in consultation with a physician. The amount of EPA and DHA in fish and fish oil is presented in the recent AHA Scientific Advisory on omega-3 fatty acids and cardiovascular disease.

An EPA + DHA supplement may be useful in patients with hypertriglyceridemia. Two to 4 g of EPA + DHA per day can lower triglycerides to 20–40%. Patients taking more than 3 g of these fatty acids from supplements should do so only under a physician's care. Very high ("Eskimo") intakes could cause excessive bleeding in some people.

American Diabetes Association

Two or more servings of fish per week (with the exception of commercially fried fish fillets) provide n-3 polyunsaturated fatty acids and are recommended.

DHA, docosahexaenoic acid; EPA, eicosapentaenoic acid; AHA, American Heart Association; ALA, alpha lipoic acid; CHD, coronary heart disease.
Source: AHA: Kris-Etherton PM, Harris WS, Appel LJ; AHA Nutrition Committee. American Heart Association. Omega-3 fatty acids and cardiovascular disease: new recommendations from the American Heart Association. *Arterioscler Thromb Vasc Biol.* 2003;23:151–152; ADA: Bantle JP, Wylie-Rosett J, Albright AL, et al; American Diabetes Association. Nutrition recommendations and interventions for diabetes: a position statement of the American Diabetes Association. *Diabetes Care.* 2008;31:S61–S78.

study found that omega - 3 – fatty acids were associated with a lower risk of sudden cardiac death in the first year after initiation of hemodialysis in ESRD patients (Friedman et al., 2013). The question as to whether omega-3 fatty acids can improve the outcomes of renal transplant allografts and their recipients is also limited by a lack of reliable data. Given that most CKD patients will have heart disease, diabetes, or both, it is logical that such patients should follow the AHA/ADA recommendations with regard to fish oil supplements. A case (purely opinion based) could be made that because mercury adversely affects the kidneys (see Chapter 3), DHA/EPA supplements should be preferred to ingestion of fish because most fish oil supplements are processed in a way to remove any contained mercury.

Fish Oil Supplements and Immunoglobulin A Nephropathy

Perhaps, the most prominent studies of omega-3 fatty acids in CKD involve their use in immunoglobulin A (IgA) nephropathy, presumably because of their immunomodulatory and anti-inflammatory effects. One study randomized 106 patients with mild to moderately advanced IgA nephropathy to approximately 3 g per day of EPA and DHA or a placebo. A slower rise in serum creatinine levels and fewer episodes of end-stage renal disease and death were noted in the fish oil group over an average of 6 years (Donadio, 1999). However, not all subsequent IgA trials have observed such beneficial effects (Friedman, 2010) and a meta-analysis was inconclusive (Chou, 2012).

MINERALS

Minerals are widely present in multivitamin preparations, including calcium, magnesium, and iron, in addition to trace minerals such as selenium and zinc.

Calcium and Magnesium

Calcium and magnesium have been discussed extensively in Chapter 8. Low serum magnesium levels have been linked to increased vascular calcifications, cardiovascular risk, and mortality in the general population and CKD patients. Patients taking proton-pump inhibitors are at risk of hypomagnesemia, and patiromer, a gut potassium-binding drug, also may lower serum magnesium levels slightly. Trials of magnesium supplementation in CKD to date have not been definitive, and further trials are needed to determine the required doses and target serum levels (Massy, 2016).

Phosphate in Oral Laxatives

In addition to being widely present as a food supplement, sodium phosphate is available as an over-the-counter laxative and bowel prep. Use of phosphate-containing bowel preparations has been linked to acute deterioration of kidney function, even in patients with baseline creatinine values in the normal range, and these should in general be avoided, as substitutes are readily available (Khurana, 2008; Schaefer, 2016).

Aluminum and Citrate

Increased aluminum has been implicated as a cause of a progressive dementia syndrome, osteomalacia, weakness of the proximal muscles of the limbs, impaired immune function, and anemia in advanced CKD patients. This is mostly applicable to maintenance dialysis patients. The KDIGO 2017 mineral bone disorder guidelines (see Chapter 8) recommend that aluminum hydroxide should not be used as a phosphate binder in predialysis CKD patients and that there is no reason to use it for its antacid properties either. Aluminum absorption is markedly increased in the presence of citrate, and at the very least, coadministration of aluminum antacids and citrate in any form should be avoided.

Fluoride

Fluoride, widely used to prevent dental caries, may affect bone micro-hardness in dialysis patients. In CKD stages 4 and 5 patients, serum fluoride levels are fourfold higher than in patients with near-normal renal function (National Kidney Foundation, 2008). The potential harm of exposure to fluoridated water in predialysis CKD patients was examined by Kidney Health Australia (Ludlow, 2007), and it was concluded that (a) "there is no evidence that consumption of optimally fluoridated drinking water poses any health risks for people with CKD, although only limited studies addressing this issue are available"; (b) "there is limited evidence that people with stage 4 or 5 CKD who ingest substances with a high concentration of fluoride may be at risk of fluorosis"; and (c) "monitoring of fluoride intake and avoidance of fluoride-rich substances would be prudent for people with stage 4 or 5 CKD, in addition to regular investigations for possible signs of fluorosis."

Selenium

Selenium is necessary for proper functioning of selenium-dependent glutathione peroxidases, and selenium participates in the defense against oxidative damage of tissues, an important problem for patients with renal failure. In limited studies, administration of selenium attenuated the development of experimental glomerulosclerosis, delayed the onset of experimental diabetic nephropathy, and decreased the oxidative stress in renal allograft recipients. Because of the touted health benefits of selenium, many patients are encountered who are taking selenium supplements for various reasons. However, selenium has a narrow toxic/therapeutic ratio, and both low and high selenium levels have adverse effects. One controlled study found that contrary to expectations, selenium supplementation increased, rather than diminished, the risk of developing type 2 diabetes (Bamias and Boletis, 2008). CARI, in its 2004 nutrition and growth guidelines (Pollock, 2005), recommends that selenium levels be monitored in predialysis CKD patients eating a low-protein diet, but this is rarely done, and other kidney guideline groups do not recommend such monitoring.

Zinc

Although the zinc content of most tissues is normal in CKD patients, serum and hair zinc levels are reported to be low. On the other hand, red blood cell zinc content is increased. Some reports indicate that poor food intake, reduced peripheral nerve conduction velocities, low sperm counts and impaired sexual function, and helper/suppressor T-cell (CD4/CD8) ratios may be improved in CKD patients by giving zinc supplements. A review of randomized trials concluded that zinc supplementation may improve testosterone levels in dialysis patients (Vecchio, 2010). The dietary requirement for zinc in CKD patients is unclear, and there is no generally accepted need for supplementation.

COMPLEMENTARY AND ALTERNATIVE MEDICINES AND CHRONIC KIDNEY DISEASE

The use of complementary and alternative medicine (CAM) is common in the United States and other developed countries. Many individuals use CAM without consulting a health care provider. Given the limited premarket safety and efficacy testing as well as the use of these supplements as mixtures, it is rather expected that CAM usage might be associated with nephrotoxicity. Table 10.5 summarizes the familiar indications and possible nephrotoxicities that may be associated with these dietary supplements.

Aristolochic Acid

Aristolochic acid is the most well-documented adulterant causing renal injury. Initially, nine Belgian women who had all consumed the same weight loss supplement presented with rapidly progressing renal failure as a result of biopsy-proven tubulointerstitial nephritis. Chromatographic analysis of the supplement revealed that the preparation had been adulterated with *Aristolochia*. Several additional case reports have demonstrated the nephrotoxic properties of aristolochic acid leading to what is called Chinese herb nephropathy. This is characterized as a rapidly progressive renal failure, which on biopsy shows extensive interstitial fibrosis with tubular atrophy and loss. In addition, exposure to aristolochic acid increases the risk for urothelial malignancies.

Balkan Nephropathy and Aristolochia Clematitis

This is a chronic tubular interstitial nephropathy that arises in residents of the rural areas in the Balkan region. It is endemic but not genetically inherited. The etiologic factor is believed to be aristolochic acid, a toxin produced by *Aristolochia* plants which grow as weeds in fields where wheat is raised. The disease onset is insidious and is often not recognized until later stages of CKD develop where patients present with weakness, pallor, lumbar pain, and anemia. Patients with Balkan nephropathy are at higher risk of developing upper urothelial cancer even after kidney transplant, and cancer is the most common cause of death in these patients (Stiborová, 2016).

Lead Contamination of Indian and Nigerian Spices, Ceremonial Powders, and Protein Shakes

Researchers in Boston (Lin, 2010) investigated lead content of Indian spices and powders in pursuing unexplained cases of lead poisoning in

	TABLE 10.5	Potentially Nephrotoxic Dietary Supplements
Common Name	**Familiar Indications**	**Nephrotoxic Manifestations**
Aristolochic acid	Contaminating Chinese herbs for weight loss	Interstitial nephritis, urogenital cancer
Cat's claw	Anti-inflammatory; GI disorder	Acute allergic interstitial nephritis
Chaparral	Antibiotic; anti-inflammatory; antioxidant	Renal cystic disease and low-grade cystic renal cell carcinoma
Chromium	Glucose control; lipid lowering; weight loss	ATN, interstitial nephritis
Cranberry	Antibiotic; urinary acidifier and deodorizer	Nephrolithiasis secondary to oxaluria
Creatine	Enhancement of muscle performance during brief, high-intensity exercise	Acute focal interstitial nephritis and focal tubular injury; nonspecific renal dysfunction; AKI secondary to rhabdomyolysis
Ephedra	Allergic rhinitis; asthma; hypotension; sexual arousal; weight loss	Nephrolithiasis secondary to ephedrine, norephedrine, and pseudoephedrine stone formation
Germanium	Anti-inflammatory; immunostimulant	Tubular degeneration with minor glomerular abnormalities
Hydrazine	Anorexia and cachexia; chemotherapeutic	Autolysis of the kidneys in the setting of hepatorenal syndrome
Licorice	Antibiotic; anti-inflammatory; GI disorders	Renal tubular injury secondary to prolonged hypokalemia; AKI secondary to hypokalemic rhabdomyolysis in the setting of pseudoaldosteronism
L-Lysine	Antiviral; wound healing	Fanconi syndrome and tubulointerstitial nephritis
Pennyroyal	Abortifacient; menstrual stimulant	Edematous hemorrhagic kidneys with ATN and proximal tubular degeneration in the setting of hepatorenal syndrome
Thunder god vine	Immunosuppressant	Unknown supplement effects in conjunction with prolonged shock
Willow bark	Analgesic, anti-inflammatory	Necrotic papillae consistent with analgesic nephropathy
Wormwood oil	Anemia; antipyretic; appetite stimulant; asthma; GI disorders	AKI secondary to rhabdomyolysis in the setting of supplement-induced tonic–clonic seizures

(*continued*)

T A B L E 10.5	Potentially Nephrotoxic Dietary Supplements (*Continued*)	
Common Name	**Familiar Indications**	**Nephrotoxic Manifestations**
Yellow oleander	Anti-inflammatory	Renal tubular necrosis with vacuolated areas in the glomerular spaces in the setting of hepatorenal syndrome
Yohimbe	Erectile dysfunction; sexual arousal	SLE with resultant renal dysfunction

GI, gastrointestinal; ATN, acute tubular necrosis; AKI, acute kidney injury; SLE, systemic lupus erythematosus.
Source: Modified from Gabardi S, Munz K, Ulbricht C. A review of dietary supplement-induced renal dysfunction. *Clin J Am Soc Nephrol.* 2007;2:757–765, with permission.

children. A majority of cultural products contained >1 mcg/g lead, and some contained extremely high bioaccessible lead levels. There is also a report (Consumer Reports Staff, 2010) that certain protein powder–based health shakes contain greater than recommended amounts of lead (>5 mcg). Nigerian spices also have been implicated (Asomugha, 2016).

FOODS THAT MAY ADVERSELY AFFECT CHRONIC KIDNEY DISEASE PATIENTS

Cortinarius Mushroom Toxicity

Orellanine, present in *Cortinarius orellanus* mushrooms, is a nephrotoxin. Patients present after a latent period, that ranges from a few days up to 3 weeks after ingestion, with thirst, diarrhea, and vomiting followed by oliguria/anuria. Acute kidney injury occurs in 30% to 75% of cases and only 30% of individuals regain full kidney function. Renal biopsy shows evidence of interstitial nephritis and tubular necrosis. Patients are managed with supportive care and renal replacement therapy as needed (Graeme, 2014).

FOODS ASSOCIATED WITH INCREASED OXALATE EXCRETION

Star Fruit

This fruit is popular in many tropical countries and contains high levels of oxalate. Several cases of acute nephropathy have been reported following consumption of a large amount of star fruit. The high content of oxalate in star fruit and the pathologic sections (obtained from patients and experimental animals) showing diffuse calcium oxalate deposition suggest that acute oxalate nephropathy is responsible for star fruit nephrotoxicity. In addition to its potential to cause acute kidney failure, outbreaks of star fruit intoxication have been reported in patients with CKD, including subjects not yet on dialysis. Patients present with persistent and intractable hiccups, vomiting, variable degrees of disturbed consciousness, psychiatric symptoms, decreased muscle power, paresthesia, paresis, insomnia, epileptic seizures, and, not uncommonly, death; the mortality rate after star fruit intoxication can range as high as 20% to 40%. Because no effective treatment has been established, star fruit consumption should be avoided in patients with CKD.

Chocolate and Tea

Both chocolate and tea have documented health benefits, and health-conscious patients may consume large amounts of these food items. However, in addition to a high phosphate load, chocolate contains a large amount of oxalate, to the point that eating a single chocolate bar increases both urinary calcium and oxalate excretion to a substantial degree. Regular tea contains a large amount of oxalate as well. Nephropathy has been reported with consumption of large amounts of iced tea (Syed, 2015). Many herbal teas contain no oxalate, and for CKD patients with hypercalciuria concerned with oxalate intake, herbal teas may be a convenient alternative beverage (Charrier, 2002).

Large amounts of green leafy vegetables and fruit ingested as juices, smoothies, and cleanses: Fruits and leafy green vegetables contain a relatively high amount of oxalate, which if ingested in a concentrated fashion in the form of juices or cleanses can cause kidney damage (Getting, 2013; Makkapati, 2018).

Other Foods

Djenkol bean or jering (*Pithecellobium jeringa*) is a traditional eastern delicacy eaten with the staple diet, rice. Jering contains 1% to 2% djenkolic acid, a sulfur-containing amino acid. Djenkolism or jering poisoning has been shown to cause mild to severe acute tubular obstruction with some glomerular cell necrosis. Djenkolism occurs within 48 hours of consumption of jering. Precipitation of djenkolic acid in urine produces a viscous sludge, which may cause obstructive nephropathy leading to acute tubular necrosis. The urine and breath of the affected individual usually have a pungent smell.

References and Selected Readings

Asomugha RN, Udowelle NA, Offor SJ, et al. Heavy metals hazards from Nigerian spices. *Rocz Panstw Zakl Hig.* 2016;67:309–314.

Bamias G, Boletis J. Balkan nephropathy: evolution of our knowledge. *Am J Kidney Dis.* 2008;52:606–616.

Bantle JP, Wylie-Rosett J, Albright AL, et al; American Diabetes Association. Nutrition recommendations and interventions for diabetes: a position statement of the American Diabetes Association. *Diabetes Care.* 2008;31:S61–S78.

Bibbins-Domingo K, Grossman DC, Curry SJ, et al. Folic acid supplementation for the prevention of neural tube defects: US Preventive Services Task Force recommendation statement. *Jama.* 2017;317:183–189.

Bostom AG, Carpenter MA, Kusek JW, et al. Homocysteine-lowering and cardiovascular disease outcomes in kidney transplant recipients: primary results from the folic acid for vascular outcome reduction in transplantation trial. *Circulation.* 2011;123:1763–1770.

Charrier MJ, Savage GP, Vanhanen L. Oxalate content and calcium binding capacity of tea and herbal teas. *Asia Pac J Clin Nutr*. 2002;11:298–301.

Chou HH, Chiou YY, Hung PH, et al. Omega-3 fatty acids ameliorate proteinuria but not renal function in IgA nephropathy: a meta-analysis of randomized controlled trials. *Nephron Clin Pract*. 2012;121:c30–c35.

Consumer Reports staff. Alert: Protein drinks. You don't need the extra protein or the heavy metals our tests found. *Consum Rep*. 2010;75:24–27.

Dali-Youcef N, Andrès E. An update on cobalamin deficiency in adults. *QJM*. 2009; 102:17–28.

de Jager J, Kooy A, Lehert P, et al. Long term treatment with metformin in patients with type 2 diabetes and risk of vitamin B-12 deficiency: randomised placebo controlled trial. *BMJ*. 2010;340:c2181.

den Elzen WP, Westendorp RG, Frölich M, et al. Vitamin B12 and folate and the risk of anemia in old age: the Leiden 85-Plus Study. *Arch Intern Med*. 2008;168:2238–2244.

Donadio JV Jr, Grande JP, Bergstralh EJ, et al. The long-term outcome of patients with IgA nephropathy treated with fish oil in a controlled trial. Mayo Nephrology Collaborative Group. *J Am Soc Nephrol*. 1999;10:1772–1777.

Friedman AN, Yu Z, Tabbey R, et al. Inverse relationship between long chain n-3 fatty acids and risk of sudden cardiac death in patients starting hemodialysis. *Kidney Int*. 2013;83:1130–1135.

Friedman AN. Omega-3 fatty acid supplementation in advanced kidney disease. *Semin Dial*. 2010;23:396–400.

Getting JE, Gregoire JR, Phul A, et al. Oxalate nephropathy due to "juicing": case report and review. *Am J Med*. 2013;126:768–772.

Graeme KA. Mycetism: a review of the recent literature. *J Med Toxicol*. 2014;10:173–189.

Holden RM, Morton AR, Garland JS, et al. Vitamins K and D status in stages 3–5 chronic kidney disease. *Clin J Am Soc Nephrol*. 2010;5:590–597.

House AA, Eliasziw M, Cattran DC, et al. Effect of B-vitamin therapy on progression of diabetic nephropathy: a randomized controlled trial. *JAMA*. 2010;303: 1603–1609.

Jamison RL, Hartigan P, Kaufman JS, et al; Veterans Affairs Site Investigators. Effect of homocysteine lowering on mortality and vascular disease in advanced chronic kidney disease and end-stage renal disease: a randomized controlled trial. *JAMA*. 2007;298:1163–1170.

Khurana A, McLean L, Atkinson S, et al. The effect of oral sodium phosphate drug products on renal function in adults undergoing bowel endoscopy. *Arch Intern Med*. 2008;168:593–597.

Kimmig LM, Karalis DG. Do omega-3 polyunsaturated fatty acids prevent cardiovascular disease? A review of the randomized clinical trials. *Lipid Insights*. 2013;6:13–20.

Kris-Etherton PM, Harris WS, Appel LJ; AHA Nutrition Committee. American Heart Association. Omega-3 fatty acids and cardiovascular disease: new recommendations from the American Heart Association. *Arterioscler Thromb Vasc Biol*. 2003;23:151–152.

Krueger T, Westenfeld R, Ketteler M, et al. Vitamin K deficiency in CKD patients: a modifiable risk factor for vascular calcification? *Kidney Int*. 2009;76:18–22.

Kwak SM, Myung SK, Lee YJ, et al; Korean Meta-analysis Study Group. Efficacy of omega-3 fatty acid supplements (eicosapentaenoic acid and docosahexaenoic acid) in the secondary prevention of cardiovascular disease: a meta-analysis of randomized, double-blind, placebo-controlled trials. *Arch Intern Med*. 2012;172:686–694.

Li Y, Chen JP, Duan L, et al. Effect of vitamin K2 on type 2 diabetes mellitus: a review. *Diabetes Res Clin Pract*. 2018;136:39–51.

Lin CG, Schaider LA, Brabander DJ, et al. Pediatric lead exposure from imported Indian spices and cultural powders. *Pediatrics*. 2010;125:e828–e835.

Lobo JC, Torres JP, Fouque D, et al. Zinc deficiency in chronic kidney disease: is there a relationship with adipose tissue and atherosclerosis? *Biol Trace Elem Res*. 2010;135:16–21.

Lok CE, Moist L, Hemmelgarn BR, et al. Effect of fish oil supplementation on graft patency and cardiovascular events among patients with new synthetic arteriovenous hemodialysis grafts: a randomized controlled trial. *Jama*. 2012;307:1809–1816.

Ludlow M, Luxton G, Mathew T. Effects of fluoridation of community water supplies for people with chronic kidney disease. *Nephrol Dial Transplant*. 2007;22:2763–2767.

Makkapati S, D'Agati VD, Balsam L. "Green smoothie cleanse" causing acute oxalate nephropathy. *Am J Kidney Dis*. 2018;71:281–286.

Massey LK, Roman-Smith H, Sutton RA. Effect of dietary oxalate and calcium on urinary oxalate and risk of formation of calcium oxalate kidney stones. *J Am Diet Assoc*. 1993;93:901–906.

Massy ZA, Nistor I, Apetrii M, et al. Magnesium-based interventions for normal kidney function and chronic kidney disease. *Magnes Res*. 2016;29:126–140.

Morcos M, Borcea V, Isermann B, et al. Effect of alpha-lipoic acid on the progression of endothelial cell damage and albuminuria in patients with diabetes mellitus: an exploratory study. *Diabetes Res Clin Pract*. 2001;52:175–183.

National Kidney Foundation. Position Paper: Fluoride intake in chronic kidney disease. 2008. Available from http://www.kidney.org/atoz/pdf/Fluoride_Intake_in_CKD. pdf. Accessed January 8, 2011.

Nigwekar SU, Bloch DB, Nazarian RM, et al. Vitamin K-dependent carboxylation of matrix gla protein influences the risk of calciphylaxis. *J Am Soc Nephrol*. 2017;28:1717–1722.

Nigwekar SU, Kang A, Zoungas S, et al. Interventions for lowering plasma homocysteine levels in dialysis patients. *Cochrane Database Syst Rev*. 2016:CD004683.

Nishida M, Sato H, Kobayashi N, et al. Wernicke's encephalopathy in a patient with nephrotic syndrome. *Eur J Pediatr*. 2009;168:731–734.

Ozkaya O, Bek K, Fişgin T, et al. Low protein Z levels in children with nephrotic syndrome. *Pediatr Nephrol*. 2006;21:1122–1126.

Pan Y, Guo L, Cai L, et al. Homocysteine-lowering therapy does not lead to reduction in cardiovascular outcomes in chronic kidney disease patients: a meta-analysis of randomised, controlled trials. *Br J Nutr*. 2012;108:400–407.

Podda GM, Lussana F, Moroni G, et al. Abnormalities of homocysteine and B vitamins in the nephrotic syndrome. *Thromb Res*. 2007;120:647–652.

Pollock C, Voss D, Hodson E, et al; Caring for Australasians with Renal Impairment (CARI). The CARI guidelines. Nutrition and growth in kidney disease. *Nephrology (Carlton)*. 2005;10:S177–S230.

Raval AD, Thakker D, Rangoonwala AN, et al. Vitamin B and its derivatives for diabetic kidney disease. *Cochrane Database Syst Rev*. 2015;1:CD009403.

Rocco M, Ikizler TA. Nutrition in dialysis patients. In: Daugirdas JT, Blake PG, Ing TS, eds. *Handbook of Dialysis*. 4th ed. Baltimore, MD: Lippincott Williams & Wilkins; 2007:462–481.

Schaefer M, Littrell E, Khan A, et al. Estimated GFR decline following sodium phosphate enemas versus polyethylene glycol for screening colonoscopy: a retrospective cohort study. *Am J Kidney Dis*. 2016;67:609–616.

Stiborová M, Arlt VM, Schmeiser HH. Balkan endemic nephropathy: an update on its etiology. *Arch Toxicol*. 2016;90:2595–2615.

Syed F, Mena-Gutierrez A, Ghaffar U. A case of iced-tea nephropathy. *N Engl J Med*. 2015;372:1377–1378.

Tatsioni A, Chung M, Sun Y, et al. Effects of fish oil supplementation on kidney transplantation: a systematic review and meta-analysis of randomized, controlled trials. *J Am Soc Nephrol*. 2005;16:2462–2470.

van Ballegooijen AJ, Beulens JW. The role of vitamin K status in cardiovascular health: evidence from observational and clinical studies. *Curr Nutr Rep*. 2017;6:197–205.

Vecchio M, Navaneethan SD, Johnson DW, et al. Treatment options for sexual dysfunction in patients with chronic kidney disease: a systematic review of randomized controlled trials. *Clin J Am Soc Nephrol*. 2010;5:985–995.

11 Acid–Base and Electrolyte Disorders

Tsering Dhondup and Qi Qian

Acid–base and electrolyte homeostasis is vital for the proper functioning of numerous metabolic processes and organ functions. The kidneys play a critical role in the maintenance and regulation of this homeostasis. Kidney diseases and dysfunction can result in alterations in electrolyte and acid–base balance.

EXCRETION OF DIETARY ACID LOAD

On a typical western diet, an adult will excrete ~0.8 to 1.0 mEq/kg body weight of nonvolatile acid (Kurtz, 1983) and 15,000 mmol of CO_2 (volatile acid) daily. The source of this acid is dietary protein, and the amount of acid excreted depends on the amount and type of protein eaten. Diets high in protein, especially animal protein, will contain a higher acid load than diets lower in protein. Vegetarian diets tend to have a lower acid load, although some cereal proteins will contain levels of noncarbonic acids that are similar to those in meat. Nonprotein dietary components also affect dietary acid load: Fruits and vegetables contain alkali-generating substances in the form of organic anions, such as citrate. These anions are metabolized to generate bicarbonate which neutralizes acid, in this way lowering the net dietary acid load. Certain fad (weight loss) diets are designed to avoid acid-rich foods. Assessment of acid–base status in a CKD patient should include a dietary history regarding the types of food eaten as well as the ingestion of any supplements that may affect the acid–base balance.

RENAL NET ACID EXCRETION

Renal net acid excretion is achieved via reclamation of filtered HCO_3^- (~4,500 mmol daily) and excretion of titratable acids and ammonium (NH_4^+).

How the Kidney Reclaims Bicarbonate

Approximately 80% of the filtered HCO_3^- is reclaimed by the proximal tubule. The remainder is reclaimed in the more distal parts of the renal tubules; 16% in the thick ascending limb of the loop of Henle (TALH) and distal convoluted tubule (DCT), and the remaining 4% in the collecting ducts. With certain disorders of the renal tubules, HCO_3^- reclamation is impaired and bicarbonate is then spilled in the urine. The lost HCO_3^- is no longer available to neutralize dietary acids, and metabolic acidosis results.

Net Secretion of Acid in the Distal Part of the Renal Tubular System

In the collecting ducts, specialized cells can excrete acid into the urine. The excreted acid must be stabilized in the tubular lumen by binding to a buffer. The major buffer is HPO_4^{2-}, which is capable of incorporating H^+ by forming $H_2PO_4^-$ which is then excreted in the urine. Other buffers which can stabilize protons excreted by specialized collecting duct cells include citrate, creatinine, and uric acid. This "titratable acid" excretion is responsible for approximately one-third of renal net acid excretion, and is a low-capacity system, limited by dietary phosphorus intake and the amount of filtered phosphorus. In chronic kidney disease, the distal tubules and their ability to secrete acid are affected to varying degrees, and this impairment of net acid excretion in the collecting duct can result in metabolic acidosis.

EXCRETION OF AMMONIUM

Approximately two-thirds of renal net acid excretion take place via renal generation and excretion of ammonium ion, NH_4^+. Renal ammoniagenesis and excretion is a high-capacity system; with normal renal function, ammoniagenesis can increase markedly in response to an increased acid load, from a baseline of ~20 to 40 mmol/day to >200 mmol/day. Ammoniagenesis and excretion of NH_4^+ in the kidney is a relatively complex process that involves various parts of the tubular system as well as the medullary interstitium. Ammoniagenesis occurs primarily in the proximal tubules, predominantly from glutamine metabolism. For each glutamine metabolized, two NH_4^+ and two HCO_3^- are generated. Generated NH_4^+ is secreted into the lumen of the proximal tubule and then reabsorbed in the TALH into the medullary interstitium. NH_4^+/NH_3 undergoes medullary recycling contributing to the medullary interstitial hypertonicity. In the distal nephron, NH_4^+/NH_3 is excreted into the lumen through both diffusion and transporter-mediated mechanisms. For every NH_4^+ excreted in the urine, an HCO_3^- is gained. Acidemia and hypokalemia promote ammoniagenesis while alkalemia and hyperkalemia cause an opposite effect. Chronic kidney disease can markedly impair the ability of the kidney to generate ammonium ion in response to an acid load, leading to metabolic acidosis.

Estimation of Urinary NH_4^+ Excretion by Urinary Anion Gap

Because direct assay for urine NH_4^+ is not widely available, urinary NH_4^+ excretion is often estimated by calculating urine anion gap. In patients with normal kidney function, urine NH_4^+ excretion is usually assessed via the urine anion gap to assist in the differential diagnosis of metabolic acidosis, to determine whether the cause is renal or extrarenal. If the cause of the acidosis is extrarenal, the renal NH_4^+ excretion will be increased. If the cause of the acidosis is renal, then the renal NH_4^+ excretion will not be increased from values found in the absence of acidosis.

$$\text{Urine anion gap} = [\text{Urine } Na^+] + [\text{Urine } K^+] - [\text{Urine } Cl^-]$$

In subjects with normal kidneys and in the absence of acidosis, urine NH_4^+ excretion, as mentioned above, is 20 to 40 mmol/day. NH_4^+ is excreted with Cl^-, and the balance between urinary Na^+, K^+, NH_4^+, and Cl^- is such that urinary Na^+ plus urinary K^+ concentrations are approximately equal to, or slightly greater (by <10 mmol/L) than, urinary Cl^-. As such, a urinary anion gap of 0 to +10 is considered normal. However, in the presence of acidosis, for example, due to diarrhea, one would expect the urinary NH_4^+ excretion to increase markedly. This causes a concomitant increase in urinary Cl^-, and as a result, urinary Cl^- excretion becomes greater than the sum of urinary Na^+ plus urinary K^+ and the urinary anion gap then becomes negative. Thus, with normal kidneys, persistence of a "normal" urine anion gap of 0 to +10 mmol/L with acidosis suggests that the kidneys are not working properly, in that NH_4^+ excretion is not being increased, and suggests the presence of renal tubular acidosis (RTA). On the other hand, a urinary anion gap of, say, −40 to −100 mmol/L or less in the presence of acidosis suggests that the kidneys are responding to the acidosis with increased NH_4^+ excretion, and that impaired acid excretion by the kidney is not the cause of the acidosis. One problem with the urinary anion gap test in patients with CKD is that as GFR and tubular function fall, the ability of the kidneys to excrete NH_4^+ is diminished, and the urinary anion gap may remain close to the "normal" 0 to 10 mmol/L range, even in the presence of acidosis (Kim, 1996), resembling findings in RTA.

METABOLIC ACIDOSIS AND THE SERUM ANION GAP

Metabolic acidosis can be broadly classified into elevated anion gap acidosis and normal anion gap acidosis. Calculation of the serum anion gap helps to determine the presence or absence of unmeasured anions, and this in turn can help point to the cause of the acidosis. The ionic environment of the blood is neutral, with the sum of cations being equal to the sum of anions. However, only certain ions (Na^+, K^+, Cl^-, and HCO_3^-) are routinely measured, and so the sum of the measured cations (Na^+ and K^+) normally exceeds the sum of the measured anions (Cl^- and HCO_3^-) resulting in an artificially positive anion gap. Serum albumin is the major contributor to the gap because negative charges on albumin account partly for the sum of measured cations being greater than the sum of measured anions. Clinically, the serum anion gap is calculated by subtracting the sum of the serum Cl^- and HCO_3^- concentrations from the serum Na^+ concentration. The serum K^+ concentration, while being a normally measured cation, is typically omitted from the anion gap calculation.

$$\text{Serum anion gap} = [Na^+] - ([Cl^-] + [HCO_3^-])$$

In healthy adults, the serum anion gap normally ranges from 8 to 12 mEq/L. In patients with hypoalbuminemia, the anion gap can be corrected for the reduced negative charges associated with albumin as follows: For every 1 g/dL drop in serum albumin, the expected serum anion gap will be lower by 2.5 mEq/L (i.e., if albumin drops from 4.5 to 3.5 g/dL, the expected anion gap should drop from 10 to 7.5 mEq/L).

TABLE 11.1 Elevated Anion Gap Acidosis

Acidosis	Clinical Scenario and Features	Other Lab Features	Management
Glycols			
1. Ethylene glycol	Antifreeze poisoning Flank pain, hematuria Renal failure, death	Serum osmolar gap >10 mOsm/kg Urine CaOx (monohydrate and dihydrate) crystals	▪ Fomepizole/ ethanol ▪ Dialysis
2. Propylene glycol	Prolonged IV infusion of benzodiazepines, phenobarbital	Acute kidney injury Serum osmolar gap >10 mOsm/kg Increased lactate	▪ Stop offending agents ▪ Dialysis
5-**O**xoproline/ pyroglutamate	Chronic acetaminophen use in malnourished females, glutathione depletion	Urine and serum 5-Oxoproline ↑	▪ Stop acetaminophen ▪ Bicarbonate ▪ N-acetyl cysteine
L-**L**actic acidosis	Type A: Septic shock, heart failure, hypovolemic shock Type B: Cancer, severe inflammation Medications such as metformin, linezolid	Lactate ↑	▪ Treat underlying cause ▪ IV bicarbonate if pH <7.1
D-Lactic acidosis	Short gut syndrome, gut bacterial overgrowth, propylene glycol poisoning	D-Lactate ↑	▪ Avoid large carbohydrate meals ▪ Bicarbonate ▪ Oral antibiotics
Methanol	Adulterated alcohol (moonshine) Accidental poisoning Headache, visual loss Coma, death	Serum osmolar gap >10 mOsm/kg	▪ Fomepizole/ ethanol ▪ Dialysis (renal failure)
Aspirin	Intentional / unintentional overdose	Salicylate level ↑ Mixed anion gap acidosis and respiratory alkalosis	▪ Urine alkalinization ▪ Dialysis (renal failure)

(*continued*)

	Elevated Anion Gap Acidosis (*Continued*)		
Acidosis	**Clinical Scenario and Features**	**Other Lab Features**	**Management**
Renal failure	Advanced stages of renal failure, uremia	BUN ↑, Cr ↑	■ NaHCO₃ ■ Dialysis
Ketoacidosis	Diabetic Starvation	↑ serum β-hydroxybutyrate, acetoacetate, glucose + urine ketones	■ Insulin ■ IV fluids ■ Nutrition

Note: Serum osmolar gap >10 mOsm/kg is considered to be elevated; Serum osmolar gap = calculated serum osmolality − measured serum osmolality; Calculated serum osmolality = $2 \times$ [Na⁺] + [glucose]/18 + [BUN]/2.8 when glucose and BUN are measured in mg/dL; Isopropyl alcohol causes increased osmolar gap but does not always cause high serum anion gap metabolic acidosis as it is metabolized to acetone.

Elevated Anion Gap Acidosis

Elevated anion gap acidosis occurs when there is an overproduction and/or underexcretion of nonvolatile acids or the presence of exogenous organic anions. Major etiology, key clinical and lab features, and management principles are summarized in Table 11.1.

Normal Anion Gap Acidosis

Normal anion gap acidosis develops when there is excessive loss of renal or gastrointestinal HCO_3^- (or HCO_3^- equivalents) or decrease in renal acid excretion or with large volume (>2 L) intravenous infusion of fluids containing a high concentration of Cl⁻. Common causes of gastrointestinal HCO_3^- loss include diarrhea, pancreatic or intestinal fistula, and ureteroileostomy, while renal loss of HCO_3^- or a defect in H⁺ excretion occurs in RTA. Type 4 RTA is the most common form of RTA. Table 11.2 summarizes the characteristics of RTAs and their management.

Another distinct entity linked to the distal RTA is incomplete distal RTA. Affected individuals develop hypocitraturia, nephrocalcinosis, and nephrolithiasis (calcium phosphate stones typically) but show a normal baseline acid–base status. Such patients typically are unable to acidify urine in response to acid loading (as tested by giving oral NH₄Cl). The underlying mechanism of this entity is unclear. Incomplete RTA is relatively common in patients with Sjögren syndrome and was present in up to 25% of such patients in one study (Both, 2015). Incomplete RTA is treated with potassium citrate.

ACIDOSIS IN CHRONIC KIDNEY DISEASE

In CKD, the prevalence of metabolic acidosis increases as renal function worsens. In a cross-sectional analysis of the baseline data from the Chronic Renal Insufficiency Cohort (CRIC) study involving 3,900 patients in CKD stages 2 to 4, the prevalence of metabolic acidosis

TABLE 11.2 Renal Tubular Acidoses

	Type 1: Distal Tubular Acidosis	Type 2: Proximal Tubular Acidosis	Type 4: Hyporeninemic Hypoaldosteronism
Defects	↓H⁺ excretion in distal tubule	↓HCO₃⁻ reabsorption in proximal tubule	↓renin and ↓ aldosterone
Etiology and clinical setting	**Acquired:** Chronic autoimmune connective tissue diseases (i.e., Sjögren syndrome, lupus, rheumatoid arthritis) **Drugs:** ■ Amphotericin ■ Lithium **Hereditary:** Loss-of-function mutations encoding the AE1 anion exchanger or subunits of H⁺-ATPase	**Acquired:** Dysproteinemia (multiple myeloma), interstitial renal diseases (less frequently), lead or mercury toxicity **Drugs:** ■ Carbonic anhydrase inhibitors (topiramate, acetazolamide) ■ Ifosfamide ■ Antiretrovirals (tenofovir) ■ Valproic acid ■ Expired tetracycline **Hereditary:** ■ Loss-of-function mutations encoding the Na⁺/3HCO₃⁻ cotransporter ■ Glycogen storage disease ■ Mitochondrial diseases ■ Cystinosis ■ Wilson disease	**Acquired:** Mild to moderate CKD (*not severe enough to explain the hyperkalemia and acidosis, often in diabetic patients*) Adrenal insufficiency due to autoimmune or infectious etiology Bilateral urinary tract obstruction (*voltage-dependent distal RTA*) **Drugs:** ■ ACE inhibitors ■ Renin inhibitors ■ ARBs ■ Aldosterone antagonists ■ K⁺-sparing diuretics ■ Calcineurin inhibitors ■ NSAIDs ■ Heparin infusion **Hereditary:** PHA1 (inactivating mutations of the *ENaC* and *NR3C2*) PHA2, aka Gordon syndrome (pathogenic mutations in *WNK1, WNK4, CUL3*, or *KLHL3*)
Acidemia	Severe if untreated	Self-limited (HCO₃⁻ at ~14–18 mmol/L)	Mild
Serum K	↓	↓	↑

(*continued*)

TABLE 11.2	Renal Tubular Acidoses (*Continued*)		
	Type 1: Distal Tubular Acidosis	**Type 2: Proximal Tubular Acidosis**	**Type 4: Hyporeninemic Hypoaldosteronism**
Urine pH	↑ (>5.3)	Variable ↓ (when HCO_3^- < Tm)	Variable
Urine NH_4^+ excretion	↓	Lack of ↑ in acidosis	↓
UAG	Positive	Variable	Positive
Urine citrate	↓	Normal or ↑	Normal
Urinary loss of nutrients (glucose, amino acids, and phosphorus)	No	Yes	No
Nephrocalcinosis	Yes	No	No
$CaPO_4$ stones	Yes	No	No
Osteomalacia	Yes	Yes	No
FE-HCO_3	<5%	Can be ↑ with alkali intake	Variable
Treatment	Alkali NaHCO₃ or citrate (approximately 1–2 mEq/kg per day)	Treat underlying causes Alkali (ineffective, not routinely used)	Treat underlying causes if possible Thiazide and/or loop diuretics (except for using salt supplementation for PHA1) Alkali (small requirement)

CKD, chronic kidney disease; FE, fractional excretion; H^+, hydrogen ion; HCO_3, bicarbonate; Tm, tubular transport maximum; $Ca^{2+}PO_4^-$, calcium phosphorus; NH_4^+, ammonium; AE1, anion exchanger 1 (Cl⁻–HCO_3^- exchanger); PHA, pseudohypoaldosteronism.

(serum HCO_3^- <22 mmol/L) was 7% for CKD stage 2, 13% for CKD stage 3, and 33% for CKD 4, with an overall acidosis occurrence of 17% (Raphael, 2014). Normal anion gap acidosis is predominant in the early stages of CKD; anion gap acidosis occurs in the late stages of CKD (GFR <30 mL/min per 1.73 m²) due to retention of anions such as sulfate, phosphate, and urate. It should be noted that net production of endogenous acids is relatively unchanged in CKD. Intrarenal ammonia and acid retention, consequences of acidosis, can cause complement activation and chronic tubulointerstitial inflammation (Nath, 1985) and increased generation of endothelin-1, angiotensin II, and aldosterone production (Wesson and Simoni, 2010), potentially promoting CKD progression. Indeed, metabolic acidosis in CKD is associated with more rapid progression of CKD (Vallet, 2015) and increased mortality (Kovesdy, 2009). Acidosis in CKD is associated with the development of sarcopenia, bone demineralization, impaired function of growth hormone and insulin, and growth retardation in children.

Correcting metabolic acidosis with alkali administration (de Brito-Ashurst, 2009; Goraya, 2014; Phisitkul, 2010) or dietary intake of alkali precursors (Goraya, 2013, 2014) slows CKD progression and improves nutritional status. The KDIGO 2012 guidelines for the evaluation and management of CKD (published in 2013) recommend the correction of metabolic acidosis. Oral $NaHCO_3$ is a commonly used alkali and may be initiated at a dosage of 650 mg (7.7 mmol of bicarbonate) two to three times daily. Dosage should be adjusted to keep serum HCO_3^- in the range of 22 to 26 mmol/L. The treatment is well tolerated and has not been shown to cause or worsen fluid retention or hypertension (Mahajan, 2010). The most common adverse effects are bloating and abdominal fullness. Sodium citrate is an alternative agent. Aluminum-containing phosphorus binders are now rarely used, but citrate should be avoided in patients on any compound containing significant amounts of aluminum (e.g., as an antacid) due to the increased gut absorption of ingested aluminum that may occur. A novel, still experimental, way of increasing serum bicarbonate in CKD patients is to give a substance that binds hydrochloric acid in the gut (Bushinsky, 2018).

METABOLIC ALKALOSIS

Metabolic alkalosis can result from a net loss of acid or a net gain of HCO_3^-. The alkalosis can be perpetuated by hypokalemia, hypovolemia, or excessive mineralocorticoid stimulation. These conditions prevent the kidney from unloading the accumulated HCO_3^-. Symptoms include confusion, lightheadedness, numbness and tingling in the extremities, and importantly, an increased risk of arrhythmias, especially when associated with hypokalemia or hypocalcemia. The major causes, pathophysiology, diagnostic features, and therapy of metabolic alkalosis in the general population are summarized in Table 11.3.

METABOLIC ALKALOSIS IN CHRONIC KIDNEY DISEASE

Although less common than metabolic acidosis, metabolic alkalosis can occur in patients with CKD. CKD patients are commonly on diuretics as well as calcium carbonate or citrate which can cause hypokalemia and alkalosis. Diagnosis is based on elevations of serum HCO_3^- and blood pH (>7.45). Measurement of urine Cl^- may not be helpful as renal Cl^- regulation may be impaired in CKD.

ELECTROLYTE DISORDERS

Electrolyte disorders are common in CKD. Hyperkalemia is among the most common electrolyte disorders. Dysnatremia often is due to

TABLE 11.3	Metabolic Alkalosis		
Causes	**Pathophysiology**	**Diagnostic Features**	**Treatment**
Vomiting and gastric suction	Loss of gastric acid	↓ urine Cl^- (<10 mmol/L)	Saline administration
Thiazide or loop diuretic therapy	↑ urine loss of Cl^-	Hypovolemia or euvolemia, ↑ urine Cl^-	Discontinue offending agents
Hypokalemia	↑ urine NH_4^+ excretion	Refractory alkalosis till serum K^+ is restored	KCl
$NaHCO_3$ administration	Exceeding the capacity of renal HCO_3^- excretion	Euvolemia or hypervolemia	Discontinue $NaHCO_3$
Chloride diarrhea	GI loss of HCO_3^- poor fluid	Hypovolemia	Treat diarrhea Saline administration
Primary hyperaldosteronism	↑ renal H^+ excretion	Hypervolemia (urine Cl^- >20 mmol/L)	Correcting hyperaldosteronism

compromised renal water regulation. The prevalence of dysmagnesemia is unclear but is likely underdiagnosed. Alterations of calcium and phosphorous balance are discussed in Chapter 8.

Potassium Regulation and Dyskalemia

Potassium (K^+) is the most abundant intracellular cation, with >98% of total body K^+ (~3,500 mmol) being intracellular and <2% (~70 mmol) extracellular. The steep intracellular to extracellular K^+ gradient is the major determinant of the plasma membrane potential. K^+ also participates in the regulation of cell volume, pH, and multiple cellular functions. In excitable tissues such as heart, nerves, and skeletal muscle, K^+ is critical for the generation of action potentials and electrical excitability. At steady state, the kidneys excrete ~95% of dietary K^+, with the small remainder excreted via the gastrointestinal tract.

Renal Potassium Regulation

K^+ is freely filtered through glomeruli. The proximal tubules reabsorb approximately 65% of the filtered K^+, while the TALH reabsorbs approximately 25%. The distal nephron (the DCT and collecting duct) is the major site of renal K^+ regulation. Depending on physiologic needs, the distal nephron can either excrete or absorb K^+.

On a typical Western diet, daily K^+ intake is higher (~90 to 120 mmol/day) than the small amount of K^+ present in the extracellular fluid (70 mmol). Normally, the distal nephron excretes K^+ to achieve balance. Key factors that determine the distal nephron K^+ secretion are (1) the serum K^+ concentration, (2) distal tubular Na^+ delivery, (3) rate of tubular fluid flow, and (4) the serum aldosterone level. In the distal nephron, aldosterone binds intracellular mineralocorticoid receptor, promoting apical ENaC-mediated Na^+ absorption. The enhanced Na^+ absorption here generates a favorable electrochemical gradient for K^+ secretion primarily via the apical membrane renal outer medullary potassium (ROMK) channels. Aldosterone also increases the basolateral Na^+/K^+-ATPase activity and promotes apical membrane expression and activity of thiazide-sensitive NCCs (sodium chloride symporters).

Acid–base perturbations affect renal K^+ excretion primarily through influencing the activity of H^+/K^+-ATPase in the distal nephron. Acidosis reduces and alkalosis enhances K^+ secretion.

Hyperkalemia

Hyperkalemia is the most common electrolyte disorder in patients with CKD. Its prevalence increases as CKD progresses. In one retrospective study ($n = 240,000$), CKD patients were more prone to hyperkalemic events ($K^+ \geq 5.5$ mmol/L) than patients without CKD, with odds ratios of 2.2 for CKD stage 3, 5.9 for CKD stage 4, and 11 for CKD stage 5 (Einhorn, 2009). Decreased glomerular filtration and ability of renal tubules to secrete K^+, often in combination with a diet generous in K^+, are the major causes of hyperkalemia. Other causes include the use of medications in CKD that further reduce the already limited capacity of distal nephron K^+ excretion, such as renin–angiotensin–aldosterone system (RAAS) inhibitors, K^+-sparing diuretics, and calcineurin inhibitors. Less common causes include transcellular K^+ shift due to insulin deficiency; mineral metabolic acidosis; tissue breakdown due to hemolysis, rhabdomyolysis, or tumor lysis syndrome; and specific disorders of renal tubular function such as hyporeninemic hypoaldosteronism (type IV) RTA.

Hyperkalemia is defined as serum K^+ concentration >5.3 mmol/L and is often arbitrarily classified as mild (5.4 to <6 mmol/L), moderate (6 to <7 mmol/L), and severe (≥ 7 mmol/L) (Ingelfinger, 2015). Symptoms and signs of hyperkalemia vary widely from nonspecific muscle weakness to paresthesia, muscle paralysis, cardiac arrhythmias, and cardiac arrest. The electrocardiogram (ECG) may show arrhythmias, peaked T waves, prolonged PR interval, loss of P waves, widening of the QRS complex, and sine waves. It is important to note that ECG changes are not sensitive in detecting hyperkalemia; CKD patients can develop life-threatening hyperkalemia without appreciable ECG changes (Khattak, 2014).

Treatment of Hyperkalemia

Treatment for hyperkalemia should be multipronged. Dietary modification with the initiation of a low K^+ diet (<75 mmol/day) is an important part of intervention. The medication regimen should be reviewed to minimize exposure of drugs that may induce hyperkalemia. Loop and thiazide diuretics can be used to promote kaliuresis. Patiromer is a nonabsorbable compound containing a Ca^{2+}–K^+ exchange polymer that selectively binds K^+, mainly in the colon. Its onset of action is 7 hours. Placebo-controlled clinical trials (Bakris, 2015; Weir, 2015) have demonstrated its efficacy and safety in lowering elevated serum K^+ levels. It is FDA-approved for treatment of chronic hyperkalemia in nondialysis CKD patients in a nonacute setting. Patiromer comes as a powder (in three strengths of 8.4, 16.2, and 25.2 g) with a recommended starting dose of 8.4 g daily. Dosage may be titrated upward weekly in increments of 8.4 g to a maximum daily dose of 25.2 g. Ingestion of patiromer should be spaced at least 3 hours away from intake of other medications due to a potential risk of drug–drug interaction. The most common known side effects are constipation and mild hypomagnesemia. Patiromer currently is not approved for treatment of acute hyperkalemia in the United States because the time course of its action is moderately delayed. An alternative agent, sodium zirconium cyclosilicate, may have a more rapid onset of action (Meaney, 2017).

Management of acute and symptomatic hyperkalemia requires monitoring in an inpatient setting. In the presence of ECG changes, intravenous calcium should be administered to stabilize the myocardium. Temporizing measures that shift K^+ into the cells, such as albuterol (10 mg) inhalation and intravenous infusion of regular insulin (10 units) combined with dextrose, are indicated. Sodium bicarbonate can be considered if there is coexistent metabolic acidosis. Definitive measures to increase excretion of K^+ include loop diuretics and/or thiazide to promote renal excretion, sodium polystyrene sulfonate to promote excretion via the gastrointestinal tract when appropriate, and hemodialysis if indicated. Hemodialysis is the most effective and definitive treatment.

Hypokalemia

Hypokalemia (serum K^+ concentration <3.5 mmol/L) is less common in CKD than hyperkalemia. It can occur due to a multitude of reasons, including the use of non–K^+-sparing diuretics, alkalosis, vomiting, diarrhea, or hypomagnesemia.

Clinical symptoms and signs of hypokalemia depend on the rate of onset and severity. These include muscle weakness, cramps, muscle paralysis and respiratory failure, cardiac arrhythmias, paralytic ileus, and rhabdomyolysis. Cardiac arrhythmias could include sinus bradycardia, A–V block, paroxysmal atrial or junctional tachycardia, ventricular tachycardia, and fibrillation. ECG changes include loss of T wave, emergence of U waves, prolonged QTc interval, and torsade de pointes (a specific form of polymorphic ventricular tachycardia in patients with a long QT interval). Hypokalemia increases renal proximal tubular ammoniagenesis and is associated with metabolic alkalosis.

Prolonged hypokalemia is associated with renal cyst formation, parenchymal fibrosis, and CKD progression. In a study of patients ($n = 2,500$) with CKD stages 1 to 4 (mean eGFR of 41 mL/min per 1.73 m^2), those with hypokalemia (serum K^+ <3.5 mmol/L) had a significantly higher risk of developing ESRD than those with serum K^+ of 4.5 to 5 mmol/L (Wang, 2013).

Management of hypokalemia in CKD patients involves correcting the underlying causes and cautious K^+ replacement.

WATER REGULATION AND DYSNATREMIA

Serum Na^+ concentration represents water balance and is the primary determinant of serum osmolality. Changes in serum osmolality drive fluid in and out of cells and affect cell volume and function. Serum Na^+ concentration is tightly regulated in a narrow range of 135 to 145 mmol/L by arginine vasopressin (AVP) and thirst. AVP is produced in the supraoptic and paraventricular nuclei of hypothalamus and is released from posterior pituitary in response to increased serum osmolality (sensed by osmoreceptors in the hypothalamus) or reduced intravascular volume (sensed by baroreceptors in the carotids and aortic arch). In the kidneys, AVP binds to V_2 receptors in the basolateral membrane of collecting ducts and activates adenylyl cyclase–mediated cAMP production and protein kinase A signaling, leading to phosphorylation and apical membrane insertion of aquaporin-2 channels. This in turn leads to free water absorption in the presence of tubulomedullary osmotic gradient.

In a retrospective study involving a cohort of veterans ($n = 655,000$) with nondialysis-dependent CKD, Kovesdy et al. found a U-shaped association between serum Na^+ concentration and mortality, with both hypernatremia (Na^+ >145 mmol/L) and hyponatremia (Na^+ <136 mmol/L) associated with increased mortality (Kovesdy, 2012).

Hyponatremia

Hyponatremia, defined as the serum Na^+ concentration <135 mmol/L, is the most common electrolyte disorder in both the community-dwelling population (Liamis, 2013) and in hospitalized patients (Holland-Bill, 2015), with occurrence rates of 8% to 15% and 44%, respectively (Hawkins, 2003). Patients with CKD are at higher risk of hyponatremia than the general population due to diminished GFR and impaired tubular regulation. In the same study noted above, among veterans with CKD (mean eGFR of 52 mL/min per 1.73 m^2) followed for a median period of 5.5 years, 26% of the subjects developed at least one episode of hyponatremia (Kovesdy, 2012).

Clinical signs and symptoms of hyponatremia are relatively nonspecific and dependent on the severity and rate of hyponatremia onset. Patients with mild to moderate hyponatremia may be asymptomatic or present with malaise, nausea, lethargy, and fatigue. The more overt neurologic symptoms often manifest when hyponatremia is severe (<120 mmol/L) and has developed rapidly. Patients can present with headache, slowing of mentation, confusion, ataxia, seizures, and coma.

Measurement of serum osmolality (normal serum osmolality = 280 to 290 mOsm/kg water) is necessary to rule out pseudohyponatremia, isotonic hyponatremia in the setting of hyperlipidemia and paraproteinemias, and hyperosmolar (>290 mOsm/kg) hyponatremia in

TABLE 11.4	Euvolemic Hyponatremia	
Cause	**Clinical and Lab Features**	**Treatment**
Severe hypothyroidism	↑ TSH ↓ T4 Myxedema, stigmata of hypothyroidism	Levothyroxine Free water restriction
Secondary adrenal insufficiency	↓ ACTH ↓ Cortisol	Hydrocortisone
Low solute intake	Elderly/malnourished (tea and toast diet) Beer potomania	Protein nutrition supplement Stop beer intake
Psychogenic polydipsia	Large water intake Dilute urine (osmolality <100 mOsm/kg)	Free water restriction
SIADH Idiopathic/aging related Nausea/vomiting Pain Cancer (small cell lung cancer) Lung: Abscess/empyema/COPD CNS: Meningitis/encephalitis Brain abscess/stroke Medications: SSRIs, TCAs, antiepileptics, barbiturates	Urine osmolality >150 mOsm/kg Urine Na^+ high or low based on Na^+ intake ↓ serum uric acid	Fluid restriction (<1 L/day) Salt tablets Loop diuretics V_2 (AVP)-receptor blockers[a] Treat the underlying cause Stop the offending medication (if possible)

[a] V_2 blockers should be initiated in the hospital setting and should not be used beyond 30 days.
SSRIs, selective serotonin reuptake inhibitors; TCAs, tricyclic antidepressants.

the setting of hyperglycemia or mannitol administration. Low serum osmolality (<280 mOsm/kg) along with hyponatremia indicates true hypotonic hyponatremia. After confirming the presence of hypotonic hyponatremia, the patient's volume status should be determined to guide treatment decisions. Volume replacement with isotonic fluids is the treatment of choice in patients with volume depletion. Restoration of volume will turn off the stimulus for vasopressin release, leading to renal water excretion and correction of hyponatremia. Causes, clinical features, and treatment for euvolemic hyponatremia are summarized in Table 11.4.

Hypervolemic hyponatremia due to liver or heart failure should be treated with loop diuretics combined with free water restriction (≤1 L/day). Vasopressin V_2-receptor blockers (vaptans) are not used routinely due to prohibitive cost and concerns of hepatotoxicity. The FDA has approved the use of tolvaptan, a selective V_2-receptor blocker, for less than 30 days for hyponatremia due to congestive heart failure but not for patients with cirrhosis. Several clinical trials have failed to show a reduction in long-term mortality and morbidity in heart failure patients treated with V_2-receptor blocker despite increasing serum Na^+ concentration (Gheorghiade, 2004; Konstam, 2007). Similarly, in a recently published TACTICS-HF study involving 257 patients hospitalized for acute heart failure, randomization to 3 days of daily tolvaptan compared to placebo failed to show any difference in length of hospital stay, 30-day mortality, and 30-day rehospitalization rates (Felker, 2017).

Patients with late-stage CKD often develop euvolemic or hypervolemic hyponatremia due to limited kidney function. Management involves free water restriction, use of loop diuretics, and, if necessary, dialysis.

Regardless of the etiology, the rate of serum Na^+ correction depends upon two key factors: (1) whether the patient is symptomatic, and (2) the rate of hyponatremia onset (<48 hours or >48 hours). For symptomatic hyponatremia, 3% saline should be administered intravenously with the goal of raising serum Na^+ by 4 to 5 mmol/L. If asymptomatic and the onset of hyponatremia is >48 hours, serum Na^+ concentration should be corrected slowly (not exceeding 6 to 8 mmol/L in the first 24 hours and not exceeding 18 mmol/L within 48 hours) to prevent neurologic damage, such as central pontine demyelination syndrome. Inadvertent overcorrection should be reversed with hypotonic fluids. Serial serum Na^+ measurements (every 2 to 6 hours) may be necessary to evaluate treatment adequacy, especially during the initial 24 hours.

Hypernatremia

Hypernatremia (serum Na^+ concentration >145 mmol/L) is relatively common, with a reported incidence of 1% to 3% in hospitalized patients (Liamis, 2013; Palevsky, 1996). In CKD, as cited above (Kovesdy, 2012), there is a reported 2% ($n = 13,289$) prevalence of hypernatremia and 7% ($n = 45,666$) occurrence of at least one episode of hypernatremia in nondialysis CKD veterans over 5.5 years of follow-up.

Hypernatremia signifies total body water deficiency relative to Na^+. It can result from either loss of water or hypotonic fluid (loss of water > loss of Na^+) or gain of sodium (and potassium), such as incidental hypertonic fluid ingestion or infusion. Diabetes insipidus, chronic hypokalemia, hypercalcemia, hyperglycemia, and medications such as loop and osmotic diuretics, lithium, and vasopressin V_2-receptor blockers can cause hypernatremia due to renal hypotonic fluid loss. Nonrenal causes of hypernatremia include osmotic diarrhea, vomiting, excessive sweating, and burns. Sustained hypernatremia typically occurs when thirst mechanism is impaired (thirst stimulates AVP secretion leading to renal water preservation) and/or due to lack of water access. Hence, intubated patients, patients with altered mental status or under sedation, elderly nursing home residents, and infants are more susceptible to hypernatremia.

Clinical symptoms and signs of hypernatremia are nonspecific and vary from asymptomatic to comatose depending on the severity and rate of onset of hypernatremia. Common manifestations include intense thirst (if thirst mechanism is intact), fatigue, lethargy, muscle weakness, slowing of mentation, confusion, and coma.

Hypernatremia is a hypertonic state. Thus, measurement of serum osmolality is in general unnecessary. Measurement of urine osmolality is useful in differentiating renal water loss, such as diabetes insipidus (inappropriately dilute urine) from extrarenal water loss (concentrated urine). In patients taking diuretics, urine osmolality may vary depending on the timing of diuretic intake.

Patients with severe hyperglycemia can be in a hyperosmolar state, but their serum $[Na^+]$ may be falsely normal or even reduced. Typically, serum $[Na^+]$ is reduced by ~1.6 mmol/L for each 100 mg/dL (5.5 mmol/L) elevation of glucose above normal range. For instance, if a patient's serum glucose is 800 mg/dL (44 mmol/L) and serum Na^+ 140 mmol/L, his/her corrected Na^+ concentration would be ~151 mmol/L, a hypertonic state. In such cases, measurement of serum osmolality should be informative.

Management of hypernatremia should focus on correction of the underlying cause and treatment of hypernatremia. The rate of water replacement depends on the onset/duration of hypernatremia. If hypernatremia is chronic (>48 hours) or unknown, serum Na^+ correction should be gradual, not exceeding 8 to 10 mmol/L in the first 24 hours to prevent cerebral edema (Adrogue and Madias, 2000). More rapid serum Na^+ correction (up to 1 mmol/L per hour) may be appropriate if onset of hypernatremia is acute (<48 hours).

Total body free water deficit in hypernatremia can be estimated with the following formula:

$$\text{Free water deficit} = \text{Total body water} \times \left(\frac{\text{serum } [Na^+]}{140} - 1\right)$$

where total body water (L) = Body weight (kg) × (0.6 for men; 0.5 for women).

The calculation provides an initial estimate of total body water deficit. The rate and amount of daily water replacement should be based not on the calculated water deficit but on the repeated measurements of serum Na^+ concentration to prevent under- or overcorrection.

Magnesium Regulation and Dysmagnesemia

Magnesium (Mg^{2+}) is the second most abundant intracellular cation with >99% located intracellularly (53% in bones, 46% in soft tissues) and ~1% or less located extracellularly. About 20% to 30% of circulating Mg^{2+} is protein bound (mainly to albumin), while 70% to 80% is freely filtered by kidneys. Mg^{2+} is a cofactor for numerous intracellular enzymes and has multiple functions in oxidative phosphorylation, DNA synthesis, repair and replication, RNA and protein synthesis, and signaling pathways.

Daily Mg^{2+} intake in an adult should be in the range of 350 to 450 mg (14.4 to 18.5 mmol). Ingested Mg^{2+} is absorbed predominantly in the distal small intestine through a paracellular process and in the cecum and colon by a transcellular process involving TRPM6 (transient receptor potential cation channel, subfamily M, member 6). Intestinal Mg^{2+} absorption can vary significantly, ranging from 25% to 75%, depending on the amount of Mg^{2+} intake. The kidneys filter ~2,400 mg (99 mmol) of Mg^{2+} daily, of which ~100 mg (4.1 mmol) is excreted in the urine. Unlike Na^+, K^+, and Ca^{2+}, bulk of the filtered Mg^{2+} (about 70%) is reabsorbed in the TALH and only about 20% is reabsorbed in the proximal tubule. The remaining 5% to 10% of filtered Mg^{2+} is reabsorbed in the distal tubule. In the TALH, Mg^{2+} is absorbed paracellularly. The major driving force is the lumen-positive transepithelial voltage generated primarily by the reabsorption of Na^+, K^+, and Cl^- in this location. In the DCT, Mg^{2+} reabsorption is transcellular via TRPM6. For more detailed information see a recent review (Li, 2017).

Both hypermagnesemia (>2.3 mg/dL [0.95 mmol/L]) and hypomagnesemia (<1.7 mg/dL [0.70 mmol/L]) are relatively common with reported prevalences of 31% and 20%, respectively, in hospitalized patients (Cheungpasitporn, 2015). Both hypo- and hypermagnesemia adversely impact patient outcomes, including increased mortality and duration of hospital stay. A complete list of causes, pathophysiology, and special features of different conditions causing hypo- and hypermagnesemia are beyond the scope of this handbook. In the early stages of CKD, decreased filtration of Mg^{2+} is balanced by reduced renal tubular reabsorption; hence, dysmagnesemia is uncommon. In advanced CKD, hypermagnesemia can be triggered by ingestion of Mg^{2+}-rich diet and/or Mg^{2+}-containing medications. Hypomagnesemia in CKD patients can occur due to inadequate intake, poor intestinal absorption (due to malabsorption syndromes or use of proton pump inhibitors [PPIs]), and renal or extrarenal loss, such as chronic diarrhea.

Symptoms of dysmagnesemia vary significantly. Mild hypo- or hypermagnesemia may be asymptomatic. Severe and chronic hypomagnesemia can present with muscle weakness, paresthesia, tetany, and seizures. It can potentiate cardiac arrhythmias. Severe hypermagnesemia can cause loss of deep tendon reflexes and paralysis.

Treatment of dysmagnesemia involves correcting the underlying causes if possible and normalizing Mg^{2+}. For severe symptomatic hypomagnesemia, parenteral magnesium administration is indicated. Oral administration of Mg^{2+} in divided doses daily, however, is the only effective method for total body Mg^{2+} repletion. In patients with adequate renal function, hypermagnesemia would mostly self-correct with urine Mg^{2+} excretion. If necessary, loop diuretics can be used to enhance renal Mg^{2+} excretion. In patients with advanced renal failure and symptomatic hypermagnesemia, intravenous calcium should be considered to stabilize the myocardium. Dialysis is the most effective and definitive treatment of hypermagnesemia in patients with renal failure.

References and Suggested Readings

Adrogue HJ, Madias NE. Hypernatremia. *N Engl J Med*. 2000;342:1493–1499.

Bakris GL, Pitt B, Weir MR, et al. Effect of patiromer on serum potassium level in patients with hyperkalemia and diabetic kidney disease: the AMETHYST-DN Randomized Clinical Trial. *JAMA*. 2015;314:151–161.

Both T, Hoorn EJ, Zietse R, et al. Prevalence of distal renal tubular acidosis in primary Sjogren's syndrome. *Rheumatology (Oxford)*. 2015;54:933–939.

Bushinsky DA, Hostetter T, Klaerner G, et al. Randomized, controlled trial of TRC101 to increase serum bicarbonate in patients with CKD. *Clin J Am Soc Nephrol*. 2018;13:26–35.

Cheungpasitporn W, Thongprayoon C, Qian Q. Dysmagnesemia in hospitalized patients: prevalence and prognostic importance. *Mayo Clin Proc*. 2015;90:1001–1010.

de Brito-Ashurst I, Varagunam M, Raftery MJ, et al. Bicarbonate supplementation slows progression of CKD and improves nutritional status. *J Am Soc Nephrol*. 2009;20:2075–2084.

Einhorn LM, Zhan M, Hsu VD, et al. The frequency of hyperkalemia and its significance in chronic kidney disease. *Arch Intern Med*. 2009;169:1156–1162.

Felker GM, Mentz RJ, Cole RT, et al. Efficacy and safety of tolvaptan in patients hospitalized with acute heart failure. *J Am Coll Cardiol*. 2017;69:1399–1406.

Gheorghiade M, Gattis WA, O'Connor CM, et al; Acute and Chronic Therapeutic Impact of a Vasopressin Antagonist in Congestive Heart Failure (ACTIV in CHF) Investigators. Effects of tolvaptan, a vasopressin antagonist, in patients hospitalized with worsening heart failure: a randomized controlled trial. *JAMA*. 2004;291:1963–1971.

Goraya N, Simoni J, Jo CH, et al. A comparison of treating metabolic acidosis in CKD stage 4 hypertensive kidney disease with fruits and vegetables or sodium bicarbonate. *Clin J Am Soc Nephrol*. 2013;8:371–381.

Goraya N, Simoni J, Jo CH, et al. Treatment of metabolic acidosis in patients with stage 3 chronic kidney disease with fruits and vegetables or oral bicarbonate reduces urine angiotensinogen and preserves glomerular filtration rate. *Kidney Int*. 2014;86:1031–1038.

Hawkins RC. Age and gender as risk factors for hyponatremia and hypernatremia. *Clin Chim Acta*. 2003;337:169–172.

Holland-Bill L, Christiansen CF, Heide-Jorgensen U, et al. Hyponatremia and mortality risk: a Danish cohort study of 279,508 acutely hospitalized patients. *Eur J Endocrinol*. 2015;173:71–81.

Ingelfinger JR. A new era for the treatment of hyperkalemia? *N Engl J Med*. 2015; 372:275–277.

Khattak HK, Khalid S, Manzoor K, et al. Recurrent life-threatening hyperkalemia without typical electrocardiographic changes. *J Electrocardiol*. 2014;47:95–97.

Kim GH, Han JS, Kim YS, et al. Evaluation of urine acidification by urine anion gap and urine osmolal gap in chronic metabolic acidosis. *Am J Kidney Dis*. 1996;27: 42–47.

Konstam MA, Gheorghiade M, Burnett JC, et al; Efficacy of Vasopressin Antagonism in Heart Failure Outcome Study With Tolvaptan (EVEREST) Investigators. Effects of oral tolvaptan in patients hospitalized for worsening heart failure: the EVEREST Outcome Trial. *JAMA*. 2007;297:1319–1331.

Kovesdy CP, Anderson JE, Kalantar-Zadeh K. Association of serum bicarbonate levels with mortality in patients with non-dialysis-dependent CKD. *Nephrol Dial Transplant*. 2009;24:1232–1237.

Kovesdy CP, Lott EH, Lu JL, et al. Hyponatremia, hypernatremia, and mortality in patients with chronic kidney disease with and without congestive heart failure. *Circulation*. 2012;125:677–684.

Kurtz I, Maher T, Hulter HN, et al. Effect of diet on plasma acid-base composition in normal humans. *Kidney Int*. 1983;24:670–680.

Li H, Sun S, Chen J, et al. Genetics of magnesium disorders. *Kidney Dis (Basel)*. 2017;3:85–97.

Liamis G, Rodenburg EM, Hofman A, et al. Electrolyte disorders in community subjects: prevalence and risk factors. *Am J Med*. 2013;126:256–263.

Mahajan A, Simoni J, Sheather SJ, et al. Daily oral sodium bicarbonate preserves glomerular filtration rate by slowing its decline in early hypertensive nephropathy. *Kidney Int.* 2010;78:303–309.

Meaney CJ, Beccari MV, Yang Y, et al. Systematic review and meta-analysis of patiromer and sodium zirconium cyclosilicate: A new armamentarium for the treatment of hyperkalemia. *Pharmacotherapy.* 2017;37:401–411.

Nath KA, Hostetter MK, Hostetter TH. Pathophysiology of chronic tubulo-interstitial disease in rats. Interactions of dietary acid load, ammonia, and complement component C3. *J Clin Invest.* 1985;76:667–675.

Palevsky PM, Bhagrath R, Greenberg A. Hypernatremia in hospitalized patients. *Ann Intern Med.* 1996;124:197–203.

Phisitkul S, Khanna A, Simoni J, et al. Amelioration of metabolic acidosis in patients with low GFR reduced kidney endothelin production and kidney injury and better preserved GFR. *Kidney Int.* 2010;77:617–623.

Raphael KL, Zhang Y, Ying J, et al. Prevalence of and risk factors for reduced serum bicarbonate in chronic kidney disease. *Nephrology (Carlton).* 2014;19:648–654.

Vallet M, Metzger M, Haymann JP, et al. Urinary ammonia and long-term outcomes in chronic kidney disease. *Kidney Int.* 2015;88:137–145.

Wang HH, Hung CC, Hwang DY, et al. Hypokalemia, its contributing factors and renal outcomes in patients with chronic kidney disease. *PLoS One.* 2013;8:e67140.

Weir MR, Bakris GL, Bushinsky DA, et al. Patiromer in patients with kidney disease and hyperkalemia receiving RAAS inhibitors. *N Engl J Med.* 2015;372:211–221.

Wesson DE, Simoni J. Acid retention during kidney failure induces endothelin and aldosterone production which lead to progressive GFR decline, a situation ameliorated by alkali diet. *Kidney Int.* 2010;78:1128–1135.

12 Dyslipidemia

Doris T. Chan, Ashley B. Irish, and Gerald F. Watts

Only a small proportion of patients with chronic kidney disease (CKD) in stages 1–4 reach end-stage renal disease (ESRD). The majority succumb to cardiovascular-related death before needing renal replacement therapy. Although the precise mechanisms for the increased risk of atherosclerotic cardiovascular complications and death in CKD are unknown, both traditional and novel cardiovascular risk factors have been implicated.

Dyslipidemia, an important modifiable cardiovascular risk factor, develops early and is prevalent in patients with CKD. Recent meta-analyses and the landmark Study of Heart and Renal Protection (SHARP) study provide robust clinical trial evidence for a cardiovascular benefit of statin therapy in nondialysis-dependent CKD patients, lending support to the notion that dyslipidemia plays a key role in the development of atherosclerotic cardiovascular disease (ASCVD) in this population (Baigent, 2011). However, uncertainty remains as to whether the benefit of statin therapy extends to those on dialysis due to differences in the epidemiology and pathophysiology of cardiovascular disease (CVD) in the setting of uremia.

REVIEW OF LIPID ABSORPTION AND METABOLISM

Lipoproteins

Lipids are insoluble in aqueous solution and must be transported in plasma as lipoprotein particles (Fig. 12.1). Lipoprotein particles consist of a central hydrophobic core in which triglyceride (TG), phospholipids, and cholesterol esters (CE) are stored. The surface contains a hydrophilic monolayer of phospholipids, free cholesterol, and apolipoproteins. Surface apolipoproteins play a crucial role in determining the fate of various lipoproteins. Apolipoproteins can direct whether a given lipoprotein will be depleted of its stored TG or cholesterol by interacting with enzymes and specific proteins on the surface of endothelial, liver, and other cells.

Lipoprotein Density

Lipoproteins are classified by their density, which is based on the relative content of fat to protein. Given that fat has a lower density than protein, lipoproteins which contain relatively more fat (as TGs, phospholipids, and CE) than protein are less dense than those which contain little fat and more protein. Chylomicrons are the least dense and typically contain 98% fat. The other less-dense lipoproteins are classified based on their density as determined by electrophoresis

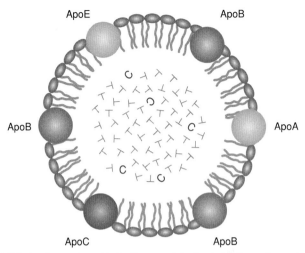

FIGURE 12.1 Lipoprotein particle (in this case, a chylomicron), showing apolipoproteins on the surface and triacylglycerol (*T*) and cholesterol esters (*C*) inside. (Reproduced with permission under the GNU Free Documentation License. http://en.wikipedia.org/wiki/File:Chylomicron.svg)

and ultracentrifugation: very–low-density lipoprotein (VLDL), intermediate-density lipoprotein (IDL), low-density lipoprotein (LDL), and high-density lipoprotein (HDL) particles. The percentage of fat content ranges from 90% with VLDL down to about 70% for HDL.

Lipoprotein Function
Chylomicrons and VLDLs contain mostly TGs (80% and 50%, respectively). Chylomicrons carry TGs absorbed from the gut to the liver, skeletal muscle, and adipose tissue. VLDLs carry TGs synthesized in the liver to adipose tissue. LDLs and HDLs contain mostly cholesterol. LDL transports cholesterol from the liver to various cells throughout the body. HDL brings cholesterol from peripheral tissues to the liver.

Exogenous Pathway. The exogenous pathway is used to distribute lipids absorbed from the gut throughout the body. Small intestine epithelial cells absorb dietary TGs, cholesterol, and phospholipids and package them into "nascent chylomicrons" lined with apolipoprotein B-48 (apoB-48). These are excreted into the lymphatic system, where they travel to the thoracic duct and from there enter the circulation. Once in the circulation, nascent chylomicrons acquire apoC-II and apoE from the surface of circulating HDL particles. ApoC-II particles on the "mature" chylomicron activate lipoprotein lipase on the surface of endothelial cells, which splits TGs carried within chylomicron into glycerol and fatty acids. These are then absorbed by muscle, fat cells, and other tissues and used for energy or storage. Having "delivered" its store of glycerol and fatty acids to tissues, the chylomicron becomes a chylomicron "remnant." These remnants, which are detected via their apoE surface receptors by the liver, are then rapidly removed from the circulation.

Endogenous Pathway. In the endogenous pathway, the source of TGs, cholesterol, and phospholipids is the liver rather than the gut. The liver assembles these into VLDLs, incorporating apoB-100 onto their surfaces. These "nascent" VLDLs are released directly into the circulation and, similar to nascent chylomicrons, acquire apoC and apoE from circulating HDL. Like chylomicrons, VLDL can activate lipoprotein lipase on endothelial cells to release part of its TGs to tissues.

After the loss of TGs and transfer of apoC to circulating HDL, VLDL now becomes the denser IDL particle. IDLs can be taken up by the liver via the LDL receptor and degraded. Alternatively, their remaining store of TGs can be hydrolyzed by hepatic lipase, which breaks down TGs into fatty acids. Further loss of TGs increases their density, converting the IDL particle to LDL.

LDL is cholesterol rich, and its contents can be taken up by the liver or delivered to peripheral tissues. When a cell requires cholesterol, it synthesizes LDL receptors and inserts them into the cell membrane. Binding of circulating LDL to the LDL receptor leads to endocytosis and release of cholesterol into the cell via lysosomal degradation.

High-Density Lipoprotein "Scavenger" Pathway. HDL particles are made in the liver. They contain a low proportion of lipids to proteins and hence have a high density. HDL particles have a high percentage of apoA-I and apoA-II on their surface. Circulating HDL accepts both cholesterol and phospholipids from various peripheral cells, transferring them back to the liver or to other apoB-containing lipoproteins. The lecithin cholesterol acyltransferase (LCAT) enzyme esterifies free cholesterol on the surface of HDL, allowing for the more hydrophobic CE to be packed into the center of the HDL particle. In addition, cholesteryl ester transfer protein (CETP) mediates the transfer of CE from HDL in exchange for TGs from TG-rich lipoprotein particles, particularly VLDL, converting VLDL to a TG-poor and cholesterol-rich LDL particle. The disc-shaped, lipid-laden HDL particle delivers its contents directly to the liver through the scavenger receptor class B type I (SRB-I) receptors. Excretion of cholesterol into the bile completes the process of reverse cholesterol transport.

MEASUREMENT OF LIPIDS AND LIPOPROTEINS

The clinically available screening tests for dyslipidemia consist of direct measurement of serum cholesterol, TGs, and HDL-cholesterol (HDL-C). Based on these values, LDL-cholesterol (LDL-C) is estimated using the Friedewald equation ([total cholesterol]-[TG/5]-[HDL-C] in mg/dL). Non–HDL-cholesterol (non–HDL-C), which reflects LDL-C plus remnants of triglyceride-rich lipoproteins (TRL) and cholesterol content of lipoprotein(a) (Lp[a]), is derived from total cholesterol minus HDL-C. Serum TG levels reflect the amount of chylomicron and VLDL particles. Normal values for lipids and lipid targets were set based on associations between lipid and lipoprotein measures and cardiovascular events in large observational databases.

FACTORS WHICH AFFECT MEASUREMENT OF LIPIDS AND LIPOPROTEINS

Although fasting samples were previously recommended, most current guidelines advocate the use of nonfasting samples for patient convenience and given the minor differences in measured LDL-C and HDL-C concentrations (Stone, 2014). In contrast, serum TG levels can differ depending on the fasting status. While TG level represents VLDL in the fasting state, there is contribution from chylomicrons following a meal.

Cholesterol is also a marker of nutrition, and patients who are malnourished or have an inflammatory state can have low levels of total cholesterol but still demonstrate an atherogenic profile of various lipoprotein and apolipoprotein components. Given that the calculated LDL-C is dependent on measured TG levels, inaccurate results can occur in the setting of significant hypertriglyceridemia (levels >400 mg/dL [4.5 mmol/L]).

ROLE OF LIPIDS AND LIPOPROTEINS IN ATHEROSCLEROSIS

Low-Density Lipoprotein

The major contribution of LDL to atherosclerosis is now indisputable, with a multitude of primary and secondary prevention studies consistently showing reduction in ASCVD events with LDL-lowering therapy, especially with statins. The reduction in ASCVD events gained by LDL lowering is determined by both the baseline cardiovascular risk and degree of the absolute reduction in LDL-C plus duration of exposure to lower LDL levels (Ference, 2017).

One postulated mechanism for this association is as follows: LDL can penetrate through endothelial cell capillary pores into the proteoglycan matrix located under the blood vessel intima. This LDL becomes oxidized, attracts inflammatory cells, especially macrophages, which then initiate a cascade of inflammatory, calcification, and coagulation events, ultimately leading to obstruction and thrombosis of the blood vessel. Small LDL particles are more atherogenic than large LDL particles, presumably because they can penetrate through endothelial pores more easily, but also because they may form stronger attachments to the arterial wall and may be more susceptible to oxidation. LDL particles can become glycated through chemical interactions with advanced glycation end products. Glycation increases LDL half-life, increasing the ability of LDL to promote atherosclerosis.

Lipoprotein(a)

Lp(a) consists of a cholesterol-rich LDL particle with a single molecule of apoB-100 that is covalently linked to the glycoprotein apolipoprotein(a) (apo[a]). Apo(a) is made by the liver, and its size is genetically determined by the apo(a) gene, which has evolved and is closely related to the plasminogen gene. Apo(a) genotype, which determines both the synthetic rate and size of the apo(a) moiety of Lp(a), alone accounts for 90% of plasma concentrations of Lp(a).

In recent years, data from genetic, epidemiologic, translational, pathophysiologic, and genetic studies have supported an independent genetic and causal link between elevated Lp(a) levels and CVD risk (Tsimikas, 2017). Lp(a) imparts its proatherogenic properties through various mechanisms including oxidative stress, antifibrinolysis, and inflammation (Tsimikas, 2017). The high concentrations of oxidized phospholipids on Lp(a) impart potent atherogenic properties to this lipoprotein particle. In addition, presence of lysine binding sites on apo(a) further potentiates its accumulation and retention in the endothelium and atherosclerotic plaque. Because Lp(a) has homology with plasminogen, there is impaired fibrinolysis through inhibition of plasminogen activation.

While Lp(a) is largely unaffected by dietary or environmental factors, it is of particular interest in CKD as it is metabolized and excreted by the kidneys. Outcome studies specifically aimed at Lp(a) lowering in CKD are worth considering.

Triglycerides

Hypertriglyceridemia marks the presence of TRLs, which in recent epidemiology, genetics, and mechanistic studies have been shown to play a causal role in the pathogenesis of ASCVD (Nordestgaard, 2016). While TGs do not accumulate in foam cells, TRLs can be taken up directly by macrophages to form foam cells without the need for modification. Plaque progression and atherosclerosis are further enhanced by inflammation derived from TG hydrolysis which releases lysolecithin and other toxic fatty acids. Confirmation of this relationship will require intervention trials specifically aimed at lowering TRLs.

ApoC-III

The presence of apoC-III on VLDL or LDL particles inhibits both lipoprotein and hepatic lipases, which in turn delays the breakdown of both VLDL and LDL particles. Thus, apoC-III may promote atherosclerosis through the accumulation of atherogenic TRLs due to impaired lipolysis, vascular inflammation, and endothelial dysfunction (Luo and Peng, 2016).

ApoC-III an important determinant of serum TG levels, has been associated with increased risk of cardiovascular events. Loss-of-function mutation in the apoC-III gene has been associated with reduced coronary risk with lower TG, higher HDL-C, and lower LDL-C concentrations, suggesting a causal relationship.

High-Density Lipoprotein

High serum HDL-C levels may protect against atherosclerosis due to HDL-mediated removal of cholesterol from lipid-laden macrophages in arterial plaque and transport to the liver for excretion in bile (reverse cholesterol transport). In addition to exhibiting protective effects on endothelial cell function, HDL particles also contain constituents which inhibit oxidation, inflammation, and activation of coagulation and platelets (Bandeali and Farmer, 2012).

Low HDL-C concentration induced by LCAT deficiency is associated with atherosclerosis and cholesterol accumulation in various body tissues. Impaired function of the HDL scavenger pathway mediates a decreased efficiency of packing CE into the HDL particle. High CETP level is also associated with lower HDL-C levels as the now TG-enriched HDL particle is more susceptible to catabolism.

ALTERATION OF LIPOPROTEIN METABOLISM IN CHRONIC KIDNEY DISEASE AND NEPHROTIC SYNDROME

Chronic Kidney Disease

Regardless of the etiology of renal disease, patients with CKD develop complex qualitative and quantitative abnormalities in lipid and lipoprotein metabolism (See Table 12.1). Uremic dyslipidemia is characterized by raised TG, low HDL-C, and normal total cholesterol concentrations. These qualitative defects become more pronounced with advancing renal failure (stages 4 and 5) and are modified by comorbid conditions (e.g., diabetes mellitus [DM]), dialysis modality (e.g., hemodialysis, peritoneal dialysis, and renal transplantation), and concurrent medications (e.g., steroids, cyclosporine). Other factors that influence these changes include diet, physical inactivity, cigarette smoking, obesity, and alcohol. Patients with CKD may also be affected by genetic dyslipidemias. This should be suspected in those who present with markedly elevated plasma cholesterol and TG levels, together with tendon xanthomas and history of premature CVD in a first-degree relative.

As renal function deteriorates in nonnephrotic patients with CKD, TG levels increase as a result of increased concentrations of TG-rich, apoB-containing lipoproteins. Delayed catabolism is the principal mechanism for the accumulation of TRLs in nonnephrotic patients with early CKD, and this may relate to decreased activity of lipolytic enzymes (i.e., lipoprotein lipase and hepatic lipase) and elevated apoC-III concentration (Chan, 2009). Total cholesterol and LDL-C concentrations are often within normal limits but there is accumulation of the more atherogenic small, dense LDL particles. Serum HDL-C level is typically reduced in nonnephrotic CKD patients due to decreased concentrations of apoA-I and apoA-II (Vaziri, 2016b). There is concurrent HDL dysfunction due to LCAT deficiency, TG enrichment of HDL, and defective reverse cholesterol transport due to oxidative modifications of apoA-I. Serum CETP concentration and activity are unchanged.

TABLE 12.1	Changes in Plasma Lipid and Lipoprotein Concentrations in Predialysis Chronic Kidney Disease and Nephrotic Syndrome	
	CKD Stages 1–4 or Predialysis Stage 5 Without Proteinuria	Nephrotic Syndrome
Total cholesterol	↔	↑↑
Triglyceride	↔ or ↑	↑↑
LDL cholesterol	↔ or ↑	↑
HDL cholesterol	↓ or ↔	↓
Small, dense LDL particles	↔ or ↑	↑
Lipoprotein(a)	↑	↑

Nephrotic Syndrome

Patients with nephrotic syndrome and preserved glomerular filtration rate also exhibit a highly atherogenic profile, characterized by elevated plasma cholesterol and TG concentrations, increased apoB-containing lipoproteins (VLDL, LDL, IDL), increased Lp(a) levels, and reduced plasma HDL-C level. These lipid and lipoprotein abnormalities are due to both impaired catabolism and increased synthesis (Vaziri, 2016a).

Hypercholesterolemia is due to a combination of increased hepatic biosynthesis through upregulation of HMG-CoA reductase and acyl coenzyme A: cholesterol acyltransferase (ACAT) activity, as well as, impaired clearance of LDL and apoB-100. Normally, the presence of high intracellular cholesterol enhances binding of the circulating serine protease, proprotein convertase subtilisin/kexin type 9 (PCSK9), to the LDL receptor, which facilitates its internalization and lysosomal degradation, thereby reducing hepatic LDL uptake. Increased cellular oxysterols also enhance the expression of another LDL receptor degrader, inducible degrader of the LDL receptor (IDOL). In nephrotic syndrome, acquired LDL receptor deficiency secondary to upregulation of PCSK9 and IDOL expressions has been described (Liu and Vaziri, 2014).

Hypertriglyceridemia in nephrotic syndrome arises from increased hepatic VLDL synthesis driven by upregulation of hepatic acyl-CoA diacylglycerol acyltransferase (DGAT) and decreased catabolism of TRLs related to reduced lipoprotein lipase, hepatic lipase, and VLDL receptor activity. Reduced activity of LCAT enzyme and upregulation of CETP activity impair maturation of HDL leading to decreased HDL-C concentration.

LIPID-LOWERING THERAPY IN NONDIALYSIS-DEPENDENT CHRONIC KIDNEY DISEASE: CARDIOVASCULAR OUTCOME STUDIES

Statins

Statins are competitive inhibitors of the HMG-CoA reductase. Statins lower LDL cholesterol and TGs, while modestly increasing HDL-C levels. Beyond their lipid-regulating effects, statins also improve inflammation, endothelial function, oxidative stress, angiogenesis, thrombosis, and plaque stability (Oesterle, 2017).

Large-scale primary and secondary prevention trials in populations without renal disease clearly show that statins reduce cardiovascular morbidity and mortality (Chou, 2016). Statins have been shown to effectively reduce LDL-C in CKD, and subgroup analyses of primary prevention trials in patients with stages 1–3 CKD have shown reduction in all-cause mortality and cardiovascular events with statin therapy (Table 12.2).

Prevention of Renal and Vascular End-Stage Disease Intervention Trial (PREVEND IT) was the first prospective randomized controlled trial (RCT) to assess the cardiovascular benefit of statins for primary prevention in early CKD (Asselbergs, 2004). In this 2×2 factorial design substudy which compared fosinopril and pravastatin to placebo in subjects with persistent microalbuminuria, pravastatin was associated with a nonsignificant 13% reduction in the primary end point of cardiovascular death and hospitalization. Unfortunately, this study was severely limited by its small sample size and low event rates.

In the largest randomized, double-blind, placebo-controlled statin trial in CKD, the SHARP study assessed the effect of simvastatin 20 mg plus ezetimibe 10 mg versus matching placebo on atherosclerotic events in 9,270 patients with CKD (predialysis CKD $n = 6,247$; dialysis $n = 3,023$) and no known history of myocardial infarction or coronary revascularization (Baigent, 2011). The combination of simvastatin plus ezetimibe was associated with LDL lowering and a significant 17% reduction in major atherosclerotic events, but had no significant effect on progression of CKD, all-cause mortality, or cancer incidence compared with placebo.

Several meta-analyses have since been conducted to affirm the effect of statins on cardiovascular outcomes in CKD. The most recent meta-analysis using individual participant data from more than 183,000 subjects reported a 21% reduction in risk of major vascular events per mmol/L reduction in LDL-C with statins (Cholesterol Treatment Trialists, 2016). Furthermore, a greater relative risk reduction was shown in earlier stage CKD with little evidence of benefit in those with advanced CKD including those on dialysis. Statin therapy had no effect on nonvascular mortality regardless of renal function. Taken together, these support the use of statin therapy for primary cardiovascular prevention in nondialysed CKD patients.

Cholesterol Absorption Inhibitors

Cholesterol absorption inhibitors (e.g., ezetimibe) effectively lower LDL-C and TG while increasing HDL-C by inhibiting the intestinal uptake of dietary and biliary cholesterol through their specific binding to the transport molecule, Niemann–Pick C1 Like-1 (NPC1L1) protein. In the Improved Reduction of Outcomes: Vytorin Efficacy International Trial (IMPROVE-IT), addition of ezetimibe to simvastatin (40 mg daily) was shown to modestly improve cardiovascular outcome (hazard ratio 0.94; 95% confidence interval [CI] 0.89–0.99, $p = 0.016$) in stable non-CKD patients with recent acute coronary syndrome and LDL-C within guideline recommendations (Cannon,

TABLE 12.2 Some Pivotal Lipid-Lowering Trials Which Assess Cardiovascular Outcomes in Nondialysis-Dependent Chronic Kidney Disease Subjects

Study (Author, Year)	Trial Design	Median Follow-Up	No. of Subjects	Patient Population	Intervention and Comparator	Primary Outcome
PREVEND IT (Asselbergs, 2004)	2×2 factorial (substudy)	46 months	864	Persistent microalbuminuria (spot urinary albumin >10 mg/L and 15–300 mg/24 hours)	Fosinopril 20 mg daily/ pravastatin 40 mg daily vs. placebo	Pravastatin showed a 13% nonsignificant reduction in composite outcome of CV mortality and hospitalization for CV morbidity.
SHARP (Baigent 2011)	RCT	4.9 years	9,270 (6,247 CKD)	CKD, HD, PD	Simvastatin 20 mg vs. simvastatin 20 mg/ezetimibe 10 mg vs. placebo	Simvastatin/ezetimibe was associated with a 17% reduction in major atherosclerotic events but had no effect on mortality.
Cholesterol Treatment Trialists (Cholesterol Treatment Trialists, 2016)	Meta-analysis	4.9 years	183,419 (28 trials)	All stages of CKD including dialysis	Statin vs. placebo or conventional therapy	Statin reduced the risk of first major vascular event (coronary events, revascularization, and stroke) by 21% per mmol/L reduction in LDL-C but had no effect on nonvascular mortality.
Jun et al. (Jun, 2012)	Meta-analysis	3 months– 5.1 years	16,869 (10 RCTs)	Subgroup analysis (eGFR >60 vs. <60 mL/min per 1.73 m²)	Fibrates vs. placebo/fish oil/dietary counseling	Fibrate therapy led to a 30% reduction in risk of major CV event and 40% reduction in CV death.
VA-HIT (Tonelli, 2004)	Post hoc subgroup analyses	5.1 years	1,046	Men with CrCl <75 mL/min, documented CVD	Gemfibrozil 1,200 mg daily vs. placebo	Gemfibrozil was associated with a significant 26% lower incidence of coronary death or nonfatal MI compared with placebo.

CKD, chronic kidney disease; CrCl, creatinine clearance by Cockcroft–Gault equation; CV, cardiovascular; CVD, cardiovascular disease; eGFR, estimated glomerular filtration rate; HD, hemodialysis; LDL-C, low-density lipoprotein-cholesterol; MI, myocardial infarction; PD, peritoneal dialysis; PPP, Prospective Pravastatin Pooling Project; RCT, randomized controlled trial; SHARP, Study of Heart and Renal Protection; VA-HIT, Veterans Affairs High-Density Lipoprotein Intervention Trial.

2015). Furthermore, a secondary analysis of the IMPROVE-IT study reported greatest relative and absolute CV risk reductions with the addition of ezetimibe in those at higher risk of recurrent CV events, as determined by a 9-point risk stratification tool which included CKD (Bohula, 2017). Whether ezetimibe has a similar independent additive effect in patients with CKD cannot be resolved by the SHARP study given the lack of a statin-only arm.

Fibric Acid Derivatives
Fibrates induce the expression of genes involved in intracellular fatty acid metabolism through activation of the peroxisome proliferator–activated receptor alpha (PPAR-α). Fibrates effectively lower TG (30% to 50%), decrease LDL-C, and raise HDL-C concentrations; potentially reversing the most common lipid abnormality associated with CKD.

The lipid-regulating effects of fibrates are mediated by:

(a) induction of lipoprotein lipolysis,
(b) stimulation of hepatic fatty acid uptake and reduction of hepatic TG production,
(c) increased removal of LDL particles,
(d) reduction of neutral lipid transfer between VLDL and HDL, and
(e) stimulation of reverse cholesterol transport (Staels, 1998).

A post hoc analysis of the Veterans Affairs High-Density Lipoprotein Intervention Trial (VA-HIT) demonstrated a 42% lower cardiovascular event rate with gemfibrozil in those with creatinine clearance <75 mL/min, diabetes, and HDL-C <40 mg/dL (1.04 mmol/L) compared with placebo (Tonelli, 2004). In a meta-analysis of 10 RCTs (not CKD specific), which included ~17,000 subjects, fibrate therapy in those with CKD (estimated glomerular filtration rate [eGFR] <60 mL/min per 1.73 m^2) was associated with improvement in lipid profile, as well as a 30% lower risk of major cardiovascular events (95% CI 0.38–0.96, $p = 0.004$) and 40% lower risk cardiovascular death (95% CI 0.38–0.96, $p = 0.03$) but had no effect on all-cause mortality (Jun, 2012). However, until similar findings are replicated in adequately powered outcome studies in CKD, broader use of fibrates will be limited by safety concerns relating to reversible increases in serum creatinine.

Nicotinic Acid
Nicotinic acid (niacin), a form of vitamin B$_3$, in higher doses has an overall favorable impact on dyslipidemia of CKD. By inhibiting adipocyte lipolysis through the nicotinic acid receptors, niacin effectively lowers TG, LDL-apoB, VLDL-C, and Lp(a), while increasing HDL-C concentration. Disappointingly, two large RCTs, the Atherothrombosis Intervention in Metabolic Syndrome with Low HDL-Cholesterol/High Triglyceride and Impact on Global Health Outcomes (AIM HIGH) and Heart Protection Study-2: Treatment of HDL to Reduce the Incidence of Vascular Events (HPS-2 THRIVE) trials and a meta-analysis of niacin in statin-treated non-CKD patients failed to show reductions in cardiovascular event and all-cause mortality despite

increasing HDL-C levels and were associated with increased risk of serious adverse events (Mani and Rohatgi, 2015). The role of niacin in CVD prevention has not systematically been assessed in patients with CKD despite its potential renoprotective properties (Streja, 2015).

Bile Acid Sequestrants

Bile acid sequestrants (BASs) (i.e., resin cholestyramine and colestipol or nonabsorbable polymer colesevelam hydrochloride) are anion exchange resins that lower LDL-C by binding bile acids in the gut and thereby blocking distal reabsorption. When used in combination with a statin, colesevelam has also been shown to lower apoB and to raise apoA-I while having a neutral effect on TG (Jones and Nwose, 2013). While not specifically studied in CKD, an early clinical trial of cholestyramine showed a 19% significant reduction in coronary heart disease (CHD) death and nonfatal myocardial infarction with LDL-C lowering in the Lipid Research Clinics Coronary Primary Prevention Trial (Jones and Nwose, 2013).

Omega-3 Polyunsaturated Fatty Acids

Omega-3 polyunsaturated fatty acids (fish oils) are essential fatty acids which consist of eicosapentaenoic acid (EPA) and docosahexaenoic acid (DHA). At pharmacologic doses (at least 2 g/day), fish oil reduces TG levels, mildly raise HDL-C, and increase LDL-C particle size (Pirillo and Catapano, 2015). Fish oil exerts their TG-lowering property by inhibiting enzymes involved in hepatic TG synthesis, reducing VLDL particle synthesis and enhancing TG removal through upregulation of lipoprotein lipase activity in extrahepatic tissues. Furthermore, fish oil affects lipid metabolism through activation of the PPAR-α receptor. Beyond TG lowering, other potential cardioprotective benefits of fish oil include blood pressure lowering, antiarrhythmic and antithrombotic properties, as well as, favorable effect on endothelial function. Higher dose fish oil supplements are available on prescription as ethyl esters (i.e., Omacor®, icosapent ethyl eicosapentaenoic acid [Vascepa®]) or carboxyl acids (Epanova®) as lipid-regulating agents.

While numerous epidemiologic, observational, and interventional studies in nonrenal populations suggest a cardioprotective role for fish oil supplementation, current RCT evidence has not consistently shown reduction in cardiovascular events in various risk groups (Siscovick, 2017). Some of these outcome studies are limited by the use of relatively low doses of fish oil (i.e., 1.8 g/day), use of agents with low EPA to DHA ratio, and intervention in low-risk nonhypertriglyceridemic subjects.

While the effect of fish oil supplementation on cardiovascular outcomes has not been specifically studied in nondialysis-dependent CKD subjects, a prospective RCT of fish oil supplementation in chronic hemodialysis patients reported significant reductions in the secondary end points of myocardial infarction and major coronary events but not the primary composite end point (Svensson, 2006). Another RCT, which assessed the effects of fish oil (1.6-g omega-3 fatty acids) on arteriovenous graft patency in Canadian hemodialysis patients, also reported significant reductions in the secondary end points of cardiovascular events and cardiac-related death (Lok, 2012). Additional prospective cardiovascular outcome studies in patients with nondialysis-dependent CKD will be required to confirm these findings.

MANAGEMENT OF DYSLIPIDEMIA IN CHRONIC KIDNEY DISEASE

There have been major changes in recent years to treatment recommendations for managing dyslipidemia in patients with CKD. Closely mirroring the lipid guidelines set by the American College of Cardiology (ACC) and the American Heart Association (AHA) (Stone, 2014), the updated 2013 Kidney Disease Improving Global Outcomes (KDIGO) Lipid guidelines presented a radical shift from a "treat to LDL target" approach to "fire and forget" with the use of fixed-dose statin therapy depending on the presence of clinical ASCVD and cardiovascular risk category (KDIGO, 2013). While statins continue to be strongly advocated, use of nonstatin lipid-lowering medications for primary or secondary CVD prevention was no longer recommended given the paucity of evidence from RCTs showing reduction in ASCVD events.

While the 2013 KDIGO guidelines received endorsement from Kidney Health Australia-Caring for Renal Impairment (KHA-CARI) (Palmer, 2014) and National Kidney Foundation–Kidney Disease Outcomes Quality Initiative (NKF-KDOQI) (Sarnak, 2015), other international organizations including the National Lipid Association (NLA) (Jacobson, 2015), Canadian Society of Cardiology (CSC) (Anderson, 2016), United Kingdom National Institute for Health and Care Excellence (UK-NICE) (NICE, 2014), European Society of Cardiology/European Atherosclerosis Society (ESC/EAS, 2011), and American Association of Clinical Endocrinologist/American College of Endocrinology (AACE/ACE) (Jellinger, 2017) published their own recommendations, with some making specific recommendations for CKD patients. Table 12.3 summarizes key similarities and differences in recommendations for patients with CKD from various international groups.

Screening, Monitoring, and Treatment Targets

Dyslipidemia is common but not universal in CKD, making it important to measure lipid profile in all newly diagnosed CKD patients. KDIGO recommends that initial lipid assessment be performed to estimate cardiovascular risk and identify those who may have secondary causes for dyslipidemia. While previous treatment guidelines by KDOQI in 2004 identified LDL-C lowering as the cornerstone of therapy, with non–HDL-C as a secondary target (Kidney Disease Outcomes Quality Initiative [K/DOQI] Group 2003), KDIGO did not define an LDL-C target but placed a greater emphasis on cardiovascular risk reduction to guide treatment decisions (KDIGO, 2013).

In contrast, other international organizations have continued to advocate LDL as a primary treatment target (see Table 12.3). Moreover, the recent NLA guideline recommends non–HDL-C as the primary target and considers this as a better measure of total of atherogenic burden (Jacobson, 2015). Measurement of serum apoB levels, which

TABLE 12.3 Comparison of Screening and Treatment Recommendations by Various International Organizations on Lipid Management in Patients With CKD

	Kidney Disease Improving Global Outcomes (KDIGO, 2013)	AACE (Jellinger, 2017)	CSC (Anderson, 2016)	United Kingdom-NICE (NICE, 2014)	NLA (Jacobson, 2015)	ESC/EAS (ESC/EAS, 2011)
Year	2013	2017	2016	2014 (update 2016)	2015	2011
Specific recommendation for CKD	Specific for CKD	CKD stage 3/4 are categorized as high (no risk factor), very high (with >1 risk factor), or extreme risk (with clinical ASCVD)	Considers CKD as statin-indicated condition	Specific recommendation for CKD	Considers CKD 3B/4 in high-risk category	CKD considered very high risk
Screening measurement	Fasting lipid profile	Fasting lipid profile	Nonfasting lipid profile	Nonfasting lipid profile	Fasting or nonfasting lipid profile	Fasting lipid profile apoB or apoB/AI as alternatives
Treatment targets	None	High risk: LDL-C <100 mg/dL Very high risk: LDL-C <70 mg/dL Extremely high risk: LDL-C <55 mg/dL	LDL-C <77.2 mg/dL or >50% reduction	Non–HDL-C: >40% reduction	Non–HDL-C <130 and LDL-C <100 mg/dL apoB <90 mg/dL optional target	LDL <70 mg/dL
Secondary lipid targets	TLC for hypertriglyceridemia	High risk: non–HDL-C <130, apoB <90 mg/dL Very high risk: non–HDL-C <100, apoB <80 mg/dL Extremely high risk: non–HDL-C <80, apoB <70 mg/dL	Non–HDL-C <100 or apoB <80 mg/dL	None	TG if >500 g/dL (risk of pancreatitis)	None

Risk Assessment Tool	Any validated risk prediction tool (FRS, SCORE, PROCAM, ASSIGN, QRISK2)	FRS MESA RRS UKPDS (T2DM)	Modified FRS CLEM	QRISK2 should not be used in CKD and/or albuminuria	Risk calculator should not be used in CKD 3B/4	SCORE
Recommended pharmacotherapy	Statin or statin/ ezetimibe: age ≥50 years with eGFR <60 Statin: age ≥50 years with eGFR ≥60; age 18–49 years with CKD with >1 of the following: CAD; DM prior CVA; estimated 10-year ASCVD risk >10%	Statins recommended to achieve target LDL-C	Statin or a statin/ ezetimibe combination indicated in CKD patients age >50 years	Atorvastatin 20 mg for the primary or secondary prevention Dose increase if >40% reduction in non–HDL-C is not achieved and eGFR >30 Consult renal specialist if higher statin dose needed for patients with eGFR <30	Moderate- to high-intensity statin	Statin (atorvastatin/ fluvastatin) In CKD 5, use low-dose statin with minimal renal excretion
Support combination therapy and use of nonstatin agents	No	Yes	Yes Consider addition of BAS, fibrate, and PCSK9 inhibitor Avoid combination with niacin	No Fibrates, nicotinic acid, BAS, omega-3 FA not routinely recommended for CVD prevention	Yes Consider combination with ezetimibe, BAS, extended-release niacin to achieve lower treatment goals Avoid fibrates in CKD 3B or greater	Consider use of prescription omega-3 fatty acids to lower TG Avoid fenofibrate if GFR <50 Reduce gemfibrozil dose to 600 mg/day if eGFR <60 and avoid if GFR <15

(continued)

TABLE 12.3 Comparison of Screening and Treatment Recommendations by Various International Organizations on Lipid Management in Patients With CKD *(Continued)*

	Kidney Disease Improving Global Outcomes (KDIGO, 2013)	AACE (Jellinger, 2017)	CSC (Anderson, 2016)	United Kingdom–NICE (NICE, 2014)	NLA (Jacobson, 2015)	ESC/EAS (ESC/EAS, 2011)
Treatment of dialysis patients	Do not initiate, but continue if on statin at dialysis initiation	Not discussed	Not discussed	No recommendation	No recommendation	No recommendation
Monitoring and surveillance	Not required for majority	Assess at 6 weeks after statin initiation then 6-weekly intervals until treatment goal achieved, then 6–12 monthly	Monitoring frequency not specified	Assess at 3 months after statin initiation to monitor degree of non–HDL-C reduction	Monitoring frequency not specified	Assess at 6–8 weeks after statin initiation or dose change, then monitor 6–12 monthly

Note: To convert from mg/dL to mmol/L: total, HDL, non-HDL, and LDL cholesterol divide mg/dL by 38.67; triglycerides divide mg/dL by 88.57. ApoB divide mg/dL by 100.

AACE/ACE, American Association of Clinical Endocrinologist/American College of Endocrinology; apoAI, apolipoprotein AI; apoB, apolipoprotein B; ASCVD, atherosclerotic cardiovascular disease; ASSIGN, CV risk estimation model from the Scottish Intercollegiate Guidelines Network; BAS, bile acid sequestrant; CAD, coronary artery disease; CSC, Canadian Society of Cardiology; CLEM, Cardiovascular Life Expectancy Model; CVD, cardiovascular disease; eGFR, estimated glomerular filtration rate in mL/min per 1.73 m²; ESC/EAS, European Society of Cardiology/European Atherosclerosis Society; FRS, Framingham Risk Score; KDIGO, Kidney Disease: Improving Global Outcomes; LDL-C, low-density lipoprotein-cholesterol; HDL-C, high-density lipoprotein-cholesterol; NLA, National Lipid Association; MESA, Multi-Ethnic Study of Atherosclerosis; PCSK9, proprotein convertase subtilisin/kexin type 9; PROCAM, Prospective Cardiovascular Munster Study; RRS, Reynolds Risk Score; SCORE, Systemic Coronary Risk Estimation; TLC, therapeutic lifestyle changes; TG, triglyceride; T2DM, type 2 diabetes mellitus; NICE, National Institute for Health and Care Clinical Excellence; UKPDS, United Kingdom Prospective Diabetes Study.

represents the number of atherogenic apoB-100–containing particles, is also thought to provide a more robust cardiovascular risk assessment than the standard plasma lipid profile. However, the measurement of apoB is limited by the lack of laboratory standardization and adds to the cost of a standard lipid measurement.

Repeated measurement of lipids in CKD following initiation of treatment is no longer recommended by the 2013 KDIGO guideline, given that LDL-C does not discriminate between high- and low-risk individuals and has not been shown to improve outcome or adherence to therapy (KDIGO, 2013). Furthermore, the association between LDL-C and adverse clinical outcome is weaker in CKD, limiting the value of ongoing monitoring once therapy is initiated. In our opinion, monitoring the plasma lipid profile should still be considered to assess adherence to therapy or when considering reducing statin dose due to adverse effects as reflected in other lipid guidelines (see Table 12.3).

Clinical Practice Guidelines and Treatment Recommendations
Therapeutic Lifestyle Changes

A wealth of epidemiologic and controlled clinical trials data strongly supports the notion that dietary recommendations can effectively lower CHD in the general population. Although there is a paucity of evidence of similar benefit in CKD, current treatment guidelines continue to emphasize the importance of adopting a healthy lifestyle in the management of dyslipidemia and prevention of ASCVD. KDIGO specifies the importance of dietary modification, weight reduction, increased physical activity, reducing alcohol intake, and control of hyperglycemia in the management of hypertriglyceridemia (KDIGO, 2013).

Dietary recommendations include adherence to a low-fat diet (<15% total calories), reduction of monosaccharide and disaccharide intake, reduction in the amount of total dietary carbohydrates, and use of fish oil to replace some long-chain TGs. Consumption of fish, especially oily fish enriched in very–long-chain omega-3 polyunsaturated fatty acids twice a week, assists in displacement of saturated and trans-fatty acids from the diet and may assist in lowering plasma TG. Dietary advice from a renal dietitian may be sought to maintain a balance between reducing dietary fat, protein, phosphorus, and potassium intake while maintaining adequate nutrition, particularly in those with more advanced CKD.

Regular exercise should also be encouraged for all because available data support favorable effects of exercise training on the lipid and lipoprotein profile (Gordon, 2014). Endurance exercise training has been shown to reduce TGs, increase apoA-I levels, and increase HDL-C concentration. Aerobic training with accompanying weight loss can lead to reductions in total cholesterol, LDL-C, VLDL-C, and TG with improvement in HDL-C levels. In recent years, resistance exercise training has also been shown to lower LDL-C and non–HDL-C levels possibly through maintenance of muscle mass, higher resting metabolic rate, better insulin control, and increased fat metabolism.

Drug Therapy

Statins. Based on current trial evidence, the latest KDIGO guidelines advocate the use of fixed-dose statin for primary prevention of ASCVD in practically all nondialyzed CKD patients who are 50 years of age or older.

For those adult nondialyzed CKD patients younger than 50 (age 18–49) statin therapy is recommended if one or more of the following risk factors is present: known coronary artery disease; diabetes mellitus; prior ischemic stroke; or estimated 10-year incidence of coronary death or nonfatal myocardial infarction >10% (KDIGO, 2013).

KDIGO recommends statin doses based on clinical trials in CKD as listed in Table 12.4. The simplified KDIGO guidelines aim to enhance implementation in CKD, a population known to be undertreated. However, concerns have been raised regarding overtreatment of older individuals given that KDIGO does not set an upper limit for age. Other guidelines also advocate the use of statins as first-line therapy with dose escalation suggested if treatment goals are not achieved (see Table 12.3).

The almost universal recommendation for statin therapy in patients with mild-to-moderate CKD puts patients at risk of unintended adverse effects, placing greater emphasis on the safety features of these agents. Although statins are considered safe for use in CKD, risk of complications, particularly myopathy and rhabdomyolysis, may increase when statins metabolized by the CYP450 3A4 system are coadministered with drugs metabolized by the same pathway (Table 12.5). When coadministration of such agents is unavoidable, it is prudent to commence CYP450-metabolized statins at a low dose to decrease the risk of myopathy and rhabdomyolysis. Alternatively, one may use statins that are not metabolized by the CYP450 3A4 pathway (e.g., fluvastatin, pravastatin, and rosuvastatin). Clinicians should also be aware that consumption of large quantities of grapefruit juice and red yeast rice, via their effect

TABLE 12.4	Recommended Statin Doses in Chronic Kidney Disease (eGFR Stages G3a–G5) (KDIGO, 2013)	
Statin	**Recommended Dose Per Day (mg)**	**Dose Adjustment With Advanced CKD**
Lovastatin	Not studied	N/A
Fluvastatin	80	No
Pravastatin	40	No
Simvastatin	40	Yes
Simvastatin/ezetimibe	20/10	Yes
Atorvastatin	20	No
Rosuvastatin	10	Yes

Source: Adapted from KDIGO with recommended doses based on clinical trials in CKD patients.

TABLE 12.5	Statins and Other Drugs Metabolized by CYP450 Isoenzymes	
CYP 3A4	**CYP 2C9**	**CYP 2C19**
Atorvastatin Simvastatin Lovastatin	Rosuvastatin Fluvastatin	Rosuvastatin
Macrolide antibiotics – Erythromycin – Clarithromycin	NSAIDs COX-2 inhibitors Phenytoin	Proton pump inhibitors – Omeprazole – Esomeprazole

Calcineurin inhibitors
– Cyclosporine
– Tacrolimus
– Sirolimus
	Angiotensin receptor
	  blockers
	– Irbesartan
	– Losartan
		Antidepressants
		– Tricyclic
		  antidepressants
		– SSRIs
		Diclofenac

Calcium channel blockers – Verapamil – Diltiazem – Amlodipine	Warfarin Sulfonylurea	Antiepileptic agents – Phenytoin – Diazepam
Azole antifungals – Ketoconazole – Itraconazole – Voriconazole		
Warfarin Amiodarone Tricyclic antidepressants SSRIs HIV protease inhibitors Proton pump inhibitors – Omeprazole – Esomeprazole Grapefruit juice (>1 quart) Red yeast rice		

CY, cytochrome; SSRIs, selective serotonin receptor inhibitors; HIV, human immunodeficiency virus; NSAIDs, nonsteroidal anti-inflammatory drugs.

on the cytochrome system, may increase the plasma levels of statins metabolized by CYP450 3A4.

Meta-analyses of large statin trials have shown an association between statins and higher risk of diabetes, prompting changes to labeling requirements to reflect this risk. Potential mechanisms include decrease in insulin levels due to attenuated beta-cell function, decreased insulin sensitivity caused by impaired insulin signaling, and dysglycemia from decrease in adiponectin levels (Rocco, 2012).

The effect of different statins on renal function has also been investigated. The Prospective Evaluation of Proteinuria and Renal Function in Diabetic and Non-Diabetic Patients with Progressive Renal Disease studies, which assessed the effect of different statin regimens (rosuvastatin 10 mg or 40 mg, or atorvastatin 80 mg) on proteinuria and eGFR over 52 weeks in diabetic (PLANET I) and non-diabetic CKD (PLANET II) patients with proteinuria, suggested that while the different statins were effective in lowering LDL, high-dose atorvastatin may reduce proteinuria without affecting eGFR when compared with rosuvastatin (de Zeeuw, 2015). However, caution must be exercised when interpreting these results given the lack of a placebo arm.

Overall, it is important to have an individualized assessment of the risk of toxicity balanced to the cardioprotective benefit when initiating statin therapy especially in lower-risk adults who will have a similar risk of side effects but have a smaller absolute risk reduction.

Cholesterol Absorption Inhibitors. Based on the SHARP study, KDIGO recommends the use of ezetimibe in combination with a statin in those aged over 50 years with an eGFR <60 mL/min per 1.73 m^2 (KDIGO, 2013). Other guidelines, also advocate the addition of ezetimibe as combination therapy (see Table 12.3). Because ezetimibe is predominantly metabolized by glucuronidation in the liver and excreted in the feces, dose adjustment is not required for patients with renal insufficiency. Data from the SHARP study indicate that ezetimibe is well tolerated with little risk of hepatotoxicity, myopathy, or renal dysfunction.

Fibrates. Fibrates are generally well tolerated and have a low incidence of serious side effects. However, use of fenofibrate has been frequently associated with a rise in serum creatinine, which is often reversible. The rise in creatinine with fenofibrate may not reflect a true decline in renal function but rather, increased endogenous production of creatinine from muscle creatine, a mechanism that may also account for the frequently observed increase in plasma homocysteine levels. Another proposed mechanism for the increase in creatinine is impaired generation of vasodilatory prostaglandins due to activation of PPARs. More studies are required to determine the mechanisms and relevance of fibrate-induced increase in creatinine.

The 2013 KDIGO guideline no longer recommends the use of fibrates in patients with mild hypertriglyceridemia given the weak evidence for safety and efficacy in patients with CKD and effective TG lowering with statins (KDIGO, 2013). However, fibrates, dose adjusted to renal function, may be considered in those with severe hypertriglyceridemia (>11.3 mmol/L or >1,000 mg/dL) to mitigate the risk of acute pancreatitis.

Nicotinic Acid. In CKD, niacin has the added benefit of lowering serum phosphate through direct inhibition of the NaPi-2a sodium-dependent phosphate cotransporter in the gut and kidneys. Renoprotection has also been postulated through attenuation of oxidative stress and inflammation in experimental models of kidney disease and small clinical trials (Streja, 2015).

Unfortunately, use of niacin is limited by poor tolerability from prostaglandin-mediated cutaneous flushing, which may be attenuated by using the extended- rather than immediate-release formulation, ingestion of aspirin, reduced consumption of saturated fat, and concomitant administration of laropiprant (potent inhibitor of the prostaglandin D_2 receptor). Other concerns relate to increased risk of myotoxicity, hyperuricemia, and dysglycemia that is due to its predominant renal elimination. Niacin also causes thrombocytopenia. Given the insufficient evidence for benefit and concerns relating to drug tolerability and toxicity in CKD, this class of drugs is not recommended in the management of hypertriglyceridemia in CKD (Anderson, 2016; KDIGO, 2013).

Bile Acid Sequestrants. The improved gastrointestinal side effect profile of second-generation BAS drugs such as colesevelam has led to a recent increase in their clinical use. Colesevelam is associated with a lower potential for drug–drug interaction particularly when drug administration is staggered by at least 4 hours (Jones and Nwose, 2013). BASs have important glucose-lowering properties, and colesevelam is now indicated for glycemic control in diabetic patients. While not well studied in patients with CKD, the favorable toxicity profile and potential to improve glycemic control have led KDIGO and other guidelines to recommend the use of BAS as second-line agents for LDL-C lowering in CKD (see Table 12.3).

Omega-3 Polyunsaturated Fatty Acids. The AHA recently published a position statement affirming that current RCTs do not support the use of fish oil supplementation for primary CVD prevention in the general population, in those who are prediabetic and with known DM (Siscovick, 2017). However, given its low toxicity risk, it may be considered for secondary prevention in those at high risk of CVD and could benefit those who have had a previous myocardial infarction or heart failure. Specific recommendation regarding the use of fish oil is not available for CKD given the paucity of clinical studies.

Practical Approach to Managing Dyslipidemia in Chronic Kidney Disease
In all newly diagnosed patients with CKD, an initial standard lipid profile is prudent to assess for baseline ASCVD risk. Secondary causes for dyslipidemia should be considered in patients with known or family history of premature CVD, significant abnormalities in standard lipid profile (i.e., LDL-C >4.5 mmol/L, TG >4.0 mmol/L, HDL-C <0.7 mmol/L, non–HDL-C >5.1 mmol/L), or when clinical clues to an inherited dyslipidemia (i.e., arcus senilis or tendon xanthoma) are noted.

Following an assessment of an individual's 10-year ASCVD risk using any of the validated tools, a discussion regarding current trial evidence, potential benefits and risk of therapy, as well as cost of lipid-lowering medications should occur to facilitate shared decision making regarding need for pharmacotherapy. Regardless, all patients must be encouraged to adopt a healthy lifestyle.

Statin-based therapy remains the cornerstone of treatment once it has been decided that pharmacotherapy is expected to be beneficial. For primary prevention, begin with low- to moderate-intensity statin (pravastatin 20 mg/day or 40 mg/day, atorvastatin 10 mg/day or 20 mg/day) and consider intensifying treatment, depending on need for greater ASCVD risk reduction and drug tolerability. For secondary prevention, one can begin with a high-intensity statin (atorvastatin 40 mg/day or 80 mg/day).

Discuss and consider the addition of evidence-based nonstatin therapy, such as ezetimibe, when additional ASCVD risk reduction is required. For those with mild to moderate intolerance to statins, consider switching to lower potency statins prior to changing to a nonstatin-based agent. Consider and discuss retesting the standard lipid profile to assess adherence to therapy and in those who develop clinical ASCVD. Regularly reassess the patient's goals for ASCVD risk reduction, tolerance to medication, and treatment plan (see Fig. 12.2).

NOVEL LIPID-MODIFYING AGENTS

Progress in our understanding of lipid and lipoprotein metabolism has led to the discovery of novel LDL-lowering therapies (Cupido, 2017). These new agents have the potential to act as adjunct therapy to reduce residual ASCVD risk in statin-treated patients who remain at high ASCVD risk, such as patients with CKD.

Inhibiting PCSK9 leads to reduction in LDL-C concentration by increasing hepatic uptake and clearance of LDL-C through reduction in degradation of LDL receptors. Two PCSK9 monoclonal antibodies (mAb), evolocumab and alirocumab, have been approved as adjunct therapy to dietary modification in those adults with familial hypercholesterolemia or clinical ASCVD who fail to achieve LDL-C targets despite being on maximum-tolerated dose of statins as monotherapy or in combination with other lipid-lowering agents, or in those who show statin intolerance or in whom statin treatment is contraindicated. Evolocumab has been shown not only to lower LDL-C level by a median of 0.78 mmol/L (30 mg/dL) in statin-treated patients but also reduce the combined end points of cardiovascular events (Sabatine, 2017). PCSK9 inhibitors are delivered as fortnightly or monthly subcutaneous injections. Experience to date has reported minimal side effects except for minor injection site reactions (5%). PCSK9 mAb have not been studied specifically in patients with eGFR <30 mL/min per 1.73 m^2 and should be used with caution in CKD patients.

CETP inhibitors have been shown to significantly raise HDL-C and lower LDL-C by inhibiting the transfer of CE from HDL-C to either VLDL or LDL. While clinical trials of several CETP inhibitors including torcetrapib, dalcetrapib, and evacetrapib have yielded disappointing results due to increased toxicity or lack of efficacy, the recently

Measure nonfasting standard lipid profile (LDL-C, non–HDL-C, and TGs) in all newly diagnosed adults with CKD for baseline risk stratification

⬇

Consider referral to specialty lipid clinic if a secondary cause for dyslipidemia is suspected (i.e., history of premature CVD and lipid profile showing LDL-C >4.5 mmol/L, TG >4.0 mmol/L, HDL-C <0.7 mmol/L, non–HDL-C >5.1 mmol/L with or without physical signs)

⬇

Assess the patient's 10-year ASCVD risk using a validated tool

Nondialyzed CKD patients in the following high-risk categories based on KDIGO:
1) age 50 years or more (stages G1–G5)
2) age 18–49 years with one or more of the following: known coronary arterydisease; diabetes mellitus; prior ischemic stroke; estimated 10-year incidence of coronarydeath or nonfatal MI >10%

⬇

Discuss evidence, benefits, risks, and cost of lipid-lowering medications in shared decision making

⬇

Encourage a healthy lifestyle for all

⬇

If the shared decision supports treatment:

For primary prevention:	For secondary prevention:
Begin with low- to moderate-intensity statin (pravastatin 20 mg/day or 40 mg/day, atorvastatin 10 mg/day or 20 mg/day)	Begin with high-intensity statin (atorvastatin 40 mg/day or 80 mg/day)
Intensify treatment depending on need for greater ASCVD risk reduction and tolerability	For those who require additional ASCVD risk reduction, discuss and consider the addition of evidence-based nonstatin therapy, such as ezetimibe

⬇

For mild-to-moderate intolerance to statins, consider switching to lower potency statin prior to changing to a nonstatin-based agent (i.e., ezetimibe or colesevelam)

⬇

Discuss retesting standard lipid profile to assess adherence to therapy and in those who develop clinical ASCVD

⬇

Regularly reassess patient's goals for ASCVD risk reduction, tolerance to medication, and treatment plan

Abbreviations: ASCVD (atherosclerotic cardiovascular disease); CKD (chronic kidney disease); eGFR (estimated glomerular filtration rate); HDL-C (high density lipoprotein-cholesterol); LDL-C (low density lipoprotein-cholesterol); TG (triglyceride)

FIGURE 12.2 Practical approach to managing dyslipidemia in chronic kidney disease for cardiovascular disease prevention.

published Randomized Evaluation of the Effects of Anacetrapib Through Lipid Modification (REVEAL) study reported a significant 10% reduction in the combined end point of coronary death, myocardial infarction, and coronary revascularization and 13% reduction in the secondary end point of myocardial infarction with no effect on coronary death with anacetrapib therapy for 4 years in 30,499 statin-treated adults aged over 50 years who were still at high risk of cardiovascular events (HPS TIMI55 REVEAL Collaborative, 2017). This positive, albeit modest, cardiovascular benefit was accompanied by a 20% lowering in LDL-C and doubling of HDL-C levels. Of interest was the small increase in blood pressure and decline in renal function. Other CETP-inhibitors (AMG-899 and K-312) are currently under investigation.

While discussions as to whether these agents, as well as others under development, hold the key to reducing the extremely high-residual CVD burden in CKD is beyond the scope of this handbook, their place in the management of dyslipidemia of CKD can only be determined by future cardiovascular outcomes trials. Until such time, the use of these novel agents in CKD cannot be justified given their extremely high cost.

SUMMARY AND CONCLUSIONS

Dyslipidemia is common in CKD and an important risk factor for CVD. The SHARP trial provided robust clinical trial evidence for a reduction in risk of ASCVD events (but not mortality) with statin therapy in those with mild-to-moderate CKD, prompting a major shift in recommendations from several international guidelines. While statin therapy is now universally advocated by some guidelines for nondialysed CKD patients regardless of LDL-C levels given their high cardiovascular risk burden, the decision to initiate pharmacotherapy must be individualized with careful discussion and consideration of the benefits, risks, and cost of treatment. Pharmacotherapy must be linked with therapeutic lifestyle changes such as improved nutrition, increased physical activity, and weight control in order to maximize benefit. Despite improved understanding of the benefits of statin therapy, patients with CKD remain at high CVD risk and novel lipid-lowering agents hold promise as future therapeutic options.

References and Suggested Readings

Anderson TJ, Gregoire J, Pearson GJ, et al. 2016 Canadian Cardiovascular Society guidelines for the management of dyslipidemia for the prevention of cardiovascular disease in the adult. *Can J Cardiol*. 2016;32:1263–1282.

Asselbergs FW, Diercks GF, Hillege HL, et al; Prevention of Renal and Vascular End-stage Disease Intervention Trial (PREVEND IT) Investigators. Effects of fosinopril and pravastatin on cardiovascular events in subjects with microalbuminuria. *Circulation*. 2004;110:2809–2816.

Baigent C, Landray MJ, Reith C, et al; SHARP Investigators. The effects of lowering LDL cholesterol with simvastatin plus ezetimibe in patients with chronic kidney disease (Study of Heart and Renal Protection): a randomised placebo-controlled trial. *Lancet*. 2011;377:2181–2192.

Bandeali S, Farmer J. High-density lipoprotein and atherosclerosis: the role of antioxidant activity. *Curr Atheroscler Rep.* 2012;14:101–107.

Bohula EA, Morrow DA, Giugliano RP, et al. Atherothrombotic risk stratification and ezetimibe for secondary prevention. *J Am Coll Cardiol.* 2017;69:911–921.

Cannon CP, Blazing MA, Giugliano RP, et al; IMPROVE-IT Investigators. Ezetimibe added to statin therapy after acute coronary syndromes. *N Engl J Med.* 2015;372:2387–2397.

Chan DT, Dogra GK, Irish AB, et al. Chronic kidney disease delays VLDL-apoB-100 particle catabolism: potential role of apolipoprotein C-III. *J Lipid Res.* 2009;50:2524–2531.

Cholesterol Treatment Trialists' (CTT) Collaboration; Herrington WG, Emberson J, Mihaylova B, et al. Impact of renal function on the effects of LDL cholesterol lowering with statin-based regimens: a meta-analysis of individual participant data from 28 randomised trials. *Lancet Diabetes Endocrinol.* 2016;4:829–839.

Chou R, Dana T, Blazina I, et al. Statins for prevention of cardiovascular disease in adults: Evidence report and systematic review for the US Preventive Services Task Force. *JAMA.* 2016;316:2008–2024.

Cupido AJ, Reeskamp LF, Kastelein JJP. Novel lipid modifying drugs to lower LDL cholesterol. *Curr Opin Lipidol.* 2017;28:367–373.

de Zeeuw D, Anzalone DA, Cain VA, et al. Renal effects of atorvastatin and rosuvastatin in patients with diabetes who have progressive renal disease (PLANET I): a randomised clinical trial. *Lancet Diabetes Endocrinol.* 2015;3:181–190.

European Association for Cardiovascular Prevention & Rehabilitation; Reiner Z, Catapano AL, De Backer G, et al. ESC/EAS guidelines for the management of dyslipidaemias: the Task Force for the management of dyslipidaemias of the European Society of Cardiology (ESC) and the European Atherosclerosis Society (EAS). *Eur Heart J.* 2011;32:1769–1818.

Ference BA, Ginsberg HN, Graham I, et al. Low-density lipoproteins cause atherosclerotic cardiovascular disease. 1. Evidence from genetic, epidemiologic, and clinical studies. A consensus statement from the European Atherosclerosis Society Consensus Panel. *Eur Heart J.* 2017;38:2459–2472.

Gordon B, Chen S, Durstine JL. The effects of exercise training on the traditional lipid profile and beyond. *Curr Sports Med Rep.* 2014;13:253–259.

HPS3/TIMI55–REVEAL Collaborative Group; Bowman L, Hopewell JC, Chen F, et al. Effects of anacetrapib in patients with atherosclerotic vascular disease. *N Engl J Med.* 2017;377:1217–1227.

Jacobson TA, Ito MK, Maki KC, et al. National lipid association recommendations for patient-centered management of dyslipidemia: part 1—full report. *J Clin Lipidol.* 2015;9:129–169.

Jellinger PS, Handelsman Y, Rosenblit PD, et al. American Association of Clinical Endocrinologists and American College of Endocrinology guidelines for management of dyslipidemia and prevention of cardiovascular disease—Executive summary complete appendix to guidelines available at http://journals.aace.com. *Endocr Pract.* 2017;23:479–497.

Jones MR, Nwose OM. Role of colesevelam in combination lipid-lowering therapy. *Am J Cardiovasc Drugs.* 2013;13:315–323.

Jun M, Zhu B, Tonelli M, et al. Effects of fibrates in kidney disease: a systematic review and meta-analysis. *J Am Coll Cardiol.* 2012;60:2061–2071.

Kidney Disease Outcomes Quality Initiative (K/DOQI) Group. K/DOQI clinical practice guidelines for management of dyslipidemias in patients with kidney disease. *Am J Kidney Dis.* 2003;41:I–IV, S1–S91.

Kidney Disease: Improving Global Outcomes Lipid Guideline Development Work Group Members. KDIGO clinical practice guideline for lipid management in chronic kidney disease. *Kidney Int Suppl.* 2013;3:259–305.

Liu S, Vaziri ND. Role of PCSK9 and IDOL in the pathogenesis of acquired LDL receptor deficiency and hypercholesterolemia in nephrotic syndrome. *Nephrol Dial Transplant.* 2014;29:538–543.

Lok CE, Moist L, Hemmelgarn BR, et al; Fish Oil Inhibition of Stenosis in Hemodialysis Grafts (FISH) Study Group. Effect of fish oil supplementation on graft patency and cardiovascular events among patients with new synthetic arteriovenous hemodialysis grafts: a randomized controlled trial. *JAMA.* 2012;307:1809–1816.

Luo M, Peng D. The emerging role of apolipoprotein C-III: beyond effects on triglyceride metabolism. *Lipids Health Dis.* 2016;15:184.

Mani P, Rohatgi A. Niacin therapy, HDL cholesterol, and cardiovascular disease: Is the HDL hypothesis defunct? *Curr Atheroscler Rep.* 2015;17:43.

National Institute for Health and Care Excellence. Cardiovascular disease: risk assessment and reduction, including lipid modification NICE guideline [CG181]. 2014. Available from http://www.nice.org.uk/guidance/cg181/resources/cardio-vascular-disease-risk-assessment-and-reduction-including-lipid-modification-pdf-35109807660997. Accessed September 5, 2017.

Nordestgaard BG. Triglyceride-rich lipoproteins and atherosclerotic cardiovascular disease: New insights from epidemiology, genetics, and biology. *Circ Res.* 2016; 118:547–563.

Oesterle A, Laufs U, Liao JK. Pleiotropic effects of statins on the cardiovascular system. *Circ Res.* 2017;120:229–243.

Palmer SC, Strippoli GF, Craig JC. KHA-CARI commentary on the KDIGO clinical practice guideline for Lipid Management in Chronic Kidney Disease. *Nephrology (Carlton).* 2014;19:663–666.

Pirillo A, Catapano AL. Update on the management of severe hypertriglyceridemia–focus on free fatty acid forms of omega-3. *Drug Des Devel Ther.* 2015;9:2129–2137.

Rocco MB. Statins and diabetes risk: fact, fiction, and clinical implications. *Cleve Clin J Med.* 2012;79:883–893.

Sabatine MS, Giugliano RP, Keech AC, et al; FOURIER Steering Committee and Investigators. Evolocumab and clinical outcomes in patients with cardiovascular disease. *N Engl J Med.* 2017;376:1713–1722.

Sarnak MJ, Bloom R, Muntner P. KDOQI US commentary on the 2013 KDIGO clinical practice guideline for lipid management in CKD. *Am J Kidney Dis.* 2015;65: 354–366.

Siscovick DS, Barringer TA, Fretts AM, et al; Council on Cardiovascular Disease in the Young; Council on Cardiovascular and Stroke Nursing; and Council on Clinical Cardiology. Omega-3 polyunsaturated fatty acid (fish oil) supplementation and the prevention of clinical cardiovascular disease: a science advisory from the American Heart Association. *Circulation.* 2017;135:e867–e884.

Staels B, Dallongeville J, Auwerx J, et al. Mechanism of action of fibrates on lipid and lipoprotein metabolism. *Circulation.* 1998;98:2088–2093.

Streja E, Kovesdy CP, Streja DA, et al. Niacin and progression of CKD. *Am J Kidney Dis.* 2015;65:785–798.

Svensson M, Schmidt EB, Jorgensen KA, et al; OPACH Study Group. N-3 fatty acids as secondary prevention against cardiovascular events in patients who undergo chronic hemodialysis: a randomized, placebo-controlled intervention trial. *Clin J Am Soc Nephrol.* 2006;1:780–786.

Tonelli M, Collins D, Robins S, et al; Veterans' Affairs High-Density Lipoprotein Intervention Trial (VA-HIT) Investigators. Gemfibrozil for secondary prevention of cardiovascular events in mild to moderate chronic renal insufficiency. *Kidney Int.* 2004;66:1123–1130.

Tsimikas S. A test in context: Lipoprotein(a): Diagnosis, prognosis, controversies, and emerging therapies. *J Am Coll Cardiol.* 2017;69:692–711.

Stone NJ, Robinson JG, Lichtenstein AH, et al. American College of Cardiology/ American Heart Association Task Force on Practice Guidelines. 2013 ACC/AHA guideline on the treatment of blood cholesterol to reduce atherosclerotic cardiovascular risk in adults: a report of the American College of Cardiology/American Heart Association Task Force on Practice Guidelines. *Circulation.* 2014;129: S1–S45.

Vaziri ND. Disorders of lipid metabolism in nephrotic syndrome: mechanisms and consequences. *Kidney Int.* 2016a;90:41–52.

Vaziri ND. HDL abnormalities in nephrotic syndrome and chronic kidney disease. *Nat Rev Nephrol.* 2016b;12:37–47.

13 Glucose Control in Diabetes Mellitus and Kidney Disease

Allison J. Hahr and Mark E. Molitch

Almost 29 million adults and children in the United States, about 9% of the population, have diabetes. Diabetes is the most common cause of kidney failure in the United States and one of the most common causes worldwide. Many people with diabetes don't know that they have it, and screening high-risk individuals. Groups most at risk are the overweight, those with relatives who have diabetes, and members of high-risk ethnic populations.

Diabetic kidney disease affects 20% to 40% of patients with diabetes (American Diabetes Association, 2018), and vigilant screening can identify diabetic kidney disease at an early stage. An American Diabetes Association Consensus Conference (Tuttle, 2014) and the Kidney Disease Outcomes Quality Initiative (KDOQI) guidelines and clinical practice recommendations for patients with diabetes and chronic kidney disease (CKD) (Kidney Disease Outcomes Quality Initiative, 2007; National Kidney Foundation, 2012) have set out a number of general principles regarding risk reduction for such patients (Table 13.1). The guidelines emphasize frequent screening; tight control of glycemia, blood pressure, and lipids; and careful attention to nutrition, exercise, and maintenance of a healthy lifestyle. CKD patients should be **screened** annually for diabetes, and those with diabetes should be screened annually for kidney disease, focusing on albuminuria detection and measurement of estimated glomerular filtration rate (eGFR). Screening patients with diabetes for eye disease as well as peripheral vascular disease and neuropathy is an important part of overall patient management. **Glycemia** should be controlled generally to an HbA_{1C} level target of 7% or lower. **Blood pressure** should be kept at 140/90 or lower using an angiotensin-converting enzyme inhibitor (ACEI) or an angiotensin receptor blocker (ARB), usually in combination with a diuretic (see Chapter 14). As detailed in Chapter 12, **lipid management** should consist of a high-intensity statin because of the high risk of cardiovascular disease (CVD) in diabetic patients with CKD (American College of Cardiology/American Heart Association, 2013; American Diabetes Association, 2018). Nutritional management includes **protein restriction** to 0.8 g/kg body weight per day as detailed in Chapter 7, as well as an emphasis on ingestion of low-glycemic index carbohydrates and unsaturated fats. Referral to a nephrologist should be considered when nephropathy progresses to an advanced stage (stage 4), especially if progression is rapid, if there is a question

TABLE 13.1	Guidelines for Patients With Chronic Kidney Disease and Diabetes	
Patient Group	**Test/Target**	**Comments**
Patients with CKD	Screen for diabetes using fasting glucose and/or HbA$_{1c}$	Yearly; more often in patients receiving immunosuppressives
Patients with diabetes	Screen for retinopathy, neuropathy, and foot ulcers	At least yearly
Patients with diabetes	Screen for microalbuminuria and estimated GFR based on serum creatinine	Yearly; begin 5 years after diagnosis in type 1 DM, at diagnosis in type 2 DM
Patients with diabetes and CKD	HbA$_{1c}$ target ≤7.0% HbA$_{1c}$ target >7.0% with advanced CKD and those at risk for hypoglycemia	Using ACEI and ARB as first choice of antihypertensive, especially when proteinuria is present
	BP target <140/90	Lower BP target not beneficial in one randomized trial
	High-intensity statin	Consider an LDL cholesterol target of <70 mg/dL (1.8 mmol/L) because high cardiovascular disease risk is present
	Protein intake 0.8 g/kg per day Target BMI <25 kg/m^2	

CKD, chronic kidney disease; GFR, glomerular filtration rate; DM, diabetes mellitus; ACEI, angiotensin-converting enzyme inhibitor; ARB, angiotensin receptor blocker; BP, blood pressure.
Source: Modified from Kidney Disease Outcomes Quality Initiative. KDOQI clinical practice guidelines and clinical practice recommendations for diabetes and chronic kidney disease. *Am J Kidney Dis.* 2007;49:S12–S154.

regarding etiology of the kidney disease, or if the clinician is unable to manage the hypertension and hyperkalemia.

SCREENING

Screening for Diabetes in Asymptomatic Adults

According to criteria set out by the American Diabetes Association (American Diabetes Association, 2018), testing should be considered in all adults who are overweight (body mass index [BMI] >25 kg/m^2 or >23 kg/m^2 in Asian Americans), who have one or more of the following risk factors: (1) a first-degree relative with diabetes, (2) ethnicity known to be at high risk for diabetes (e.g., African American, Latino, Native American, Asian American, Pacific Islander), (3) history of CVD or hypertension, (4) women with polycystic ovary syndrome, (5) physical inactivity, or (6) other conditions known to be associated with insulin resistance (severe obesity, acanthosis nigricans).

Patients with prediabetes (A$_{1C}$ ≥5.7% [39 mmol/mol], impaired glucose tolerance, or impaired (elevated, see below) fasting glucose) should be tested yearly. Women who have been diagnosed with gestational diabetes mellitus should have lifelong testing at least every 3 years. For all other patients, testing should begin at age 45 years. If results are normal, testing should be repeated at a minimum of 3-year intervals, with consideration of more frequent testing depending on initial results and risk status.

Screening Patients With Chronic Kidney Disease for Diabetes

Because of insulin resistance and other associated conditions, in addition to the high-risk patients listed above, patients with stages 3 to 5 CKD also should be screened annually for diabetes (Kidney Disease Outcomes Quality Initiative, 2007). Patients who have had a kidney transplant or who are receiving immunosuppressive drugs for other reasons may need to be screened more often as they are at particular risk; glucocorticoids are known to cause insulin resistance, and tacrolimus (and, to a lesser extent, cyclosporine and sirolimus) can exhibit toxicity to pancreatic islet cells (Wallia, 2016).

Detection of Diabetes Mellitus

To diagnose diabetes, several methods may be employed. Since 2010, the American Diabetes Association has included the use of HbA_{1c} for diagnosis (American Diabetes Association, 2018). Fasting plasma glucose (>126 mg/dL or 7.0 mmol/L) or HbA_{1c} ($\geq 6.5\%$) is preferred because they are easy, quick, and economical. The oral glucose tolerance test (OGTT) is more sensitive but also more time consuming. The OGTT can be used to look for diabetes in those with mildly increased fasting glucose or when diabetes is suspected in a patient with a normal fasting glucose (e.g., a woman with a history of gestational diabetes).

Screening Patients With Diabetes for Kidney Disease

Diabetic patients should be screened annually for evidence of kidney disease. In those with type 1 diabetes, annual screening should begin 5 years after initial diagnosis. The onset of type 1 diabetes is usually known, as it is characterized by high blood glucose levels leading to symptoms such as polyuria and polydipsia, bringing the affected individual to medical attention fairly quickly. Typically, microvascular disease as reflected by microalbuminuria starts to manifest 5 years or more after the initial diagnosis of type 1 diabetes because of cumulative excessive exposure to hyperglycemia. In contrast, with type 2 diabetes, screening for kidney disease should begin at the time of initial diagnosis. The exact date of onset of type 2 diabetes often will be unknown. Patients usually will have had hyperglycemia for a number of years before diagnosis and may have already developed nephropathy at the time that diagnosis is first made.

Recommended Screening Tests for Kidney Disease

The first sign of diabetic kidney disease typically is the onset of elevated albumin levels in the urine. Those who have albuminuria have greater rates of CKD progression than those who do not. However, about one-third of patients with both type 1 and type 2 diabetes may progress to CKD stage 3 and worse without ever developing albuminuria; whether these patients have the same pathology as those who develop albuminuria is not known (Krolewski, 2015). Thus, in addition to annual screening for albuminuria, annual measurement of serum creatinine with calculation of eGFR using the (Chronic Kidney Disease Epidemiology Collaboration) formula (Levey, 2009) should be performed.

Detection of Micro- and Macroalbuminuria

The detection of micro- and macroalbuminuria has been reviewed in Chapter 1. The current KDOQI recommended method is to analyze the ratio of albumin (mg) to creatinine (g) in a random (spot) urine sample. This is called the **albumin–creatinine ratio** or **ACR**. The amount of albumin can also be measured in a timed (24 hour or other period, such as 4 hour) urine collection; this was formerly the advised method, but most guideline recommendations have since been updated to favor the spot urine, which is more reliably useful in the clinical setting. An abnormal urine screen is defined as the presence of elevated albumin levels in the urine on at least two of three measurements done over a 6-month interval. **Microalbuminuria** is defined as a spot ACR of ≥30 to 299 mg/g, or ≥30 to 299 mg/24 h in a timed collection. **Albuminuria** or **macroalbuminuria** is defined as a spot ACR of ≥300 mg/g, or ≥300 mg/24 h in a timed collection. Recently, the National Kidney Foundation has also used the terms high albuminuria and very high albuminuria to describe microalbuminuria and macroalbuminuria (Levey, 2011). As discussed in Chapter 1, when evaluating urinary protein excretion, concurrent conditions and illnesses that can increase urinary albumin excretion should be considered and treated or avoided. These include urinary tract infections, postural proteinuria, exercise, blood (e.g., menstrual), and extreme hypertension.

Is the Kidney Disease the Result of Diabetes?

According to KDOQI diabetes/CKD guidelines (Kidney Disease Outcomes Quality Initiative, 2007), in most patients with diabetes, CKD usually can be attributed to diabetes if macroalbuminuria is present or if microalbuminuria has been found in the presence of diabetic retinopathy or in a patient who has had type 1 diabetes for at least 10 years. Many diseases other than diabetes can affect the kidneys to cause albuminuria and reduction of GFR (Sharma, 2013). A cause other than diabetes for the kidney disease should be suspected if there is no diabetic retinopathy; if there is very rapidly increasing proteinuria or decreasing GFR; if there is refractory hypertension, active urinary sediment, or signs or symptoms of another systemic disease known to affect the kidneys; or if there is a >30% reduction in GFR within 2 to 3 months of starting an ACEI or ARB (American Diabetes Association, 2018; Kidney Disease Outcomes Quality Initiative, 2007).

Screening for Eye Disease

A thorough assessment of other associated comorbidities should be pursued in any individual with diabetic kidney disease. All patients should have ongoing evaluation for other micro- and macrovascular complications. This includes screening for retinopathy at least annually with a dilated eye examination by a qualified eye care professional (American Diabetes Association, 2018).

Screening for Peripheral Vascular Disease and Neuropathy

Patients with diabetic kidney disease are at high risk for lower-extremity ulcers and amputations, and patients should be educated to inspect their own feet. In addition, on a regular basis, health care providers should perform a foot inspection, testing for vibratory sensation, monofilament testing for loss of protective sensation, and an assessment of pedal pulses (American Diabetes Association, 2018). Screening for peripheral vascular disease is discussed in Chapter 16.

GLYCEMIC CONTROL AND CHRONIC KIDNEY DISEASE

Glycemic Goal of HbA$_{1c}$ <7.0%

An overall glycemic goal for persons with diabetes is an HbA$_{1c}$ <7.0% (American Diabetes Association, 2018). This is strongly supported by data obtained from both patients with type 1 and type 2 diabetes examining the benefits of "tight glycemic control" in large, prospective randomized studies. The Diabetes Control and Complications Trial (DCCT) Research Group and the Epidemiology of Diabetes Interventions and Complications (EDIC) studies focused on development and progression of the long-term complications of type 1 diabetes with intensive glucose control (Nathan, 1993). Intensive therapy reduced the occurrence of microalbuminuria, albuminuria, and fall in GFR (de Boer, 2011, 2014; Nathan, 1993). Several studies in patients with type 2 diabetes have demonstrated the beneficial effect of intensive glucose control on development and progression of nephropathy (Coca, 2012; Perkovic, 2013; Wong, 2016).

Many of the studies focused on nonrenal major complications of diabetes, especially retinopathy. With respect to kidney outcomes, data are very strong for tight control slowing the development of microalbuminuria. With improved glycemic control, the numbers of patients going on to more advanced outcomes, such as albuminuria and decrease in GFR, are significantly reduced; much of this benefit is related to a smaller number of patients who have been tightly controlled developing microalbuminuria to begin with. Nonetheless, even for these more advanced outcomes, evidence is supportive for health benefits when attaining an HbA$_{1c}$ target in the 7% range (de Boer, 2011, 2014; Perkovic, 2013; Wong, 2016).

Benefits of Lowering HbA$_{1c}$ to Levels Above 7%

Improvement in glycemic control results in a reduction of adverse retinopathy outcomes, albuminuria, and neuropathy, even when HbA$_{1c}$ is reduced to levels above 7% when the comparison level is an even higher HbA$_{1c}$ value (Skupien, 2014). Therefore, efforts should always be put forth to attain better glycemic control even if, in a given patient, an HbA$_{1c}$ level of 7% cannot be practically achieved.

Potential Risks of HbA$_{1c}$ Targets in the Range of 7%

Achieving an HbA$_{1c}$ of <7% is difficult and generally limited by an increased risk of hypoglycemia. The HbA$_{1c}$ target needs to be tailored to the individual. A target HbA$_{1c}$ >7% should be considered in children and in those with a history of severe hypoglycemia, in patients with shorter life expectancies, in the presence of certain comorbidities, advanced age, or in patients who have had a long history of diabetes with minimal complications (American Diabetes Association, 2018; Inzucchi, 2015). *Because of the potential fragility of patients with more advanced CKD, given their increased risks of coronary artery disease and fracture, avoidance of hypoglycemia should be a high priority and may necessitate higher glucose and HbA$_{1c}$ goals* (Inzucchi, 2015).

Lack of Cardiovascular Benefit of Lowering HbA$_{1c}$ Targets Below 7%

The Action to Control Cardiovascular Risk in Diabetes Study Group (ACCORD) showed increased risks of hypoglycemia, weight gain, and mortality in a group assigned to an HbA$_{1c}$ target <6.0% and achieving an A$_{1c}$ of 6.4% compared with a group assigned to an HbA$_{1c}$ target of 7.0% to 7.9% and achieving a target of 7.5% (Gerstein, 2008). In the similarly designed ADVANCE trial, mortality was not increased in a group that had a mean achieved A$_{1c}$ of 6.5% compared with a less intensively treated group, in which the achieved mean A$_{1c}$ was 7.3% (Patel, 2008). In neither the ACCORD nor the ADVANCE studies was there a benefit of reduced adverse cardiovascular outcomes with very tight glucose control. Thus, the target HbA$_{1c}$ is now generally recommended to be <7.0% rather than 6.5%. It should be pointed out; however, that such a further reduction in A$_{1c}$ has associated with improved kidney outcomes (Perkovic, 2013).

Accuracy of HbA$_{1c}$ in Chronic Kidney Disease

There is some inaccuracy of the HbA$_{1c}$ measurement in reflecting ambient glucose levels in patients with CKD stages 4 to 5. Factors that may contribute to falsely decreased values include a reduced red blood cell life span, hemolysis, and iron deficiency. **Fructosamine** and **glycated albumin** are alternative integrated measures of glucose loads but reflect the previous 2 weeks rather than 3 months of ambient glucose levels. Whether they correlate better or worse with time-averaged glucose in CKD patients is controversial. Studies suggest that glycated albumin is superior to HbA$_{1c}$ in estimating glucose control in dialysis patients but this measurement is not well-standardized across laboratories (Freedman, 2010; Molitch, 2018; Peacock, 2008).

HbA$_{1c}$ and Home Glucose Monitoring and Targets

The HbA$_{1c}$ should be measured on average twice yearly in those with stable glucose control and at goal; it should be measured every 3 months if the goal is not being met or if therapy has been altered. Preprandial capillary glucose levels should ideally be 80 to 130 mg/dL (4.4 to 6.7 mmol/L), and postprandial capillary glucose levels 1 to 2 hours after the meal, if measured, should be <180 mg/dL (10.0 mmol/L)

(American Diabetes Association, 2018). However, as noted above, patients with advanced CKD are at greater risk for hypoglycemia and higher goals may be appropriate in such patients to avoid hypoglycemia (Inzucchi, 2015).

MEDICAL THERAPY FOR DIABETES: INSULIN

Long-Acting Insulins

Glargine
Insulin glargine (Lantus, Basaglar; U100) is soluble at an acidic pH, but less soluble when at a physiologic pH, so subcutaneous injection leads to precipitation and slower absorption. Glargine does not have a clear peak concentration and lasts about 22 to 24 hours after injection (Table 13.2). Recently, a more concentrated version of 300 U/mL U300 (Toujeo) has become available in pen form only and provides an even smaller peak and less day-to-day variability.

Detemir
Insulin detemir (Levemir) binds to albumin after injection. This is what gives detemir its prolonged action, extending its half-life in the circulation and delaying its entrance into cells. This also causes lower peak concentration values. Detemir lasts approximately 18 to 22 hours.

Degludec
Insulin degludec (Tresiba) is another very–long-acting insulin with a half-life of about 25 hours and comes in both U100 and U200 forms.

TABLE 13.2	Onset, Peak Effect, and Duration of Various Insulin Compounds		
Insulin	**Onset**	**Peak**	**Duration (hours)**
Long acting			
Glargine (Lantus, Basaglar)	2–4 hours	none	22–24
Detemir (Levemir)	1–3 hours	6–8 hours	18–22
Glargine U300 (Toujeo)	6 hours	None	36
Degludec (Tresiba)	1 hour	None	42
Intermediate acting			
NPH	2–4 hours	4–10 hours	10–18
Short acting			
Regular	0.5–1 hour	2–3 hours	5–8
Rapid acting			
Aspart (NovoLog)	5–15 minutes	0.5–2 hours	3–5
Lispro (Humalog)	5–15 minutes	0.5–2 hours	3–5
Glulisine (Apidra)	5–15 minutes	0.5–2 hours	3–5
Premixed			
70% NPH/30% regular	0.5–1 hour	3–12 hours (dual)	10–16
50% NPH/50% regular	0.5–1 hour	2–12 hours (dual)	10–16
75% NPL/25% lispro	5–15 minutes	1–4 hours (dual)	10–16
50% NPL/50% lispro	5–15 minutes	1–4 hours (dual)	10–16
70% NPA/30% aspart	5–15 minutes	1–4 hours (dual)	10–16

NPH, neutral protamine Hagedorn; NPL, neutral protamine lispro; NPA, neutral protamine aspart.

It also has a minimal peak and low day-to-day variability; it is also available only in a pen.

Intermediate-Acting Insulins: NPH
Isophane insulin (neutral protamine Hagedorn [NPH]) is an intermediate-acting insulin, resulting from the addition of protamine to regular insulin. Its onset of action is estimated to be at 2 to 4 hours, with a peak at 4 to 10 hours. Effects can last for 10 to 18 hours and it generally is given twice daily. One problem with NPH insulin is the high amount of variability in terms of its absorption.

Short-Acting (Regular) Insulin
Regular crystalline insulin has an onset of action of 30 to 60 minutes, a peak action at 2 to 3 hours, and duration of action of 5 to 8 hours after injection. Regular insulin should be given about 30 minutes before meals.

Rapid-Acting Insulins
The rapid-acting insulin analogs aspart (Novolog), lispro (Humalog, U100, and U200), and glulisine (Apidra) are absorbed more quickly than regular insulin, with earlier achievement of peak levels and shorter durations of action. They more closely mimic physiologic insulin secretion than regular insulin. The rapid-acting insulins can be given immediately before meals, which is more convenient for the patient. Peak concentrations of all three rapid-acting insulins occur at about 30 to 90 minutes, and duration of action is about 5 hours. Giving rapid-acting insulins in patients with gastroparesis *after* a meal sometimes results in better matching of peak insulin levels with the timing of glucose absorption from the meal. In patients with poor appetites who do not end up eating all the food they thought they might eat at a meal, giving the rapid-acting insulin after the meal allows for more targeted adjustment of the insulin dose in proportion to the amount of food that was eaten.

Premixed Combinations
There are various premixed preparations of insulin, which contain a fixed percentage of two different types of insulin.

U100 Versus U200, U300, and U500 Dosages
Almost all insulins are U100, defined as 100 units of insulin per 1 mL. U500 contains 500 units per 1 mL and is available only as regular insulin. The high concentration of U500 alters its kinetics, making it act more like NPH insulin when injected subcutaneously. The U300 form of glargine (Toujeo) and the U200 form of degludec are discussed above. These concentrated forms of insulin are useful for patients with severe insulin resistance who require large doses of insulin as well as patients with minimal fat depots. As an example, the U200 form of Humalog offers the advantage of the same amount of insulin delivered in a smaller volume. It is also useful for those with high insulin requirement and will allow the pens to last longer (each pen contains 600 units per pen instead of the standard 300 units).

Prolongation of Insulin Action in Chronic Kidney Disease

About one-third of insulin degradation is carried out by the kidney, and reduction in kidney function is associated with a prolonged half-life of insulin. The insulin preparations described above can all be used to treat diabetes in CKD. Doses used should be those that attain goal glycemic control and minimize hypoglycemia. The insulin types and doses used must be individualized to each patient and level of CKD. For example, one study compared usual doses to halving of the usual doses of insulin (glargine plus prandial glulisine) in inpatients with an eGFR <45 mL/min per 1.73 m^2, finding comparable levels of glycemic control but much less hypoglycemia (Baldwin, 2012). The longer durations of action of glargine U300 and degludec are due to a prolongation of their absorption time from the subcutaneous injection sites and not due to decreased renal clearance. Therefore, despite their longer duration of action, their pharmacokinetics are not changed with advancing CKD (Blair and Keating, 2016; Kiss, 2014) and no specific additional changes are needed for them in addition to the general need for dose reduction for all insulins as kidney function declines.

ORAL AGENTS AND NONINSULIN INJECTABLE DRUGS

There are currently six classes of oral medications and two classes of noninsulin injectable drugs approved for the treatment of type 2 diabetes.

Sulfonylureas

Sulfonylureas increase insulin secretion by binding to a sulfonylurea receptor on the β cells of the pancreas. These are the oldest available oral agents. So-called first-generation sulfonylureas include acetohexamide, chlorpropamide, tolazamide, and tolbutamide. Later developed second-generation compounds include glipizide, glimepiride, glyburide, and gliclazide (not available in the United States). Sulfonylureas are given once or twice daily. On average, they lower HbA$_{1c}$ by 1.5% to 2.0%. Hypoglycemia is a common problem, and with chlorpropamide or glyburide, prolonged hypoglycemia can occur.

Sulfonylurea Use in Chronic Kidney Disease

First-generation sulfonylureas should be avoided in CKD because they are eliminated by the kidney and thus have longer half-lives leading to a greater risk of hypoglycemia. Caution should also be used with the second-generation sulfonylureas glyburide and glimepiride. With glipizide and gliclazide, a decrease in dose is not necessary because they do not have active metabolites and are not renally excreted, but they should be used with caution (Table 13.3).

Glinides

Repaglinide and nateglinide increase insulin secretion by closing an adenosine triphosphate (ATP)-dependent potassium channel on pancreatic β cells. It is necessary for glucose to be present for the glinides

TABLE 13.3	Dose Adjustment for Insulin Compounds and Oral Medications for Diabetes in Chronic Kidney Disease
Medication Class	**CKD Stages 3 and 4 and Predialysis 5**
Insulins	No advised dose adjustment[a]
First-generation sulfonylureas	
Acetohexamide	Avoid use
Chlorpropamide	GFR 50–80 mL/min per 1.73 m^2: reduce dose 50%
	GFR <50 mL/min per 1.73 m^2: avoid
Tolazamide	Avoid use
Tolbutamide	Avoid use
Second-generation sulfonylureas	
Glipizide	No dose adjustment
Glimepiride	Start conservatively at 1 mg daily
Glyburide	Avoid use
Gliclazide	No dose adjustment
Glinides	
Repaglinide	No dose adjustment
Nateglinide	Start conservatively at 60 mg with meals. Do not use if eGFR <60 mL/min per 1.73 m^2
Biguanides	
Metformin	Maximum dose 1,000 mg/day for eGFR <45 mL/min per 1.73 m^2 and discontinue for eGFR <30 mL/min per 1.73 m^2
Thiazolidinediones	
Pioglitazone	No dose adjustment
Rosiglitazone	No dose adjustment
α-Glucosidase inhibitors	
Acarbose	Avoid if GFR <26 mL/min per 1.73 m^2
Miglitol	Avoid use
DPP-4 inhibitor	
Sitagliptin	GFR ≥50 mL/min per 1.73 m^2: 100 mg daily
	GFR 30 to <50 mL/min per 1.73 m^2: 50 mg daily
	GFR <30 mL/min per 1.73 m^2: 25 mg daily
Saxagliptin	GFR ≥45 mL/min per 1.73 m^2: 5 mg daily
	GFR <45 mL/min per 1.73 m^2: 2.5 mg daily
Alogliptin	GFR ≥60 mL/min per 1.73 m^2: 25 mg daily
	GFR 30 to <60 mL/min per 1.73 m^2: 12.5 mg daily
	GFR <30 mL/min per 1.73 m^2: 6.25 mg daily
Linagliptin	No restrictions
GLP-1 agonists	
Exenatide	Not recommended if GFR <30 mL/min per 1.73 m^2
Liraglutide	No dose adjustment
Dulaglutide	No dose adjustment
Semaglutide	No dose adjustment
Lixisenatide	Not recommended if eGFR <15 mL/min per 1.73 m^2
Amylin analog	
Pramlintide	No dose adjustment

(*continued*)

TABLE 13.3	Dose Adjustment for Insulin Compounds and Oral Medications for Diabetes in Chronic Kidney Disease (*Continued*)
Medication Class	**CKD Stages 3 and 4 and Predialysis 5**
SGLT2 Inhibitors	
Canagliflozin	eGFR 45 to <60 mL/min per 1.73 m^2: max dose 100 mg once daily
	eGFR <45 mL/min per 1.73 m^2: avoid use
Dapagliflozin	eGFR <60 mL/min per 1.73 m^2: avoid use
Empagliflozin	eGFR <45 mL/min per 1.73 m^2: avoid use
Ertugliflozin	eGFR <60 mL/min per 1.73 m^2: do not use chronically
	eGFR <30 mL/min per 1.73 m^2: avoid use

[a]Adjust dose based on patient response.
CKD, chronic kidney disease; GFR, glomerular filtration rate.

to work, and they result in quick- and short-duration insulin release. Because they have a quicker onset of action and briefer duration than sulfonylureas, the meglitinides ideally are given before each meal. They too can cause hypoglycemia.

Glinide Use in Chronic Kidney Disease
Increased serum levels of active metabolites have been found in patients with CKD taking nateglinide. This has not been shown with repaglinide and it can be used with caution.

Biguanides (Metformin)
Biguanides (metformin) act by decreasing hepatic gluconeogenesis and they also increase insulin sensitivity. Metformin lowers HbA$_{1c}$ on average by 1.0% to 2.0%. Metformin does not cause hypoglycemia when used alone. Also, it does not cause weight gain and is associated with modest reductions in low-density lipoprotein (LDL) and triglyceride levels. The most common side effects are bloating, abdominal cramping, and diarrhea. Vitamin B$_{12}$ deficiency has been reported with prolonged use (Wile, 2010). Lactic acidosis is a very rare but serious side effect that may be precipitated when metformin blood levels are too high, such as in patients with advanced CKD.

Metformin Use in Chronic Kidney Disease
Metformin is renally cleared and levels may build up with renal impairment, putting patients at risk for lactic acidosis, although the incidence of lactic acidosis with metformin use is very rare (Bakris and Molitch, 2016; Inzucchi, 2014). The FDA guidelines have recently been revised so that metformin should not be given to patients with an eGFR <30 mL/min per 1.73 m^2; it seems prudent to reduce the maximum dose to 1,000 mg/day with an eGFR <45 mL/min per 1.73 m^2 (Bakris and Molitch, 2016; Inzucchi, 2014). Furthermore, metformin should be held when patients are in unstable conditions, such as hypotension, hypoxia, and following radiocontrast administration (Bakris and Molitch, 2016; Inzucchi, 2014).

Thiazolidinediones

Thiazolidinediones (pioglitazone, rosiglitazone) are peroxisome proliferator–activated receptor γ (PPARγ) agonists that increase peripheral insulin sensitivity. On average, they decrease HbA_{1c} by 0.5% to 1.5% (Yki-Jarvinen, 2004). The major side effects are weight gain and edema. They should not be used in patients with heart failure and other edema-forming states. Although there was a concern several years ago about an increased risk of ischemic heart disease with rosiglitazone, subsequent analyses did not support this conclusion and a prior warning from the FDA was lifted.

Thiazolidinediones in Chronic Kidney Disease

Rosiglitazone and pioglitazone are cleared by the liver, and doses do not have to be reduced in patients with renal impairment. Therefore, rosiglitazone and pioglitazone do not present an increased risk for hypoglycemia in patients with developing CKD; however, they do have the potential to worsen fluid retention. Recently, this class of drugs has been found to decrease bone resorption and to cause an increase in fracture rate. Whether this effect on bone resorption will worsen renal osteodystrophy is not known but it is of potential concern.

α-Glucosidase Inhibitors

α-Glucosidase inhibitors (acarbose, miglitol) decrease the breakdown of oligo- and disaccharides in the small intestine, thereby delaying the digestion of carbohydrates and slowing the absorption of glucose after a meal. The major side effects are bloating, flatulence, and abdominal cramping. The average effect on HbA_{1c} is a decrease of 0.5% to 1.0%.

Acarbose and Miglitol in Chronic Kidney Disease

Acarbose is only minimally absorbed, but with reduced renal function, serum levels of the drug and its metabolites increase significantly. Although no adverse effects have been reported, its use in patients with a GFR <26 mL/min per 1.73 m^2 is not recommended (Snyder, 2004). Miglitol has greater systemic absorption and undergoes renal excretion, and it should not be used in patients with decreased GFR (Snyder, 2004).

Dipeptidyl Peptidase Inhibitors

The dipeptidyl peptidase-4 (DPP-4) inhibitors (sitagliptin [Januvia], saxagliptin [Onglyza], alogliptin [Nesina], and linagliptin [Tradjenta]) decrease the breakdown of the incretin hormones such as glucagon-like peptide 1 (GLP-1). GLP-1 is normally secreted by the gastrointestinal tract in response to food and promotes insulin secretion from the pancreas while decreasing glucagon release. GLP-1 also slows gastric emptying. DPP-4 inhibitors improve both fasting and postprandial glucose levels.

DPP-4 Inhibitors in Chronic Kidney Disease

All of the DPP-4 inhibitors can be used in CKD patients, but sitagliptin, saxagliptin, and alogliptin are cleared by the kidney and therefore need downward dose adjustments as detailed in Table 13.3. Linagliptin is not cleared by the kidney and does not need any dose adjustment as the GFR falls. Although some studies have found an increased risk of congestive heart failure with DPP-4 inhibitors, others have not and this area remains controversial (Filion and Suissa, 2016).

Sodium Glucose Cotransporter 2 Inhibitors

Sodium glucose cotransporter 2 (SGLT2) inhibitors (canagliflozin [Invokana], dapagliflozin [Farxiga], empagliflozin [Jardiance], and ertugliflozin [Steglatro]) reduce glucose reabsorption in the proximal tubule, leading to an increase in glucose excretion, a reduction in HbA_{1c} of ~0.8%, and weight loss, and do not cause hypoglycemia. The EMPA-REG and CANVAS studies recently demonstrated significant benefits in reduction of cardiovascular outcomes and mortality and eGFR progression with empagliflozin and canagliflozin use, respectively (Neal, 2017; Wanner, 2016; Zinman, 2015). Renal outcomes, as defined by decline in GFR, requirement for renal replacement therapy, or renal death, was decreased in subjects given canagliflozin as compared to placebo in the CANVAS study (Mahaffey, 2018). Genital yeast infections occur in up to 10% or women and older patients may experience symptoms due to volume contraction. In addition, there have been recent reports of "euglycemic" diabetic ketoacidosis, primarily in those with type 1 diabetes (in whom these drugs sometimes are used "off-label" but also in very rare patients with type 2 diabetes). Of some concern is a recent analysis suggesting that the risk of amputations may be increased with this category of medication (Udell, 2018).

SGLT2 Inhibitors in Chronic Kidney Disease

The amount of reduction in HbA_{1c} becomes much lower as the eGFR dips below 60 mL/min per 1.73 m^2, but interestingly, the modest reduction in blood pressure remains (Gilbert, 2016). Because of a small increase in adverse events related to intravascular volume contraction, no more than 100 mg once daily of canagliflozin should be used in patients with an eGFR of 45 to <60 mL/min per 1.73 m^2. Canagliflozin and empagliflozin should be stopped if the eGFR is <45 mL/min per 1.73 m^2 and dapagliflozin stopped at 60 mL/min per 1.73 m^2, primarily because of a decrease in efficacy. Ertugliflozin should be stopped if the eGFR is <30 mL/min per 1.3 m^2 and its prolonged use is not recommended if the eGFR is <60 mL/min per 1.73 m^2.

GLP-1 Receptor Agonists

Exenatide (Byetta), liraglutide (Victoza), dulaglutide (Trulicity), lixisenatide (Adlyxin), and semaglutide (Ozempic) are injectable incretin mimetics. They are approved by the FDA as adjunctive treatments in patients using a sulfonylurea and/or metformin. In practice, they have also been used with insulin. In fact, there are now fixed-dose combinations of insulin degludec/liraglutide (IDegLira) and insulin glargine/lixisenatide (IGlarLixi) that can be titrated upward in dose to achieve glycemic control. The GLP-1 receptor agonists effectively reduce HbA_{1c} and also body weight. In addition, they contribute to satiety by a central nervous system mechanism that decreases appetite and contributes to their effectiveness in weight loss. Although their use has been associated with pancreatitis in some patients, the overall frequency of pancreatitis with their use is not greater than in diabetic patients using other agents. Exenatide is available in a twice-daily dosing form (Byetta) and also as a weekly depot injection (Bydureon). Both albiglutide and dulaglutide are available only as weekly injections. The LEADER and SUSTAIN-6 studies demonstrated significant reductions in cardiovascular mortality with liraglutide and semaglutide (Marso, 2016a; Marso, 2016b).

GLP-1 Receptor Agonists in Chronic Kidney Disease

Exenatide is not recommended for use with a GFR <30 mL/min per 1.73 m^2 (Linnebjerg, 2007). Furthermore, exenatide has been found to cause renal failure in a number of cases (U.S. Food and Drug Administration, 2009). Liraglutide is completely metabolized in the body, and the kidney is not a major organ of elimination (Jacobsen, 2009); however, because of similar reports of acute kidney injury (AKI) with liraglutide, it should be used with caution when the eGFR is <30 mL/min per 1.73 m^2. There are also no dose restrictions with dulaglutide or semaglutide, but lixisenatide should not be used when the GFR is <15 mL/min per 1.73 m^2.

Pramlintide

Pramlintide is an injectable amylin analog available as a complement to insulin therapy. Normally it is given with each meal. Amylin is cosecreted by the β cells of the pancreas along with insulin, and amylin is deficient in patients with diabetes. Amylin decreases glucagon release, slows gastric emptying, and also has an effect on suppressing appetite.

Pramlintide in Chronic Kidney Disease

Pramlintide is metabolized and eliminated predominantly by the kidneys. However, because pramlintide has a wide therapeutic index, dosage adjustments are not usually required in the presence of mild to moderate renal insufficiency.

GLYCEMIC THERAPY FOR DIABETES: STRATEGY

Insulin therapy for patients with type 1 and type 2 diabetes differs greatly.

Type 1 Diabetes

Patients with type 1 diabetes need a regimen that mimics endogenous insulin secretion. This is best achieved with combination insulin therapy, with use of a long-acting basal insulin, and with multiple daily injections of a short- (i.e., regular) or rapid-acting insulin with meals (Wallia and Molitch, 2014).

Twice-Daily NPH and Regular Insulin

Before the availability of insulin analogs, a combination of twice-daily NPH and regular insulin was used in an attempt to mimic endogenous insulin secretion. Typically, the two were given together before breakfast and before dinner. Because both types of insulin serve to treat fasting and postprandial glucose levels, such a regimen can be difficult to use to attain target glycemic control. Such fixed insulin combinations require that patients maintain similar mealtimes and meal sizes each day, and they also do not mimic normal physiologic insulin secretion (Wallia and Molitch, 2014). The only advantage of using NPH and regular insulin is their much lower cost compared to the newer analog insulins.

Glargine Insulin or Detemir Instead of NPH

Glargine insulin does not have a distinct peak, is superior to twice-daily NPH in reducing fasting glucose levels with less hypoglycemia, and results in more stable fasting glucose values. Reductions in HbA$_{1c}$ have been reported in studies comparing glargine and NPH (Wallia and Molitch, 2014). Compared with NPH, glargine and detemir have been shown to have less intra- and interindividual variability with greater predictability and reproducibility. Few studies have compared detemir with glargine in a clinical practice setting. The two newer very–long-acting basal insulins, insulin glargine U300 (Toujeo), and insulin degludec (Tresiba) have even less intra- and interindividual variability and less hypoglycemia than insulin glargine U100 and detemir.

Rapid-Acting Insulin Analogs Instead of Regular Insulin

In a number of studies, use of the rapid-acting insulins lispro, aspart, or glulisine compared with regular insulin showed better postprandial glucose control, decreases in hypoglycemia, and in some but not all studies, lower HbA$_{1c}$ (Wallia and Molitch, 2014).

Type 1 Diabetes Insulin Regimen: Summary

The insulin regimen for each individual with type 1 needs to be customized. As a basal insulin, once-daily glargine would be an optimal first-choice agent, followed by twice-daily detemir, then NPH, with any of the rapid-acting insulin analogs used for mealtime insulin supplemental doses. In some individuals, the use of glargine U300 and degludec may provide more even glycemic control with less hypoglycemia. As noted above, doses usually need to be reduced as the GFR falls and careful home glucose monitoring is needed to guide this and prevent hypoglycemia.

Glycemia Management of Type 2 Diabetes

Initial Use of Oral Agents

There are several options for treatment in type 2 diabetes. When medical therapy is initiated in type 2 diabetes, if the diabetes is mild, starting with an oral agent is ideal because of ease of administration and a lower risk of hypoglycemia. Metformin is an ideal first choice given the lack of associated hypoglycemia and may lead to weight loss but the dose may need to be reduced depending upon the level of kidney function (see above). An ideal starting dose is 500 mg once daily with gradual titration to 2,000 mg daily depending on glucose response and gastrointestinal tolerance. Any of the other oral agents can be used as a second agent when control is not achieved with lifestyle change and metformin (Inzucchi, 2015; Qaseem, 2017). The DPP-4 inhibitors can be considered as there is no associated hypoglycemia; doses need to be reduced for sitagliptin, saxagliptin, and alogliptin but not linagliptin for patients with decreased GFR (Table 13.3). Pioglitazone is a reasonable choice as it decreases insulin resistance, but weight gain and fluid retention are major undesirable side effects. The SGLT2 inhibitors are also now used as a second agent commonly, given their proven cardiovascular and CKD benefits, but they are not particularly useful when the eGFR is <60 mL/min per 1.73 m^2. GLP-1 receptor agonists are also increasingly used as second agents, given the substantial weight loss that sometimes can be achieved. Lastly, the second-generation sulfonylureas are effective, although they carry a risk of hypoglycemia and therefore require more vigilant monitoring on the part of the physician and patient; glyburide, in particular, should be avoided in patients with CKD. The use of three drugs is not uncommon but at that point consideration is also given to adding insulin to the treatment regimen.

Adding Insulin to Compensate for Progressive Pancreatic β-Cell Failure

In type 2 diabetes, there is a defect in insulin action leading to insulin resistance combined with progressive pancreatic β-cell failure. In those with severe insulin resistance or deficiency, insulin is often necessary to achieve optimal glycemic control that cannot be attained by the use of oral hypoglycemic medications alone. There is no clear consensus on which regimen to use in which patient. The insulin regimen needs to be customized to the patient and time of day when hyperglycemia is occurring.

Insulin Use in Combination With Oral Agents

A long-acting insulin can be added to oral hypoglycemic agents. A typical regimen includes insulin at bedtime to treat suboptimal fasting blood glucose levels; these may be due to hepatic gluconeogenesis that has been inadequately treated with the oral agent.

Initial Basal Insulin Dose and How to Adjust It

To start, the basal insulin can be initiated at a dose of 10 to 15 U administered at bedtime. The basal insulin can be glargine, detemir, glargine U300, degludec, or NPH, but the risk of nocturnal hypoglycemia may be higher with NPH. Subsequently, no more frequently than every 3 days, the insulin dose can be increased by 1 to 2 U until the fasting goal is reached while, at the same time, avoiding hypoglycemia (Wallia and Molitch, 2014).

Mealtime Insulin Supplemental Doses

Individuals may also need the addition of prandial insulin if they are hyperglycemic during the day but have controlled fasting blood sugar levels. Premixed insulins in vials and pens are more convenient for use but patients need to follow a similar diet from day to day. Because the insulin ratio is fixed, there is less freedom with titration of basal and prandial doses, and often tight control without frequent hypoglycemia is difficult to achieve. Prandial insulin can be added initially to the largest meal of the day but often prandial insulin is needed for each meal, with the dose guided by the carbohydrate content of the meal as well as the premeal glucose level (Wallia and Molitch, 2014).

In individuals affected only by hyperglycemia during the day, prandial insulin may be all that is needed.

RISK OF HYPOGLYCEMIA

The major limitation for patients in obtaining HbA$_{1c}$ levels <7.0% is the increasing development of hypoglycemia with lower glucose levels. This is particularly true for those with type 1 diabetes being treated with insulin. Although the risk of hypoglycemia is increased in those with type 2 diabetes being treated with insulin, the magnitude of the risk is considerably less. The UKPDS (which studied type 2 diabetic patients) showed that sulfonylureas are associated with a very small risk of hypoglycemia (Shichiri, 2000; UK Prospective Diabetes Study [UKPDS] Group, 1998).

Increased Risk of Hypoglycemia in Chronic Kidney Disease

Patients with type 1 diabetes receiving insulin who had significant creatinine elevations (mean 2.2 mg/dL [195 mcmol/L]) had a fivefold increase in the frequency of severe hypoglycemia (Hasslacher and Wittmann, 2003; Muhlhauser, 1991). Therefore, it is imperative that patients being treated intensively must monitor their glucose levels closely and adjust doses of medications accordingly. Patients with progressing kidney disease with substantial decreases in GFR (CKD stages 3 to 5) have increased risks for hypoglycemia for three reasons: (a) decreased clearance of insulin as noted above; (b) decreased clearance of some of the oral agents used to treat diabetes, as shown in Table 13.3; and (c) impaired renal gluconeogenesis (Alsahi and Gerich, 2014). With decreased kidney mass, the amount of gluconeogenesis carried out by the kidney is decreased. This decline in gluconeogenesis may reduce the ability of a patient who is becoming hypoglycemic as the result of excessive insulin/oral agents or lack of food intake to defend against hypoglycemia. In some patients, anorexia and weight loss associated with uremia may also play a role in increased insulin sensitivity.

PANCREAS–KIDNEY TRANSPLANT

Cure of diabetes by successful pancreas transplantation has been demonstrated, after 10 years of normoglycemia, to be associated with a reversal of the established lesions of diabetic nephropathy, including glomerular and tubular basement membrane thickening and mesangial expansion (Wallia and Molitch, 2014). However, the benefits of pancreas transplantation must be balanced against the surgical and lifelong immunosuppression risks and the potential serious injurious impact of calcineurin inhibitors on renal structure and function (Wallia and Molitch, 2014) (see also Chapter 28).

IMPORTANCE OF REDUCING CARDIOVASCULAR AND METABOLIC RISK FACTORS

Diabetes is a strong risk factor for CVD, and CVD is the leading cause of death in patients with CKD. Thus, the combination of diabetes and

CKD is particularly serious in terms of increased CVD risk. When patients with CKD are divided into those with and without diabetes, the annual mortality rate is increased substantially in those with diabetes. Conversely, when individuals with diabetes are divided into those with and without evidence of CKD, the CVD risk is far higher in those with evidence of diabetic kidney disease, even at the early stage of just micro-albuminuria, and the risk increases as the kidney disease progresses to clinical albuminuria and then decreased GFR (Afkarian, 2013; Fox, 2012). Thus, control of CVD risk factors is particularly important in any individual who has both diabetes and CKD. There are many risk factors for CVD in people with diabetes and CKD, including smoking, dyslipid-emias, hypertension, and obesity, and intensive efforts to lower as many risk factors as possible should be pursued.

In the Steno-2 study, the effect of tight glycemic control, blood pressure, and cholesterol control in type 2 diabetes and established microalbuminuria on microvascular disease, CVD, and mortality was assessed (Gaede, 2003, 2008). In the initial study, patients with inten-sive treatment had lower rates of nephropathy (relative hazard ratio, 0.39) and CVD (relative hazard ratio, 0.47) (Gaede, 2003). Patients were then followed for more than 13 years. Those in the intensive treatment group had significantly lower rates of cardiovascular events, cardiovascular-related deaths, and death from any cause (Gaede, 2008). The benefit attributable to glycemic control versus blood pressure and cholesterol control was unable to be determined exactly. However, through the use of a risk calculator, the authors concluded the use of blood pressure control agents and statins may have had the largest effect, followed by the use of diabetic therapies and aspirin (Gaede, 2008).

Diabetic Dyslipidemias

As detailed in Chapter 12, dyslipidemias are a major risk factor for CVD in nondiabetic and diabetic populations. Because of the very high risk of CVD, the LDL goal in most patients with this combination should be <70 mg/dL (1.8 mmol/L), if a target LDL is used. It has been recommended that high-intensity statin treatment should be used in patients at such high risk for CVD (American College of Cardiology/ American Heart Association, 2014; American Diabetes Association, 2018). Please also refer to Chapter 12.

Blood Pressure Control

Hypertension is commonly seen in patients with diabetes and is a major risk factor in the development of CVD. In type 1 diabetes, hyper-tension is usually a consequence of nephropathy, whereas in type 2 diabetes, hypertension may be present independent of nephropa-thy. Elevated blood pressure is associated with progression of CKD in diabetes, and optimizing blood pressure control is important in decreasing the progression of nephropathy. Several studies have dem-onstrated the association between progression of nephropathy and elevation in blood pressure.

Blood Pressure Targets

Blood pressure should be taken at every office visit, although home blood pressure measurement may have special utility, as described in Chapter 14. The recommended blood pressure target is a systolic blood pressure (SBP) ≤140 mm Hg and a diastolic blood pressure ≤90 mm Hg (American Diabetes Association, 2018; Tuttle, 2014). The Systolic Blood Pressure Intervention Trial (Wright, 2015) which evaluated 9,361 nondiabetic persons randomized to SBP targets of <140 versus <120 mm Hg showed a 25% reduction in major adverse cardiac events and a 27% reduction in all-cause mortality with the more intensive treatment (Wright, 2015). There were significant increases in rates of hypotension, syncope, electrolyte abnormalities, and acute kidney injury or failure in the more intensively treated group (SPRINT). A recent meta-analysis that incorporated SPRINT and 122 other studies supported an SBP target <130 mm Hg (Ettehad, 2016).

It should be emphasized, however, that SPRINT did not include patients with diabetes. Evidence from the ACCORD study showed no cardiovascular benefit of lowering the SBP target in patients with diabetes to an even lower value: <120 mm Hg (Cushman, 2010), as there was no reduction in the rate of major cardiovascular events, although the risk of stroke was reduced. Systematic reviews and meta-analyses of studies of patients with diabetes and hypertension have shown that an SBP treatment goal of 130 to 40 mm Hg is optimal and that a goal of <130 mm Hg is associated with a drop of stroke risk but no further benefit (and even higher risk [J curve] in some reviews) on other CVD outcomes and mortality and with higher adverse effects (Arguedas, 2013; Bangalore, 2011; Brunström and Carlberg, 2016; Emdin, 2015; McBrien, 2012; Reboldi, 2012).

The Diabetes and Hypertension Position Statement of the American Diabetes Association supported a target of <140/90 mm Hg for "fitter" older individuals but a higher SBP (145 to 160 mm Hg) for individuals with loss of autonomy or major functional limitations (de Boer, 2017). However, the guideline from the American College of Cardiology (ACC)/American Heart Association (AHA) Task Force on clinical practice guidelines redefined hypertension as being a BP of 130/80 and recommended a target of <130/80 mm Hg for all adults, including those with DM because of the increased cardiovascular risk in such patients while acknowledging the lack of randomized trial data supporting this target in those with diabetes (Whelton, 2017).

Thus, although most studies and guidelines have recommended the BP target of <140/90 mm Hg, the recent ACC/AHA guideline recommends a target of <130/80 mm Hg, even in older patients with DM (Whelton, 2017). Thus, treatment approaches and goals are controversial. Many clinicians may opt for this lower target in patients at high CVD risk after careful discussion of the pros and cons of such increased intensity of treatment with the patient. The ACC/AHA guideline also recommended that for adults with a high burden of comorbidity and limited life expectancy, such as those with advanced CKD, clinical judgment, patient preference, and a team-based approach, to assess risk/benefit is reasonable for decisions regarding intensity of BP lowering and the choice of antihypertensive drugs (Whelton, 2017).

Use of Angiotensin-Converting Enzyme Inhibitors
or Angiotensin Receptor Blockers

ACEIs or ARBs are advised as initial therapy when pharmacologic treatment of high BP is needed. Several studies in type 1 diabetes show benefit of BP control with ACEIs on slowing the progression from micro- to macroalbuminuria and delaying decline in GFR. In patients with type 2 diabetes and macroalbuminuria, ARBs are effective in slowing decline in GFR and progression to kidney failure. They also delay the progression from micro- to macroalbuminuria (see Kidney Disease Outcomes Quality Initiative, 2007, for a review). In individuals with type 2 diabetes and hypertension, ACEIs slow onset of microalbuminuria. As diabetic kidney disease progresses, generally two or more antihypertensive medications are needed to control blood pressure. Please also refer to Chapter 14.

Nutrition and Weight Control

Lifestyle modification is an integral part of diabetes management. Management of nutrition in a patient with both diabetes and CKD is complex because intake of protein, potassium, sodium, and phosphorus, among other nutrients, must be considered carefully (Tuttle, 2014). For diabetes in general, weight loss can reduce insulin resistance, thus a goal BMI <25 kg/m^2 is desirable. This can be achieved by the use of low-calorie, carbohydrate-restricted, or fat-restricted diets. In either diet, it is important to restrict saturated fat and trans fats as well as high-glycemic index carbohydrates. Carbohydrate intake needs to be assessed in any individual with diabetes and followed closely. As previously mentioned, protein restriction to 0.8 g/kg body weight per day may help delay progression of nephropathy (Kidney Disease Outcomes Quality Initiative, 2007; Tuttle, 2014). Popular high-protein weight-loss diets such as Atkins, South Beach, Protein Power, Sugar Busters, and the Zone should be followed with caution or avoided. With a decrease in protein intake, there must naturally be an increase in carbohydrate and fat intake for equal caloric consumption. Thus, the diet in an individual with CKD and diabetes presents challenges, and referral to a dietitian is essential (Tuttle, 2014).

References and Suggested Readings

Afkarian M, Sachs MC, Kestenbaum B, et al. Kidney disease and increased mortality risk in type 2 diabetes. *J Am Soc Nephrol.* 2013;24:302–308.

Alsahi M, Gerich JE. Hypoglycemia, chronic kidney disease, and diabetes mellitus. *Mayo Clin Proc.* 2014;89:1564–1571.

American Diabetes Association. Standards of medical care in diabetes—2018. *Diabetes Care.* 2018;41:S1–S153.

Arguedas JA, Leiva V, Wright JM. Blood pressure targets for hypertension in people with diabetes mellitus. *Cochrane Database Syst Rev.* 2013:CD008277.

Bakris GL, Molitch ME. Should restrictions be relaxed for metformin use in chronic kidney disease? Yes, they should be relaxed! What's the fuss? *Diabetes Care.* 2016;39:1287–1291.

Baldwin D, Zander J, Munoz C, et al. A randomized trial of two weight-based doses of insulin glargine and glulisine in hospitalized subjects with type 2 diabetes and renal insufficiency. *Diabetes Care.* 2012;35:1970–1974.

Bangalore S, Kumar S, Lobach I, et al. Blood pressure targets in subjects with type 2 diabetes mellitus/impaired fasting glucose: observations from traditional and bayesian random-effects meta-analyses of randomized trials. *Circulation.* 2011;123:2799–2810.

Blair HA, Keating GM. Insulin Glargine 300 U/mL: A review in diabetes mellitus. *Drugs.* 2016;76:363–374.

Brunström M, Carlberg B. Effect of antihypertensive treatment at different blood pressure levels in patients with diabetes mellitus: systematic review and meta-analyses. *BMJ.* 2016;352:i717.

Coca SG, Ismail-Beigi F, Haq N, et al. Role of intensive glucose control in development of renal end points in type 2 diabetes mellitus: systematic review and meta-analysis intensive glucose control in type 2 diabetes. *Arch Intern Med.* 2012;172:761–769.

Cushman WC, Evans GW, Byington RP, et al; ACCORD Study Group. Effects of intensive blood-pressure control in type 2 diabetes mellitus. *N Engl J Med.* 2010;362: 1575–1585.

de Boer IH; DCCT/EDIC Research Group. Kidney disease and related findings in the The Diabetes Control and Complications Trial/Epidemiology of Diabetes Interventions and Complications Study. *Diabetes Care.* 2014;37:24–30.

de Boer IH, Bangalore S, Benetos A, et al. Diabetes and hypertension: a position statement by the American Diabetes Association. *Diabetes Care.* 2017;40:1273–1284.

de Boer IH, Sun W, Cleary PA, et al; DCCT/EDIC Research Group. Intensive diabetes therapy and glomerular filtration rate in type 1 diabetes. *N Engl J Med.* 2011;365:2366–2376.

Emdin CA, Rahimi K, Neal B, et al. Blood pressure lowering in type 2 diabetes. A systematic review and meta-analysis. *JAMA.* 2015;313:603–615.

Ettehad D, Emdin CA, Kiran A, et al. Blood pressure lowering for prevention of cardiovascular disease and death: a systematic review and meta-analysis. *Lancet.* 2016;387:957–967.

Filion KB, Suissa S. DPP-4 inhibitors and heart failure: some reassurance, some uncertainty. *Diabetes Care.* 2016;39:735–737.

Fox CS, Matsushita K, Woodward M, et al; Chronic Kidney Disease Prognosis Consortium. Associations of kidney disease measures with mortality and end-stage renal disease in individuals with and without diabetes: a meta-analysis. *Lancet.* 2012;380:1662–1673.

Freedman BI, Shenoy RN, Planer JA, et al. Comparison of glycated albumin and hemoglobin A1c concentrations in diabetic subjects on peritoneal and hemodialysis. *Perit Dial Int.* 2010;30:72–79.

Gaede P, Lund-Andersen H, Parving HH, et al. Effect of a multifactorial intervention on mortality in type 2 diabetes. *N Engl J Med.* 2008;358:580–591.

Gaede P, Vedel P, Larsen N, et al. Multifactorial intervention and cardiovascular disease in patients with type 2 diabetes. *N Engl J Med.* 2003;348:383–393.

Gerstein HC, Miller ME, Byington RP, et al; Action to Control Cardiovascular Risk in Diabetes Study Group. Effects of intensive glucose lowering in type 2 diabetes. *N Engl J Med.* 2008;358:2545–2559.

Gilbert RE, Weir MR, Fioretto P, et al. Impact of age and estimated glomerular filtration rate on the glycemic efficacy and safety of canagliflozin: a pooled analysis of clinical studies. *Can J Diabetes.* 2016;40:247–257.

Hasslacher C, Wittmann W. [Severe hypoglycemia in diabetics with impaired renal function]. *Dtsch Med Wochenschr.* 2003;128:253–256.

Herrington WG, Levy JB. Metformin: effective and safe in renal disease? *Int Urol Nephrol.* 2008;40:411–417.

Inzucchi SE, Bergenstal RM, Buse JB, et al. Management of hyperglycemia in type 2 diabetes 2015: a patient-centered approach. Update to a Position Statement of the American Diabetes Association and the European Association for the Study of Diabetes. *Diabetes Care.* 2015;38:140–149.

Inzucchi SE, Lipska KJ, Mayo H, et al. Metformin in patients with type 2 diabetes and kidney disease: a systematic review. *JAMA.* 2014;312: 2668–2675.

Ismail-Beigi F, Craven T, Banerji MA, et al; ACCORD trial group. Effect of intensive treatment of hyperglycaemia on microvascular outcomes in type 2 diabetes: an analysis of the ACCORD randomised trial. *Lancet.* 2010;376:419–430.

Jacobsen LV, Hindsberger C, Robson R, et al. Effect of renal impairment on the pharmacokinetics of the GLP-1 analogue liraglutide. *Br J Clin Pharmacol.* 2009;68: 898–905.

Kidney Disease Outcomes Quality Initiative. KDOQI clinical practice guidelines and clinical practice recommendations for diabetes and chronic kidney disease. *Am J Kidney Dis.* 2007;49:S12–S154.

Kiss I, Arold G, Roepstorff C, et al. Insulin degludec: pharmacokinetics in patients with renal impairment. *Clin Pharmacokinet.* 2014;53:175–183.

Krolewski AS. Progressive renal decline: the new paradigm of diabetic nephropathy in type 1 diabetes. *Diabetes Care.* 2015;38:954–962.

Levey AS, de Jong PE, Coresh J, et al. The definition, classification, and prognosis of chronic kidney disease: a KDIGO Controversies Conference report. *Kidney Int.* 2011;80:17–28.

Levey AS, Stevens LA, Schmid CH, et al; CKD-EPI (Chronic Kidney Disease Epidemiology Collaboration). A new equation to estimate glomerular filtration rate. *Ann Intern Med.* 2009;150:604–612.

Linnebjerg H, Kothare PA, Park S, et al. Effect of renal impairment on the pharmacokinetics of exenatide. *Br J Clin Pharmacol.* 2007;64:317–327.

Mahaffey KW, Neal B, Perkovic V, et al. Canagliflozin for primary and secondary prevention of cardiovascular events: results from the CANVAS program (Canagliflozin Cardiovascular Assessment Study). *Circulation.* 2018;137:323–334.

Marso SP, Bain SC, Consoli A, et al; SUSTAIN-6 Investigators. Semaglutide and cardiovascular outcomes in patients with type 2 diabetes. *N Engl J Med.* 2016a;375:1834–1844.

Marso SP, Daniels GH, Brown-Frandsen K, et al; LEADER Trial Investigators. Liraglutide and cardiovascular outcomes in type 2 diabetes. *N Engl J Med.* 2016b;375:311–322.

McBrien K, Rabi DM, Campbell N, et al. Intensive and standard blood pressure targets in patients with type 2 diabetes mellitus: Systematic review and meta-analysis. *Arch Inter Med.* 2012;172:1296–1303.

Molitch ME. Glycemic control assessment in the dialysis patient: Is glycated albumin the answer? *Am J Nephrol.* 2018;47:18–20.

Molitch ME, Adler AI, Flyvbjerg A, et al. Diabetic kidney disease: a clinical update from the Kidney Disease: Improving Global Outcomes (KDIGO). *Kidney Int.* 2015;87: 20–30.

Muhlhauser I, Toth G, Sawicki PT, et al. Severe hypoglycemia in type I diabetic patients with impaired kidney function. *Diabetes Care.* 1991;14:344–346.

Nathan DM, Buse JB, Davidson MB, et al; American Diabetes Association; European Association for Study of Diabetes. Medical management of hyperglycemia in type 2 diabetes: a consensus algorithm for the initiation and adjustment of therapy: a consensus statement of the American Diabetes Association and the European Association for the Study of Diabetes. *Diabetes Care.* 2009;32:193–203.

Nathan DM, Genuth S, Lachin J, et al; Diabetes Control and Complications Trial Research Group. The effect of intensive treatment of diabetes on the development and progression of long-term complications in insulin-dependent diabetes mellitus. *N Engl J Med.* 1993;329:977–986.

National Kidney Foundation. KDOQI clinical practice guideline for diabetes and CKD: 2012 update. *Am J Kidney Dis.* 2012;60:850–886.

Neal B, Perkovic V, Mahaffey KW, et al; CANVAS Program Collaborative Group. Canagliflozin and cardiovascular and renal events in type 2 diabetes. *N Engl J Med.* 2017;377:644–657.

Patel A, MacMahon S, Chalmers J, et al; ADVANCE Collaborative Group. Intensive blood glucose control and vascular outcomes in patients with type 2 diabetes. *N Engl J Med.* 2008;358:2560–2572.

Peacock TP, Shihabi ZK, Bleyer AJ, et al. Comparison of glycated albumin and hemoglobin A(1c) levels in diabetic subjects on hemodialysis. *Kidney Int.* 2008;73:1062–1068.

Perkovic V, Heerspink HL, Chalmers J, et al; ADVANCE Collaborative Group. Intensive glucose control improves kidney outcomes in patients with type 2 diabetes. *Kidney Int.* 2013;83:517–523.

Peters AL, Buschur EO, Buse JB, et al. Euglycemic diabetic ketoacidosis: a potential complication of treatment with sodium-glucose cotransporter 2 inhibition. *Diabetes Care*. 2015;38:1687–1693.

Qaseem A, Barry MJ, Humphrey LL, et al; Clinical Guidelines Committee of the American College of Physicians. Oral pharmacologic treatment of type 2 diabetes mellitus: a clinical practice guideline update from the American College of Physicians. *Ann Intern Med*. 2017;166:279–290.

Reboldi G, Gentile G, Manfreda VM, et al. Tight blood pressure control in diabetes: evidence-based review of treatment targets in patients with diabetes. *Curr Cardiol Rep*. 2012;14:89–96.

Sharma SG, Bomback AS, Radhakrishnan J, et al. The modern spectrum of renal biopsy findings in patients with diabetes. *Clin J Am Soc Nephrol*. 2013;8:1718–1724.

Shaw JS, Wilmot RL, Kilpatrick ES. Establishing pragmatic estimated GFR thresholds to guide metformin prescribing. *Diabet Med*. 2007;24:1160–1163.

Shichiri M, Kishikawa H, Ohkubo Y, et al. Long-term results of the Kumamoto Study on optimal diabetes control in type 2 diabetic patients. *Diabetes Care*. 2000;23:B21–B29.

Skupien J, Warram JH, Smiles A, et al. Improved glycemic control and risk of ESRD in patients with type 1 diabetes and proteinuria. *J Am Soc Nephrol*. 2014;25:2916–2925.

Snyder RW, Berns JS. Use of insulin and oral hypoglycemic medications in patients with diabetes mellitus and advanced kidney disease. *Semin Dial*. 2004;17:365–370.

Stone NJ, Robinson JG, Lichtenstein AH, et al; American College of Cardiology/American Heart Association Task Force on Practice Guidelines. 2013 ACC/AHA guideline on the treatment of lood cholesterol to reduce atherosclerotic cardiovascular risk in adults: a report of the American College of Cardiology/American Heart Association Task Force on Practice Guidelines. *J Am Coll Cardiol*. 2014;63:2889–2934.

Tuttle KR, Bakris GL, Bilous RW, et al. Diabetic kidney disease: a report from an ADA Consensus Conference. *Diabetes Care*. 2014;37:2864–2883.

UK Prospective Diabetes Study (UKPDS) Group. Intensive blood-glucose control with sulphonylureas or insulin compared with conventional treatment and risk of complications in patients with type 2 diabetes (UKPDS 33). *Lancet*. 1998;352:837–853; erratum in: *Lancet*. 1999;354:602.

U.S. Food and Drug Administration. Information for Healthcare Professionals. Reports of altered kidney function in patients using exenatide (marketed as Byetta). 2009. Available from http://www.fda.gov/Drugs/DrugSafety/PostmarketDrugSafetyInformationforPatientsandProviders/DrugSafetyInformationforHeathcareProfessionals/ucm188656.htm. Accessed January 11, 2011.

U.S. Food and Drug Administration. FDA Drug Safety Communication: FDA revises warnings regarding use of the diabetes medicine metformin in certain patients with reduced kidney function. Available from http://www.fda.gov/Drugs/DrugSafety/ucm493244.htm. Accessed April 8, 2016.

Udell JA, Yuan Z, Rush T, et al. Cardiovascular outcomes and risks after initiation of a sodium glucose cotransporter 2 inhibitor. *Circulation*. 2018;137:1450–1459.

Wallia A, Illuri V, Molitch ME. Diabetes care after transplant: definitions, risk factors, and clinical management. *Med Clin North Am*. 2016;100:535–550.

Wallia A, Molitch ME. Insulin therapy for type 2 diabetes mellitus. *JAMA*. 2014;311:2315–2325.

Wanner C, Inzucchi SE, Lachin JM, et al; EMPA-REG OUTCOME Investigators. Empagliflozin and progression of kidney disease in type 2 diabetes. *N Engl J Med*. 2016;375:323–334.

Wanner C, Lachin JM, Inzucchi SE, et al. Empagliflozin and clinical outcomes in patients with type 2 diabetes mellitus, established cardiovascular disease, and chronic kidney disease. *Circulation*. 2018;137:119–129.

Wile DJ, Toth C. Association of metformin, elevated homocysteine, and methylmalonic acid levels and clinically worsened diabetic peripheral neuropathy. *Diabetes Care*. 2010;33:156–161.

Whelton PK, Carey RM, Aronow WS, et al. 2017 ACC/AHA/AAPA/ABC/ACPM/AGS/APhA/ASH/ASPC/NMA/PCNA guideline for the prevention, detection, evaluation, and management of high blood pressure in adults. Executive summary: A report of the American College of Cardiology/American Heart Association Task Force on clinical practice guidelines. *Hypertension.* 2017: pii: HYP.0000000000000066.

Wong MG, Perkovic V, Chalmers J, et al; ADVANCE-ON Collaborative Group. Long-term benefits of intensive glucose control for preventing end-stage kidney disease: ADVANCE-ON. *Diabetes Care.* 2016;39:694–700.

Wright JT Jr, Williamson JD, Whelton PK, et al; Sprint Research Group. A randomized trial of intensive versus standard blood-pressure control. *N Engl J Med.* 2015;373:2103–2116.

Yki-Jarvinen H. Thiazolidinediones. *N Engl J Med.* 2004;351:1106–1118.

Zinman B, Wanner C, Lachin JM, et al; EMPA-REG OUTCOME Investigators. Empagliflozin, cardiovascular outcomes, and mortality in type 2 diabetes. *N Engl J Med.* 2015;373:2117–2128.

14

Optimizing Blood Pressure and Reducing Proteinuria

Rigas G. Kalaitzidis and George L. Bakris

HYPERTENSION AND PROGRESSION OF CHRONIC KIDNEY DISEASE

Hypertension is a risk factor for chronic kidney disease (CKD) and CKD progression. It is a strong predictor of end-stage renal disease (ESRD) development as well. The second most common cause of ESRD after diabetic nephropathy is hypertensive nephrosclerosis. In an individual with CKD, many of the abnormalities present or certain agents used could be responsible for blood pressure elevation (Table 14.1).

Interventions that lower blood pressure in patients with CKD consistently slow the rate of kidney function loss. In patients with diabetic or nondiabetic kidney disease, the lower the achieved blood pressure (down to levels in the range of 130 to 133 mm Hg), the greater the preservation of kidney function (Fig. 14.1) (Bakris, 2000).

There now have been three randomized trials powered to evaluate CKD progression in hypertensive kidney disease, and none supports a blood pressure target of <130/80 mm Hg to further slow CKD progression. However, all three demonstrated reduced cardiovascular events at BP levels below 130/80 mm Hg.

Importance of Proteinuria on the Hypertension-Progression Relationship

Urinary protein excretion of >300 mg/day is strongly predictive of a more rapid decline in kidney function. The impact of blood pressure reduction on slowing progression of CKD is greatest in those patients with proteinuria well above 300 mg/day (Jafar, 2003). While reductions in albuminuria of at least 30% or more are consistent with a slowed decline in kidney function, this is not apparent when urinary protein excretion is less than 300 mg/day.

HYPERTENSION, CHRONIC KIDNEY DISEASE, AND CARDIOVASCULAR DISEASE RISK

Blood Pressure Targets

New guidelines released in 2017 by the American College of Cardiology/American Heart Association recommend a blood pressure goal, <130/80 mm Hg, for patients with CKD and/or diabetes (Whelton, 2017). This is in keeping with the recent American Diabetes Association (ADA) BP guidelines (2018) and other international guidelines (KDOQI, 2012; Mancia, 2013).

TABLE 14.1	Factors Potentially Related to Hypertension in Chronic Kidney Disease

Pre-existing essential hypertension
Extracellular fluid volume expansion
Renin–angiotensin–aldosterone system stimulation
Increased sympathetic activity
Endogenous digitalis-like factors
Prostaglandin/bradykinin
Alterations in endothelium-derived factors (nitric oxide/endothelin)
Increased body weight
Erythropoietin administration
Parathyroid hormone secretion/increased intracellular calcium/hypercalcemia
Calcification of arterial tree
Cyclosporine, tacrolimus, or other immunosuppressive and corticosteroid therapy
Renal artery disease

Source: Adapted from Mailloux LU, Haley WE. Hypertension in the ESRD patient: pathophysiology, therapy, outcomes, and future directions. *Am J Kidney Dis.* 1998;32:705–719.

There is some evidence in patients with 1 g/day or higher albuminuria to support a blood pressure target of less than 130/80 mm Hg (KDOQI, 2012). The ADA has recommended that lower systolic blood pressure (SBP) and diastolic blood pressure (DBP) targets, such as 130/80 mm Hg, may be appropriate for individuals at high risk of cardiovascular

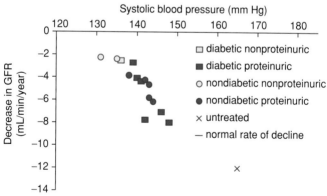

FIGURE 14.1 Relationship between achieved blood pressure control and declines in GFR in clinical trials of diabetic (*squares*) and nondiabetic (*circles*) kidney disease. Trials studying mostly proteinuric patients are marked as *solid squares* or *circles*; those studying patients with minimal proteinuria are shown as *hollow squares* or *circles*. The "*x*" shows data from an untreated group of hypertensives for comparison.
(Adapted from and updated from Bakris GL, Williams M, Dworkin L, et al. Preserving renal function in adults with hypertension and diabetes: a consensus approach. National Kidney Foundation Hypertension and Diabetes Executive Committees Working Group. *Am J Kidney Dis.* 2000;36:646–661.

disease, if such targets can be achieved without undue treatment burden (ADA, 2018; de Boer, 2018).

The Systolic Blood Pressure Intervention Trial (SPRINT) demonstrated that those with pre-existing CKD randomized to a BP <120 mm Hg had lower CV event rates but no difference in CKD progression (Wright, 2015).

In the Action in Diabetes and Vascular Disease: Preterax and Diamicron Controlled Evaluation (ADVANCE) study, the active blood pressure intervention arm (a single-pill, fixed-dose combination of perindopril and indapamide) compared with the placebo group, experienced an average reduction of 5.6 mm Hg in SBP and 2.2 mm Hg in DBP. The final blood pressure in the treated group was 136/73 mm Hg. The study showed a significant reduction in the risk of the primary composite end point (major macro- or microvascular event) and significant reductions in the risk of death from any cause and of death from cardiovascular causes. A 6-year follow-up of the ADVANCE trial, (ADVANCE-ON), reported a benefit on CKD progression in the treatment group, which was noted after 4 years (Zoungas, 2014).

THE SPECTRUM OF ALBUMINURIA

High albuminuria (formerly microalbuminuria) is defined as urine albumin excretion (UAE) between 30 and 299 mg/day and very high albuminuria (formerly macroalbuminuria) as UAE >300 mg/day, if measured in a 24-hour urine collection, or the same ranges measured in spot urine collections, in units of mg/g of creatinine. The presence of high albuminuria is associated with an increased risk for cardiovascular events and has been identified to be a cardiovascular risk marker (Bakris and Molitch, 2014; KDOQI, 2012).

The presence of very high albuminuria is associated with more rapid progression to kidney failure and increased risk of cardiovascular disease. Reductions in very high albuminuria correlate with preservation of kidney function and reductions in cardiovascular mortality. The goal of therapy in patients with very high albuminuria is reducing the rate of kidney disease progression and the risk of cardiovascular disease.

In individuals with very high albuminuria, current guidelines mandate the use of angiotensin-converting enzyme inhibitors (ACEIs) or angiotensin receptor blockers (ARBs) as part of an antihypertensive regimen, coupled with a low-sodium diet to reduce albuminuria and blood pressure. This initial selection of antihypertensives is no longer mandated in those individuals with normotension or with high albuminuria.

Effect of Angiotensin-Converting Enzyme Inhibitors and Angiotensin Receptor Blockers

ACEIs and ARBs are agents shown to slow the rate of decline in kidney function in both diabetic and nondiabetic kidney disease.

Dual RAAS Blockade

There is evidence of harm as evidenced by accelerated decline in kidney function when ACEIs and ARBs are combined, even though albuminuria is further reduced. Thus, current guidelines recommend against the combination of ARBs with ACEIs.

Aldosterone Receptor Antagonists

Aldosterone blockade can further reduce proteinuria in patients already receiving a RAAS-blocking agent. Use of aldosterone receptor antagonists such as spironolactone, eplerenone, or finerenone may be indicated in patients with very high albuminuric CKD. However, when using spironolactone or eplerenone, the serum potassium must be followed closely because levels rise in a dose-dependent fashion, and a dose adjustment of concomitantly given conventional (loop or thiazide) diuretic therapy should be always considered to help counterbalance this hyperkalemia.

In patients, already on an ACEI or an ARB, further blockade of the RAAS with an aldosterone receptor antagonist such as spirono-lactone or eplerenone is beneficial in the setting of heart failure and albuminuria reduction. However, there is no evidence of effect on slowing of CKD progression.

MANAGEMENT OF HYPERTENSION

The achievement of a goal of blood pressure <140/90 mm Hg in patients with kidney disease requires lifestyle modifications, the most important of which are dietary sodium restriction to <2,300 mg/day as well as a minimum of 6 hours of uninterrupted sleep at night. As noted previously, there is no prospective evidence to support a BP target lower than <130/80 mm Hg versus lower than <140/90 mm Hg to slow CKD progression. However, there are multiple post hoc analyses showing a further slowing of CKD progression at the lower BP targets in those subjects with >1 g/day of albuminuria.

Blood Pressure Measurement

Automated office blood pressure measurement (AOBPM) is the preferred method for recording blood pressure and is reflected in the latest AHA/ACC BP guidelines. This technique was used in both the SPRINT and ACCORD trials. The method requires 5 minutes of rest in a quiet room followed by BP measurement in triplicate with a programmed device. Such values are lower than routine BP measured in clinic by 5 to 10 mm Hg.

There is increasing emphasis on the usefulness of out-of-office blood pressures, obtained primarily by the patient at home on a regular basis or 24-hour ambulatory blood pressure monitoring. There is considerable evidence that **so-called "masked" hypertension**, normal office BP with increased ambulatory BP, has prognostic value in nondialysis CKD patients. Its diagnosis should be confirmed by repeating office and out-of-office BP measurements using ambulatory or home measurements, and treatment decisions should be based on out-of-office measurements. In patients with CKD, masked hypertension, rather than white coat hypertension, is associated with increased risks of all-cause mortality, major adverse cardiac events, and cerebrovascular events. Masked hypertension is also associated with adverse outcomes in terms of increased proteinuria and/or progression of CKD.

Ambulatory BP measurement has prognostic value as well; including the nighttime ambulatory BP. Lack of a nocturnal decrease in BP on ambulatory monitoring is associated with increased risk of progression of CKD and increased mortality. The indications for ambulatory BP monitoring in CKD patients include suspected white coat hypertension, resistant hypertension, presence of unexplained hypotensive symptoms, and patients with autonomic dysfunction (KDOQI, 2004).

Home Blood Pressure Monitoring
The use of home BP monitoring is convenient and is being increasingly recommended by various guideline bodies (ADA, 2018; KDOQI, 2004; KDOQI, 2012; Parati, 2016). When home BP monitoring is used, care must be taken to purchase a system validated to give accurate BP readings (Kollias, 2018).

Blood Pressure Variability
Home and ambulatory BP monitoring is the best way to evaluate blood pressure variability. Twenty-four hour BP variability is higher in subjects with white coat hypertension, and a blunted nocturnal BP decrease is observed more frequently in subjects with masked hypertension. Higher SBP visit-to-visit variability has been associated with the development of proteinuria and with increased risk of adverse events in patients with CKD. The magnitude of the association of SBP variability with renal outcomes is nearly as large as that of mean SBP, a well-established risk factor for renal outcomes. Individuals with more severe CKD have greater BP variability, and this seems to be related in part to poor sleep quality (Yeh, 2017).

Low-Sodium Diet
Salt reduction in individuals with CKD will reduce BP considerably and consistently, and also is associated with decreases in UAE. Furthermore, salt reduction magnifies the effects of ACEI/ARB treatment on albuminuria reduction, and also can be very helpful in controlling resistant hypertension.

Angiotensin-Converting Enzyme Inhibitors and Angiotensin Receptor Blockers
The evidence for preferential use of ACEI/ARBs is strongest for patients with nephropathy, regardless of cause, in whom there is very high albuminuria and CKD (Table 14.2). The evidence of benefit is strongest at moderate to high doses of these RAAS inhibitors, and may be minimal at low doses of these agents. In general, dose of RAAS blockers does not markedly affect the side-effect profile of these drugs.

			Other Agents to Reduce Cardiovascular
Type of Kidney Disease	**Blood Pressure Target (mm Hg)**	**Preferred Agents for CKD, With Hypertension**	**Disease Risk and Reach Blood Pressure Target**
Diabetic kidney disease[a]	<140/90	ACE inhibitor or ARB	CCB preferred, then diuretic or BB
Diabetic kidney disease with high cardiovascular risk[a] or moderate/severe albuminuria	SBP <130–125 DBP <80 (auscultatory measurements)	ACE inhibitor or ARB	CCB preferred, then diuretic or BB
Nondiabetic kidney disease without proteinuria	<130/80	None preferred	ACE inhibitor or ARB, CCB or diuretic
Nondiabetic kidney disease with protein excretion 500–1,000 mg/day or more	<130/80[b]	ACE inhibitor or ARB	CCB preferred, then diuretic or BB

TABLE 14.2 Recommendations for Blood Pressure Control in Chronic Kidney Disease

[a]Per American Diabetes Association Guidelines 2018.
[b]Modification of Diet in Renal Disease (MDRD)/African American Study of Kidney Disease and Hypertension (AASK) trials.
CKD, chronic kidney disease; ACE, angiotensin-converting enzyme; ARB, angiotensin receptor blocker; CCB, calcium channel blocker; BB, β-blocker.
Source: Adapted from National Kidney Foundation. KDOQI clinical practice guideline for diabetes and CKD: 2012 update. *Am J Kidney Dis.* 2012;60:850–886.

In contrast to their beneficial effects in albuminuria and CKD, the use of ACEI/ARBs does not appear to be more effective compared to other antihypertensive agents in CKD patents without proteinuria. There currently is no strong evidence that would suggest a preference for ACEIs versus ARBs. When ACEI versus ARB comparisons have been done, equivalent efficacy was found. ARBs are extremely well tolerated and do not have the side effect of cough often seen with ACEIs.

ACEIs, ARBs, and aldosterone receptor antagonists are contraindicated in pregnancy. ACEIs can precipitate angioedema and so are contraindicated in patients with a history of angioedema. ARBs also must be used with caution in patients with angioedema as a 10% cross-reactivity has been reported in those individuals who have had ACEI- induced angioedema.

Increases in Serum Creatinine With RAAS Blockers
Analysis of long-term clinical trial data confirms that ACEI-induced reduction in kidney function plateaus within 2 months (Bakris and Weir, 2000). If serum creatinine increases by >30% or continues to

rise after 3 months of therapy with a RAAS-blocking agent, volume depletion, unsuspected left ventricular dysfunction, or bilateral renal artery stenosis should be considered.

These data have made their way into guidelines. All major U.S. blood pressure guidelines note that at serum creatinine values of <3.0 mg/dL (265 mcmol/L) and age <65 years, a 30% to 35% increase in serum creatinine above the starting point is acceptable within the first 3 to 4 months of starting blood pressure lowering treatment. This is true if creatinine does not continue to rise and hyperkalemia does not occur. Therefore, ACEIs or ARBs should be withdrawn only when the rise of serum creatinine exceeds baseline by 30% to 35% within the first 3 to 4 months of therapy or when hyperkalemia (serum potassium >5.2 mmol/L) occurs.

Concomitant use of diuretics and nonsteroidal anti-inflammatory drugs (NSAIDs) with ACEI/ARB increases the risk of creatinine increases. In patients receiving ACEIs/ARBs, NSAIDs should be avoided if possible, and if deemed necessary, used for the shortest time possible. To limit the combined adverse effects of diuretics and ACEIs/ARBs, it is best to not start these drugs concurrently, but rather to adjust the dose of ACEIs/ARBs first, and then to add diuretics as needed.

Hyperkalemia With RAAS Blockers

ACEIs, ARBs, and aldosterone receptor antagonists often are discontinued because of a resulting increase in serum potassium above 5.2 mmol/L. If detected early, elevations in serum potassium can be rectified by starting, or increasing the dose of, a loop diuretic. One also should always stop, if feasible, any concomitantly administered drugs known to increase the serum potassium, especially potassium-sparing diuretics (triamterene, amiloride, and aldosterone antagonists), NSAIDs, heparin, and trimethoprim. Dietary education regarding potassium-containing foods is also important. Patients at highest risk for developing hyperkalemia after aldosterone antagonist administration are those with a baseline estimated glomerular filtration date (GFR)/1.73 m^2 < 45 mL/min and baseline serum potassium > 4.5 mmol/L who were already on an appropriate diuretic and who were being maximally dosed with an ACEI or ARB (Khosla, 2009; Lazich and Bakris, 2014).

The introduction of a novel ion exchange resin represents the first new pharmacologic therapy for hyperkalemia. Patiromer is a calcium-based resin that works in the distal colon and is effective for decreasing serum potassium in patients with CKD. It is safe when taken daily for at least up to 1 year (Bakris, 2016). Moreover, its better tolerability and similar cost and restrictions to sodium polystyrene make patiromer a more palatable choice for long-term management of hyperkalemia. Sodium zirconium cyclosilicate is a sodium-based "sorbent" compound that has been designed to bind potassium in the gut and increase its fecal excretion (Meaney, 2017).

Diuretics

The use of a diuretic restores the antiproteinuric effect of an ACEI when a high-sodium diet is consumed. Thiazide and thiazide-like diuretics (chlorthalidone and indapamide) become less effective when GFR falls below 30 mL/min per 1.73 m². Adequate blood pressure control in patients with more severe CKD thus, very likely will require concomitant administration of a loop diuretic (e.g., furosemide, torsemide, bumetanide) as part of the blood pressure–lowering regimen, because these compounds have higher intrinsic efficacy compared with thiazides.

Thiazide diuretics are associated with increased serum uric acid levels as well as increased serum glucose and low-density lipoprotein (LDL) cholesterol. They can cause both hypokalemia and hypomagnesemia, both of which are associated with increased cardiovascular risk. Thiazide-like diuretics (chlorthalidone or indapamide) are preferable to the thiazides based on outcomes data. Thiazide-like diuretics have a substantially longer duration of action and this may result in a greater fall in nighttime blood pressure.

Potassium-sparing diuretics (triamterene, amiloride) should be avoided in patients with pre-existing hyperkalemia, that is, serum potassium >5.2 mmol/L.

COMBINATION THERAPY

RAAS Blocker Plus a Calcium Channel Blocker

Combination therapy of two or more antihypertensive agents should be used initially to achieve blood pressure goals if blood pressure is >20/10 mm Hg above the goal of <140/90 mm Hg. To achieve blood pressure goal in most patients with CKD, a calcium antagonist should be considered as an add-on therapy to the ACEI or ARB regimen plus an appropriate type of long-acting diuretic, dosed correctly, regardless of CKD etiology. This approach has been tested in clinical trials (ACCOMPLISH) (Fig. 14.2).

β-Blockers

β-Blockers are often used to treat patients with recent myocardial infarction or coronary artery disease. Certain members of this drug class (carvedilol, extended-release metoprolol, or bisoprolol) have been shown to prevent secondary adverse cardiovascular events in patients with heart failure with systolic dysfunction.

In the absence of such indications β-blockers are not indicated as first-line therapy in the treatment of hypertension (Whelton, 2017). One important additional utility for β-blockers: patients with hypertension being treated with vasodilators commonly develop tachycardia and require β-blockers to mitigate this side effect of vasodilators.

β-Blockers are associated with reduced cardiovascular events in patients with CKD but have not been consistently shown to slow the rate of CKD progression.

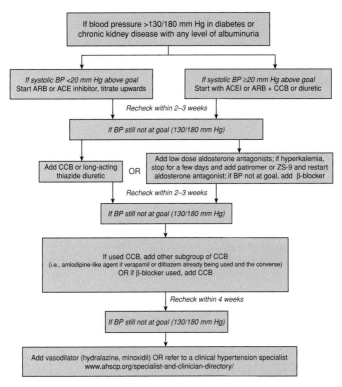

FIGURE 14.2 Blood pressure management algorithm. Note carvedilol has the best data in CKD for proteinuria and BP reduction. ACE Inhibitor, angiotensin-converting enzyme inhibitor; ARB, angiotensin II receptor blocker; BP, blood pressure; CCB, calcium channel blocker.

Calcium Channel Blockers

Calcium channel blockers (CCBs) are effective BP-lowering agents and within this class of antihypertensive drugs, various subclasses have different effects on proteinuria independent of their blood pressure–lowering effects. These differences are due to differing effects of these subclasses on glomerular permeability. Non-dihydropyridine CCBs (verapamil, diltiazem) reduce proteinuria among patients with advanced very high albuminuric nephropathy, whereas dihydropyridine CCBs (nifedipine, felodipine, and amlodipine) have a minimal or neutral effect unless used in combination with a RAAS blocker. Hence, dihydropyridine CCBs should not be used as monotherapy in CKD patients with very high albuminuria. Additionally, dihydropyridine CCBs are less efficacious in slowing progression of CKD compared to ACEIs or ARBs.

Central α-Adrenergic Agonists

The most commonly used drug in this group is clonidine. Other members of the class include guanfacine and methyldopa. The rationale for their use is to mitigate the increase in sympathetic activity commonly observed in CKD. Clonidine causes sedation, dry mouth, bradycardia, and can worsen depression. These agents have never been shown to slow CKD progression and have a very high side-effect profile. They are effective if used appropriately to lower BP.

Vasodilators

Minoxidil or hydralazine is sometimes required when other antihypertensive treatments have failed. They are drugs of last resort. Reduction of hypertension using vasodilator therapy has not been shown to improve renal outcomes. Vasodilator use is associated with reflex tachycardia that can worsen angina pectoris, and these powerful vasodilators should always be combined with a β-adrenergic blocker. Minoxidil has a niche indication in the subgroup of patients with resistant hypertension and CKD. Hydralazine is a leading cause of drug-induced lupus syndrome, and its use should be avoided in any patient with a history of autoimmune disease.

α-Adrenergic Blockers

α-Blockers have not been shown to slow CKD progression or consistently reduce UAE in patients with type 2 diabetes and albuminuria. Moreover, this class of agents also failed to reduce cardiovascular events in the Antihypertensive and Lipid-Lowering Treatment to Prevent Heart Attack Trial (ALLHAT); the α-blocker arm of the ALLHAT was stopped early for safety reasons because of a relatively increased incidence of heart failure in patients taking doxazosin.

RENOVASCULAR DISEASE

Prevalence and Clinical Features

Renovascular disease is a potentially correctable cause of secondary hypertension and renal dysfunction. Renovascular disease can be due to atherosclerotic renal artery stenosis or to fibromuscular dysplasia. Atherosclerotic renal artery stenosis represents >90% of cases. The disease is common among smokers and those with hyperlipidemia that is not controlled. Patients are generally over 55 years of age and the condition often coexists with other vascular diseases and associated atherosclerotic comorbidities. The presence of renovascular disease is significantly and independently associated with ischemic heart disease and increased cardiovascular morbidity and mortality (Zanoli, 2014). Fibromuscular dysplasia most often affects women under the age of 50 years and typically involves the distal main renal artery or its intrarenal branches.

Renovascular disease can result in hypertension that is relatively resistant to therapy and consequently can induce accelerated target organ injury; including left ventricular hypertrophy, proteinuria, reduced glomerular filtration rate, and stroke.

The most common clues to renovascular hypertension include severe and/or resistant hypertension; onset at a young age with a negative family history; and an acute rise in blood pressure above a previously stable value (Table 14.3).

	Common Evidence for an Increased Suspicion of Renovascular Hypertension
TABLE 14.3	

Severe or refractory hypertension
Abdominal bruit
Unexplained acute increase in serum creatinine of more than 30% after initiating a renin–angiotensin system inhibitor or angiotensin receptor blocker
Unexplained kidney asymmetry (i.e., a unilateral small kidney)
Recurrent episodes of flash pulmonary edema
Renal dysfunction following initiation of a diuretic
Uncontrolled hypertension in younger-aged women or older men with severe atherosclerotic disease

Diagnostic Evaluation

Evaluation should be initiated with noninvasive studies such as Doppler ultrasonography. Duplex Doppler ultrasonography is useful to diagnose both unilateral and bilateral disease as well as to determine disease progression and to detect recurrent stenosis in previously treated patients. This may be followed by two-dimensional imaging, including angiography, computed tomographic angiography, or magnetic resonance angiography. Magnetic resonance angiography can detect proximal renal artery stenosis and provide excellent vascular imaging; however, in patients with reduced kidney function, lingering concerns about gadolinium-associated complications have reduced its application in this setting.

Clinically significant stenosis, that is, stenosis related to an increase in blood pressure or to decreased renal perfusion, usually occurs only when at least 70% to 80% stenosis can be demonstrated, with a 15% to 20% gradient post stenosis.

Angiography, continues to be considered the gold standard for estimating luminal stenosis in cases where the noninvasive test is inconclusive and the clinical suspicion remains high. Blood oxygen level–dependent (BOLD) magnetic resonance imaging is a promising new technique that allows a direct evaluation of oxygenation at the renal tissue level using the paramagnetic characteristics of deoxyhemoglobin (Sag, 2016). In patients with renal insufficiency, renography (nuclear medicine testing) is also indicated to determine the relative function of each kidney.

Medical Treatment

Improvement in systemic arterial blood pressure as well as the preservation of renal function are the main goals of treatment. Several randomized clinical trials such as the Cardiovascular Outcomes for Renal Artery Lesions (CORAL) trial or/and Angioplasty and Stenting for Renal Atherosclerotic Lesions (ASTRAL) trial failed to show superiority of revascularization over optimal medical therapy in terms of BP control (Ritchie, 2014). However, if kidney function deteriorates within a month of initiating medical therapy, angiographic stenting should be pursued.

ACEIs and ARBs are effective in treating hypertension in patients with renal artery stenosis. RAAS blockade diminishes progressive nephrosclerosis due to suppression of renal cell proliferation and infiltration of mononuclear cells that trigger expression of extracellular matrix proteins. Kidney function should be checked frequently within 1 to 2 weeks after initiation of therapy. Starting at a low dose may be helpful.

Surgical Treatment or Stenting
Surgical revascularization is rarely done today for correcting renal artery stenosis. Stenting of the renal artery is far more common to correct this problem; however, there is a substantial risk of causing atheroembolic disease distal to the lesion. This can even result in renal failure, albeit rarely (Lerman, 2009).

In patients with fibromuscular dysplasia, angioplasty rather than stenting is indicated, and more than 60% of the patients have been reported to be cured of their hypertension after such treatment (Slovut and Olin, 2004).

DOSAGE ADJUSTMENT OF ANTIHYPERTENSIVE DRUGS IN PATIENTS WITH REDUCED GLOMERULAR FILTRATION RATE

Dose adjustments for certain classes of antihypertensive drugs are recommended for patients with CKD. The primary classes of antihypertensive agents needing dose adjustment, mostly in stages 4 to 5 CKD, are those β-blockers and ACEIs that are primarily excreted by the kidneys. Please see Chapter 23 for details.

References and Suggested Readings

Al Dhaybi O, Bakris GL. Renal targeted therapies of antihypertensive and cardiovascular drugs for patients with stages 3 through 5d kidney disease. *Clin Pharmacol Ther.* 2017;102:450–458.

American Diabetes Association. Standards of medical care in diabetes. *Diabetes Care.* 2018;41:S1–S156.

Bakris GL. The implications of blood pressure measurement methods on treatment targets for blood pressure. *Circulation.* 2016;134:904–905.

Bakris GL, Molitch M. Microalbuminuria as a risk predictor in diabetes: the continuing saga. *Diabetes Care.* 2014;37:867–875.

Bakris GL, Pitt B, Weir MR, et al; Amethyst-DN Investigators. Effect of patiromer on serum potassium level in patients with hyperkalemia and diabetic kidney disease: The AMETHYST-DN randomized clinical trial. *JAMA.* 2015;314:151–161.

Bakris GL, Sarafidis PA, Weir MR, et al; ACCOMPLISH Trial investigators. Renal outcomes with different fixed-dose combination therapies in patients with hypertension at high risk for cardiovascular events (ACCOMPLISH): a prespecified secondary analysis of a randomised controlled trial. *Lancet.* 2010;375:1173–1181.

Bakris GL, Weir MR. Angiotensin-converting enzyme inhibitor-associated elevations in serum creatinine: is this a cause for concern? *Arch Intern Med.* 2000;160:685–693.

Bakris GL, Weir MR, Secic M, et al. Differential effects of calcium antagonist subclasses on markers of nephropathy progression. *Kidney Int.* 2004;65:1991–2002.

Bakris GL, Williams M, Dworkin L, et al. Preserving renal function in adults with hypertension and diabetes: a consensus approach. National Kidney Foundation Hypertension and Diabetes Executive Committees Working Group. *Am J Kidney Dis.* 2000;36:646–661.

de Boer IH, Bakris G, Cannon CP. Individualizing blood pressure targets for people with diabetes and hypertension: comparing the ADA and the ACC/AHA recommendations. *JAMA.* 2018;319:1319–1320.

Grams ME, Juraschek SP, Selvin E, et al. Trends in the prevalence of reduced GFR in the United States: a comparison of creatinine- and cystatin C-based estimates. *Am J Kidney Dis.* 2013;62:253–260.

Hansen KJ, Edwards MS, Craven TE, et al. Prevalence of renovascular disease in the elderly: a population-based study. *J Vasc Surg.* 2002;36:443–451.

Jafar TH, Stark PC, Schmid CH, et al; AIPRD Study Group. Progression of chronic kidney disease: the role of blood pressure control, proteinuria, and angiotensin-converting enzyme inhibition: a patient-level meta-analysis. *Ann Intern Med.* 2003;139:244–252.

Kane GC, Xu N, Mistrik E, et al. Renal artery revascularization improves heart failure control in patients with atherosclerotic renal artery stenosis. *Nephrol Dial Transplant.* 2010;25:813–820.

Khosla N, Kalaitzidis R, Bakris GL. Predictors of hyperkalemia risk following hypertension control with aldosterone blockade. *Am J Nephrol.* 2009;30:418–424.

Kidney Disease Outcomes Quality Initiative (K/DOQI). K/DOQI clinical practice guidelines on hypertension and antihypertensive agents in chronic kidney disease. *Am J Kidney Dis.* 2004;43:S1–S290.

Kidney Disease Outcomes Quality Initiative (K/DOQI). KDOQI clinical practice guideline for diabetes and CKD: 2012 update. *Am J Kidney Dis.* 2012;60:850–886.

Kollias A, Andreadis E, Agaliotis G, et al. The optimal night-time home blood pressure monitoring schedule: agreement with ambulatory blood pressure and association with organ damage. *J Hypertens.* 2018;36:243–249.

Lazich I, Bakris GL. Prediction and management of hyperkalemia across the spectrum of chronic kidney disease. *Semin Nephrol.* 2014;34:333–339.

Lerman LO, Textor SC, Grande JP. Mechanisms of tissue injury in renal artery stenosis: ischemia and beyond. *Prog Cardiovasc Dis.* 2009;52:196–203.

Mancia G, Fagard R, Narkiewicz K, et al; Task Force Members. 2013 ESH/ESC Guidelines for the management of arterial hypertension: the Task Force for the management of arterial hypertension of the European Society of Hypertension (ESH) and of the European Society of Cardiology (ESC). *J Hypertens.* 2013;31:1281–1357.

Meaney CJ, Beccari MV, Yang Y, et al. Systematic review and meta-analysis of patiromer and sodium zirconium cyclosilicate: A new armamentarium for the treatment of hyperkalemia. *Pharmacotherapy.* 2017;37:401–411.

Parati G, Ochoa JE, Bilo G, et al; European Renal and Cardiovascular Medicine (EURECA-m) working group of the European Renal Association-European Dialysis Transplantation Association (ERA-EDTA). Hypertension in chronic kidney disease part 2: Role of ambulatory and home blood pressure monitoring for assessing alterations in blood pressure variability and blood pressure profiles. *Hypertension.* 2016;67:1102–1110.

Ritchie J, Alderson HV, Kalra P A. Where now in the management of renal artery stenosis? Implications of the ASTRAL and CORAL trials. *Curr Opin Nephrol Hypertens.* 2014;23:525–532.

Sag AA, Inal I, Okcuoglu J, et al. Atherosclerotic renal artery stenosis in the post-CORAL era part 1: the renal penumbra concept and next-generation functional diagnostic imaging. *J Am Soc Hypertens.* 2016;10:360–367.

Slovut DP, Olin JW. Fibromuscular dysplasia. *N Engl J Med.* 2004;350:1862–1871.

Whelton PK, Carey RM, Aronow WS, et al. 2017 ACC/AHA/AAPA/ABC/ACPM/AGS/APhA/ASH/ASPC/NMA/PCNA Guideline for the prevention, detection, evaluation, and management of high blood pressure in adults: A Report of the American College of Cardiology/American Heart Association Task Force on clinical practice guidelines. *Hypertension.* 2017; doi: 10.1161/HYP.0000000000000065.

Wright JT Jr, Williamson JD, Whelton PK, et al; SPRINT Research Group. A randomized trial of intensive versus Standard Blood-Pressure Control. *N Engl J Med.* 2015;373:2103–2116.

Yeh CH, Yu HC, Huang TY, et al. The risk of diabetic renal function impairment in the first decade after diagnosed of diabetes mellitus is correlated with high variability of visit-to-visit systolic and diastolic blood pressure: a case control study. *BMC Nephrol.* 2017;18:99.

Zanoli L, Rastelli S, Marcantoni C, et al. Non-hemodynamically significant renal artery stenosis predicts cardiovascular events in persons with ischemic heart disease. *Am J Nephrol.* 2014;40:468–477.

Zoungas S, Chalmers J, Neal B, et al; ADVANCE-ON Collaborative Group. Follow-up of blood-pressure lowering and glucose control in type 2 diabetes. *N Engl J Med.* 2014;371:1392–1406.

15

Resistant Hypertension

Eric K. Judd and David A. Calhoun

Resistant hypertension is defined as blood pressure that remains above goal in spite of the concurrent use of three antihypertensive agents of different classes (Calhoun, 2008). Ideally, one of the three agents should be a diuretic, and all agents should be prescribed at optimal doses. Patients whose blood pressure is controlled but who require four or more medications to do so are also considered resistant to treatment. Identifying a patient as resistant allows for screening for secondary causes of hypertension and initiation of specific management strategies like mineralocorticoid receptor antagonism and evaluation of modifiable lifestyle factors.

PREVALENCE, PATIENT CHARACTERISTICS, AND PROGNOSIS

Among treated adults with hypertension, resistant hypertension prevalence has been reported at 10% to 18% (Egan, 2013; Judd and Calhoun, 2014; Muntner, 2014). Prevalence is higher within groups at risk for resistant hypertension, with rates up to 40% in patients with chronic kidney disease (CKD) and 25% in patients with a history of stroke (Howard, 2015; Thomas, 2016). Patient characteristics that predict resistant hypertension include African-American race, obesity, CKD, albuminuria, older age, diabetes mellitus, and obstructive sleep apnea (Persell, 2011; Sim, 2013). Of these, CKD has the strongest association with resistant hypertension (adjusted odds ratio 1.84, 95% confidence interval 1.78 to 1.90) (Sim, 2013). More than 50% of patients reaching CKD stage 4 have resistant hypertension (Thomas, 2016).

Resistant hypertension portends a poor prognosis. Compared to adults treated for hypertension, patients with resistant hypertension are at a higher risk for end-stage kidney disease, ischemic heart disease, heart failure, stroke, and mortality (Sim, 2015). Among individuals with CKD, resistant hypertension increases the risk of death by 30% and the risk of heart failure by 59% (Thomas, 2016).

DIFFERENTIAL DIAGNOSIS

A patient with uncontrolled blood pressure may meet initial criteria for resistant hypertension, but after further scrutiny the patient may be found to have **pseudoresistant hypertension**. Suboptimal treatment, antihypertensive medication nonadherence, white-coat effect, or inaccurate blood pressure measurement, each can result in pseudoresistance. Pseudoresistance is common, being present in approximately one-third of patients initially identified as resistant to treatment (Judd and Calhoun, 2014).

A **suboptimal or inappropriate medical regimen** may be the most significant modifiable factor contributing to pseudoresistance. In one large Southern California health system, blood pressure control rates improved from 54% in 2004 to 84% after implementing a multidisciplinary model of care with a stepwise treatment algorithm (Sim, 2014). Individuals who meet criteria for resistant hypertension are typically prescribed a diuretic; however antihypertensive medications are commonly dosed below 50% of their maximally recommended dose (Egan, 2013). Overall, ideal regimens take into account efficacy and medication adherence by *utilizing fewer numbers of medications at maximum dosing, consolidating dosing frequency to once or twice per day, incorporating combination pills or capsules, and considering out-of-pocket costs.*

Despite an ideal regimen, some patients are **nonadherent**. Because resistant hypertension is defined by blood pressure control and number of medications prescribed, the resistant population is enriched with those individuals who are nonadherent. In one study that measured antihypertensive metabolites in the urine, 53% of individuals identified as resistant to treatment were shown to be nonadherent (Gupta, 2017; Jung, 2013). Nonadherence is difficult to recognize, but can be discovered through a frank discussion with the patient about potential barriers to therapy.

Inaccurate blood pressure measurement due to poor technique and a significant **white-coat effect** (e.g., persistently elevated clinic blood pressures while out-of-office blood pressure readings are normal or significantly lower) may also result in pseudoresistance and a false diagnosis of resistant hypertension. While 24-hour ambulatory blood pressure monitoring can identify a white-coat effect and minimizes inaccurate measurement, it may not be widely available for clinical use. Self-measured home blood pressure measurement and automated office blood pressure (AOBP) measurement, however, have become popular in the United States and have been employed in clinical trials (Williams, 2015; Wright, 2015). An AOBP measurement is obtained by an oscillometric device that cycles through multiple blood pressure measurements in the absence of an operator. For a comprehensive review of blood pressure measurement technique, the reader is referred to the American Heart Association's recommendation for blood pressure measurement in humans (Pickering, 2005).

When evaluating a patient with potential resistant hypertension, it is important to first exclude pseudoresistance. Patients with uncontrolled hypertension due to nonadherence, inappropriate treatment regimen, or white-coat effect often do not need further evaluation for secondary causes.

SECONDARY HYPERTENSION

A secondary cause of hypertension can be identified in 10% to 40% of patients with resistant hypertension. Hyperaldosteronism, CKD, and renal artery stenosis are the most common, whereas pheochromo-cytoma, Cushing syndrome, genetic disorders (e.g., Liddle syndrome, familial hyperkalemic hypertension [formerly, pseudohypoaldoste-ronism type II or Gordon syndrome], and glucocorticoid remediable aldosteronism), primary hyperparathyroidism, aortic coarctation, and intracranial tumors are some uncommon secondary causes.

Primary Aldosteronism

Primary aldosteronism, which was historically believed to be a rare cause of hypertension, has been shown to be common in patients with resistant hypertension, with a prevalence of ~20% (Calhoun, 2002). Because of its relatively high prevalence, all patients with resistant hypertension should be evaluated for hyperaldosteronism.

Screening for primary aldosteronism consists of measuring a serum aldosterone level and plasma renin activity, ideally in a patient with a normal blood potassium level (i.e., after potassium has been repleted in the setting of hypokalemia) and who has been seated for at least 30 minutes prior to sampling. A ratio of aldosterone (ng/dL) to plasma renin activity (ng/mL/h) >30:1 or >20:1 with an aldosterone level $\geq$16 ng/dL is a positive screening test. Concomitant use of a mineralocorticoid antagonist like spironolactone or eplerenone may cause a false-positive screening aldosterone-to-renin ratio, and these medications should be held for at least 4 weeks before testing. A diagnostic aldosterone-to-renin ratio typically prompts an endo-crinology or hypertension specialist referral for confirmatory testing and evaluation for an adrenal adenoma that might be amenable to surgical removal (Fig. 15.1).

Renal Parenchymal Disease

CKD is both a cause and consequence of uncontrolled hypertension. Reduced kidney function results in impaired salt excretion, dys-regulation of the renin–angiotensin–aldosterone system, increased sympathetic nervous system activity, and blunted antihypertensive medication efficacy. Patients with CKD are more likely to have salt sensitivity, where blood pressure rises following a dietary salt load. A positive salt balance limits efficacy of angiotensin-converting enzyme inhibitors (ACEIs) and angiotensin receptor blockers (ARBs). Fur-thermore, salt has a direct effect on function of the vasculature and blunting vasodilation (Titze and Luft, 2017). Because the majority of patients with advanced kidney disease (e.g., CKD stage 4 or 5) have resistant hypertension, screening for additional underlying causes of hypertension is reserved for patients with a high clinical suspicion in this population.

Renovascular Disease

When evaluated by renal arteriogram, renal artery stenosis is pres-ent in ~20% of older patients with resistant hypertension (Benjamin, 2014). The vast majority of renal artery lesions are atherosclerotic in etiology, and prevalence increases with greater patient age, known

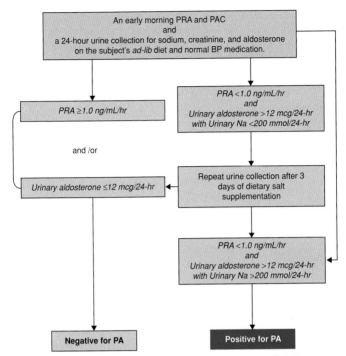

FIGURE 15.1 Flowchart for confirmatory testing for primary aldosteronism (PA). Na, sodium; PAC, plasma aldosterone concentration; PRA, plasma renin activity.
(Adapted with permission from Nishizaka M, Pratt-Ubunama M, Zaman MA, et al. Validity of plasma aldosterone-to-renin activity ratio in African American and white subjects with resistant hypertension. *Am J Hypertens*. 2005;18:805–812.)

atherosclerotic disease, and presence of unexplained renal insufficiency. Bilateral renal artery stenosis should be suspected in patients with a history of "flash" or episodic pulmonary edema, especially when echocardiography indicates preserved systolic heart function. Multiple randomized clinical trials argue against an advantage of revascularization procedures over medical treatment for atherosclerotic-related renal artery stenosis (Cooper, 2014). However, renal artery stenosis due to fibromuscular dysplasia does respond favorably to balloon angioplasty. Fibromuscular dysplasia is a congenital collagen vascular disorder that classically presents as severe hypertension in a young female with an abdominal bruit on physical examination. Renovascular disease is discussed in more detail in Chapter 14.

Pheochromocytoma

Pheochromocytoma is an uncommon but important secondary cause of resistant hypertension, occurring in 0.1% to 0.6% of hypertensives in a general ambulatory population. Pheochromocytoma is characterized by increased blood pressure variability, headaches, palpitations, and pallor with piloerection (i.e., "cold sweat"), typically occurring in an episodic fashion. Pheochromocytomas are associated with certain genetic disorders, including neurofibromatosis type 1, Von Hippel–Lindau disease, and multiple endocrine neoplasia (MEN) type II. Plasma-free metanephrine levels are an effective screening test with a sensitivity of 96% to 100% (Schwartz, 2011).

Obstructive Sleep Apnea

Obstructive sleep apnea is a common finding in patients with resistant hypertension, with a reported prevalence of more than 80% of patients (Logan, 2001). However, as opposed to other conditions associated with secondary hypertension, obstructive sleep apnea may not be a cause of resistant hypertension, but instead, due to a shared physiology of excess central fluid, particularly in hyperaldosteronism. In patients with resistant hypertension, treatment of obstructive sleep apnea with continuous positive airway pressure reduces blood pressure by an average of 3 mm Hg (Martinez-Garcia, 2013).

Evaluation

Figure 15.2 illustrates a schematic for evaluating a patient with resistant hypertension. A thorough history includes asking about duration of hypertension; treatment adherence; response to prior medications, including adverse events; current medication use, including herbal and over-the-counter medications; and symptoms of possible secondary causes of hypertension. An expanded social history may reveal heavy alcohol ingestion, regular cocaine use, and/or high dietary salt intake. Pharmacologic and lifestyle factors that contribute to treatment resistance are summarized in Table 15.1. A family history of early death or stroke supports genetic causes like glucocorticoid remediable aldosteronism. Physical examination findings of abdominal striae support Cushing syndrome and an abdominal bruit in a young individual may indicate fibromuscular dysplasia.

Blood Pressure Measurement

Appropriate blood pressure measurement technique is needed to accurately identify resistant hypertension. Blood pressure measurement begins by preparing the individual. Individuals should empty their urinary bladder (if full) and be seated in a quiet room, ideally for 5 minutes before measurement. A blood pressure cuff with a bladder length of at least 80% of the arm circumference and a width of at least 40% of the arm circumference is placed directly on the skin on the upper arm, at the level of the heart. During measurement the individual is seated with support for his/her feet, back, and arm. A minimum of two readings 1 minute apart are obtained (Pickering, 2005). As discussed above, AOBP measurement and self-measured home blood pressure monitoring minimize the white-coat effect and are recommended for patients with uncontrolled hypertension.

Confirm Treatment Resistance
Office blood pressure >40/90 or 130/80 mm Hg in patients with diabetes or CKD

and

Patient prescribed 3 or more antihypertensive medications at optimal doses, including
if possible a diuretic

or

Office blood pressure at goal but patient requiring 4 or more antihypertensive medications

↓

Exclude Pseudoresistance
Is patient adherent with prescribed regimen?
Obtain home, work, or ambulatory blood pressure readings to exclude white-coat effect

Identify and Reverse Contributing Lifestyle Factors
Obesity
Physical inactivity
Excessive alcohol ingestion
High-salt, low-fiber diet

↓

Discontinue or Minimize Interfering Substances
Nonsteroidal anti-inflammatory agents
Sympathomimetics (diet pills, decongestants)
Stimulants
Oral contraceptives
Licorice
Ephedra

↓

Screen for Secondary Causes of Hypertension
Obstructive sleep apnea (snoring, witnessed apnea, excessive daytime sleepiness)
Primary aldosteronism (elevated aldosterone/rennin ratio)
CKD (creatinine clearance <30 mL/min)
Renal artery stenosis (young female, known atherosclerotic disease, worsening renal function)
Pheochromocytoma (episodic hypertension palpitations, diaphoresis, headache)
Cushing syndrome (moon facies, central obesity, abdominal striae, interscapular fat deposition)
Aortic coarctation (differential in brachial or femoral pulses, systolic bruit)

↓

Pharmacologic Treatment
Maximize diuretic therapy, including possible addition of mineralocorticoid receptor antagonist
Combine agents with different mechanisms of action
Use of loop diuretics in patients with CKD and/or patients receiving potent vasodilators
(e.g., minoxidil)

↓

Refer to Specialist
Refer to appropriate specialist for known or suspected secondary cause(s) of hypertension
Refer to hypertension specialist if blood pressure remains uncontrolled after 6 months of
treatment

FIGURE 15.2 Resistant hypertension: diagnostic and treatment recommendations.
(Adapted with permission from Calhoun DA, Jones D, Textor S, et al. Resistant hyperten-
sion: diagnosis, evaluation, and treatment: a scientific statement from the American
Heart Association Professional Education Committee of the Council for High Blood
Pressure Research. *Hypertension.* 2008;51:1403–1419.)

Laboratory Tests

Biochemical evaluation of patients with resistant hypertension
should include a routine metabolic profile, urinalysis, and paired
morning blood samples for serum aldosterone and plasma renin

TABLE 15.1	Pharmacologic and Lifestyle Factors That Can Interfere With Blood Pressure Control

Obesity
Physical inactivity
Heavy alcohol intake (>30–50 g/day)
High dietary salt intake
Medications:
   Nonsteroidal anti-inflammatory agents, including selective COX-2 inhibitors
   Sympathomimetic agents (e.g., pseudoephedrine, ephedrine, phentermine, cocaine)
   Stimulants (e.g., methylphenidate, dexmethylphenidate, dextroamphetamine, amphetamine, methamphetamine)
   Oral contraceptives (estrogen containing)
   Immunosuppressive agents (e.g., calcineurin inhibitors like cyclosporine and tacrolimus, VEGF inhibitors)
   Erythropoietin
Monoamine oxidase inhibitors (effect exacerbated by foods containing tyramine)
Natural licorice
Herbal compounds (e.g., ephedra, ma-huang)

activity to screen for primary aldosteronism (see primary aldosteronism above). In patients in whom pheochromocytoma is being considered, plasma-free metanephrine levels are an appropriate initial screening test, due to its high negative predictive value.

Imaging Studies

Imaging studies are not recommended in the initial evaluation of resistant hypertension. However, if the clinical suspicion for fibromuscular dysplasia is high, then renal artery imaging can be part of the initial evaluation. When screening for fibromuscular dysplasia, due to the need to detect an irregular and beaded pattern of artery narrowing, angiography either by computed tomography or magnetic resonance is recommended over duplex ultrasonography. In patients at risk for atherosclerotic-related renal artery stenosis (e.g., older individuals with a history of tobacco use), duplex ultrasonography can establish the diagnosis but might not alter management (Cooper, 2014). Abdominal imaging of the adrenal gland by computed tomography with and without contrast is only indicated following positive biochemical laboratory studies (e.g., elevated aldosterone, metanephrines, cortisol).

TREATMENT

Lifestyle changes including weight loss, regular exercise, ingestion of low-salt diet, and moderation of alcohol intake (to no more than two or three drinks per day) should be encouraged when appropriate. Drugs, stimulants, and other substances known to increase blood pressure (Table 15.1) should be withdrawn as clinically allowable. The amount of blood pressure lowering with each of these approaches is often modest but clinically important (Whelton, 2018). Accurate diagnosis and appropriate treatment of secondary causes of hypertension and effective multidrug regimens are essential for adequate treatment of resistant hypertension. Particular attention to factors related to poor adherence, such as medication cost and adverse effects, can improve patient adherence and efficacy of treatment. A multidisciplinary approach with nurses, pharmacists, and nutritionists working together and following standardized protocols for blood pressure management can improve treatment results.

Use of Diuretics

Individuals with resistant hypertension commonly have an excess of salt and intravascular volume expansion (Pimenta, 2009). A physiologic state of overperfusion is supported by the observation that the majority (~67%) of patients with resistant hypertension have suppressed renin levels (Eide, 2004). In a randomized crossover study, low-sodium intake (50 mEq/24 h) compared to high-sodium intake (250 mEq/24 h) decreased office systolic and diastolic blood pressure by 22.7 and 9.1 mm Hg, respectively. Plasma renin activity increased whereas brain natriuretic peptide and creatinine clearance decreased during low-salt intake, suggesting intravascular volume reduction as a likely mechanism (Pimenta, 2009). A diuretic is essential to maximize blood pressure control unless contraindicated or not tolerated. The longer-acting thiazide-like diuretic chlorthalidone is preferred over hydrochlorothiazide due to improved efficacy. Chlorthalidone 25 mg daily provides greater 24-hour ambulatory blood pressure reduction than hydrochlorothiazide 50 mg (Ernst, 2006). In patients with advanced CKD (e.g., estimated glomerular filtration rate [eGFR] <30 mL/min per 1.73 m^2), the addition of loop diuretics may be necessary for effective volume and blood pressure control.

Combination Drug Therapy

Individuals with resistant hypertension will, by definition, be receiving at least three antihypertensive medications. The use of combination pills with two or more medications per pill/capsule reduces overall pill burden, potentially improving adherence. In addition, certain medication combinations have complementary effects. For example, the use of a potassium-sparing diuretic like amiloride with a thiazide diuretic was found to improve blood pressure control and prevent glucose intolerance (Brown, 2016). However, there are limitations to combination therapy. For example, the use of β-blockers in combination with nondihydropyridine calcium channel blockers (e.g., verapamil or diltiazem) often results in bradycardia. The concomitant use of ACEIs and ARBs is associated with acute kidney injury and hyperkalemia (Fried, 2013). See Chapter 14 for a broader discussion of multidrug regimens.

Aldosterone Antagonists

Low doses (e.g., 25 to 50 mg) of spironolactone provide significant blood pressure reduction when added to existing multidrug regimens, and the effect is independent of aldosterone and renin levels. Among 1,411 participants in the Anglo-Scandinavian Cardiac Outcomes Trial who received spironolactone as a fourth-line agent, blood pressure was reduced by 21.9/9.5 mm Hg after a median of 1.3 years of treatment (Chapman, 2007). When evaluated in a double-blind, placebo-controlled, crossover trial (PATHWAY-2), spironolactone at 25 to 50 mg dosing was superior to doxazosin or bisoprolol as a fourth-line antihypertensive medication. Home systolic blood pressure was reduced with spironolactone by a mean of 8.7 mm Hg compared to placebo, 4.0 mm Hg compared to doxazosin, and 4.5 mm Hg compared to bisoprolol ($p < 0.0001$ for all three comparisons) (Williams, 2015). Based on these data and others, spironolactone is recommended as the first medication to add if blood pressure is not controlled using the three foundational classes of antihypertensive medications: (1) ACEI or ARB, (2) dihydropyridine calcium channel blocker, and (3) thiazide or thiazide-like diuretic.

Although, well tolerated at low doses, aldosterone antagonists can be associated with hyperkalemia, gynecomastia in men, and reduced libido. More specific mineralocorticoid receptor antagonists like eplerenone reduce the occurrence of sexual side effects. However, eplerenone has been studied primarily as treatment for systolic heart failure and primary aldosteronism as opposed to a fourth-line agent for the treatment of resistant hypertension. Early clinical trials using a highly selective mineralocorticoid receptor antagonist, finerenone, have shown only modest reductions in blood pressure (<3 mm Hg), suggesting that off-target effects of spironolactone may contribute to blood pressure lowering (Filippatos, 2016).

An elevation of serum potassium levels is seen with all aldosterone antagonists. Among individuals with CKD stage 3, spironolactone raised the serum potassium level by an average of 0.4 mEq/L when added to lisinopril 80 mg (Van Buren, 2014). Administration of spironolactone in combination with a thiazide-like diuretic minimizes the risk of hyperkalemia and also enhances the antihypertensive benefit. Serum potassium and creatinine levels should be monitored closely after prescribing spironolactone, and due to the risks of hyperkalemia and acute kidney injury, caution is advised with spironolactone use in advanced CKD (e.g., eGFR <30 mL/min per 1.73 m^2).

Amiloride

Unlike aldosterone antagonists, which exert their kidney effects via interaction on the blood-side or basolateral side of distal nephron cells, amiloride is secreted into the tubular fluid in the proximal nephron. Once the tubular fluid reaches the distal nephron, amiloride concentrations have increased to ~100 times that of plasma, which is desirable since this is amiloride's site of action. Amiloride blocks the epithelial sodium channel in the distal nephron, and is classified, along with the aldosterone antagonists, as a potassium-sparing diuretic. Amiloride specifically treats Liddle syndrome, a monogenic cause of hypertension due to overactive epithelial sodium channels. However, amiloride may also be effective in treating African Americans with a suppressed plasma renin activity (Saha, 2005).

Potassium-Binding Agents

The kidneys excrete ~90% of dietary potassium intake to maintain homeostasis (Palmer and Clegg, 2016). Potassium balance is typically maintained up until the late stages of CKD (e.g., eGFR <15 mL/min per 1.73 m^2). However, the presence of agents that interrupt renin–angiotensin–aldosterone signaling can lead to hyperkalemia. The use of gastrointestinal tract potassium binders, like patiromer and sodium zirconium cyclosilicate (ZS-9), has been proposed to offset potassium-raising effects of aldosterone antagonists and ACEI/ARBs (Epstein and Pitt, 2016). However, the clinical utility of potassium binders in resistant hypertension is limited. (1) Hyperaldosteronism and associated hypokalemia are common in resistant hypertension. (2) Maximizing diuretic therapy often lowers serum potassium levels. (3) Aldosterone antagonists are not currently recommended for use in advance stages of CKD, where hyperkalemia is prevalent. (4) Patiromer can bind other drugs (i.e., ciprofloxacin, levothyroxine, metformin) in the gastrointestinal tract necessitating separation in dosing by 3 hours. However, if potassium lowering is needed in resistant hypertension, both ZS-9 and patiromer are effective. Sodium zirconium cyclosilicate may be better suited to treat acute hyperkalemia (Meaney, 2017).

Device-Based Therapies (e.g., Renal Denervation)

At present, device-based treatment for resistant hypertension remains investigational. Large reductions in clinic blood pressure were seen in early trials that used an arterial catheter to deliver radiofrequency energy through the walls of the renal arteries aimed at renal nerve ablation. However, in the first sham-controlled, randomized trial SYMPLICITY HTN-3, catheter-based renal denervation was no different than the sham-control in blood pressure reduction for individuals with resistant hypertension (change in 24-hour ambulatory systolic blood pressure at 6 months: −6.75 ± 15.11 mm Hg in the denervation group vs. −4.79 ± 17.25 mm Hg in the sham-procedure group, $p = 0.98$ for superiority with a margin of 2 mm Hg) (Bhatt, 2014). Following methodologic concerns with SYMPLICITY HTN-3, investigation has continued using catheters designed for more extensive denervation. Proof-of-principle trial results using different catheters have shown blood pressure reduction compared to sham-control (Azizi, 2018; Townsend, 2017). Other devices undergoing therapeutic testing for resistant hypertension include carotid baroreceptor activation and central arteriovenous fistula formation.

Acknowledgments

Dr. Calhoun is the recipient of NHLBI Grant HL113004. Dr. Judd is the recipient of NIDDK Grant K23 DK102660.

References and Suggested Readings

Azizi M, Schmieder RE, Mahfoud F, et al. Endovascular ultrasound renal denervation to treat hypertension (RADIANCE-HTN SOLO): a multicentre, international, single-blind, randomised, sham-controlled trial [epub ahead of print May 23, 2018]. *Lancet*. doi: https://doi.org/10.1016/S0140-6736(18)31082-1.

Benjamin MM, Fazel P, Filardo G, et al. Prevalence of and risk factors of renal artery stenosis in patients with resistant hypertension. *Am J Cardiol*. 2014;113:687–690.

Bhatt DL, Kandzari DE, O'Neill WW, et al; SYMPLICITY HTN-3 Investigators. A controlled trial of renal denervation for resistant hypertension. *N Engl J Med*. 2014;370:1393–1401.

Brown MJ, Williams B, Morant SV, et al; British Hypertension Society's Prevention and Treatment of Hypertension with Algorithm-Based Therapy (PATHWAY) Studies Group. Effect of amiloride, or amiloride plus hydrochlorothiazide, versus hydrochlorothiazide on glucose tolerance and blood pressure (PATHWAY-3): a parallel-group, double-blind randomised phase 4 trial. *Lancet Diabetes Endocrinol*. 2016;4:136–147.

Calhoun DA, Jones D, Textor S, et al. Resistant hypertension: diagnosis, evaluation, and treatment. A scientific statement from the American Heart Association Professional Education Committee of the Council for High Blood Pressure Research. *Hypertension*. 2008;51:1403–1419.

Calhoun DA, Nishizaka MK, Zaman MA, et al. Hyperaldosteronism among black and white subjects with resistant hypertension. *Hypertension*. 2002;40:892–896.

Chapman N, Dobson J, Wilson S, et al; Anglo-Scandinavian Cardiac Outcomes Trial Investigators. Effect of spironolactone on blood pressure in subjects with resistant hypertension. *Hypertension*. 2007;49:839–845.

Cooper CJ, Murphy TP, Cutlip DE, et al; CORAL Investigators. Stenting and medical therapy for atherosclerotic renal-artery stenosis. *N Engl J Med*. 2014;370:13–22.

Dudenbostel T, Calhoun DA. Use of Aldosterone antagonists for treatment of uncontrolled resistant hypertension. *Am J Hypertens*. 2017;30:103–109.

Egan BM, Zhao Y, Li J, et al. Prevalence of optimal treatment regimens in patients with apparent treatment-resistant hypertension based on office blood pressure in a community-based practice network. *Hypertension*. 2013;62:691–697.

Eide IK, Torjesen PA, Drolsum A, et al. Low-renin status in therapy-resistant hypertension: a clue to efficient treatment. *J Hypertens*. 2004;22:2217–2226.

Epstein M, Pitt B. Recent advances in pharmacological treatments of hyperkalemia: focus on patiromer. *Expert Opin Pharmacother*. 2016;17:1435–1448.

Ernst ME, Carter BL, Goerdt CJ, et al. Comparative antihypertensive effects of hydrochlorothiazide and chlorthalidone on ambulatory and office blood pressure. *Hypertension*. 2006;47:352–358.

Filippatos G, Anker SD, Bohm M, et al. A randomized controlled study of finerenone vs. eplerenone in patients with worsening chronic heart failure and diabetes mellitus and/or chronic kidney disease. *Eur Heart J*. 2016;37:2105–2114.

Fried LF, Emanuele N, Zhang JH, et al. Combined angiotensin inhibition for the treatment of diabetic nephropathy. *N Engl J Med*. 2013;369:1892–1903.

Gupta P, Patel P, Strauch B, et al. Biochemical screening for nonadherence is associated with blood pressure reduction and improvement in adherence. *Hypertension*. 2017;70:1042–1048.

Howard VJ, Tanner RM, Anderson A, et al. Apparent treatment-resistant hypertension among individuals with history of stroke or transient ischemic attack. *Am J Med*. 2015;128:707–714.e2.

Judd E, Calhoun DA. Apparent and true resistant hypertension: definition, prevalence and outcomes. *J Hum Hypertens*. 2014;28:463–468.

Jung O, Gechter JL, Wunder C, et al. Resistant hypertension? Assessment of adherence by toxicological urine analysis. *J Hypertens*. 2013;31:766–774.

Logan AG, Perlikowski SM, Mente A, et al. High prevalence of unrecognized sleep apnoea in drug-resistant hypertension. *J Hypertens*. 2001;19:2271–2277.

Martinez-Garcia MA, Capote F, Campos-Rodriguez F, et al; Spanish Sleep Network. Effect of CPAP on blood pressure in patients with obstructive sleep apnea and resistant hypertension: the HIPARCO randomized clinical trial. *JAMA*. 2013;310:2407–2415.

Meaney CJ, Beccari MV, Yang Y, et al. Systematic review and meta-analysis of patiromer and sodium zirconium cyclosilicate: A new armamentarium for the treatment of hyperkalemia. *Pharmacotherapy*. 2017;37:401–411.

Muntner P, Davis BR, Cushman WC, et al; ALLHAT Collaborative Research Group. Treatment-resistant hypertension and the incidence of cardiovascular disease and end-stage renal disease: results from the Antihypertensive and Lipid-Lowering Treatment to Prevent Heart Attack Trial (ALLHAT). *Hypertension*. 2014;64:1012–1021.

Palmer BF, Clegg DJ. Physiology and pathophysiology of potassium homeostasis. *Adv Physiol Educ*. 2016;40:480–490.

Persell SD. Prevalence of resistant hypertension in the United States, 2003–2008. *Hypertension*. 2011;57:1076–1080.

Pickering TG, Hall JE, Appel LJ, et al. Recommendations for blood pressure measurement in humans and experimental animals: part 1: blood pressure measurement in humans: a statement for professionals from the Subcommittee of Professional and Public Education of the American Heart Association Council on High Blood Pressure Research. *Circulation*. 2005;111:697–716.

Pimenta E, Gaddam KK, Oparil S, et al. Effects of dietary sodium reduction on blood pressure in subjects with resistant hypertension: results from a randomized trial. *Hypertension*. 2009;54:475–481.

Saha C, Eckert GJ, Ambrosius WT, et al. Improvement in blood pressure with inhibition of the epithelial sodium channel in blacks with hypertension. *Hypertension*. 2005;46:481–487.

Schwartz GL. Screening for adrenal-endocrine hypertension: overview of accuracy and cost-effectiveness. *Endocrinol Metab Clin North Am*. 2011;40:279–294, vii.

Sim JJ, Bhandari SK, Shi J, et al. Characteristics of resistant hypertension in a large, ethnically diverse hypertension population of an integrated health system. *Mayo Clin Proc*. 2013;88:1099–1107.

Sim JJ, Bhandari SK, Shi J, et al. Comparative risk of renal, cardiovascular, and mortality outcomes in controlled, uncontrolled resistant, and nonresistant hypertension. *Kidney Int*. 2015;88:622–632.

Sim JJ, Handler J, Jacobsen SJ, et al. Systemic implementation strategies to improve hypertension: the Kaiser Permanente Southern California experience. *Can J Cardiol*. 2014;30:544–552.

Thomas G, Xie D, Chen HY, et al; CRIC Study Investigators. Prevalence and prognostic significance of apparent treatment resistant hypertension in chronic kidney disease: Report from the chronic renal insufficiency cohort study. *Hypertension*. 2016;67:387–396.

Titze J, Luft FC. Speculations on salt and the genesis of arterial hypertension. *Kidney Int*. 2017;91:1324–1335.

Townsend RR, Mahfoud F, Kandzari DE, et al; SPYRAL HTN-OFF MED Trial Investigators. Catheter-based renal denervation in patients with uncontrolled hypertension in the absence of antihypertensive medications (SPYRAL HTN-OFF MED): a randomised, sham-controlled, proof-of-concept trial. *Lancet*. 2017;390:2160–2170.

Van Buren PN, Adams-Huet B, Nguyen M, et al. Potassium handling with dual renin-angiotensin system inhibition in diabetic nephropathy. *Clin J Am Soc Nephrol*. 2014;9:295–301.

Whelton PK, Carey RM, Aronow WS, et al. 2017 ACC/AHA/AAPA/ABC/ACPM/AGS/APhA/ASH/ASPC/NMA/PCNA Guideline for the prevention, detection, evaluation, and management of high blood pressure in adults: a report of the American College of Cardiology/American Heart Association Task Force on Clinical Practice Guidelines. *J Am Coll Cardiol*. 2018;71:e127–e248.

Williams B, MacDonald TM, Morant S, et al; British Hypertension Society's PATHWAY Studies Group. Spironolactone versus placebo, bisoprolol, and doxazosin to determine the optimal treatment for drug-resistant hypertension (PATHWAY-2): a randomised, double-blind, crossover trial. *Lancet*. 2015;386:2059–2068.

Wright JT Jr, Williamson JD, Whelton PK, et al; SPRINT Research Group. A randomized trial of intensive versus standard blood-pressure control. *N Engl J Med*. 2015;373:2103–2116.

PERIPHERAL ARTERY DISEASE

Peripheral artery disease (PAD) affects 5% of adults in the general population; globally, over 200 million adults have PAD. Individuals with kidney disease have an increased prevalence of PAD and are at an increased risk of developing clinically significant disease. Exact numbers of those affected depend on how PAD is defined. According to the latest National Health and Nutrition Examination Survey (NHANES), it is estimated that 24% of patients with chronic kidney disease (CKD) have PAD as defined by an ankle brachial index (ABI) of <0.9 (O'Hare, 2004). Intermittent claudication affects 1% to 5% of adults in the general population compared with 7% with CKD. Patients with CKD are more likely to present with more advanced PAD, requiring revascularization and subsequent amputation. Much of the increased incidence of PAD may be due to the high prevalence of traditional risk factors in this group, such as advanced age, diabetes mellitus, dyslipidemia, tobacco use, and hypertension; however, CKD is an independent risk factor.

Prevention

Risk Factor Modification

PAD is a coronary artery disease (CAD) risk equivalent condition ("risk equivalent condition" means that the cardiovascular event risk in patients with PAD but without CAD is equivalent to that in patients with CAD). The preventive measures are similar to those for CAD risk factor modification. Preventive measures target control of diabetes, hypertension, dyslipidemias, and smoking cessation, with goals being similar to those for patients with cardiovascular disease (CVD) and CKD, as described in other chapters of this handbook. Risk reduction therapy is underutilized in patients with PAD. Successful implementation of medical therapy to target cardiovascular risk is critical to reducing the cardiovascular morbidity and mortality. Studies showing a benefit of achieving these targets in terms of improving PAD outcomes are lacking. For example, current evidence does not support that strict glycemic or blood pressure control favorably affects the course of PAD. In the general population with PAD, statin therapy may increase pain-free walking. In one large study in U.S. Veterans, in which 7% of participants had CKD, statin use, esp. at higher doses, was associated with both limb preservation and increased survival (Arya, 2018); however, no studies have examined the effects of statin therapy on prevention or progression of PAD specifically in the CKD population. With regard ti PAD in patients with diabetes, the EASEL trial found an elevated risk of below the knee amputation associated with use of SGLT2 inhibitors (Udell, 2018). The mechanism is uncertain and the results need to be confirmed.

An important risk factor for PAD is tobacco use. High priority should be given to counseling patients with PAD regarding smoking cessation and offering them pharmacotherapy (e.g., antidepressants and nicotine replacement) as needed to assist with their efforts. Smoking cessation slows PAD progression, resulting in lower amputation rates.

Diabetic Foot Care
Diabetes is a major risk factor for PAD. Diabetic patients are also at risk for neuropathy, which can result in foot ulceration. Untreated or nonhealing foot ulcers often lead to limb amputation. Although there have been no prospective studies of the effects of foot care on PAD and reducing risk for limb loss in the CKD population, in the general population, studies have shown that patient education and proper foot care can reduce amputation rates. Diabetic foot care should involve hygiene, regular inspection of the feet by both the patient and by health care providers, use of proper footwear, and early referral for vascular evaluation for ulcers that fail to heal properly within 2 weeks. Once an ulcer has developed, the diabetic patient with significant PAD often will require revascularization to improve wound healing.

Peripheral Artery Disease Screening
Currently no organization recommends routine screening for PAD in asymptomatic patients. The following is a summary of national and international guidelines. In 2013, the U.S. Preventive Services Task Force (USPSTF) changed its recommendation against screening to an indeterminate recommendation, due to insufficient evidence to assess the balance of benefits and harms. In individuals with known CVD or diabetes, the USPSTF recommends risk reduction interventions, including antiplatelet or lipid-lowering therapies. Trans-Atlantic Inter-Society Consensus (TASC II, 2015) recommends screening for PAD in (1) patients with exertional leg symptoms, (2) patients aged 50 to 69 years with cardiovascular risk factors, (3) all patients aged 70 years, and (4) patients with a 10-year risk of a cardiovascular event of 10% to 20%, determined by SCORE or Framingham Heart Association guidelines. The American College of Cardiology/American Heart Association (ACC/AHA) guidelines recommend screening for PAD in the following high-risk groups: age 70 years and older; age 50 to 69 years and history of smoking and/or diabetes; age 40 to 49 years and diabetes and one other atherosclerosis risk factor; and anyone with intermittent claudication, rest pain, or abnormal lower-extremity vascular examination or known atherosclerosis at other sites (e.g., carotid, coronary, or renal artery disease). According to these guidelines, CKD patients with high-risk categories or claudication symptoms should be screened. Individuals with an appropriate clinical history and physical

examination findings along with defined risk factors should undergo measurement of limb blood pressures and calculation of the ABI, the standard noninvasive diagnostic test for PAD, as described below.

Ankle Brachial Index

The standard noninvasive test for screening is the ABI. The ABI is the ratio of the pressure in the leg to the pressure in the arm. First the blood pressure is measured in both arms, and, assuming a difference <10 mm Hg, the higher of the two arm pressures is used as the arm pressure. Then pressure is measured in the left leg using a Doppler probe placed over the posterior tibial artery. A cuff is inflated over the calf until the Doppler artery flow signal disappears. Then the cuff is deflated until the signal reappears, marking the level of the leg pressure reading. The leg blood pressure is then remeasured using the dorsalis pedis artery. The higher of the two leg artery pressures is chosen, and then the ratio of the leg-to-arm pressures is calculated as the ABI. Typical ABI values in healthy person range from 1.0 to 1.10. Values between 0.9 and 1.3 represent a broader, acceptable range. PAD is defined by an ABI <0.9. In patients with vascular calcifications, and particularly medial artery calcification (e.g., diabetic patients), ABI values can be supranormal (>1.3) because of noncompressible vessels. Recent studies suggest that these supranormal ABI values are as predictive of CVD as low values.

Toe Brachial Index

Another means to screen patients with calcified vessels is to measure a toe brachial index (TBI), which is calculated similar to the ABI, but using the pressure in the big toe instead of the foot as the numerator. The pressure in the big toe can be measured by placing a small cuff around the big toe and attaching a plethysmography probe at the pulp of the big toe tip. A TBI of <0.6 (at our institution, <0.7) is diagnostic and may be more accurate for diagnosing PAD than a low value of the ABI. Many primary care physicians' offices are equipped to perform ABI measurements. If not available in these settings, patients should be referred to a specialized vascular laboratory.

Diagnosis of Peripheral Artery Disease

Patients with an abnormal ABI, TBI, or other noninvasive test usually go on to have lower-extremity arteriography for more detailed vascular mapping. Most often, mapping is performed with iodinated contrast, which can be of concern for patients with advanced CKD, especially those with diabetes, because of the risk for contrast nephropathy. The potential benefits of the examination should be weighed against the risk for worsening renal function.

Increasingly, magnetic resonance angiography (MRA) is the preferred imaging study for patients with CKD. However, MRA is not without risk. For patients with advanced CKD (estimated glomerular filtration rate [eGFR] <30 mL/min), gadolinium-based contrast, which is commonly used for MRA, may increase the risk for nephrogenic systemic fibrosis, and in patients with advanced CKD, use of gadolinium should be done only after carefully balancing the risks versus benefits of the procedure. Use of MRA contrast agents has been reported to be relatively safe in terms of this complication, even in patients with far-advanced renal failure (Martin, 2018).

Medical/Noninvasive Therapies for Peripheral Artery Disease

The management of PAD includes strategies to prevent progression of PAD and to reduce the risk for catastrophic cardiovascular events. Risk factor modification is recommended to prevent cardiovascular events. Patients with intermittent claudication usually are managed initially with antiplatelet therapy and structured exercise programs.

The role of **antiplatelet agents** in reducing PAD progression has not been studied in patients with CKD, but in the general population, aspirin and clopidogrel have been demonstrated to reduce cardiovascular risk and improve graft patency after limb revascularization surgery. Patients with intermittent claudication who have inadequate relief with exercise and are not candidates for revascularization may benefit from the use of cilostazol. Cilostazol is a phosphodiesterase inhibitor that reduces platelet aggregation and also acts as a mild vasodilator. It has not been studied specifically in the CKD population, but subjects with CKD were not excluded from most cilostazol trials. According to the package insert, caution is advised for use in patients with a creatinine clearance <25 mL/min.

Exercise therapy often is used along with medical therapy as first-line treatment for intermittent claudication. Structured exercise programs have been demonstrated to reduce symptoms and improve pain-free walking times. Typical exercise programs are supervised and have patients engage in aerobic exercise for 45 to 60 minutes three or more times per week. The benefits and safety of such programs have not been studied in CKD patients.

Invasive Therapies for Peripheral Artery Disease

Critical limb ischemia is characterized by rest pain, ulcers, and gangrene. Patients with critical limb ischemia should be referred immediately for vascular evaluation. Revascularization, either by endovascular treatment or by open surgery, is indicated for patients with intermittent claudication that is unresponsive to medical therapy and for those with disabling intermittent claudication as long as they have a reasonable life expectancy, and would be expected to benefit from the procedure. There are two established classification schemes to describe PAD severity. The first is a functional assessment (Fontaine or Rutherford classification [RC]). The second classification scheme is an anatomic lesion classification (TASC II, 2015). If the patient is a candidate for either endovascular or open surgery, the less invasive option is the current standard of care.

There has been a shift in practice over the past 25 years for treatment of aortoiliac disease with a transition from open surgery with aorto-bi-iliac or aorto-bifemoral bypass to **endovascular treatments** for complex and diffuse disease (TASC D). This preference for less invasive strategy is evidence based and driven by shorter length of stay and lower periprocedural morbidity and mortality rates, while achieving comparable patency rates (4- to 5-year primary patency of 60% to 86%, with secondary patency rates of 80% to 98%). In 2011, the European Society of Cardiology (ESC) and ACC/AHA PAD guidelines recommended the following: (1) an endovascular-first approach for aortoiliac lesions, (2) borderline lesions be assessed with hemodynamic gradients, and (3) supported primary stent placement in the aortoiliac arteries. The 2014 expert consensus document from the Society for Cardiac Angiography and Interventions on appropriate use criteria for aortoiliac intervention (Klein, 2014) is in agreement with the current guidelines.

Vascular surgery is considered for patients with lesions not amenable to precutaneous transluminal angioplasty (PTA). Surgery is a higher-risk procedure compared with PTA, and patients with CKD should undergo appropriate preoperative screening. Amputation is reserved for patients who have failed revascularization or who were not candidates for such procedures. In retrospective analyses, mortality is lower among patients who undergo revascularization procedures compared with those who receive amputation. However, such observational data are subject to selection bias, and a randomized trial would be needed to more conclusively demonstrate benefits of revascularization.

The incidence of **amputation** is higher among CKD patients compared with the general population. This may be due to the fact that CKD patients more often present with more severe forms of PAD, such as critical limb ischemia. As with revascularization, after amputation CKD patients experience a higher rate of postoperative mortality compared with non-CKD patients.

CEREBROVASCULAR DISEASE IN CHRONIC KIDNEY DISEASE: SCOPE OF THE PROBLEM

Stroke is the third leading cause of death in the United States. Patients with CKD may face up to a 43% increased risk for stroke compared with the general population. According to NHANES data, microalbuminuria and decreased glomerular filtration rate (GFR) are independently associated with stroke among U.S. adults older than 55 years (Ani and Ovbiagele, 2010; Wu, 2010). The overrepresentation of traditional risk factors in this group accounts for most of the increased risk of stroke. After adjustment for traditional risk factors, incidence of stroke still remains high.

Strokes can be either hemorrhagic (20%) or ischemic (80%). Hemorrhagic strokes can be either intracerebral (hypertension, amyloid, arteriovenous malformations) or subarachnoid. Ischemic strokes are far more prevalent and can result from occlusion (plaque rupture, lacunar), embolism (arterial, cardiogenic, air, amniotic fluid, fat), or vasculitis. With the increased availability of computed tomography (CT) and magnetic resonance imaging (MRI), silent brain infarcts are more commonly diagnosed. Silent brain infarcts are incidental findings on neuroimaging often without an accompanying clinical history of stroke but are associated with cognitive impairment. Impaired kidney function is associated with increased risk for silent brain infarcts (Kobayashi, 2009).

Primary Prevention

Strategies for preventing stroke among patients with CKD usually target modifying cardiovascular risk factors, including hypertension, smoking, diabetes, obesity, dyslipidemia, and sedentary lifestyle (Bilha, 2018). Medical therapies should always be given in conjunction with lifestyle modification, including weight loss, regular aerobic exercise, and the limiting of alcohol intake.

Blood Pressure Control

Control of blood pressure probably is the most important therapy for stroke prevention. Isolated systolic hypertension, prevalent among elderly patients, is highly associated with stroke risk. Blood pressure variability, particularly the visit-to-visit variability of systolic blood pressure, has also recently been identified as a strong risk factor for subsequent stroke (Rothwell, 2010). Studies have demonstrated the benefits of blood pressure lowering on stroke reduction with various antihypertensive therapies, including angiotensin-converting enzyme inhibitors (ACEIs), angiotensin receptor blockers (ARBs), and calcium channel blockers (CCBs). There is some evidence that ARBs may be superior to ACEIs in stroke prevention, largely because of effects of ARB that go beyond blood pressure lowering. For example, losartan blocks platelet aggregation and reduces serum uric acid. Both platelet aggregation and hyperuricemia have been linked to increased stroke risk. Telmisartan, losartan, and valsartan have all been linked to a lower risk for new-onset diabetes compared with other antihypertensive agents, such as CCBs and β-blockers. However, CCBs are associated with reduced blood pressure variability compared with other classes of antihypertensives, which may provide unique benefits for stroke risk reduction (Webb, 2010).

Blood Pressure Target

Regardless of the antihypertensive agent chosen, the key is to lower the blood pressure to the suggested targets as per the Joint National Committee on Prevention, Detection, Evaluation, and Treatment of High Blood Pressure (JNC8) guidelines. JNC8 also recommended, for patients aged 18 years and older with CKD, initial or additional therapy should include an ACEI or ARB, regardless of race or diabetic status.

In the blood pressure–lowering arm of the Action to Control Cardiovascular Risk in Diabetes (ACCORD) study, which evaluated the benefits of lowering systolic blood pressure to <120 mm Hg in diabetic patients, although there was no overall cardiovascular advantage, and although there were increased adverse events in the lower blood pressure target group, stroke risk, a prespecified secondary outcome, was reduced (ACCORD, 2010). Nevertheless, in the elderly (>80 years) and in patients with bilateral severe carotid stenosis, particular effort should be expended to minimize orthostatic changes. Blood pressure targets <130 mm Hg systolic in the elderly have not been conclusively demonstrated to have an acceptable benefit/risk ratio and should be used cautiously in the elderly. Even relatively conservative blood pressure reduction targets (e.g., <150 mm Hg systolic) have substantially reduced risk of stroke in elderly patients (Beckett, 2008).

Lipid-Lowering Drugs

Therapy with lipid-lowering agents, particularly statins, has been demonstrated to be efficacious for primary and secondary prevention of stroke in the general population (Everett, 2010). The benefits of statin therapy for reducing stroke risk in CKD patients are less clear. A post hoc analysis of the Cholesterol and Recurrent Events (CARE) trial, in which patients with CKD were treated with pravastatin, did not demonstrate a significant reduction in stroke risk (Tonelli, 2003). However, in the Treating to New Targets Study, in which patients with CKD were enrolled, major cardiovascular events (i.e., death from coronary heart disease, nonfatal myocardial infarction, resuscitation after cardiac arrest, or fatal or nonfatal stroke) were reduced in subjects receiving long-term high-dose statin therapy compared with those receiving a lower dose. The Study of Heart and Renal Protection (SHARP), which is a prospective study on the effects of statin therapy on prevention of heart disease and stroke in CKD patients, demonstrated a significant reduction in the primary composite end point of atherosclerotic events in the low-density lipoprotein (LDL) lowering arm. This was driven by reduction in ischemic stroke and coronary revascularization procedures; there was no significant difference in coronary deaths or nonfatal myocardial infarction.

Aspirin

The use of aspirin for primary prevention of stroke is controversial. According to recommendations from the USPSTF, in patients with low risk for coronary heart disease (absolute 10-year risk <10% according to Framingham risk score), the benefits for reducing cardiovascular events may not exceed the risk for aspirin-associated bleeding. However, among those with moderate to high risk, the benefits for aspirin therapy are clearer. The American Diabetes Association (ADA) and the AHA from 2014 also state that aspirin is useful for primary stroke prevention in patients with diabetes mellitus but low 10-year risk of CVD is unclear. In those individuals in whom the 10-year risk is >10%, the AHA suggests to consider aspirin. The AHA also suggests aspirin use in persons with CKD (eGFR <45 mL/min per 1.73 m^2 but not <30 mL/min per 1.73 m^2) for primary stroke prevention.

The ESC also suggests the consideration of aspirin for primary prevention of CVD in both sexes if risk of major cardiovascular events (death, stroke, or myocardial infarction) is >2 per 100 subject-years if there is no evidence of an increased risk for bleeding. A joint statement from the ADA/AHA/ACCF was consistent with the above primary prevention guidelines. They recommend for intermediate-risk patients (younger patients with ≥1 risk factor, older patients with no risk factors, or patients with 10-year CVD risk 5% to 10%), that low-dose (75 to 162 mg/day) aspirin may be considered for prevention. To reduce the risks of bleeding-related adverse events, a dose of aspirin ≤100 mg daily should be used, as studies have demonstrated no additional cardiovascular benefits above this dose.

Anemia Correction

Unlike the general population, CKD patients are more likely to have anemia, which is also associated with an increased risk for stroke. Anemia in CKD is often treated with erythropoietin-stimulating agents (ESAs). Correction of anemia with ESAs to levels of hemoglobin >12.5 g/dL is associated with increased risk for cardiovascular events, including stroke. It is postulated that increases in blood pressure associated with ESA therapy, greater blood viscosity, relative thrombocytosis, and decreased bleeding tendency associated with greater hemoglobin levels result in the increased incidence of stroke.

Atrial Fibrillation

The prevalence of atrial fibrillation in CKD is two to three times higher compared to the general population according to a report from the Chronic Renal Insufficiency Cohort Study (Soliman, 2010). Optimal management in this group is unclear. Warfarin is indicated for those with a history of stroke and cardiogenic embolism, often in the setting of atrial fibrillation. However, the recent retrospective cohort study of CKD patients on hemodialysis with atrial fibrillation who were receiving warfarin therapy found an increased incidence of stroke compared with nonusers (Chan, 2009). These results will need to be verified with a prospective analysis. For patients unable to tolerate warfarin, full-strength aspirin (325 mg) is an acceptable alternative. The direct thrombin inhibitor dabigatran is as good, if not better than warfarin, in the general population with atrial fibrillation, but has not been well studied in CKD patients. Dabigatran is renally excreted, and so dose would need to be reduced in CKD (Stangier, 2010). Other studies that included other new anticoagulants (dabigatran, rivaroxaban, and apixaban) show promising results in the trials both in patients with stage 3 CKD and those without CKD (Kimachi, 2017). Severe CKD (CrCl <30 mL/min) has been an exclusion criteria in most trials. These novel anticoagulants are not only more efficient than warfarin but have significantly less risk of bleeding with apixaban having bleeding risk as low as aspirin with no significant drug–food interactions. However, these agents are renally excreted; thus in patients they have a prolonged half-life and high-drug levels in this patient population, increasing their risk of bleeding. Further research is essential to describe the efficacy and safety of these drugs in moderate to severe renal disease before they can be used effectively (see Ashley, 2018; Jain, 2018).

Additionally, mechanical exclusion of the left atrial appendage, a common source of thromboembolism, may be another option for anticoagulation intolerant patients (Cruz-Gonzalez, 2010). There are preliminary encouraging data regarding the efficacy of catheter ablation for atrial fibrillation (Marrouche, 2018) in CKD patients (Ullall, 2017).

Secondary Prevention

Once a patient has suffered a stroke, the risk for recurrence is as high as 20%. Therefore, secondary stroke prevention is also important. Risk factor modification is critical. Strategies should again focus on control of hypertension, diabetes, dyslipidemia, and smoking cessation.

Blood Pressure Control

Multiple studies have examined the benefits of antihypertensive therapies in secondary prevention of stroke. For example, the Perindopril pROtection aGainst REcurrent Stroke Study (PROGRESS) trial demonstrated that combination antihypertensive therapy (specifically an ACEI and a thiazide diuretic) affords superior protection against recurrent stroke and cardiovascular events compared with monotherapy (PROGRESS Collaborative Group, 2001). Patients with CKD, particularly those with diabetes, often require multiple agents for adequate blood pressure control. ACEIs and ARBs are preferred in the patient with diabetic or other forms of proteinuric renal diseases, given the added benefits of reducing progression of kidney disease.

Dyslipidemia

Regarding dyslipidemias, statins are the only class of lipid-lowering agents demonstrated to reduce the risk of recurrent stroke. The Stroke Prevention by Aggressive Reduction of Cholesterol Levels (SPARCL) trial demonstrated that atorvastatin reduces the incidence of recurrent stroke and cardiovascular events. This effect is independent of cholesterol level and suggests that properties aside from the lipid-lowering effects of statins explain their protective benefits. For patients who have hyperlipidemia, the LDL goal is <100 mg/dL (2.6 mmol/L) and <70 mg/dL (1.8 mmol/L) in high-risk individuals. The benefits of statin therapies for reducing recurrent stroke in CKD patients are unknown.

Antiplatelet Therapies

Antiplatelet therapies are recommended in secondary prevention of stroke. There are no data on the safety or efficacy of aspirin for primary or secondary prevention of stroke in CKD; therefore, recommendations are largely extrapolated from the general population. Aspirin with dipyridamole or clopidogrel is superior to aspirin alone. One randomized controlled trial demonstrated that aspirin plus dipyridamole compared to clopidogrel offered equivalent protection against recurrent stroke (Sacco, 2008). Clopidogrel is also a good choice for aspirin-allergic patients. Aspirin monotherapy may be an option for patients for whom clopidogrel or aspirin with dipyridamole imposes a financial burden. Choice of antiplatelet therapy should be individualized based on each patient's risk of stroke or bleeding risk. Several bleeding scores such as HAS-BLED, HEMORR(2)HAGES, and ATRIA have included kidney disease to predict the risk of bleeding.

Diagnosis

Patients with a clinical presentation or history suggestive of stroke (e.g., new neurologic deficits or altered level of consciousness) should be referred emergently for diagnostic testing. A noncontrast CT scan is usually the first diagnostic test of choice. CT scans are rapid tests that can quickly identify hemorrhagic strokes (intracerebral hemorrhage, subarachnoid hemorrhage). Ischemic strokes may not be apparent early in the course by either CT or MRI. Once the diagnosis has been made and the patient stabilized in the course of the acute episode, further diagnostic testing may be required to determine the etiology of the stroke. If an embolic stroke is suspected, testing is needed to determine the source of emboli. Cardiac monitoring usually is recommended during the first 24 hours of observation to check for presence of atrial fibrillation. Duplex ultrasound of the carotid arteries may be done to evaluate for clinically significant carotid stenosis. A transthoracic echocardiogram may be also needed to further establish a source of emboli (e.g., intracardiac thrombus). A transesophageal echocardiogram is particularly well suited to diagnose intra-atrial thrombi and patent foramen ovale.

Treatment of Acute Stroke
Thrombolytics
Once the diagnosis is made, treatment is initiated to prevent worsening of neurologic damage. Thrombolytics (tissue-type plasminogen activator [t-PA], recombinant tissue–type plasminogen activator [rt-PA], Activase) are recommended for patients with an acute ischemic stroke who have a measurable neurologic deficit if treatment can be started quickly enough and the patient has no contraindications. Guidelines suggest alteplase is beneficial for carefully selected patients with acute ischemic stroke when given up to 3 to 4.5 hours after stroke onset. Thombolytic therapy for stroke in patients with CKD has been associated with a higher risk of bleeding, but this may be due to non-CKD associated risk factors (Ovbiagele, 2014). Contraindications include intracranial hemorrhage, severe stroke, minor stroke, seizure with stroke, thrombocytopenia or hypercoagulable state, hypo- or hyperglycemia, arterial or venous puncture within 7 days, recent stroke or myocardial infarction within the past 3 months, serious trauma in the past 2 weeks, significant head trauma in the past 3 months, hypertension >185/110, active cancer, severe liver disease, and history of bleeding in the past 3 weeks.

Blood Pressure Control
Blood pressure often is elevated following an acute ischemic stroke. This may be in part a physiologic response to attempt to maintain perfusion distal to the obstructed vessel. Therefore, permissive hypertension is allowed in this setting and guidelines recommend treating hypertension only if blood pressure exceeds 220/120 mm Hg. They suggest if the blood pressures are above 220/110, to lower systolic blood pressure by 15% over the first 24 hours. After the first 24 hours, antihypertensive agents can be restarted with gradual lowering of the blood pressure over 7 to 10 days. However, if a patient is a candidate for thrombolytic therapy, then blood pressure must be lowered to <180/110 mm Hg before initiation of tissue plasminogen activator. The antihypertensive

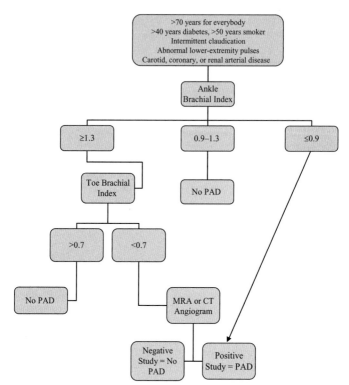

FIGURE 16.1 Diagnostic algorithm for peripheral arterial disease per the ACC/AHA guidelines, including patients with chronic kidney disease with risk factors.

drug of choice in the setting of an acute stroke is labetalol. Decompressive surgery is recommended for malignant edema of the cerebral hemispheres or a space occupying cerebellar infarction. Aspirin should be started 24 to 48 hours after an ischemic stroke to reduce the risk of death, dependency, and recurrent stroke.

Nonmedical/Invasive Therapies for Secondary Prevention
Patients with a history of stroke and moderate to severe carotid stenosis may be candidates for carotid endarterectomy performed by an experienced surgeon. CKD patients have high rates of perioperative stroke and mortality from these procedures. Therefore, carotid artery stenting or medical therapy with antiplatelet therapy may be preferred in this setting. Data are lacking regarding benefit/risk of carotid stenting in CKD.

References and Suggested Readings

ACCORD Study Group; Cushman WC, Evans GW, Byington RP, et al. Effects of intensive blood-pressure control in type 2 diabetes mellitus. *N Engl J Med.* 2010;362:1575–1585.

Adams RJ, Albers G, Alberts MJ, et al; American Heart Association; American Stroke Association. Update to the AHA/ASA recommendations for the prevention of stroke in patients with stroke and transient ischemic attack. *Stroke.* 2008;39:1647–1652.

Amarenco P, Goldstein LB, Szarek M, et al; SPARCL Investigators. Effects of intense low-density lipoprotein cholesterol reduction in patients with stroke or transient ischemic attack: the stroke prevention by aggressive reduction in cholesterol levels (SPARCL) trial. *Stroke.* 2007;38:3198–3204.

Ani C, Ovbiagele B. Relation of baseline presence and severity of renal disease to long-term mortality in persons with known stroke. *J Neurol Sci.* 2010;288:123–128.

Arya S, Khakharia A, Binney ZO, et al. Association of statin dose with amputation and survival in patients with peripheral artery disease. *Circulation.* 2018;137: 1435–1446.

Ashley J, Sood MM. Novel oral anticoagulants in chronic kidney disease: ready for prime time? *Curr Opin Nephrol Hypertens.* 2018;27:201–208.

Baber U, Mann D, Shimbo D, et al. Combined role of reduced estimated glomerular filtration rate and microalbuminuria on the prevalence of peripheral arterial disease. *Am J Cardiol.* 2009;104:1446–1451.

Beckett NS, Peters R, Fletcher AE, et al; HYVET Study Group. Treatment of hypertension in patients 80 years of age or older. *N Engl J Med.* 2008;358:1887–1898.

Bilha SC, Burlacu A, Siriopol D, et al. Primary prevention of stroke in chronic kidney disease patients: a scientific update. *Cerebrovasc Dis.* 2018;45:33–41.

Chan KE, Lazarus JM, Thadhani R, et al. Warfarin use associates with increased risk for stroke in hemodialysis patients with atrial fibrillation. *J Am Soc Nephrol.* 2009;20:2223–2233.

Chou R, Dana T, Blazina I, et al. Statin use for the prevention of cardiovascular disease in adults: A systematic review for the U.S. preventive services task force. Evidence Syntheses. November 2016; No. 139.

Cruz-Gonzalez I, Yan BP, Lam YY, et al. Left atrial appendage exclusion: state-of-the-art. *Catheter Cardiovasc Interv.* 2010;75:806–813.

DeLoach SS, Mohler ER 3rd. Peripheral arterial disease: a guide for nephrologists. *Clin J Am Soc Nephrol.* 2007;2:839–846.

Everett BM, Glynn RJ, MacFadyen JG, et al. Rosuvastatin in the prevention of stroke among men and women with elevated levels of C-reactive protein: Justification for the Use of Statins in Prevention: an Intervention Trial Evaluating Rosuvastatin (JUPITER). *Circulation.* 2010;121:143–150.

Garimella PS, Hart PD, O'Hare A, et al. Peripheral artery disease and CKD: a focus on peripheral artery disease as a critical component of CKD care. *Am J Kidney Dis.* 2012;60:641–654.

Gerard-Herman MD. 2016 AHA/ACC Guideline on the management of patients with lower extremity peripheral artery disease: executive summary: a report of the American College of Cardiology/American Heart Association Task Force on Clinical Practice Guidelines. *J Am Coll Cardiol.* 2017;69:1465–1508.

Jain N, Reilly RF. Clinical pharmacology of oral anticoagulants in patients with kidney disease. *Clin J Am Soc Nephrol.* 2018, in press. doi: 10.2215/CJN.02170218.

Jones DW, Dansey K, Hamdan AD. Lower extremity revascularization in end-stage renal disease. *Vasc Endovascular Surg.* 2016;50:582–585.

Kernan WN, Ovbiagele B, Black HR, et al; American Heart Association Stroke Council, Council on Cardiovascular and Stroke Nursing, Council on Clinical Cardiology, and Council on Peripheral Vascular Disease. Guidelines for the prevention of stroke in patients with stroke and transient ischemic attack: a guideline for healthcare professionals from the American Heart Association/American Stroke Association. *Stroke.* 2014;45:2160–2236.

Kimachi M, Furukawa TA, Kimachi K, et al. Direct oral anticoagulants versus warfarin for preventing stroke and systemic embolic events among atrial fibrillation patients with chronic kidney disease. *Cochrane Database Syst Rev.* 2017;11:CD011373.

Klein AJ, Feldman DN, Aronow HD, et al; Peripheral Vascular Disease Committee for the Society for Cardiovascular Angiography and Interventions. SCAI expert consensus statement for aorto-iliac arterial intervention appropriate use. *Catheter Cardiovasc Interv.* 2014;84:520–528.

Kobayashi M, Hirawa N, Yatsu K, et al. Relationship between silent brain infarction and chronic kidney disease. *Nephrol Dial Transplant.* 2009;24:201–207.

Lau YC, Proietti M, Guiducci, et al. Atrial fibrillation and thromboembolism in patients with chronic kidney disease. *J Am Coll Cardiol.* 2016;68:1452–1464.

Marrouche NF, Brachmann J, Andresen D, et al for the CASTLE- AF Investigators. Catheter ablation for atrial fibrillation with heart failure. *N Engl J Med*. 2018; 378:417–427.

Martin DR, Kalb B, Mittal A, et al. No incidence of nephrogenic systemic fibrosis after gadobenate dimeglumine administration in patients undergoing dialysis or those with severe chronic kidney disease. *Radiology*. 2018;286:113–119.

O'Hare AM, Sidawy AN, Feinglass J, et al. Influence of renal insufficiency on limb loss and mortality after initial lower extremity surgical revascularization. *J Vasc Surg*. 2004;39:709–716.

Olin JW, White CJ, Armstrong EJ, et al. Peripheral artery disease: evolving role of exercise, medical therapy and endovascular options. *J Am Coll Cardiol*. 2016;67:1338–1357.

Ovbiagele B, Smith EE, Schwamm LH, et al. Chronic kidney disease and bleeding complications after intravenous thrombolytic therapy for acute ischemic stroke. *Circ Cardiovasc Qual Outcomes*. 2014;7:929–935.

Pande RL, Perlstein TS, Beckman JA, et al. Secondary prevention and mortality in peripheral artery disease: National Health and Nutrition Examination Study, 1999 to 2004. *Circulation*. 2011;124:17–23.

PROGRESS Collaborative Group. Randomised trial of a perindopril-based blood pressure-lowering regimen among 6,105 individuals with previous stroke or transient ischemic attack. *Lancet*. 2001;358:1033–1041.

Rothwell PM, Howard SC, Dolan E, et al. Prognostic significance of visit-to-visit variability, maximum systolic blood pressure, and episodic hypertension. *Lancet*. 2010;375:895–905.

Sacco RL, Diener HC, Yusuf S, et al; PRoFESS Study Group. Aspirin and extended-release dipyridamole versus clopidogrel for recurrent stroke. *N Engl J Med*. 2008; 359:1238–1251.

Shepherd J, Kastelein JJ, Bittner V, et al; TNT (Treating to New Targets) Investigators. Intensive lipid lowering with atorvastatin in patients with coronary heart disease and chronic kidney disease: the TNT (Treating to New Targets) study. *J Am Coll Cardiol*. 2008;51:1448–1454.

Soliman EZ, Prineas RJ, Go AS, et al; Chronic Renal Insufficiency Cohort (CRIC) Study Group. Chronic kidney disease and prevalent atrial fibrillation: the Chronic Renal Insufficiency Cohort (CRIC). *Am Heart J*. 2010;159:1102–1107.

Stangier J, Rathgen K, Stähle H, et al. Influence of renal impairment on the pharmacokinetics and pharmacodynamics of oral dabigatran etexilate: an open-label, parallel-group, single-centre study. *Clin Pharmacokinet*. 2010;49:259–268.

TASC Steering Committee; Jaff MR, White CJ, Hiatt WR, et al. An update on methods for revascularization and expansion of the TASC lesion classification to include below-the-knee arteries: a supplement to the inter-society consensus for the management of peripheral arterial disease (TASC II). *Vasc Med*. 2015;20:465–478.

Tonelli M, Moye L, Sacks FM, et al; Cholesterol and Recurrent Events (CARE) Trial Investigators. Pravastatin for secondary prevention of cardiovascular events in persons with mild chronic renal insufficiency. *Ann Intern Med*. 2003;138:98–104.

Townsend RR. Stroke in chronic kidney disease: prevention and management. *Clin J Am Soc Nephrol*. 2008;3:S11–S16.

Udell JA, Yuan Z, Rush T, et al. Cardiovascular outcomes and risks after initiation of a sodium glucose cotransporter 2 inhibitor: results from the EASEL population-based cohort study (evidence for cardiovascular outcomes with sodium glucose cotransporter 2 inhibitors in the real world). *Circulation*. 2018;137:1450–1459.

Ullal AJ, Kaiser DW, Fan J, et al. Safety and clinical outcomes of catheter ablation of atrial fibrillation in patients with chronic kidney disease. *J Cardiovasc Electrophysiol*. 2017;28:39–48.

Webb AJ, Fischer U, Mehta Z, et al. Effects of antihypertensive-drug class on interindividual variation in blood pressure and risk of stroke: a systematic review and meta-analysis. *Lancet*. 2010;375:906–915.

Wu CK, Yang CY, Tsai CT, et al. Association of low glomerular filtration rate and albuminuria with peripheral arterial disease: the National Health and Nutrition Examination Survey, 1999–2004. *Atherosclerosis*. 2010;209:230–234.

Diagnosis and Management of Acute Coronary Syndromes

Henry An Tran and Christopher R. deFilippi

A 62-year-old white woman with a history of hypertension presents to the emergency department with the chief symptom of 6 hours of epigastric discomfort without radiation and unrelieved by antacids. She has no functional limitations but does not exercise regularly. She has no prior cardiac hospital admissions. Her electrocardiogram (ECG) shows voltage criteria for left ventricular hypertrophy with nonspecific ST- and T-wave abnormalities interpreted as consistent with repolarization abnormalities seen with left ventricular hypertrophy. Her creatinine is 1.6 mg/dL (140 mcmol/L, estimated glomerular filtration rate [eGFR] 34 mL/min per 1.73 m^2) and her initial cardiac troponin (cTn) T level is 0.06 ng/mL (upper limit of normal is 0.03 ng/mL). What further diagnostic and therapeutic measures should be considered?

Nomenclature:

ACS Acute coronary syndrome
MI Myocardial infarction
STEMI ST-segment elevation *myocardial infarction*
NSTEMI Non–ST-segment elevation *myocardial infarction*
UA Unstable angina

INTRODUCTION

Large population-based studies and registry data demonstrate that the prevalence of coronary artery disease is higher in subjects who have reduced levels of kidney function. Medicare data demonstrate that prevalence of any cardiovascular disease (CVD) in chronic kidney disease (CKD) patients is double that of patients without CKD (69% vs. 34%). Furthermore, unadjusted survival of patients with CVD progressively worsens as renal function deteriorates (USRDS, 2018) (Gupta, 2004). CKD serves as a significant, adverse predictor of cardiovascular events and mortality. Risk rises substantially once the eGFR decreases below 60 mL/min per 1.73 m^2 (Go, 2004; Han, 2015; Mann, 2001; McCullough, 2000). Among those with moderate to severe CKD (stage 3 and higher), the most common cause of death is CVD related, and most patients with CKD die of cardiovascular causes before progressing to end-stage renal disease (ESRD).

In addition to predicting adverse CVD events, CKD portends a worse clinical outcome after a CVD event. For example, a retrospective study of Medicare recipients reviewed the clinical outcomes of more than 130,000 patients after suffering a myocardial infarction (MI). For individuals with normal renal function, the 1-year mortality rate was 24%, but risk almost doubled, to 46%, for patients with mild CKD, and tripled, to 66%, for patients with moderate to severe CKD (Shlipak, 2002). While overall mortality may have decreased more recently, these ratios for risk of death remain intact. In a different population of 14,500 acute MI survivors with heart failure or left ventricular dysfunction and serum creatinine levels ≤2.5 mg/dL (220 mcmol/L), a subgroup analysis demonstrated that for each decrease in eGFR of 10 mL/min per 1.73 m^2 below 80, there was a 10% increase in the relative risk for all-cause mortality and nonfatal cardiovascular complications (Anavekar, 2004b). In patients with non–ST-segment elevation acute coronary syndrome (NSTEMI), there was a 16% increase in 6-month mortality for each decrease in eGFR/1.73 m^2 of 10 mL/min (Gibson, 2004). Proposed explanations for the increased risk of adverse cardio-vascular outcomes in CKD patients with acute coronary syndrome (ACS) are a greater prevalence of baseline cardiac risk factors and decreased use of traditional treatment strategies to modify cardiovascular risk before and during ACS onset.

OVERVIEW OF ACUTE CORONARY SYNDROME

ACSs comprise a group of clinical conditions that reflect a spectrum of myocardial ischemia and share a common pathophysiology, namely the disruption of vulnerable or high-risk atherosclerotic plaques.

The diagnosis of an **ST-segment elevation MI (STEMI)** is defined by symptoms of myocardial ischemia in the setting of persistent ST-segment elevations and the subsequent release of biomarkers of myocardial necrosis involves with a characteristic rise and fall (O'Gara, 2013; Thygesen, 2012). The diagnosis of **NSTEMI** is based on clinical symptoms suggestive of myocardial ischemia combined with electrocardiographic findings of ST depression or prominent T-wave inversion and/or rise and/or fall markers of myonecrosis (e.g., cTn I or T). Elevated biomarkers of myocardial necrosis distinguish an NSTEMI from an unstable angina (UA) event (Amsterdam, 2014). In the absence of symptoms, additional factors that can be included with cardiac biomarkers to make the diagnosis of a NSTEMI include: new pathologic Q waves on ECG, or imaging evidence of new loss of viable myocardium or new regional wall motion abnormality (Thygesen, 2012). NSTEMI often is diagnosed even in the absence of diagnostic ECG findings, as long as a rise and subsequent fall in cTn occurs in the presence of suggestive symptoms.

PATHOPHYSIOLOGY

The pathophysiologic condition that results in ACS is an imbalance between myocardial oxygen supply and demand. ACS commonly results from the disruption or erosion of an atherosclerotic plaque that promotes thrombus formation and resultant diminished coronary blood flow. Atherosclerosis is in large part an inflammatory disorder (Teague, 2017). Activated macrophages and T lymphocytes, located at the fibrous cap of the atherosclerotic plaque, promote expression of proteolytic enzymes such as matrix metalloproteinases, which degrade plaque integrity, creating fissures, erosions, or rupture. The associated endothelial damage combined with exposure of atheromatous contents to the bloodstream promotes release of substances that engender platelet activation, adhesion, and aggregation, neutrophil activation and thrombin generation, and ultimately thrombus formation. Thrombus formation combined with distal microembolization of platelet aggregates and components of the disrupted plaque are thought to be responsible for any ensuing myocardial necrosis. Other causes that reduce myocardial oxygen supply include dynamic obstruction (which means reversible obstruction, usually because of focal spasm of a segment of coronary artery), progressive narrowing of atherosclerotic plaques without spasm or plaque rupture, and coronary artery dissection.

So-called MI type 2 is due to an unfavorable balance of myocardial oxygen supply and demand that occurs when the precipitating condition is extrinsic to the coronary arterial bed, although the latter often has some degree of atherosclerotic narrowing. MI type 2 can be caused by increases in myocardial oxygen requirements, such as with fever, tachycardia, or thyrotoxicosis; by reversible decreases in coronary perfusion, such as with hypotension; or by reduced myocardial oxygen delivery, such as with anemia or hypoxemia (Roffi, 2016; Thygesen, 2012).

STEMI arises from the same mechanism of atherosclerotic plaque disruption as found in NSTEMI. However, the resultant thrombus typically will have occluded the coronary artery that was supplying the infarcted portion of the myocardium. Depending on the extent of collateral flow and factors affecting myocardial oxygen consumption and delivery, myocardial necrosis may develop as soon as 15 minutes after coronary artery occlusion, spreading from the endocardium to epicardium (Reimer, 1977). **Coronary thrombus** formation is seen in more than 90% of patients with STEMI and in 35% to 75% of patients with NSTEMI versus only 1% of patients with stable angina.

Coronary Arteries in Chronic Kidney Disease

Postmortem examination of coronary arteries in ESRD patients finds increased medial thickness and a smaller cross-sectional area of the arterial lumen compared with age- and sex-matched controls. Whereas coronary artery plaques in patients with normal kidney function are mostly fibroatheromatous in nature, plaques in CKD patients are more commonly calcified. For example, an electron beam computed tomography study showed coronary calcification in 92% of individuals with ESRD, with coronary artery calcium scores exceeding by 10-fold the 95th percentile. Evidence suggests that coronary calcium in CKD patients is several millimeters thick and its location cannot be distinguished between the intimal and medial layers of the vessel. Therefore the identification of calcium deposits in atherosclerotic plaques rather than arteriosclerosis is very limited. Thus although coronary calcium could be a predictor for coronary disease and CVD events in patients with all severities of CKD, the results from several small studies have been conflicting regarding the predictive value of coronary calcification (Bashir, 2015; Haydar, 2004; McCullough, 2009; Shantouf, 2010).

CLINICAL PRESENTATION OF ACUTE CORONARY SYNDROME

Classic angina is described as a deep and poorly localized chest or arm discomfort that is reproducibly associated with physical exertion or emotional stress. Anginal discomfort is relieved promptly (in <5 minutes) with rest and/or the use of sublingual nitroglycerin (NTG). It is important to note that atypical features, such as reproducible chest discomfort upon palpation and pleuritic chest pain, do not necessarily exclude the presence of ACS. Patients experiencing myocardial ischemia as a result of ACS may not present with chest discomfort.

In fact, the presentation of ACS is affected by the presence and severity of CKD (Roffi, 2016). Compared to patients with out CKD, patients with most advanced stages of CKD have chest pain less often upon presentation and will have other atypical features. The Framingham Study originally showed that up to half of all individuals with MIs had disease that was clinically silent (i.e., asymptomatic) (Kannel, 1986). Observations from the SWEDEHEART registry found that up to one-third of dialysis patients did not have chest pain during ACS (Szummer, 2010). Therefore other symptoms which are regarded as **anginal equivalents** need to be screened for: **dyspnea; fatigue; diaphoresis; syncope or near syncope; discomfort located in the jaw, neck, ear, arm, shoulder, back, or epigastrium.** In CKD patients, the specificity of chest discomfort for ACS may be reduced because of concomitant anemia, poorly controlled hypertension, or left ventricular hypertrophy. Dyspnea may be related to volume overload, anemia, or diastolic dysfunction rather than to an anginal equivalent. Symptoms reported by patients with CKD that are even partially suggestive of a cardiac etiology must be considered seriously and investigated thoroughly.

Evaluation

Patients with symptoms of suspected ACS must be evaluated and triaged rapidly to clinically distinguish between an acute STEMI and UA/NSTEMI according to the American College of Cardiology (ACC) and American Heart Association (AHA) guidelines (Fig. 17.1) (Amsterdam, 2014). Based on a combination of history, examination findings, ECG, and cardiac biomarker data, physicians must determine whether a patient's presentation is most consistent with a noncardiac process, UA, or with possible or definite ACS.

History

The most important factor is the character of chest discomfort, followed by any prior history of coronary artery disease, age, sex, and number of traditional risk factors present.

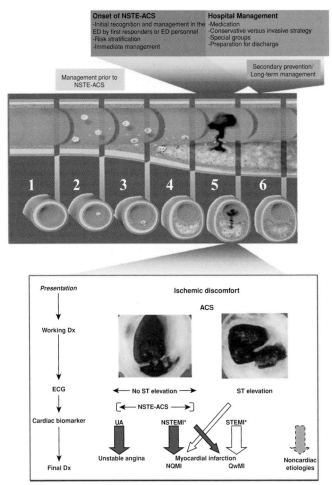

FIGURE 17.1 Acute coronary syndromes. *Elevated cardiac biomarker (e.g., troponin). ACS, acute coronary syndrome; CPG, clinical practice guideline; Dx, diagnosis; ECG, electrocardiogram; ED, emergency department; MI, myocardial infarction; NQMI, non–Q-wave myocardial infarction; NSTE-ACS, non–ST-elevation acute coronary syndromes; QwMI, Q-wave myocardial infarction. (Amsterdam, 2014).

Physical Examination

The goals of the physical examination are threefold: (a) assess the severity of the cardiovascular event; (b) identify potential secondary causes of myocardial ischemia that will affect therapeutic management, such as uncontrolled hypertension, thyrotoxicosis, or gastrointestinal bleeding; and (c) identify alternative nonischemic or noncardiac causes for symptoms at presentation. Every patient with suspected ACS should receive a thorough cardiovascular and chest examination with particular attention to vital signs, presence of left ventricle dysfunction (rales, S_3 gallop), organ hypoperfusion, murmurs, and bruits.

Electrocardiogram

A goal should be to obtain an ECG within 10 minutes of presentation. The ECG serves as the single most important data point in the evaluation of ACS because of its ability to identify patients who benefit from immediate reperfusion therapy via percutaneous coronary intervention (PCI) or thrombolytics. This population includes those with ST-segment elevations ≥1 mm (0.1 mV) in at least two contiguous leads, new-onset left bundle branch block (LBBB), or those with evidence of true posterior MI, manifested by ST depressions in leads V1 to V2 or ST elevations in the posterior ECG leads. These findings accurately predict an MI in more than 90% of cases as confirmed by serial cardiac biomarkers. ECG changes that are presumably new and obtained during presenting symptoms demonstrating ST depressions >0.5 mm (0.05 mV) or marked, symmetrical precordial T-wave inversions >2 mm (0.2 mV) that resolve when the patient is asymptomatic are strongly suggestive of acute myocardial ischemia. A completely normal ECG may represent an evolving MI in 1% to 6% of cases, and up to 15% may develop UA (Rouan, 1989). Therefore, if the initial ECG is not diagnostic of ACS and the patient remains symptomatic, serial ECGs should be performed.

The same strategy regarding ECG interpretation to support evidence of ACS applies to individuals with CKD. However, given the high incidence of hypertension and left ventricular hypertrophy in the CKD population, ECGs in individuals with CKD presenting with suspected ACS often exhibit confounding baseline ST depression, T-wave inversions, or an LBBB that may decrease the specificity for ACS. Patients with advanced CKD also may have electrolyte abnormalities causing ECG findings of peaked T waves or ST elevations. Certainly in this population, baseline and serial ECGs are required to support an ACS diagnosis. Further information regarding interpretation of ECG changes in ACS is available in the ACC/AHA guidelines for UA/NSTEMI and STEMI (Amsterdam, 2014; O'Gara, 2013).

Cardiac Biomarkers

The presence of cTn is essential for confirmation of an MI as well as risk stratification in patients with NSTEMI. In the evaluation of ACS, troponins are the accepted biomarkers of choice as opposed to CK-MB and myoglobin (Thygesen, 2012). Troponins can be detected in the blood as early as 2 to 4 hours after the onset of symptoms, although elevations can be delayed for up to 6 to 12 hours. Increased levels may persist in the blood for up to 5 to 14 days, but often return to close to baseline for smaller NSTEMI by this time period. Although the presence of cTn identifies myocardial necrosis, it does not specify the cause or acuity of necrosis. Troponins may be elevated because of cardiac injury resulting from arrhythmia, trauma, acute decompensated heart

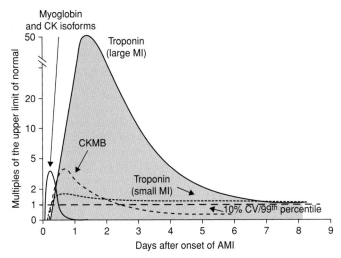

FIGURE 17.2 Timing of release of various biomarkers after acute myocardial infarction. (Anderson JL, Adams CD, Antman EM, et al. ACC/AHA 2007 guidelines for the management of patients with unstable angina/non-ST-elevation myocardial infarction. *J Am Coll Cardiol.* 2007;50:e1–e157.)

failure, inflammation or infection, neurologic injury, sepsis, drug toxicity, pulmonary embolism with right ventricular strain, or as a result of chronic causes, including left ventricular hypertrophy, stable heart failure, or renal insufficiency (Fig. 17.2).

Newer high-sensitive (hs) assays for cTnI and cTnT have been used throughout most of the world for most of the decade and have recently been approved for use in the United States. Advantages include the potential for accelerated ACS evaluation protocols with serial testing using intervals as short as an hour between troponin measurements (Roffi, 2016). A "normal" value is defined as less than the 99th percentile value found in a healthy general population. It has long been recognized with conventional cTn assays that asymptomatic ESRD patients will have elevated values and these elevations are associated with increased risk of death. More recently, levels of hs–cTnT were found to be elevated in the large majority of asymptomatic patients with CKD not on dialysis within the NIH Chronic Renal Insufficiency Cohort (CRIC). Higher levels are associated with a greater burden of CVD pathology including left ventricular hypertrophy and to a lesser extent, a decreased left ventricular ejection fraction (LVEF <50%) (Bansal, 2015). Clinicians should anticipate an initially elevated level of cTn in patients with CKD, particularly when using an hs assay, with or without a final diagnosis of ACS. Fortunately, both sensitive and hs–cTn assays maintain a high accuracy for the diagnosis of NSTEMI (Twerenbold, 2015). For patients with CKD, serial changes in cTn levels are even more important for diagnosis. Ultimately, a higher initial cutoff value may be appropriate compared to those without CKD, but this hasn't been implemented clinically or recommended in guidelines. The exact change in serial cTn levels for diagnosis of an NSTEMI isn't explicit and whether this should be an absolute change or percent change remains up for debate. A change of at least >20% has been recommended (Thygesen, 2012).

ESTIMATION OF RISK

The initial and most critical risk stratification in the evaluation of suspected ACS patients focuses on the identification of STEMI based on ECG findings, as STEMI requires immediate treatment with PCI or thrombolysis. Given the risk of serious, adverse clinical outcomes, the possible occurrence of NSTEMI also needs to be assessed, and this is done based on history, exam findings, ECG, and biochemical marker data.

Recent Medical History

Components of the history that are associated with a higher short-term risk of death or a nonfatal MI include an accelerating tempo of ischemic symptoms in the preceding 48 hours or prolonged ongoing rest pain for >20 minutes; recent use of aspirin; age; prior history of documented coronary artery disease, MI, or heart failure; or presence of multiple coronary artery disease risk factors. As discussed previously, renal dysfunction serves as an independent predictor of adverse mortality outcomes in ACS patients (Anavekar, 2004b; Gibson, 2004; Shlipak, 2002).

Examination Findings

Examination findings that portend worse prognosis for an ACS event and constitute a medical emergency include signs compatible with cardiogenic shock (e.g., hypotension, decreased urine output, elevated jugular venous pressure, cold clammy skin), new or worse rales compatible with acute pulmonary edema, new or worsening mitral regurgitation murmur, or presence of an S_3 gallop heart sound.

High-Risk Electrocardiogram Findings

Several studies have demonstrated that a gradient of risk for death and further ischemic events exists based on the nature of the ECG abnormality. For example, patients with NSTEMI and new LBBB represented the highest risk of mortality or MI at 1 year, then ST deviation >2 mm, then those with significant T-wave inversions >2 mm (0.02 mV), and last those with nonspecific isolated T-wave inversions <2 mm (0.02 mV) and normal ECG patterns (Cannon, 1997). In addition, the magnitude of ST-segment deviations and presence of T-wave inversions have prognostic utility. Although ST elevations predict the highest early risk of death, ST-segment depression on admission ECG portends the highest risk of death at 6 months, with the magnitude of ST depressions strongly associated with the outcome. Lastly, an increasing number of leads demonstrating ST-segment elevations are associated with higher risk of mortality (O'Gara, 2013).

Prognostic Value of Cardiac Troponins

cTns provide important prognostic utility for both CKD and non-CKD populations based on the evidence that there is a clear, quantitative relationship between the amount of cTn elevation during an acute MI, the size of the infarct, and the overall risk of death. The GUSTO IV trial demonstrated further that the prognostic value of cTnT with respect to mortality was actually greater in patients with CKD and suspected ACS compared with those with more normal renal function (Aviles, 2002).

Risk Prediction Algorithms

Several risk assessment tools have been developed to assist in estimating overall risk of death and ischemic events in patients with NSTE-ACS with the goal of guiding further therapeutic interventions to decrease cardiovascular morbidity and mortality. These algorithms are helpful in their predictive accuracy for death and MI at 1 year and therefore in identifying patients who might be likely to benefit from aggressive therapy, including early myocardial revascularization. The thrombolysis in myocardial infarction **(TIMI) risk score** created by Antman et al. calculates risk for all-cause mortality, new or recurrent MI, or severe recurrent ischemia requiring urgent revascularization at 14 days based on seven criteria that may be obtained at presentation (Antman, 2000). Although widely used, the TIMI risk score does not account for renal function and therefore may underestimate the risk for adverse outcomes in those with CKD. Alternatively, the **Global Registry of Acute Coronary Events (GRACE) risk model** was developed to predict in-hospital mortality or MI for patients with STEMI and NSTE-ACS and this model does incorporate creatinine (Eagle, 2004; Fox, 2010).

BASIC PRINCIPLES OF MANAGEMENT

Patients with definite ACS are triaged based on the pattern of the 12-lead ECG. In general, patients with ST-segment elevation should be evaluated for immediate pharmacologic or PCI-based reperfusion therapy to restore flow promptly in the occluded epicardial infarct-related artery and treated according to the ACC/AHA guidelines for the management of patients with STEMI (O'Gara, 2013). Individuals without ST-segment elevation (NSTE-ACS) may be either observed further in a specialized facility (e.g., chest pain unit or emergency department) or hospital setting.

Given the increased CVD risk and worse outcomes of patients with CKD, recent guidelines from both the European Society of Cardiology (ESC) and AHA/ACC favor an invasive strategy of coronary catheterization and revascularization in patients presenting with NSTEMI. The ESC guidelines make a more specific recommendation that these patients should undergo cardiac catheterization via radial artery access within 72 hours of presentation (Roffi, 2016). The basis of revascularization (PCI vs. coronary artery bypass graft surgery

Class I Recommendations for Anti-Ischemic Therapy: Continuing Ischemia/Other Clinical High-Risk Features Present[a]
Bed/chair rest with continuous ECG monitoring.
Supplemental oxygen with an arterial saturation less than 90%, respiratory distress, or other high-risk features for hypoxemia. Pulse oximetry can be useful for continuous measurement of SaO_2.
NTG 0.4 mg sublingually every 5 minutes for a total of three doses; afterward, assess need for IV NTG.
NTG IV for first 48 hours after UA/NSTEMI for treatment of persistent ischemia, HF, or hypertension.
Decision to administer NTG IV and dose should not preclude therapy with other mortality-reducing interventions such as β-blockers or ACE inhibitors.
β-Blockers (via oral route) within 24 hours without a contraindication (e.g., HF) irrespective of concomitant performance of PCI.
When β-blockers are contraindicated, a nondihydropyridine calcium antagonist (e.g., verapamil or diltiazem) should be given as initial therapy in the absence of severe LV dysfunction or other contraindications.
ACE inhibitor (via oral route) within first 24 hours with pulmonary congestion, or LVEF less than or equal to 0.40, in the absence of hypotension (systolic blood pressure less than 100 mm Hg or less than 30 mm Hg below baseline) or known contraindications to that class of medications.
ARB should be administered to UA/NSTEMI patients who are intolerant of ACE inhibitors and have either clinical or radiologic signs of heart failure or LVEF less than or equal to 0.40.

[a]Recurrent angina and/or ischemia-related ECG changes (0.05 mV or greater ST-segment depression or bundle-branch block) at rest or with low-level activity; or ischemia associated with HF symptoms, S 3 gallop, or new or worsening mitral regurgitation; or hemodynamic instability or depressed LV function (LVEF less than 0.40 on noninvasive study); or serious ventricular arrhythmia.
Source: Adapted from Anderson JL, Adams CD, Antman EM, et al. 2012 ACCF/AHA focused update incorporated into the ACCF/AHA 2007 guidelines for the management of patients with unstable angina/non-ST-elevation myocardial infarction. *J Am Coll Cardiol.* 2013;61:e179–e347.

[CABG]) should be determined by clinical status, comorbidities, and coronary disease severity.

Although NSTE-ACS patients are not candidates for immediate pharmacologic reperfusion, treatment is directed toward resolution of symptoms with anti-ischemic therapy (Table 17.1), and prevention of adverse cardiovascular events with antithrombotic therapy and invasive catheter–based therapy, as needed. Patients determined to be at low risk for ACS (e.g., those with low-risk ECG findings, negative cardiac biomarkers, and negative stress test or cardiac computed tomographic angiography study) may be discharged with appropriate outpatient follow-up (Fig. 17.1) (Amsterdam, 2014). Antithrombin therapy and antiplatelet therapy should be administered to all patients with ACS in the absence of contraindication regardless of the presence or absence of ST-segment elevation.

Impact of Chronic Kidney Disease

Management of individuals with CKD who have been diagnosed definitively with ACS is challenging for many reasons. Most clinical ACS trials have excluded patients with moderate to severe renal impairment, and thus use of established ACS therapies in the CKD population is not based on solid evidence. According to an analysis by Charytan and Kuntz, 75% of the major therapeutic ACS studies in the 1990s and 2000s excluded patients with moderate to severe CKD (Charytan and Kuntz, 2006; Han, 2006). The presence of moderate to severe CKD in patients with ACS has been associated with decreased use of antithrombotic, antiplatelet, and anti-ischemic medications, diagnostic coronary angiography, thrombolytic therapy, and PCIs (Berger, 2003; Charytan and Kuntz, 2006; Freeman, 2003; Wright, 2002). This underutilization is likely reflective of other high-risk characteristics in this population. Other explanations for this broad failure to adhere to ACC/AHA guidelines for managing UA/NSTEMI events include a concern for increased bleeding complications from antithrombotic and antiplatelet therapies, a higher risk of temporary or permanent contrast-induced renal failure, the need for renal dosing for many ACS medications, and the unclear benefit of these therapies in the CKD population. Pharmacotherapy in CKD patients with ACS has been summarized in an AHA scientific statement (Washam, 2015). See also Jain and Reilly, 2018 and Table 23.16.

ANTI-ISCHEMIC AND ANALGESIC THERAPY

Nitrates

NTG is an endothelium-independent vasodilator that relieves myocardial ischemia via several mechanisms. NTG increases myocardial blood flow via dilatation of epicardial coronary arteries. It decreases myocardial oxygen demand that is due to peripheral venodilation, which results in decreased preload and ultimately ventricular wall stress. Also, NTG reduces myocardial oxygen demand (modestly) by systemic arterial vasodilation, which results in decreased systolic wall stress (decreased afterload). Large randomized trials for patients with suspected ACS have not shown any mortality benefit of nitrates when given to either NSTEMI or STEMI patients; nevertheless, nitrates are routinely given for persistent myocardial ischemia, heart failure, or hypertension unless contraindicated because of hypotension, severe bradycardia or tachycardia, cardiogenic shock, or recent use of sildenafil or related compounds.

β-Adrenergic Receptor Blockers

Limited data are available regarding the efficacy and safety of short-term β-blockade in CKD patients with ACS. Post hoc and retrospective cohort analyses have shown that β-blockade in the presence of CKD compared with non-CKD offers a similar mortality benefit (Berger, 2003; Chonchol, 2008). In summary, oral β-blockers are recommended early in the care of ACS patients, including those with CKD, in the absence of the following high-risk features: hypotension, bradycardia, advanced atrioventricular block, evidence of acute pulmonary edema, history of asthma or emphysema, risk of cardiogenic shock, or evidence of a low-output state.

Calcium Channel Blockers

Aside from the short-acting dihydropyridine nifedipine, which has been shown to be dangerous for ACS patients in the absence of concomitant β-blockade (Furberg, 1995), meta-analyses of calcium channel blockers (CCBs) as a class show them to be safe and useful for symptom control although providing no mortality or reinfarction benefits (Held, 1989). There are limited data evaluating the role of CCBs in patients with ACS and CKD. Until such studies are performed, nondihydropyridine CCBs appear reasonable to use in treating persistent ischemic symptoms in ACS patients with variant angina, or in individuals who have symptoms despite already receiving adequate doses of nitrates and β-blockade, or in those who are unable to tolerate either nitrates or β-blockers, as long as there are no contraindications to CCB treatment, such as hemodynamic instability, cardiogenic shock, pulmonary edema, or moderate to severe left ventricular dysfunction (LVEF ≤40%).

Inhibitors of the Renin–Angiotensin–Aldosterone System

Angiotensin-converting enzyme inhibitors (ACEIs) have been shown to improve short-term mortality rates in all acute MI patients as well as long-term mortality rates in acute MI patients with left ventricular systolic dysfunction by about 23% (ACE Inhibitor Myocardial Infarction Collaborative Group, 1998; Pfeffer, 1992). A meta-analysis of four major ACEI trials in 100,000 ACS patients, including many with preserved left ventricular systolic function, showed a 7% reduction in mortality at 30 days, although in absolute terms the mortality reduction was not very impressive, from 7.6% to 7.1% (ACE Inhibitor Myocardial Infarction Collaborative Group, 1998). In the VALIANT study, angiotensin receptor blockers (ARBs) were equally effective as ACEIs with respect to mortality reduction in acute MI patients complicated by left ventricular systolic dysfunction, heart failure, and creatinine levels ≤2.5 mg/dL (220 mcmol/L) (Pfeffer, 2003). Furthermore, ACEIs/ARBs were well tolerated in the subgroup of patients with an eGFR/1.73 m^2 <45 mL/min, with only 5% discontinuing the drug for renal reasons; hyperkalemia accounted for drug discontinuation in only 0.7% (Anavekar, 2004a). **Eplerenone**, a selective aldosterone receptor blocker, was found to significantly reduce morbidity and mortality in MI patients complicated by left ventricular dysfunction and heart failure (Pitt, 2003). For patients with a creatinine ≥1.1 mg/dL (100 mcmol/L), there was no significant mortality benefit, and in those with a creatinine clearance <50 mL/min, hyperkalemia developed in 10% versus 6% in the placebo group. Current guidelines recommend use of ACEIs, or ARBs (if patients are intolerant of ACEIs), for ACS patients with pulmonary congestion or LVEF ≤40% in the absence of hypotension or known contraindications to these classes of medications. These recommendations may reasonably be applied to individuals with mild to moderate CKD based on results from the VALIANT study (Pfeffer, 2003); however, efficacy of these medications is unknown in those with more advanced renal dysfunction.

ANTIPLATELET AND ANTICOAGULANT THERAPY

Antiplatelet and antithrombotic therapy is an essential ACS treatment that modifies the pathophysiologic process of thrombus formation and alters the natural progression to death or recurrent MI. A combination of aspirin, an anticoagulant, and additional antiplatelet therapy has been established as the most effective antithrombotic approach for ACS (Amsterdam, 2014).

Aspirin

The benefits of aspirin are well known in the prevention of death and nonfatal recurrent MI in all ACS patients. A meta-analysis of 11 randomized trials of patients with a history of MI, UA, stroke, or transient ischemic attack (TIA) reported a 25% reduction in death, recurrent MI, or stroke for those receiving 75 to 325 mg/day of aspirin (1994). Analyses of registry and observational data have shown that following an MI, the benefits of aspirin with regard to reduction of mortality are similar in CKD and non-CKD patients (Berger, 2003; McCullough, 2002). As a cautionary note, aspirin may increase the bleeding risk in patients with severe to advanced renal dysfunction by prolonging bleeding times in the setting of uremia (Livio, 1986). A more contemporary study showed that low-dose (100-mg) aspirin was associated with an increased risk of minor, but not major bleeding (vs. placebo) across a spectrum of renal function (Baigent, 2005). Although there are no randomized, controlled efficacy or safety trials to date, retrospective data suggest that there is no significant difference in the relative risk reduction for 30-day mortality in ESRD versus non-ESRD patients (Berger, 2003). As such, aspirin is still recommended as first-line treatment in CKD patients with ACS unless contraindicated.

Thienopyridines: Clopidogrel, Prasugrel, and Ticagrelor

Thienopyridines are antagonists of the P2Y12 receptor which binds adenosine diphosphate on the surface of platelets. For many years, dual antiplatelet therapy with aspirin and clopidogrel had been the default combination. However, more recent studies have suggested superior clinical outcomes with ticagrelor or prasugrel. Thus, the most recent guidelines from both the ACC/AHA and ESC preferentially recommend either ticagrelor or prasugrel instead of clopidogrel in patients with ACS treated with an early invasive strategy and/or stenting (Roffi, 2016).

Ticagrelor reversibly binds with the P2Y12 receptor. Compared to clopidogrel, it has a shorter plasma half-life and a more consistent onset of action. In the PLATO (PLATelet inhibition and patient outcomes) trial, patients with ACS treated with ticagrelor had a significant reduction in the composite primary outcome of death from vascular causes, MI, or stroke (hazard ratio [HR] 0.84, $p < 0.0001$) (Wallentin, 2009). There was also a significant reduction in mortality in the overall cohort, although there was regional heterogeneity in this finding. In a prespecified subgroup analysis of patients with eGFR <60 mL/min, there was a more robust reduction in the primary cardiovascular outcome (17.3% vs. 22.0%; HR 0.77; 95% CI, 0.65–0.90) compared with clopidogrel (James, 2010). This was driven by a 4% decrease in total mortality (10.0% vs. 14.0%; HR 0.72; 95% CI, 0.58–0.89). Notably there was no significant increase in major bleeding.

In the TRITON-TIMI (Trial to assess improvement in therapeutic outcomes by optimizing platelet inhibition with prasugrel–thrombolysis in myocardial infarction) 38 trial, prasugrel was found to reduce the composite of cardiovascular death, nonfatal MI, and stroke (HR 0.81; $p = 0.001$) compared to clopidogrel. However, these benefits were limited by a significant increase in bleeding especially in patients >75 years of age or of low body weight (<60 kg) (Wiviott, 2007). Therefore, the ACA/AHA guidelines recommend prasugrel over clopidogrel only in patients who are not at high risk for bleeding complications. Prasugrel is contraindicated in patients with prior TIA.

There is no dose adjustment recommended for any of the P2Y12 inhibitors in CKD patients. It is important to note that these landmark trials excluded patients with ESRD, as have most trials of ACS therapy.

Anticoagulation With Unfractionated Heparin or Low–Molecular-Weight Heparin

Heparin is another cornerstone of therapy for NSTE-ACS. Unfractionated Heparin (UFH) has been shown to provide a significant short-term benefit as an add-on to aspirin therapy for ACS patients, halving the mortality and MI rate after 1 week (Petersen, 2004).

A subgroup analysis of 12,000 patients with NSTEMI and mild to severe CKD from the GRACE registry demonstrated that the use of low–molecular-weight heparin (LMWH) alone compared with UFH alone was better tolerated with respect to major bleeding and more effective in reducing risk of death at 30 days (4.2% vs. 6.2%), irrespective of renal function. However, major bleeding complication rates doubled, regardless of which heparin was used, for those with severe CKD (Collet, 2005). Although the evidence suggests that there is a comparable efficacy of LMWH compared with UFH in patients with mild CKD presenting with ACS, physicians should exercise caution when administering LMWH to those with more severe degrees of renal impairment as there is no clear benefit, with a potential for increased minor and major bleeding complications (Montalescot, 2004).

Platelet Glycoprotein IIb/IIIa Inhibitors

Platelet glycoprotein (GP) IIb/IIIa inhibitors are primarily indicated for individuals with high-risk NSTE-ACS in whom a possible PCI is planned. Despite the wealth of data on GP IIb/IIIa inhibitor use in the general population for ACS events, the safety and efficacy data regarding GP IIb/IIIa inhibitor use in those with CKD is limited (Januzzi, 2002; Reddan, 2003). A subgroup analysis of 12,000 patients with NSTE-ACS and mild to severe CKD from the GRACE registry demonstrated that bleeding rates with GP IIb/IIIa use increased

			Return of Platelet Function	Renal Clearance (%)	Renal Dose Adjustment
Class	Half-Life	Reversibility			
Abciximab chimeric human-murine monoclonal antibody	10–30 minutes, but remains in circulation platelet-bound for 10 days	Slow	Slow (>48 hours)	None	None
Eptifibatide synthetic peptide	2.5 hours	Fast	Fast	50	Yes
Tirofiban synthetic nonpeptide	2.0 hours	Fast	Fast	65	Yes

TABLE 17.2 Comparison of the Platelet GP IIb/IIIa Inhibitors

significantly with progressive renal dysfunction (Collet, 2005). Although the available evidence suggests that there is a clinical benefit of GP IIb/IIIa inhibitor use in patients with mild to moderate renal dysfunction and concomitant NSTE-ACS, physicians must weigh this advantage against the increased bleeding risks involved, especially in those with thrombocytopenia, progressive renal impairment, severe hypertension, recent major surgery, or stroke. Doses of some of these agents must be adjusted in the presence of moderate to severe CKD (Table 17.2).

REPERFUSION THERAPY

Reperfusion strategies have evolved over the past several decades into the most critical and fundamental ACS therapy to reduce the risk of future adverse events, especially in the STEMI population.

Reperfusion therapy is underutilized in patients with CKD; patients with advanced renal impairment are four times less likely to receive reperfusion therapy compared with patients with normal renal function (Wright, 2002), a trend observed at all levels of CKD severity. In addition, patients with MI and renal dysfunction are evaluated with coronary angiography almost one-third less frequently than individuals with normal renal function and are revascularized half as often as their non-CKD counterparts (Charytan and Kuntz, 2006). The reluctance to proceed with reperfusion in patients with renal impairment certainly is in part due to the significantly higher rates of complication involving bleeding, stroke, restenosis, and progression of renal dysfunction that is due to contrast-induced nephropathy (Table 17.3).

As expected, there is very little evidence regarding the efficacy and safety of reperfusion strategies in the CKD population despite

TABLE 17.3	Incidence of Hospital Stroke and Major Bleeding Stratified by Renal Function		
	Normal Renal Function (n = 8,937)	Moderate Renal Dysfunction (n = 2,924)	Severe Renal Dysfunction (n = 459)
Primary PCI (n = 3,350)			
Stroke, %	0.2 (p = 0.04)	1.3 (p = 0.71)	1.4 (p = 0.77)
Major bleeding, %	2.7 (p < 0.001)	6.8 (p < 0.001)	7.3 (p = 0.23)
Fibrinolysis (n = 3,723)			
Stroke, %	1.2 (p = 0.004)	1.7 (p = 0.53)	2.7 (p = 0.64)
Major bleeding, %	1.9 (p = 0.02)	3.4 (p = 0.11)	8.2 (p = 0.12)
No reperfusion (n = 5,247)			
Stroke, %	0.6	1.3	1.9
Major bleeding, %	1.4	2.5	4.2

Note: N = 12,320. p-values are given with "no reperfusion" as the reference group and are adjusted for GRACE risk score.

the high risk of mortality and reinfarction in these patients. What limited data exist are complex and appear mixed. A retrospective cohort analysis of more than 4,000 ACS patients with at least mild CKD demonstrated relative mortality reductions of 11% and 15% with fibrinolytic and PCI strategies, respectively (Keough-Ryan, 2005). In contrast, a recent post hoc analysis of the GRACE registry, which included 2,974 patients with moderate CKD and 467 patients with severe CKD, showed no mortality reduction with fibrinolysis in patients with STEMI or new LBBB and concomitant CKD. In fact, for moderate CKD patients with STEMI, the in-hospital risk of mortality was worse with fibrinolysis, although this was offset by a trend toward reduced 6-month mortality.

Evidence for pharmacotherapy for ACS patients with CKD has been summarized in detail (see Washam, 2015 and also Table 23.16).

CORONARY REVASCULARIZATION

Traditionally CABG for multivessel coronary artery disease has been associated with superior outcomes in patients with both ESRD and CKD not on dialysis compared to PCI (Herzog, 2002). In an analysis of 22,000 ESRD patients on maintenance dialysis by the U. S. Renal Data System, revascularization by CABG had superior adjusted mortality compared to PCI (HR 0.87, 95% CI, 0.84–0.90) and the composite of death or MI (HR 0.88, 95% CI, 0.86–0.91) (Chang, 2012). Therefore CABG is preferred instead of PCI in patients with multivessel disease and expected survival >1 year (Roffi, 2016).

SECONDARY PREVENTION

Long-term secondary prevention therapies are as important as in-hospital ACS treatment, given the markedly increased risk of death and cardiovascular morbidity in patients with CKD. Patients with the greatest degree of renal dysfunction, who carry the highest risk for serious long-term adverse events post-MI, are routinely prescribed the least amount of guideline-recommended medical therapy. This is similar to the disproportionate underutilization of antiplatelet, anti-ischemic, anticoagulant, and reperfusion therapies in patients with renal dysfunction and ACS compared with patients with normal renal function (Fox, 2010; Keough-Ryan, 2005; McCullough, 2002). Again, much of this therapeutic nihilism stems probably from unfavorable risk/benefit profiles with respect to bleeding, contraindications that are due to other comorbidities (e.g., heart failure), and absence of prospective randomized controlled evidence to support use of these long-term therapies.

Although the majority of secondary prevention prospective randomized trials typically excluded patients with CKD, retrospective and subgroup analyses suggest that the benefits of antiplatelet therapy, β-blockade, statins, and especially ACEIs may be reasonably extrapolated to the CKD population in the absence of contraindications (Dargie, 2001; Ellis, 2003; Harper and Jacobson, 2008; Keltai, 2007). Additional integral measures for secondary prevention include lifestyle risk-factor modification, including smoking cessation, weight management, and aerobic exercise or cardiac rehabilitation, as meta-analyses have shown that all of these provide clear and sustained mortality benefits in the general population (Clark, 2005). Prospective randomized trials involving current secondary preventive treatments are required for confirmation of benefit across the spectrum of CKD.

Based on the results of the SHARP study, practice guidelines from the Kidney Disease Improving Global Outcomes (KDIGO) recommend the use of statins and statin/ezetimibe for all patients with CKD excluding patients treated with chronic hemodialysis. In chronic dialysis patients, the initiation of statin therapy is not recommended however it should be continued in those patients previously on lipid-lowering therapy (Baigent, 2011; Khan, 2005; Tonelli and Wanner, 2014).

CONCLUSION

In the past several years, there have been significant advances in the treatment of ACS. These treatments are more important in the CKD populations given the higher risk of disease and complications. In the clinical case presented at the beginning of this chapter, the patient should be observed and have repeat troponins drawn to determine if there was an MI. If troponin elevations are observed, this patient would be diagnosed with an NSTEMI since her initial ECG did not demonstrate ST-segment elevation. Risk stratification should be calculated with either the TIMI or GRACE risk scores to assist management decisions. Given her CKD, she should be managed with an invasive strategy. Cardiac catheterization (if available in the hospital) is recommended within 72 hours. She would be treated with antiplatelet agents, a statin, and antihypertensive medications for secondary prevention.

References and Suggested Readings

ACE Inhibitor Myocardial Infarction Collaborative Group. Indications for ACE inhibitors in the early treatment of acute myocardial infarction: systematic overview of individual data from 100,000 patients in randomized trials. *Circulation.* 1998;97:2202–2212.

Amsterdam EA, Wenger NK, Brindis RG, et al. 2014 AHA/ACC guideline for the management of patients with non-ST-elevation acute coronary syndromes: a report of the American College of Cardiology/American Heart Association Task Force on practice guidelines. *J Am Coll Cardiol.* 2014;64:e139–e228.

Anavekar NS, Gans DJ, Berl T, et al. Predictors of cardiovascular events in patients with type 2 diabetic nephropathy and hypertension: a case for albuminuria. *Kidney Int Suppl.* 2004a:S50–S55.

Anavekar NS, McMurray JJ, Velazquez EJ, et al. Relation between renal dysfunction and cardiovascular outcomes after myocardial infarction. *N Engl J Med.* 2004b;351:1285–1295.

Anderson JL, Adams CD, Antman EM, et al. 2012 ACCF/AHA focused update incorporated into the ACCF/AHA 2007 guidelines for the management of patients with unstable angina/non–ST-elevation myocardial infarction: a report of the American College of Cardiology Foundation/American Heart Association Task Force on Practice Guidelines. *Circulation.* 2013;127:e863–e864.

Antman EM, Cohen M, Bernink PJ, et al. The TIMI risk score for unstable angina/non-ST elevation MI: a method for prognostication and therapeutic decision making. *JAMA.* 2000;284:835–842.

Aviles RJ, Askari AT, Lindahl B, et al. Troponin T levels in patients with acute coronary syndromes, with or without renal dysfunction. *N Engl J Med.* 2002;346:2047–2052.

Baigent C, Landray M, Leaper C, et al. First United Kingdom Heart and Renal Protection (UK-HARP-I) study: biochemical efficacy and safety of simvastatin and safety of low-dose aspirin in chronic kidney disease. *Am J Kidney Dis.* 2005;45:473–484.

Baigent C, Landray MJ, Reith C, et al. The effects of lowering LDL cholesterol with simvastatin plus ezetimibe in patients with chronic kidney disease (Study of Heart and Renal Protection): a randomised placebo-controlled trial. *Lancet.* 2011;377:2181–2192.

Bansal N, Hyre Anderson A, Yang W, et al. High-sensitivity troponin T and N-terminal pro-B-type natriuretic peptide (NT-proBNP) and risk of incident heart failure in patients with CKD: the Chronic Renal Insufficiency Cohort (CRIC) study. *J Am Soc Nephrol.* 2015;26:946–956.

Bashir A, Moody WE, Edwards NC, et al. Coronary artery calcium assessment in CKD: Utility in cardiovascular disease risk assessment and treatment? *Am J Kidney Dis.* 2015;65:937–948.

Berger AK, Duval S, Krumholz HM. Aspirin, beta-blocker, and angiotensin-converting enzyme inhibitor therapy in patients with end-stage renal disease and an acute myocardial infarction. *J Am Coll Cardiol.* 2003;42:201–208.

Cannon CP, McCabe CH, Stone PH, et al. The electrocardiogram predicts one-year outcome of patients with unstable angina and non-Q wave myocardial infarction: results of the TIMI III Registry ECG Ancillary Study. Thrombolysis in myocardial ischemia. *J Am Coll Cardiol.* 1997;30:133–140.

Chang TI, Shilane D, Kazi DS, et al. Multivessel coronary artery bypass grafting versus percutaneous coronary intervention in ESRD. *J Am Soc Nephrol.* 2012;23:2042–2049.

Charytan D, Kuntz RE. The exclusion of patients with chronic kidney disease from clinical trials in coronary artery disease. *Kidney Int.* 2006;70:2021–2030.

Chonchol M, Benderly M, Goldbourt U. Beta-blockers for coronary heart disease in chronic kidney disease. *Nephrol Dial Transplant.* 2008;23:2274–2279.

Clark AM, Hartling L, Vandermeer B, et al. Meta-analysis: secondary prevention programs for patients with coronary artery disease. *Ann Intern Med.* 2005;143:659–672.

Collaborative overview of randomised trials of antiplatelet therapy–I: Prevention of death, myocardial infarction, and stroke by prolonged antiplatelet therapy in various categories of patients. Antiplatelet Trialists' Collaboration. *BMJ*. 1994;308: 81–106; erratum in: *BMJ*. 1994;308:1540.

Collet JP, Montalescot G, Agnelli G, et al; GRACE Investigators. Non–ST-segment elevation acute coronary syndrome in patients with renal dysfunction: benefit of low-molecular-weight heparin alone or with glycoprotein IIb/IIIa inhibitors on outcomes. The Global Registry of Acute Coronary Events. *Eur Heart J.* 2005;26:2285–2293.

Dargie HJ. Effect of carvedilol on outcome after myocardial infarction in patients with left-ventricular dysfunction: the CAPRICORN randomised trial. *Lancet.* 2001;357:1385–1390.

Eagle KA, Lim MJ, Dabbous OH, et al; GRACE Investigators. A validated prediction model for all forms of acute coronary syndrome: estimating the risk of 6-month postdischarge death in an international registry. *JAMA.* 2004;291: 2727–2733.

Ellis K, Tcheng JE, Sapp S, et al. Mortality benefit of beta blockade in patients with acute coronary syndromes undergoing coronary intervention: pooled results from the Epic, Epilog, Epistent, Capture and Rapport Trials. *J Interv Cardiol.* 2003;16:299–305.

Fox CS, Muntner P, Chen AY, et al. Use of evidence-based therapies in short-term outcomes of ST-segment elevation myocardial infarction and non–ST-segment elevation myocardial infarction in patients with chronic kidney disease: a report from the National Cardiovascular Data Acute Coronary Treatment and Intervention Outcomes Network registry. *Circulation.* 2010;121:357–365.

Freeman RV, Mehta RH, Al Badr W, et al. Influence of concurrent renal dysfunction on outcomes of patients with acute coronary syndromes and implications of the use of glycoprotein IIb/IIIa inhibitors. *J Am Coll Cardiol.* 2003;41:718–724.

Furberg CD, Psaty BM, Meyer JV. Nifedipine. Dose-related increase in mortality in patients with coronary heart disease. *Circulation.* 1995;92:1326–1331.

Gibson CM, Dumaine RL, Gelfand EV, et al; TIMI Study Group. Association of glomerular filtration rate on presentation with subsequent mortality in non–ST-segment elevation acute coronary syndrome; observations in 13,307 patients in five TIMI trials. *Eur Heart J.* 2004;25:1998–2005.

Go AS, Chertow GM, Fan D, et al. Chronic kidney disease and the risks of death, cardiovascular events, and hospitalization. *N Engl J Med.* 2004;351:1296–1305.

Gupta R, Birnbaum Y, Uretsky BF. The renal patient with coronary artery disease: current concepts and dilemmas. *J Am Coll Cardiol.* 2004;44:1343–1353.

Han JH, Chandra A, Mulgund J, et al. Chronic kidney disease in patients with non–ST-segment elevation acute coronary syndromes. *Am J Med.* 2006;119:248–254.

Han Y, Guo J, Zheng Y, et al; BRIGHT Investigators. Bivalirudin vs heparin with or without tirofiban during primary percutaneous coronary intervention in acute myocardial infarction: the BRIGHT randomized clinical trial. *JAMA.* 2015;313: 1336–1346.

Harper CR, Jacobson TA. Managing dyslipidemia in chronic kidney disease. *J Am Coll Cardiol.* 2008;51:2375–2384.

Haydar AA, Hujairi NM, Covic AA, et al. Coronary artery calcification is related to coronary atherosclerosis in chronic renal disease patients: a study comparing EBCT-generated coronary artery calcium scores and coronary angiography. *Nephrol Dial Transplant.* 2004;19:2307–2312.

Held PH, Yusuf S, Furberg CD. Calcium channel blockers in acute myocardial infarction and unstable angina: an overview. *BMJ.* 1989;299:1187–1192.

Herzog CA, Ma JZ, Collins AJ. Comparative survival of dialysis patients in the United States after coronary angioplasty, coronary artery stenting, and coronary artery bypass surgery and impact of diabetes. *Circulation.* 2002;106:2207–2211.

Indications for ACE inhibitors in the early treatment of acute myocardial infarction: systematic overview of individual data from 100,000 patients in randomized trials. ACE Inhibitor Myocardial Infarction Collaborative Group. *Circulation.* 1998;97:2202–2212.

Jain N, Reilly RF. Clinical pharmacology of oral anticoagulants in patients with kidney disease. *Clin J Am Soc Nephrol.* 2018 May 25, in press.

James S, Budaj A, Aylward P, et al. Ticagrelor versus clopidogrel in acute coronary syndromes in relation to renal function: results from the Platelet Inhibition and Patient Outcomes (PLATO) trial. *Circulation.* 2010;122:1056–1067.

Januzzi JL Jr, Snapinn SM, DiBattiste PM, et al. Benefits and safety of tirofiban among acute coronary syndrome patients with mild to moderate renal insufficiency: results from the Platelet Receptor Inhibition in Ischemic Syndrome Management in Patients Limited by Unstable Signs and Symptoms (PRISM-PLUS) Trial. *Circulation.* 2002;105:2361–2366.

Kannel WB. Silent myocardial ischemia and infarction: insights from the Framingham Study. *Cardiol Clin.* 1986;4:583–591.

Keltai M, Tonelli M, Mann JF, et al. Renal function and outcomes in acute coronary syndrome: impact of clopidogrel. *Eur J Cardiovasc Prev Rehabil.* 2007;14:312–318.

Keough-Ryan TM, Kiberd BA, Dipchand CS, et al. Outcomes of acute coronary syndrome in a large Canadian cohort: impact of chronic renal insufficiency, cardiac interventions, and anemia. *Am J Kidney Dis.* 2005;46:845–855.

Khan NA, Hemmelgarn BR, Tonelli M, et al. Prognostic Value of Troponin T and I among asymptomatic patients with end-stage renal disease: a meta-analysis. *Circulation.* 2005;112:3088–3096.

Livio M, Viganò G, Benigni A, et al. Moderate doses of aspirin and risk of bleeding in renal failure. *The Lancet.* 1986;327:414–416.

Mann JF, Gerstein HC, Pogue J, et al. Renal Insufficiency as a Predictor of cardiovascular outcomes and the impact of ramipril: The HOPE randomized trial. *Ann Intern Med.* 2001;134:629–636.

McCullough PA, Agarwal M, Agrawal V. Review article: risks of coronary artery calcification in chronic kidney disease: Do the same rules apply? *Nephrology (Carlton).* 2009;14:428–436.

McCullough PA, Sandberg KR, Borzak S, et al. Benefits of aspirin and beta-blockade after myocardial infarction in patients with chronic kidney disease. *Am Heart J.* 2002;144:226–232.

McCullough PA, Soman SS, Shah SS, et al. Risks associated with renal dysfunction in patients in the coronary care unit. *J Am Coll Cardiol.* 2000;36:679–684.

Montalescot G, Collet JP, Tanguy ML, et al. Anti-Xa activity relates to survival and efficacy in unselected acute coronary syndrome patients treated with enoxaparin. *Circulation.* 2004;110:392–398.

O'Gara PT, Kushner FG, Ascheim DD, et al. 2013 ACCF/AHA guideline for the management of ST-elevation myocardial infarction: a report of the American College of Cardiology Foundation/American Heart Association Task Force on practice guidelines. *Circulation.* 2013;127:e362–e425.

Petersen JL, Mahaffey KW, Hasselblad V, et al. Efficacy and bleeding complications among patients randomized to enoxaparin or unfractionated heparin for antithrombin therapy in non–ST-segment elevation acute coronary syndromes: a systematic overview. *JAMA.* 2004;292:89–96.

Pfeffer MA, Braunwald E, Moye LA, et al. Effect of captopril on mortality and morbidity in patients with left ventricular dysfunction after myocardial infarction. Results of the survival and ventricular enlargement trial. The SAVE Investigators. *N Engl J Med.* 1992;327:669–677.

Pfeffer MA, McMurray JJ, Velazquez EJ, et al; Valsartan in Acute Myocardial Infarction Trial Investigators. Valsartan, captopril, or both in myocardial infarction complicated by heart failure, left ventricular dysfunction, or both. *N Engl J Med.* 2003;349:1893–1906.

Pitt B, Remme W, Zannad F, et al; Eplerenone Post-Acute Myocardial Infarction Heart Failure Efficacy and Survival Study Investigators. Eplerenone, a selective aldosterone blocker, in patients with left ventricular dysfunction after myocardial infarction. *N Engl J Med.* 2003;348:1309–1321.

Reddan DN, O'Shea JC, Sarembock IJ, et al. Treatment effects of eptifibatide in planned coronary stent implantation in patients with chronic kidney disease (ESPRIT Trial). *Am J Cardiol.* 2003;91:17–21.

Reimer KA, Lowe JE, Rasmussen MM, et al. The wavefront phenomenon of ischemic cell death. 1. Myocardial infarct size vs duration of coronary occlusion in dogs. *Circulation*. 1977;56:786–794.

Roffi M, Patrono C, Collet JP, et al. 2015 ESC Guidelines for the management of acute coronary syndromes in patients presenting without persistent ST-segment elevation. Task force for the management of acute coronary syndromes in patients presenting without persistent ST-segment elevation of the European Society of Cardiology (ESC). *Eur Heart J*. 2016;37:267–315.

Rouan GW, Lee TH, Cook EF, et al. Clinical characteristics and outcome of acute myocardial infarction in patients with initially normal or nonspecific electrocardiograms (a report from the Multicenter Chest Pain Study). *Am J Cardiol*. 1989;64:1087–1092.

Shantouf RS, Budoff MJ, Ahmadi N, et al. Total and individual coronary artery calcium scores as independent predictors of mortality in hemodialysis patients. *Am J Nephrol*. 2010;31:419–425.

Shlipak MG, Heidenreich PA, Noguchi H, et al. Association of renal insufficiency with treatment and outcomes after myocardial infarction in elderly patients. *Ann Intern Med*. 2002;137:555–562.

Szummer K, Lindahl B, Sylven C, et al. Relationship of plasma erythropoietin to long-term outcome in acute coronary syndrome. *Int J Cardiol*. 2010;143:165–170.

Teague HL, Ahlman MA, Alavi A, et al. Unraveling vascular inflammation: from immunology to imaging. *J Am Coll Cardiol*. 2017;70:1403–1412.

Thygesen K, Alpert JS, Jaffe AS, et al. Third universal definition of myocardial infarction. *J Am Coll Cardiol*. 2012;60:1581–1598.

Tonelli M, Wanner C; Kidney Disease: Improving Global Outcomes Lipid Guideline Development Work Group Members. Lipid management in chronic kidney disease: synopsis of the kidney disease: improving global outcomes 2013 clinical practice guideline. *Ann Intern Med*. 2014;160:182.

Twerenbold R, Wildi K, Jaeger C, et al. Optimal cutoff levels of more sensitive cardiac troponin assays for the early diagnosis of myocardial infarction in patients with renal dysfunction. *Circulation*. 2015;131:2041–2050.

USRDS. United States Renal Data Systems. 2017 USRDS annual data report: Epidemi of kidney disease in the United States. Chapter 4: Cardiovascular disease in patients with CKD. *Am J Kidney Dis*. 2018;71:S77–S94. https://www.usrds.org/2017/view/v1_04.aspx.

Wallentin L, Becker RC, Budaj A, et al. Ticagrelor versus clopidogrel in patients with acute coronary syndromes. *N Engl J Med*. 2009;361:1045–1057.

Washam JB, Herzog CA, Beitelshees AL, et al. Pharmacotherapy in chronic kidney disease patients presenting with acute coronary syndrome: a scientific statement from the American Heart Association. *Circulation*. 2015;131:1123–1149.

Wiviott SD, Braunwald E, McCabe CH, et al; TRITON-TIMI 38 Investigators. Prasugrel versus clopidogrel in patients with acute coronary syndromes. *N Engl J Med*. 2007;357:2001–2015.

Wright RS, Reeder GS, Herzog CA, et al. Acute myocardial infarction and renal dysfunction: a high-risk combination. *Ann Intern Med*. 2002;137:563–570.

18 Heart Failure in Chronic Kidney Disease

Ruth F. Dubin

Up to 50% of heart failure patients with either preserved or reduced ejection fraction (EF) have chronic kidney disease (CKD) (Lofman, 2017); renal insufficiency worsens prognosis for heart failure regardless of EF (Smith, 2013). Patients with concomitant CKD and heart failure present numerous challenges to nephrology, cardiology, and primary providers involved in their care. There have been few interventional trials designed specifically to study clinical outcomes in this population, but subgroup analyses of heart failure trials that have included CKD patients do yield important data. At this time, neither Kidney Disease Outcomes Quality Initiative (KDOQI) nor Kidney Disease Improving Global Outcomes (KDIGO) provides specific guidelines for management of heart failure in CKD.

CARDIORENAL PHYSIOLOGY

The terms cardiorenal and renocardiac syndromes are intended to classify patients who have both cardiac and renal disease and in whom there is a clear temporal sequence of which organ system was affected first, the heart or kidneys (Ronco, 2010). Either syndrome may occur in the acute or chronic setting. For example, when a patient with decompensated heart failure presents with volume overload and acutely worsened renal function, one may suspect acute cardiorenal syndrome. If the patient has cold extremities and hypotension, it is likely that lower cardiac output is causing a reduction of blood flow to the kidney and thus a reduction in estimated glomerular filtration rate (eGFR). Alternatively, worsened cardiac output may have resulted in venous congestion, causing higher pressure in the venous system, reaching all the way back to the glomerulus and causing higher intraglomerular pressure, which can cause kidney injury. In this latter type of patient, diuresis may relieve venous congestion and result in improved kidney function. In the vast majority of stable patients that present in clinic to a new primary care provider, nephrologist, or cardiologist, medical records are only available over the short term, so it is difficult to determine which came first—the heart failure or the CKD. Furthermore, in some cases, an incipient systemic disease such as diabetes may be responsible for both cardiac and renal disease and having caused the two organ systems to deteriorate simultaneously.

Whether or not we know which came first, cardiac or renal disease, it is useful to understand the dysfunctional biologic pathways involved in cardiorenal disease. Decreased cardiac output and higher preload together cause decreased perfusion pressure at glomerulus, leading to RAAS (renin angiotensin aldosterone system) activation. Angiotensin II has several effects that are compensatory for reduced cardiac output in normal physiology, but are detrimental when chronically activated, including sympathetic stimulation, vasoconstriction to compensate for reduced cardiac output, and increased venous tone and venous congestion. Aldosterone causes fibrosis via several pathways, including the release of galectin-3, which acts as a paracrine signal on fibroblasts, leading to fibroblast proliferation and procollagen deposition in the heart and kidney. Cardiac fibrosis is an underlying mechanism for the development of left ventricular hypertrophy (LVH), a common feature of heart failure in patients with CKD. As fibrotic tissue replaces healthy tissue in the kidney, kidney function worsens, and lower urine output may result in volume overload that adversely affects cardiac output. In advanced kidney disease, uremic toxins accumulate that adversely affects endothelial function and further instigate inflammation and fibrosis. In a vicious circle, aldosterone also increases salt retention, worsening volume overload and heart failure.

Left Ventricular Hypertrophy

For over a century, LVH has been recognized as a *sine qua non* of cardiac disease in the setting of CKD (Bright, 1836). Studies in the Chronic Renal Insufficiency Cohort show that renal insufficiency is associated with higher left ventricular mass index at all stages of CKD even after adjustment for hypertension and anemia (Park, 2012), and that patients with higher left ventricular mass have higher rates of incident heart failure (Dubin, 2017). LVH has traditionally been understood as a physiologic maladaptation to anemia and hypertension; now, we know that there are additional associated factors in patients with CKD. For example, the phosphaturic hormone, fibroblast growth factor 23 (FGF23), as a potential causal mediator of LVH (Faul, 2011) and predictor of heart failure in CKD (Scialla, 2014) although causality in terms of cardiovascular risk has been questioned (Marthi, 2018).

Diagnostic Guidelines for Heart Failure Based on Serum Markers

Current American College of Cardiology (ACC) and American Heart Association (AHA) guidelines (Yancy, 2017a, 2017b) emphasize the utility of the biomarkers brain natriuretic peptide (**BNP**) and N-terminal prohormone of brain natriuretic peptide (**NT-proBNP**) for diagnosing acute heart failure and establishing prognosis in chronic heart failure. However, in the setting of CKD, these biomarkers are less useful. Both BNP and NT-proBNP are renally cleared (van Kimmenade, 2009), and particularly in patients with eGFR <30, renal dysfunction may significantly contribute to serum levels of these markers. While a normal BNP (<100 pg/mL) could rule out heart failure in a CKD patient, a high BNP or NT-proBNP serum level may reflect a noncardiac cause of elevated serum levels of these natriuretic peptides, including age, or reduced eGFR. Using age-specific cutoffs for NT-proBNP may help adjust for lower eGFR; for example, for persons 50 to 75 years, an

NT-proBNP >900 pg/mL suggests heart failure, whereas for those older than 75 years, an NT-proBNP >1,800 pg/mL may be a more appropriate cutoff value (Kim and Januzzi, 2011). Biomarkers of myocardial fibrosis such as soluble suppression of tumorigenicity 2 (ST2) receptor, **galectin-3**, or **high-sensitivity cardiac troponin**, predict adverse outcomes in CKD, but currently there are no clinical guidelines for their use in diagnosis or prognosis in heart failure patients with or without CKD.

Staging Guidelines for Heart Failure

Although most clinical trials and treatment guidelines still refer to heart failure with reduced ejection fraction (HFrEF) (EF <40%) or heart failure with preserved ejection fraction (HFpEF) (EF >50%), in 2016, the European Society of Cardiology introduced heart failure with midrange ejection fraction (HFmrEF) as a subclass of HFpEF, with EF 40% to 49% (Ponikowski, 2016). The authors of these guidelines emphasize that a patient's symptoms and/or EF may change over time. This is especially true in patients with CKD who have variable urine output and volume status, and thus it makes sense that clinical staging of heart failure does not depend on specific cutoffs for EF.

In 2001, the staging of heart failure was expanded (Hunt, 2001) to include patients at risk for heart failure, and to incorporate symptomatology with structural cardiac disease.

Patients in **stage A** are at risk for heart failure due to comorbidities but do not have symptoms or structural disease. Predisposing comorbidities include coronary artery disease, diabetes, and hypertension; since the writing of those guidelines, much evidence has accumulated that CKD is also a risk factor for heart failure (Dubin, 2017; Park, 2017).

Patients in **stage B** have structural heart disease (including LVH or left atrial enlargement), but have never had symptoms. Given the prevalence of LVH in CKD (Park, 2012), many CKD patients fall into stage B.

Patients in **stage C** have symptoms and structural heart disease, and those in **stage D** have end-stage heart failure that has failed medical management. The New York Heart Association (NYHA) guidelines stages developed in 1994 are based solely on the patient's symptoms related to physical exertion, and NYHA II–IV apply to patients who are in stage C of the newer classification.

Treatment of Heart Failure in the Context of CKD

Heart Failure With Reduced Ejection Fraction

The cornerstones for treatment of HFrEF are still angiotensin-converting enzyme inhibitors (ACEIs) or angiotensin receptor blockers (ARBs), β-blockers, and diuretics. Newer treatment recommendations for symptomatic HFrEF include using an **angiotensin receptor neprilysin inhibitor (ARNI)** instead of ACEI or ARB (Yancy, 2017a). Neprilysin inhibitors impede the breakdown of BNP. Although used as a biomarker of heart failure, BNP is a compensatory hormone released in response to volume expansion that causes vasodilation and natriuresis (Jhund and McMurray, 2016). Several post hoc analyses of ARNI trials show similar benefits of these agents in patients with and without renal dysfunction. In the Prospective comparison of ARNI with ACEI to Determine Impact on Global Mortality and morbidity in Heart Failure (PARADIGM-HF) study, 8,000 HFrEF patients were randomized to the neprilysin inhibitor **LCZ696** or enalapril, and the study was stopped early due to lower incidence of the primary outcome of death in the LCZ696 arm; additionally, patients in this arm also had lower rates of renal injury and hyperkalemia (McMurray, 2014). Results of the Prospective Comparison of ARNI with ARB on Management of HFpEF (PARAMOUNT) trial showed that LCZ696 was more effective than valsartan in lowering levels of NT-proBNP in patients with HFpEF (Solomon, 2012), and a post hoc analysis showed better preservation of eGFR in the patients on LCZ696 (Voors, 2015). A multicenter trial is underway in the United Kingdom to compare the effect of treatment with ARNI plus ARB (sacubitril plus valsartan) versus ARB alone (irbesartan) on the outcome of change in eGFR over 12 months and to evaluate safety of the combination treatment in CKD (UK HARP-III Collaborative Group, 2017). Sacubitril/valsartan, U.S. trade name Entresto, does still have the potential for causing renal injury or hyperkalemia and is given at reduced dose to patients with eGFR <30 mL/min per 1.73 m^2.

Another new recommendation for HFrEF is to add **ivabradine** to the regimen of HFrEF patients in sinus rhythm in whom the heart rate remains elevated despite β-blockers. Ivabradine reduces heart rate by inhibition of the pacemaker current, or so-called "funny current" —l a mixed Na–K channel active in spontaneously active regions of the heart. A post hoc analysis of a trial of ivabradine in HFrEF indicated that benefits of adding ivabradine were similar in patients with and without CKD (Voors, 2014). Ivabradine does not require dose reduction in patients with reduced eGFR.

Cardiac resynchronization therapy (CRT) is recommended in the most recent European Society of Cardiology guidelines for patients with HFrEF (EF <35%) who have a QRS interval >150 ms and LBBB morphology, and who remain symptomatic after optimal medical therapy (Ponikowski, 2016). CRT is thought to have similar benefits for patients with predialysis CKD as for non-CKD patients. Subgroup analysis of three randomized control trials showed reduced death and hospitalization rates in subgroups of HFrEF patients with CKD treated with CRT, and a meta-analysis of these and 14 observational studies indicate that CRT can improve EF as well as eGFR in these patients (Garg, 2013). An analysis of the recent Get With The Guidelines study showed that the survival benefits of CRT were similar among patients with or without CKD, but CRT is underprescribed for CKD and particularly dialysis patients (Pun, 2017).

Heart Failure With Preserved Ejection Fraction

HFpEF is difficult to treat—no therapy has been shown to have a survival benefit in patients with HFpEF. Spironolactone, added to existing therapy, was shown in Treatment of Preserved Cardiac Function

Heart Failure With an Aldosterone Antagonist (TOPCAT) to reduce hospitalizations in HFpEF, although treatment was associated with worsening renal function and hyperkalemia (Pitt, 2014). Although current guidelines state that spironolactone may be used in CKD patients with eGFR >30 and potassium <5 with careful monitoring (Yancy, 2017a), the risk of hyperkalemia in patients with CKD may outweigh potential benefits, unless the patient tends to be hypokalemic. HFpEF guidelines acknowledge the importance of diuretics in managing symptoms, especially in CKD. Target systolic blood pressure (SBP) is <130 for HFpEF patients and ACEI/ARBs are favored antihypertensives for HFpEF (Yancy, 2017a).

Admittedly, it is discouraging that few drugs have significant mortality benefit in HFpEF, and that patients with CKD may not be able to tolerate medications that have modest benefit in HFpEF, such as spironolactone or ACEIs, due to risk of hyperkalemia. However, I have found that patients' symptoms can be greatly relieved with judicious use of diuretics, and moderating fluid and salt intake. Mild hyperkalemia often resolves with sensible limitations on potassium-containing food such as potatoes or giving a loop diuretic. Occasionally, for a patient who has completely cut salt out of their diet, a slightly more liberal salt intake may encourage sodium/potassium exchange in the distal tubule and allow for better excretion of potassium. Patiromer, described below, may enable more patients with CKD to tolerate RAAS inhibition.

ANTICOAGULATION FOR ATRIAL FIBRILLATION

According to current European guidelines, for patients without kidney disease, non vitamin K–dependent oral anticoagulant agents (NOACs) are preferred over warfarin for valvular and nonvalvular atrial fibrillation (Ponikowski, 2016). This newer class of medicine has higher efficacy in stroke prevention, lower incidence of hemorrhage, and the convenience of not needing to be monitored with frequent laboratory checks. Post hoc analyses of NOAC trials indicate they are effective and safe in patients with mild to moderate CKD, but the safety of NOACs in patients with advanced renal dysfunction is less certain. All NOACs are renally cleared to some extent; apixaban has the least renal clearance (27% of clearance is through the kidneys). In patients with eGFR 25 to 50, the dose of apixaban is reduced from 5 mg BID to 2.5 mg BID (Chan, 2016). However, for patients with eGFR <30 mL/min per 1.73 m^2, concerns remain about over- or under-dosing of apixaban, as these could increase bleeding or stroke risk, respectively (Yao, 2017). AHA and European Heart Rhythm guidelines suggest that warfarin is safer than NOACs in patients with atrial fibrillation and eGFR <30 (Yancy, 2017a).

SLEEP APNEA AND HEART FAILURE

Sleep apnea disorders are common in patients with end-stage renal disease (ESRD) (Abuyassin, 2015; Lyons, 2015); several studies suggest high prevalence of obstructive sleep apnea (OSA) in predialysis CKD (Sakaguchi, 2011). OSA and central sleep apnea (CSA) are risk factors for atrial fibrillation, ventricular arrhythmias, and worsening heart failure. Patients with OSA and CKD tend to have a burden of comorbidities such as diabetes, older age, or obesity that are known to be related to CKD progression as well as cardiovascular disease, so it is difficult to show whether OSA and CKD are causally related to each other or simply share a common etiology. However, it has been hypothesized that CKD and sleep apneic disorders may have a bidirectional causal relationship. Transient hypoxemic episodes may result in small ischemic insults to the kidney that accumulate over time. Pharyngeal edema may itself cause narrowing of airways, and in ESRD patients, more intensive dialysis to relieve volume overload might alleviate OSA (Abuyassin, 2015). Sequelae of kidney disease such as chronic renal acidosis and higher sympathetic tone might cause the CKD patient to be more sensitive to transient hypercarbia, which could contribute to hypocapnic CSA (Dharia, 2015).

Small short-term studies indicate that among patients with diagnosed OSA, continuous positive airway pressure (CPAP) may improve renal function. Current AHA guidelines cite evidence that treatment of OSA is particularly beneficial for heart failure patients with atrial fibrillation (Yancy, 2017a). It is reasonable to have a high suspicion for sleep apnea in patients with CKD, and to refer patients who have symptoms of sleep apnea for a sleep study, particularly those with atrial fibrillation.

Nitrates in the Setting of Heart Failure

In an effort to avoid the adverse effects of RAAS inhibitors on renal function and potassium, well-intentioned providers may reach for nitrates +/– hydralazine in patients with CKD. The current consensus is that unless the patient has angina, nitrates are not beneficial in HFrEF (Ural, 2017) or HFpEF (Lim, 2017) and in HFpEF nitrates may reduce exercise tolerance (Redfield, 2015). The combination of **Isordil/hydralazine** was shown to have a mortality benefit for African Americans, but only when added to a regimen consisting of ACE/ARB (Taylor, 2004). A mechanistic study of Isordil/hydralazine in patients with HFpEF found that it may have deleterious effects on cardiac remodeling and exercise tolerance (Zamani, 2017).

HYPERKALEMIA AND THE NEW POTASSIUM-LOWERING AGENT, PATIROMER

In the Candesartan in Heart Failure-Assessment of Reduction in Mortality and Morbidity (CHARM) study, patients with heart failure and creatinine between 2 and 3 had higher rates of hyperkalemia, independent of treatment (Desai, 2007). Understandably, providers may avoid ACE/ARB in patients with heart failure and CKD to mitigate this risk of hyperkalemia. Patiromer is a polymer that binds calcium in exchange for potassium, and this new drug may enable more patients with CKD to tolerate RAAS inhibitors without the adverse effect of hyperkalemia. Patiromer lowered potassium in patients with moderate or advanced CKD on RAAS inhibitors in the Evaluating the Efficacy and Safety of Patiromer for the Treatment of Hyperkalemia (OPAL-HK) trial, in which almost half of the 237 participants had baseline heart failure (Pitt, 2015; Weir, 2015). Results of the Evaluation of Patiromer in Heart Failure Patients (PEARL-HF) trial showed that patiromer was effective in helping patients tolerate spironolactone, and included a small number of patients with baseline CKD (Pitt, 2011). Patiromer has a relatively slow onset of action (7 hours), and thus is recommended for chronic maintenance of normokalemia; it also adsorbs other medications and should be given 3 hours before or after other oral meds. Possible adverse effects include constipation, hypomagnesemia, and binding of other drugs (Rafique, 2017). Dose titration of patiromer in patients with CKD may be of benefit (Pitt, 2018).

SODIUM GLUCOSE COTRANSPORTER 2 INHIBITORS

Sodium glucose cotransporter 2 (SGLT2) inhibitors are a promising therapy for patients with diabetes and CKD, as they have recently been shown to reduce incident heart failure in patients with or without CKD, as well as to slow progression of kidney disease. The sodium glucose cotransporter in the proximal renal tubule normally causes reabsorption of sodium and glucose, a process that results in lower sodium delivery to the distal tubule and macula densa. The macula densa senses this as low perfusion, and via tubuloglomerular feedback the afferent renal arteriole dilates. The resulting hyperfiltration can cause nephron injury and loss. SGLT2 inhibitors restore sodium delivery to the macula densa, improving tubuloglomerular feedback, allowing the afferent arteriole to constrict and lessening glomerular hyperfiltration (Anders, 2016).

In the Empagliflozin Cardiovascular Outcome Event Trial in Type 2 Diabetes Mellitus Patients (EMPA-REG OUTCOME), 7,000 patients with diabetes were treated with **empagliflozin** 10 mg or 25 mg or placebo. Those treated with empagliflozin had reduced risk of heart failure hospitalization, cardiovascular mortality, and all-cause mortality, and these results were consistent among patients with or without heart failure (Zinman, 2015). In a subgroup analysis of the 2,250 EMPA-REG participants with either eGFR between 30 and 59 or urine albumin to creatinine ratio >300 mg/g, empagliflozin reduced the risk of heart failure hospitalizations by 39% (HR, 0.61; 95% CI, 0.42–0.87) (Wanner, 2018). The mechanisms underlying this effect on heart failure are not completely understood, but may include blood pressure lowering, fluid loss, or dampening of the renin–angiotensin system (Butler, 2017). In an analysis of the entire EMPA-REG trial cohort, patients treated with empagliflozin had lower risk of incident CKD or CKD progression (Wanner, 2016); these effects are likely attributed to the direct effect of empagliflozin on reducing glomerular hyperfiltration.

PRACTICAL SUGGESTIONS FOR DIURESIS FOR THE PATIENT WITH HEART FAILURE AND CKD

If you see a patient with CKD and heart failure as an *outpatient* and your question is "to diurese or not to diurese," rest assured that even the most experienced nephrologists or cardiologists cannot tell with 100% certainty whether a patient's creatinine will improve, worsen, or stay the same with diuresis. Your guess is much more likely to be correct if you *ask the patient about symptoms* (both cardiac—dyspnea, orthopnea, orthostasis, and uremic symptoms—loss of appetite, decreased urine output, asterixis). *Checking labs every 2 weeks after changing the diuretic regimen* allows one to detect over-diuresis before any permanent injury to the kidneys occurs. "Good" diuresis results in the patient feeling better (presumably due to better heart function), regardless of creatinine. A lab check 1 to 2 weeks after the diuretic change may show lowering of Cr, or slight increase (≤0.5 mg/dL [44 mcmol/L] increase in the frail or normal weight patient, or ≤0.8 mg/dL [70 mccmol/L] in a larger patient). The BUN may rise moderately (<20 mg/dL [7 mmol/L] and not exceeding 100 mg/dL [36 mmol/L]). However, these changes are often acceptable if the patient feels better *and* the BUN/Cr stabilizes (do not increase further). Frequent lab checks are helpful in monitoring stability of kidney function.

Before starting or increasing diuretics, inquire about fluid and salt intake. Some patients with CKD are under the impression they should drink gallons of water each day to flush out the kidney. Higher fluid intake may be important for specific kidney disorders such as kidney stones, but if the patient also has heart failure, moderate fluid intake is advisable. If the patient feels well, but is elderly and has some lower-extremity edema, consider whether venous insufficiency may be the cause of lower-extremity edema, rather than intravascular volume or reduced cardiac output. Patients with lower-extremity edema due to venous insufficiency tend to become intravascularly dry and may develop acute kidney injury when diuretics are increased. This type of patient may either be able to live with mild edema, or trying high socks or compression stockings could improve the edema and reduce the need for high-dose diuretics. If the patient has low SBP (<120 mm Hg), ask the patient about orthostatic symptoms and consider lowering one of the antihypertensives before initiating aggressive diuresis. If the creatinine is already high, consider stopping ACE before aggressive diuresis. The truly hypotensive patient (SBP <110, off medication) with CKD and new or acute heart failure or volume overload likely needs to be seen by a specialist or hospitalized.

If the patient is becoming resistant to his or her current furosemide dose, there are several questions I consider, including timing, dose, and whether or not to change to a different diuretic. Ask the patient if he or she is actually taking the medicine; some may avoid taking it so as not to have to find a public restroom during the day or to avoid worsening nocturia. In the latter case, patients with benign prostatic hyperplasia and nocturia may have an easier time with furosemide dosed as early in the day as possible, at least 2 hours prior to going to work or other activities, and then 6 to 8 hours later, well before they go to bed, to avoid worsening of nocturia. In general, patients with CKD require higher doses of furosemide (60 to 80 mg BID), largely due to the fact that the medicine has to reach the inside of the tubule to be effective, and in the setting of lower glomerular filtration, a higher serum level may be required for enough to be filtered through the glomerulus. However, it is important to keep in mind that high doses of furosemide may cause ototoxicity; while this has primarily been documented as an adverse effect of rapid IV administration, the risk is present for oral administration if the oral furosemide dose exceeds 200 mg/day.

The loop diuretic **bumetanide** (Bumex) may be preferable to furosemide if the patient has advanced kidney disease and heart failure. Bumetanide is thought to have a lower risk of ototoxicity and better gastrointestinal absorption. Bumetanide 1-mg dose is equivalent to 40-mg dose of furosemide, and typical dosing in CKD with heart failure is 1 to 3 mg BID. **Torsemide** is another loop diuretic that may be used instead of furosemide for patients with CKD and heart failure; torsemide has lower risk of ototoxicity than furosemide, and since it has a longer half-life than furosemide, torsemide can be given once a day. Torsemide 20 mg is equivalent to furosemide 40 mg. When the patient is not responding adequately even to strong loop diuretics such as bumetanide or torsemide, a thiazide diuretic is sometimes added to the loop diuretic regimen. The addition of metolazone may effectively increase urine output, but this medicine does carry a high risk of over-diuresis and electrolyte abnormality. It is wise to start metolazone at a low dose (2.5 mg) and low frequency (once or twice a week, then advancing to every other day) with frequent lab checks (every 2 weeks).

NEPHROLOGY CARE FOR THE PATIENT WITH ADVANCED CKD

As a patient nears ESRD, it is important for the patient to receive education about dialysis, which is one of the main reasons KDOQI recommends that patients with eGFR <30 should be referred to a nephrologist (National Kidney Foundation, 2015). The following sections pertain to issues specific to nephrology care, but a general understanding may be helpful to the cardiologist or primary care following these patients.

How near the patient is to needing dialysis is a judgment based on both eGFR as well as assessment of uremic signs and symptoms (such as decreased urine output, weight loss due to poor appetite, weakness, volume overload resistant to diuretics, and impairment of cognitive function). As a rough guide, dialysis initiation is usually considered at an eGFR <15 mL/min per 1.73 m^2 + uremic symptoms, eGFR <20 mL/min per 1.73 m^2 + symptoms for diabetics, or eGFR <6 mL/min per 1.73 m^2 regardless of symptoms (Tattersall, 2011). Creatinine-based equations are usually adequate unless the patient is very frail or malnourished, in which case cystatin-based equations may give a more accurate calculation of eGFR. There is no evidence to show that starting dialysis earlier (at higher eGFR) leads to better outcomes (Tattersall, 2011).

Occasionally patients who are very elderly or who have a terminal illness, or who adamantly oppose dialysis for personal reasons, may decide they would not want dialysis under any condition. Patients who do wish to have dialysis when it becomes necessary should receive education about peritoneal dialysis (PD), in-center hemodialysis, and if it is available, home hemodialysis. Each patient will decide with his or her nephrologist whether PD or hemodialysis is the best option; this decision is often based on whether the patient is willing or able to perform dialysis at home. If a patient nearing ESRD has heart failure, the nephrologist may take the patient's heart failure status into consideration when advising on which dialysis modality is most appropriate. Even among nephrologists, opinions differ as to whether peritoneal or hemodialysis is superior in the setting of heart failure. We know that rapid fluid removal during hemodialysis can cause myocardial stunning, and that the gradual fluid removal during PD does not causing stunning (Burton, 2009). However, this slower rate of fluid removal may not be as effective in treating volume overload, especially in patients who are anuric. Peritoneal dialysis for refractory congestive heart failure using icodextrin to optimize osmotic fluid removal has been associated with a moderate worsening of hyponatremia (Kunin, 2018). The most common scenario for a heart failure patient who has become resistant to diuretics is to plan for hemodialysis.

It is preferable to plan for either peritoneal or vascular access at least 2 months prior to needing dialysis, and for hemodialysis, a fistula or graft is preferred over tunneled catheter due to the high rate of infection of catheters. Fistulas do have multiple hemodynamic effects (Agarwal, 2015) including increasing preload, and could place a patient with severely reduced EF at risk for worsening heart failure; in patients with EF <30%, a tunneled catheter may be safer despite its higher rate of infection (Roca-Tey, 2016). Fistulas are expected to have flow rates of 1 to 2 L/min; if a fistula expands over time and develops flows >2 L/min, and/or the fistula flow rate exceeds 30% of cardiac output, this could cause a patient to develop either worsened or *de novo* high-output cardiac failure (MacRae, 2004). Whether or not the patient has started dialysis, if a fistula appears to be expanded or visibly aneurysmal, refer the patient to see a vascular surgeon who can evaluate whether the fistula needs partial or total ligation to narrow or obliterate such a high-output fistula.

References and Suggested Readings

Abuyassin B, Sharma K, Ayas NT, et al. Obstructive sleep apnea and kidney disease: a potential bidirectional relationship?. *J Clin Sleep Med*. 2015;11:915–924.

Agarwal AK. Systemic effects of hemodialysis access. *Adv Chronic Kidney Dis*. 2015; 22:459–465.

Anders HJ, Davis JM, Thurau K. Nephron protection in diabetic kidney disease. *N Engl J Med*. 2016;375:2096–2098.

Bright R. Tubular view of the morbid appearances in 100 cases connected with albuminous urine: with observations. *Guy's Hosp Rep.* 1836;1:380–400.

Burton JO, Jefferies HJ, Selby NM, et al. Hemodialysis-induced cardiac injury: determinants and associated outcomes. *Clin J Am Soc Nephrol.* 2009;4:914–920.

Butler J, Hamo CE, Filippatos G, et al; EMPEROR Trials Program. The potential role and rationale for treatment of heart failure with sodium-glucose co-transporter 2 inhibitors. *Eur J Heart Fail.* 2017;19:1390–1400.

Chan KE, Giugliano RP, Patel MR, et al. Nonvitamin K anticoagulant agents in patients with advanced chronic kidney disease or on dialysis with AF. *J Am Coll Cardiol.* 2016;67:2888–2899.

Desai AS, Swedberg K, McMurray JJ, et al; CHARM Program Investigators. Incidence and predictors of hyperkalemia in patients with heart failure: an analysis of the CHARM Program. *J Am Coll Cardiol.* 2007;50:1959–1966.

Dharia SM, Unruh ML, Brown LK. Central sleep apnea in kidney disease. *Semin Nephrol.* 2015;35:335–346.

Dubin RF, Deo R, Bansal N, et al. Associations of conventional echocardiographic measures with incident heart failure and mortality: the Chronic Renal Insufficiency Cohort. *Clin J Am Soc Nephrol.* 2017;12:60–68.

Faul C, Amaral AP, Oskouei B, et al. FGF23 induces left ventricular hypertrophy. *J Clin Invest.* 2011;121:4393–4408.

Garg N, Thomas G, Jackson G, et al. Cardiac resynchronization therapy in CKD: a systematic review. *Clin J Am Soc Nephrol.* 2013;8:1293–1303.

Hunt SA, Baker DW, Chin MH, et al. ACC/AHA guidelines for the evaluation and management of chronic heart failure in the adult: executive summary. A report of the American College of Cardiology/American Heart Association Task Force on Practice Guidelines (Committee to revise the 1995 Guidelines for the Evaluation and Management of Heart Failure). *J Am Coll Cardiol.* 2001;38:2101–2113.

Jhund PS, McMurray JJ. The neprilysin pathway in heart failure: a review and guide on the use of sacubitril/valsartan. *Heart.* 2016;102:1342–1347.

Kim HN, Januzzi JL Jr. Natriuretic peptide testing in heart failure. *Circulation.* 2011; 123:2015–2019.

Kunin M, Ganon L, Holtzman EJ, et al. Hyponatremia in refractory congestive heart failure patients treated with icodextrin-based peritoneal dialysis: a case series. *Nefrologia.* 2018;38:87–91.

Lim SL, Benson L, Dahlstrom U, et al. Association between use of long-acting nitrates and outcomes in heart failure with preserved ejection fraction. *Circ Heart Fail.* 2017;10:pii:e003534.

Lofman I, Szummer K, Dahlstrom U, et al. Associations with and prognostic impact of chronic kidney disease in heart failure with preserved, mid-range, and reduced ejection fraction. *Eur J Heart Fail.* 2017;19:1606–1614.

Lyons OD, Bradley TD, Chan CT. Hypervolemia and sleep apnea in kidney disease. *Semin Nephrol.* 2015;35:373–382.

MacRae JM, Pandeya S, Humen DP, et al. Arteriovenous fistula-associated high-output cardiac failure: a review of mechanisms. *Am J Kidney Dis.* 2004;43:e17–e22.

Marthi A, Donovan K, Haynes R, et al. Fibroblast Growth Factor-23 and risks of cardiovascular and noncardiovascular diseases: A meta-analysis. *J Am Soc Nephrol.* 2018, in press. doi: 10.1681/ASN.2017121334.

McMurray JJ, Packer M, Solomon SD. Neprilysin inhibition for heart failure. *N Engl J Med.* 2014;371:2336–2337.

National Kidney Foundation: KDOQI. Update of the KDOQI clinical practice guideline for hemodialysis adequacy. 2015. Available from https://www.kidney.org/sites/default/files/KDOQI-Clinical-Practice-Guideline-Hemodialysis-Update_Public-Review-Draft-FINAL_20150204.pdf. Accessed March, 2017.

Park M, Hsu CY, Go AS, et al. Urine kidney injury biomarkers and risks of cardiovascular disease events and all-cause death: the CRIC study. *Clin J Am Soc Nephrol.* 2017;12:761–771.

Park M, Hsu CY, Li Y, et al; Chronic Renal Insufficiency Cohort (CRIC) Study Group. Associations between kidney function and subclinical cardiac abnormalities in CKD. *J Am Soc Nephrol.* 2012;23:1725–1734.

Pitt B, Anker SD, Bushinsky DA, et al; PEARL-HF Investigators. Evaluation of the efficacy and safety of RLY5016, a polymeric potassium binder, in a double-blind, placebo-controlled study in patients with chronic heart failure (the PEARL-HF) trial. *Eur Heart J*. 2011;32:820–828.

Pitt B, Bakris GL, Bushinsky DA, et al. Effect of patiromer on reducing serum potassium and preventing recurrent hyperkalaemia in patients with heart failure and chronic kidney disease on RAAS inhibitors. *Eur J Heart Fail*. 2015;17:1057–1065.

Pitt B, Bushinsky DA, Kitzman DW, et al for the Patiromer-204 Investigators. Evaluation of an individualized dose titration regimen of patiromer to prevent hyperkalaemia in patients with heart failure and chronic kidney disease. *ESC Heart Fail*. 2018;5:257–266.

Pitt B, Pfeffer MA, Assmann SF, et al; TOPCAT Investigators. Spironolactone for heart failure with preserved ejection fraction. *N Engl J Med*. 2014;370:1383–1392.

Ponikowski P, Voors AA, Anker SD, et al. 2016 ESC Guidelines for the diagnosis and treatment of acute and chronic heart failure: the task force for the diagnosis and treatment of acute and chronic heart failure of the European Society of Cardiology (ESC). Developed with the special contribution of the Heart Failure Association (HFA) of the ESC. *Eur J Heart Fail*. 2016;18:891–975.

Pun PH, Sheng S, Sanders G, et al. Prescription of guideline-recommended implantable cardioverter defibrillator and cardiac resynchronization therapy among patients hospitalized with heart failure and varying degrees of renal function. *Am J Cardiol*. 2017;119:886–892.

Rafique Z, Weir MR, Onuigbo M, et al. Expert panel recommendations for the identification and management of hyperkalemia and role of patiromer in patients with chronic kidney disease and heart failure. *J Manag Care Spec Pharm*. 2017;23:S10–S19.

Redfield MM, Anstrom KJ, Levine JA, et al; NHLBI Heart Failure Clinical Research Network. Isosorbide mononitrate in heart failure with preserved ejection fraction. *N Engl J Medicine*. 2015;373:2314–2324.

Roca-Tey R. Permanent arteriovenous fistula or catheter dialysis for heart failure patients. *J Vasc Access*. 2016;17:S23–S29.

Ronco C, McCullough P, Anker SD, et al. Cardio-renal syndromes: report from the consensus conference of the acute dialysis quality initiative. *Eur Heart J*. 2010;31:703–711.

Sakaguchi Y, Shoji T, Kawabata H, et al. High prevalence of obstructive sleep apnea and its association with renal function among nondialysis chronic kidney disease patients in Japan: a cross-sectional study. *Clin J Am Soc Nephrol*. 2011;6:995–1000.

Scialla JJ, Xie H, Rahman M, et al; Chronic Renal Insufficiency Cohort (CRIC) Study Investigators. Fibroblast growth factor-23 and cardiovascular events in CKD. *J Am Soc Nephrol*. 2014;25:349–360.

Smith DH, Thorp ML, Gurwitz JH, et al. Chronic kidney disease and outcomes in heart failure with preserved versus reduced ejection fraction: the Cardiovascular Research Network PRESERVE Study. *Circ Cardiovasc Qual Outcomes*. 2013;6:333–342.

Solomon SD, Zile M, Pieske B, et al; Prospective comparison of ARNI with ARB on Management Of heart failUre with preserved ejectioN fracTion (PARAMOUNT) Investigators. The angiotensin receptor neprilysin inhibitor LCZ696 in heart failure with preserved ejection fraction: a phase 2 double-blind randomised controlled trial. *Lancet*. 2012;380:1387–1395.

Tattersall J, Dekker F, Heimburger O, et al; ERBP Advisory Board. When to start dialysis: updated guidance following publication of the Initiating Dialysis Early and Late (IDEAL) study. *Nephrol Dial Transplant*. 2011;26:2082–2086.

Taylor AL, Ziesche S, Yancy C, et al; African-American Heart Failure Trial Investigators. Combination of isosorbide dinitrate and hydralazine in blacks with heart failure. *N Engl J Med*. 2004;351:2049–2057.

UK HARP-III Collaborative Group. Randomized multicentre pilot study of sacubitril/valsartan versus irbesartan in patients with chronic kidney disease: United Kingdom Heart and Renal Protection (HARP)-III-rationale, trial design and baseline data. *Nephrol Dial Transplant*. 2017;32:2043–2051.

Ural D, Kandemir AS, Karauzum K, et al. Effect of oral nitrates on all-cause mortality and hospitalization in heart failure patients with reduced ejection fraction: a propensity-matched analysis. *J Card Fail.* 2017;23:286–292.

van Kimmenade RR, Januzzi JL Jr, Bakker JA, et al. Renal clearance of B-type natriuretic peptide and amino terminal pro-B-type natriuretic peptide a mechanistic study in hypertensive subjects. *J Am Coll Cardiol.* 2009;53:884–890.

Voors AA, Gori M, Liu LC, et al; PARAMOUNT Investigators. Renal effects of the angiotensin receptor neprilysin inhibitor LCZ696 in patients with heart failure and preserved ejection fraction. *Eur J Heart Fail.* 2015;17:510–517.

Voors AA, van Veldhuisen DJ, Robertson M, et al. The effect of heart rate reduction with ivabradine on renal function in patients with chronic heart failure: an analysis from SHIFT. *Eur J Heart Fail.* 2014;16:426–434.

Wanner C, Inzucchi SE, Zinman B. Empagliflozin and progression of kidney disease in type 2 diabetes. *N Engl J Med.* 2016;375:1801–1802.

Wanner C, Lachin JM, Inzucchi SE, et al; EMPA-REG OUTCOME Investigators. Empagliflozin and clinical outcomes in patients with type 2 diabetes mellitus, established cardiovascular disease, and chronic kidney disease. *Circulation.* 2018;137:119–129.

Weir MR, Bakris GL, Bushinsky DA, et al; OPAL-HK Investigators. Patiromer in patients with kidney disease and hyperkalemia receiving RAAS inhibitors. *N Engl J Med.* 2015;372:211–221.

Yancy CW, Jessup M, Bozkurt B, et al. 2017 ACC/AHA/HFSA focused update of the 2013 ACCF/AHA guideline for the management of heart failure: a report of the American College of Cardiology/American Heart Association Task Force on Clinical Practice Guidelines and the Heart Failure Society of America. *J Am Coll Cardiol.* 2017;2017a;70:776–803.

Yancy CW, Januzzi JL Jr, Allen LA, et al. 2017 ACC expert consensus decision pathway for optimization of heart failure treatment: Answers to 10 pivotal issues about heart failure with reduced ejection fraction: A report of the American College of Cardiology Task Force on Expert Consensus Decision Pathways. *J Am Coll Cardiol.* 2018b;71:201–230.

Yao X, Shah ND, Sangaralingham LR, et al. Non-Vitamin K antagonist oral anticoagulant dosing in patients with atrial fibrillation and renal dysfunction. *J Am Coll Cardiol.* 2017;69:2779–2790.

Zamani P, Akers S, Soto-Calderon H, et al. Isosorbide dinitrate, with or without hydralazine, does not reduce wave reflections, left ventricular hypertrophy, or myocardial fibrosis in patients with heart failure with preserved ejection fraction. *J Am Heart Assoc.* 2017;6:pii:e004262.

Zinman B, Wanner C, Lachin JM, et al; EMPA-REG OUTCOME Investigators. Empagliflozin, cardiovascular outcomes, and mortality in type 2 diabetes. *N Engl J Med.* 2015;373:2117–2128.

19 Hematuria Investigation and Management

Timothy Mathew

Hematuria is defined as the presence of an abnormal number of red blood cells (RBCs) in the urine and can be either visible bleeding (macroscopic hematuria) or invisible and detected only by microscopy or dipstick (microscopic hematuria) (Kelly, 2009). Irrespective of whether the hematuria is macroscopic or microscopic, it may be a sign of serious underlying disease, such as bladder or other uroepithelial cancer or kidney parenchymal disease. The prevalence of microscopic hematuria in adult population–based studies (microscopy and dipstick analyses) varies from 2% to 31% (American Urological Association Guideline, 2016) though the true prevalence of persistent isolated microscopic hematuria is likely to be much lower, around 0.3% (Vivante, 2011). The prevalence of microscopic hematuria rises with age in both sexes (Chadban, 2003).

SCREENING

Screening for microscopic hematuria is by dipstick testing of the urine, described in detail below. Is screening for microscopic hematuria justifiable? Screening for detection of urinary tract cancers in asymptomatic adult patients has not been recommended because of perceived lack of cost benefit (Davis, 2012; Nielsen and Qaseem, 2016). A case has been made for screening populations at high risk for bladder cancer, particularly older men (Messing, 1995); however, it has not been demonstrated that screen-detected cases of bladder cancer have an improved outcome compared with cases presenting in the usual fashion. A case for screening young asymptomatic adults for hematuria by urine dipstick testing has been made, but rests in large part on the concomitant screen for proteinuria that yields additional potential benefit (Brown, 2011). The consensus view remains that opportunistic or routine screening of adults and children for microscopic hematuria is not recommended on grounds of not being cost effective.

TESTING FOR HEMATURIA

The finding of a few red cells in the urine is a normal finding in healthy adults. In guidelines and reviews, the number of red blood cells/high-power field (RBC/HPF) that defines microscopic hematuria surprisingly lacks agreement and varies from 2 to 5 (Cohen and Brown, 2003; Grossfeld, 2001; Mariani, 1989). The reliability of microscopy in detecting hematuria depends on examining a fresh sample immediately after collection. In practice this means performing microscopy "on site" for any delay in getting the sample to a laboratory allows lysis of RBCs to occur, frequently leading to an underestimation of the hematuria.

Dipstick Test

Dipstick testing of the urine for blood is the most frequent means of detection of microscopic hematuria in clinical practice. The typical dipstick is designed to be sensitive to 1 to 2 RBC/HPF and therefore may overdiagnose. Testing the urine by dipstick for blood and protein remains part of routine life insurance and employment medical exams, and when the findings are positive, patients are referred for diagnosis and management.

The dipstick test for hemoglobin relies on oxidation of organic peroxide on the test strip by the peroxidase-like activity of hemoglobin. Intact red cells cause punctate color change on the strip. Free hemoglobin or myoglobin, if present, causes uniform staining of the strip; the occurrence of hemolysis or rhabdomyolysis in patients being screened for hematuria is quite uncommon. The urine dipstick test for blood may be falsely negative in the presence of a high urinary concentration of vitamin C. False-negative results are more common than false-positive results (Fraser, 1985).

A positive dipstick test for hematuria should be confirmed (at least once) by careful and timely urine microscopy (American Urological Association Guideline, 2016).

Phase-Contrast Microscopy

The gold standard test that defines the presence of microscopic hematuria is phase-contrast microscopy of a freshly collected, midstream, clean-catch unspun urine specimen that shows >2 RBC/HPF. It is essential that the specimen not be contaminated by debris or infection. Regular bright-field microscopy can easily undercount or completely fail to detect urine RBCs.

Dysmorphic Red Blood Cells (Acanthocytes)

In the course of using phase-contrast microscopy to count red cells in the urine, valuable information can be obtained from the appearance of the cells. Glomerular hematuria usually is characterized by a high proportion of bizarrely shaped cells (acanthocytes), with each one different to the other. In contrast, red cells in the urine from nonglomerular sources usually are seen as smooth disks, with each red cell appearing similar to the other. It must be emphasized that for red cell morphology to be reliably determined, use of phase-contrast microscopy is essential.

IS THE MICROSCOPIC HEMATURIA PERSISTENT?

Transient microscopic hematuria is common and may be caused by urinary infection, exercise, sexual intercourse, menstrual contamination, or mild trauma. Before proceeding with further investigations, it is thus appropriate to repeat urine testing once or twice to confirm that hematuria is persistent. If not confirmed on a repeat dipstick 1 to 2 weeks later, then the initial finding of hematuria usually needs no further investigation. Hematuria can persist for up to 72 hours after vigorous exercise (not necessarily involving contact sports), and this usually is glomerular in origin. Exercise-related microscopic hematuria is underrecognized and is considered a benign condition. Microscopic hematuria may be caused by urinary tract infection and may persist for some weeks after urinary tract infection. For this reason, urinary tract infection needs to be excluded by urine culture, and, if present, a dipstick test for hematuria should be repeated about 6 weeks after eradication of infection.

INVESTIGATING PERSISTENT MICROSCOPIC HEMATURIA

Once it has been established that microscopic hematuria is persistent, the following should be done:

1. *A careful history and physical examination.* The patient may recall having had previous urine tests that will clarify the length of time this abnormality has been present. Symptoms suggestive of urinary infection should be sought. A history of medication use is important—past analgesic abuse (even from 20 to 30 years ago) and past exposure to cyclophosphamide are relevant. Other known risks for bladder cancer or transitional cell cancer of the urinary tract should be ascertained, for example, smoking or exposure to toxins (e.g., employment in leather, dye, or tire industries). A careful review of drugs that might be causing interstitial nephritis (Table 19.1) is appropriate. Anticoagulation therapy in the therapeutic range usually does not per se cause microscopic hematuria, and previous experience has demonstrated that cases of microscopic hematuria occurring in patients taking oral anticoagulants should undergo a full investigation.

2. *Serum creatinine measurement.* Kidney function should be assessed by a serum creatinine measurement to find the estimated glomerular filtration rate (eGFR).

3. *Quantification of proteinuria.* If urine protein is found on dipstick, it should be quantitated either by determining a urine protein/creatinine ratio on a spot sample or by a 24-hour urine collection. In those with microscopic hematuria and low-grade proteinuria (0.3 to 2.5 g/day), renal biopsy reveals major and potentially progressive nephropathies in 70% of patients (Hall, 2004), and in another study, the concurrent findings of microscopic hematuria and low-grade proteinuria were a better marker for glomerular versus nonglomerular bleeding than the presence of acanthocytes on phase-contrast microscopy (Ohisa, 2008). In a study of 1,800 nondiabetic CKD (stages 3 to 5) patients, microscopic hematuria with minor

| TABLE 19.1 | Recognized Causes of Microscopic Hematuria |

Renal
Glomerular Causes

Acute nephritic injury
Fabry disease
Focal glomerular sclerosis
Goodpasture syndrome
Hemolytic uremic syndrome
Henoch–Schönlein purpura
Hereditary nephritis (Alport syndrome)
Immunoglobulin A nephropathy
Mesangiocapillary glomerulonephritis
Mesangial proliferative glomerulonephritis
Microscopic polyarteritis
Other forms of glomerulonephritis
Postinfectious glomerulonephritis
Systemic lupus erythematosus
    Thin basement membrane disease (benign familial hematuria)
Wegener granulomatosis

Nonglomerular Causes

Acute kidney injury (acute tubular necrosis)
Familial
    Medullary cystic disease
    Multicystic kidney disease
    Polycystic kidney disease
Infection
    Pyelonephritis
    Tuberculosis
    Cytomegalovirus
    Epstein–Barr virus
Interstitial nephritis
    Drug induced
        Penicillins, cephalosporins, diuretics, nonsteroidal anti-inflammatory drugs,
            proton pump inhibitors, cyclophosphamide, anticonvulsants, combination
            analgesics
    Systemic disease causing interstitial nephritis
        Sarcoidosis, Sjögren syndrome, lymphoma
    Loin pain hematuria syndrome
    Metabolic
        Hypercalciuria
        Hyperuricosuria
    Renal cell carcinoma
    Renal cysts (simple)
    Vascular disease
        Arteriovenous malformation
        Renal artery embolism/thrombosis
        Renal venous thrombosis
        Sickle cell disease

(continued)

| | Recognized Causes of Microscopic Hematuria (*Continued*) |

Extrarenal

Benign prostatic hypertrophy
Calculi
Coagulation disorders
    Primary
    Secondary to anticoagulation
Endometriosis
Factitious
Foreign bodies
Infection—bladder, prostate, urethra
Inflammation—drug or radiation induced
Perineal irritation
Strictures
Transitional cell carcinoma of bladder/ureter
Trauma—catheter or closed injury

Other Causes

Exercise
Menstrual contamination
Sexual intercourse

proteinuria was associated with a significant increase in risk for end-stage renal disease (ESRD) (Lin, 2015).
   4. *Ultrasound of bladder and kidneys.* All patients with persistent microscopic hematuria should have an ultrasound.

INITIAL WORKUP

The object of this first series of simple tests is to determine whether the microscopic hematuria is glomerular or nonglomerular in origin (Fig. 19.1). In clinical practice, this determines whether the problem is nephrologic or urologic in nature. Blood in the urine can originate from any site in the kidneys and urinary tract from the glomeruli down to the urethra. Any glomerular disease can cause microscopic hematuria. Acute nephritis usually is associated with large numbers of RBCs and casts. Conditions characterized by heavy proteinuria (e.g., nephrotic syndrome and membranous nephritis) usually are associated with fewer numbers of RBCs. Other common nephrologic causes include immunoglobulin A (IgA) nephropathy, thin basement membrane disease, and hereditary nephritis. Common urologic causes include tumors of the urinary tract, stone disease, urinary tract infection, and bleeding from benign prostate conditions (Ezz el Din, 1996). Figure 19.2 shows common causes of hematuria by age, and a more complete list of causes is shown in Table 19.1.

   One clinical concern in properly evaluating microscopic hematuria has been the risk of missing a urinary tract cancer. However, missing serious kidney parenchymal disease that can be prevented from progressing to kidney failure may be just as important or more so.

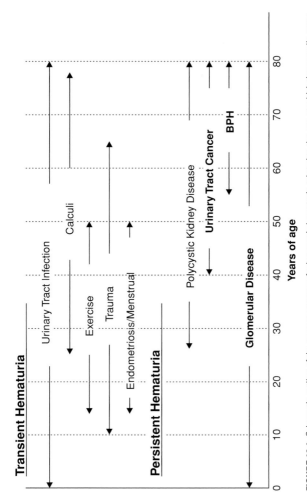

FIGURE 19.1 Schematic outline of the common causes of microscopic hematuria related to the age at which they usually occur (horizontal axis). The most common conditions are highlighted in bold text. BPH, benign prostatic hypertrophy.

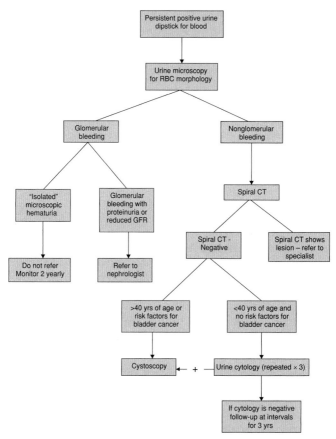

FIGURE 19.2 Simplified algorithm for management of persistent microscopic hematuria. It is recommended that all patients should have an ultrasound early in the diagnostic pathway.

The literature dealing with microscopic hematuria is weighted heavily toward urologic causes, such as cancer and stones, and little attention has been paid to renal parenchymal causes of microscopic hematuria, which in fact contribute most of the cases, particularly in those patients who are younger than 40 to 50 years of age. In two large series (combined total of about 6,000 patients), the incidence of urinary tract cancer in patients with microscopic hematuria was about 5%, with bladder cancer accounting for the vast majority of these. Macroscopic hematuria was associated with about a four times greater risk of renal and urinary tract cancer than microscopic hematuria. Both these series report about 55% of patients as "normal" and "no diagnosis"; scant mention was made of the likelihood of the majority of these having a nephrologic cause of urinary bleeding (Edwards, 2006; Khadra, 2000). Thus, the view held by some that isolated microscopic hematuria is benign and needs no follow-up must be questioned, but the risk appears to be more nephrologic than urologic.

Does the Presence of Microscopic Hematuria Predict End-Stage Renal Disease?

Over the long term, screen-detected microscopic hematuria has been shown to be a significant predictor of end-stage renal failure, increasing the risk by 18% over a 17-year follow-up period. Hematuria also amplifies the predictive value of proteinuria for development of kidney failure (Iseki, 2003). Follow-up of a cohort referred with isolated microscopic hematuria showed 19% developed proteinuria, hypertension, or kidney failure over a 5-year period (Chow, 2004). The largest and most comprehensive study is of 1.2 million Israeli military recruits followed for over 20 years in whom 3,690 (0.3%) were shown to have persistent isolated microscopic hematuria. Of those with persistent microscopic hematuria 0.7% developed ESRD. The risk of ESRD while small was increased 30-fold over those with no hematuria (Vivante, 2011). In contrast a smaller population–based study at the time of a "health check" with an older age at recruitment (mean 40 years) showed no significant association of a single-positive dipstick hematuria finding with ESRD in long-term follow-up (Hsu, 2009). In a study of 8,700 subjects from Korea where the endpoint was incident CKD, defined as an eGFR <60 mL/min per 1.73 m^2, the relative risk for CKD in those with microscopic hematuria without proteinuria was 1.83, and increased more than five-fold in those with both hematuria and proteinuria (Kim, 2018).

Work-Up of Nonglomerular or Indeterminate Source of Bleeding

In patients with persistent microscopic hematuria of nonglomerular origin, no proteinuria, and normal kidney function, it is essential to determine if there is a structural lesion present in the urinary tract causing urinary tract bleeding. Urothelial cancer is the main consideration.

Spiral Computed Tomography

For the detection of renal cancer and/or stone disease, spiral computed tomography (CT) (with or without contrast), particularly with use of thin slices, has superseded both intravenous pyelography (because of the increased diagnostic yield) and ultrasonography (because of the lack of ability of ultrasound to detect small tumors [<3 cm in diameter]). CT without the use of contrast agent is recommended if stone disease is suspected, but in other cases, a CT with contrast should follow to provide full information about tumors and cysts. In patients allergic to contrast media, one can use ultrasound and a plain x-ray of the urinary tract followed by cystoscopy and a retrograde pyelogram.

In adults with asymptomatic microscopic hematuria, particularly in those with a lesser degree of bleeding, the need for routine imaging of the upper tract has been questioned. Recent emphasis has been on the increased cost and small additional yield of cancer detection associated with guideline-driven use of CT to investigate asymptomatic microscopic hematuria (Halpern, 2017; Subak and Grady, 2017). The case has been made for individualizing the decision to image the upper tracts, with emphasis on limiting investigations to the combination of ultrasound and cystoscopy even in those aged >40 years unless there are additional risk factors or high numbers of urinary RBC/HPF. While the consensus view is in favor of routine imaging, there is disparity between the American Urological Association guidelines which recommend routine CT as opposed to the Canadian and Dutch guidelines that recommend ultrasound as the primary and definitive investigation (Grossfeld, 2001; Van der Molen and Hovius, 2012; Wollin, 2009).

Cystoscopy

For patients older than 40 years of age in whom the risk of bladder cancer is increased (particularly men), if diagnostic imaging proves to be negative, then cystoscopy is recommended. For patients younger than the age of 40 years, the diagnostic yield from cystoscopy is very low, particularly in younger women (Grossfeld, 2001). Cystoscopy should be performed at any age if there are risk factors evident on history, such as heavy smoking, prolonged use of analgesics, exposure to certain dyes, or past exposure to cyclophosphamide.

Urine Cytology

The role of urine cytology in those with negative diagnostic imaging is less well established. The yield from urine cytology varies with the grade of the tumor, the number of samples examined, and the experience of the cytopathologist. The reported sensitivity of urine cytology has ranged from 40% to 76%, but with low-grade transitional cell cancer, sensitivity may be as low as 15% to 25%. A negative result from three consecutive daily early-morning urine specimens can be used as an alternative to cystoscopy in those at low risk of transitional cell urinary tract cancer. Any positive cytologic finding necessitates further evaluation by cystoscopy (Grossfeld, 2001).

Monitoring and Follow-Up of Nonglomerular Bleeding

If the investigative pathway has been followed and no cause for persistent nonglomerular microscopic hematuria has been detected, it is recommended that urinalysis, cytology, and blood pressure be rechecked at 6, 12, 24, and 36 months. If new symptoms develop at any time during follow-up or gross (macroscopic) hematuria occurs, then prompt urologic referral should follow.

Glomerular Bleeding

If the microscopic hematuria is predominantly glomerular in origin (more than 80% of red cells appear dysmorphic), if red cell casts are seen on microscopy, or if proteinuria is shown to be present, then the source of the hematuria is highly likely to be in the renal parenchyma. In one study of diabetic patients with microscopic hematuria, the presence of acanthocytes was a marker for glomerular disease other than that due to diabetes (Heine, 2004), although microscopic hematuria due to diabetic nephropathy does occur (Zhou, 2008).

With glomerular bleeding, the risk of urinary tract cancer is low. Thus, in this situation, there is generally no indication for proceeding with detailed imaging and urologic investigation unless the risk profile of the patient is high for urinary tract cancer (Wollin, 2009).

Kidney Biopsy and Nephrology Referral

In patients with isolated microscopic hematuria, renal biopsy usually is not considered to be indicated. Series in which biopsy has been done find something in about 50%, and when pathology is found, IgA nephropathy and thin basement membrane disease are the most common abnormalities (Tiebosch, 1989; Topham, 1994). Similarly, if the glomerular hematuria is isolated (normal renal function, no proteinuria or red cell casts, no other sign of kidney disease), then specialist referral usually is not required, and follow-up can be performed by the generalist.

Follow-Up and Monitoring of Glomerular Bleeding

A repeat of the kidney performance tests—serum creatinine concentration (with eGFR), urine protein quantification, and blood pressure check—6 months later and thereafter every 2 years is indicated to watch for hypertension (an increased risk in this group is well documented) and to ensure that a more serious parenchymal lesion is not evolving. Any development of new abnormalities should trigger nephrologic referral.

References and Suggested Readings

American Urological Association Guidelines. Diagnosis, evaluation and follow-up of asymptomatic microhematuria in adults. Available from http://www.auanet.org/Documents/education/clinical-guidance/Asymptomatic-Microhematuria.pdf. Accessed June 3, 2018.

Brown RS. Has the time come to include urine dipstick testing in screening asymptomatic young adults? *JAMA.* 2011;306:764–765.

Chadban SJ, Briganti EM, Kerr PG, et al. Prevalence of kidney damage in Australian adults: the AusDiab kidney study. *J Am Soc Nephrol.* 2003;14:S131–S138.

Chow KM, Kwan BC, Li PK, et al. Asymptomatic isolated microscopic hematuria: long-term follow-up. *QJM.* 2004;97:739–745.

Cohen RA, Brown RS. Clinical practice. Microscopic hematuria. *N Engl J Med.* 2003;348:2330–2338.

Davis R, Jones JS, Barocas DA, et al; American Urological Association. Diagnosis, evaluation and follow up of asymptomatic hematuria in adults: AUA guideline. *J Urol.* 2012;188:2473–2481.

Edwards TJ, Dickinson AJ, Natale S, et al. A prospective analysis of the diagnostic yield resulting from the attendance of 4020 patients at a protocol-driven hematuria clinic. *BJU Int.* 2006;97:301–305.

Ezz el Din K, Koch WF, de Wildt MJ, et al. The predictive value of microscopic haematuria in patients with lower urinary tract symptoms and benign prostatic hyperplasia. *Eur Urol.* 1996;30:409–413.

Fraser CG. Urine analysis: current performance and strategies for improvement. *Br Med J (Clin Res Ed).* 1985;291:321–323.

Grossfeld GD, Wolf JS Jr, Litwin MS, et al. Asymptomatic microscopic hematuria in adults: summary of AUA best practice recommendations. *Am Fam Physician.* 2001;63:1145–1154.

Hall CL, Bradley R, Kerr A, et al. Clinical value of renal biopsy in patients with asymptomatic microscopic hematuria with and without low-grade proteinuria. *Clin Nephrol.* 2004;62:267–272.

Halpern JA, Chughtai B, Ghomrawi H. Cost-effectiveness of common diagnostic approaches for the evaluation of asymptomatic microscopic hematuria. *JAMA Intern Med.* 2017;177:800–807.

Heine GH, Sester U, Girndt M, et al. Acanthocytes in the urine: useful tool to differentiate diabetic nephropathy from glomerulonephritis? *Diabetes Care.* 2004;27: 190–194.

Hsu CY, Iribarren C, McCulloch CE, et al. Risk factors for end-stage renal disease: 25-year follow-up. *Arch Intern Med.* 2009;169:342–350.

Iseki K, Ikemiya Y, Iseki C, et al. Proteinuria and the risk of developing end-stage renal disease. *Kidney Int.* 2003;63:1468–1474.

Kelly JD, Fawcett DP, Goldberg LC. Assessment and management of nonvisible haematuria in primary care. *BMJ.* 2009;338:a3021.

Khadra MH, Pickard RS, Charlton M, et al. A prospective analysis of 1930 patients with hematuria to evaluate current diagnostic practice. *J Urol.* 2000;163:524–527.

Kim H, Lee M, Cha MU, et al. Microscopic hematuria is a risk factor of incident chronic kidney disease in the Korean general population: a community-based prospective cohort study. *QJM.* 2018, in press. doi: 10.1093/qjmed/hcy054.

Lang EK, Thomas R, Davis R, et al. Multiphasic helical CT for the assessment of microscopic hematuria: a prospective study. *J Urol.* 2004;171:237–243.

Lin HYH, Yen CY, Lim LM, et al. Microscopic haematuria and clinical outcomes in patients with stage 3-5 non-diabetic chronic kidney disease. *Sci Rep.* 2015;5:15242.

Mariani AJ, Mariani MC, Macchioni C, et al. The significance of adult hematuria: 1,000 hematuria evaluations including a risk-benefit and cost-effectiveness analysis. *J Urol.* 1989;141:350–355.

Messing EM, Young TB, Hunt VB, et al. Hematuria home screening: repeat testing results. *J Urol.* 1995;154:57–61.

Nielsen M, Qaseem A; High Value Care Task Force of the American College of Physicians. Hematuria as a marker of occult urinary tract cancer: Advice for high-value care from the American College of Physicians. *Ann Intern Med.* 2016;164:488–497.

Ohisa N, Yoshida K, Matsuki R, et al. A comparison of urinary albumin-total protein ratio to phase-contrast microscopic examination of urine sediment for differentiating glomerular and nonglomerular bleeding. *Am J Kidney Dis.* 2008;52:235–241.

Subak LL, Grady D. Asymptomatic microscopic hematuria—rethinking the diagnostic algorithm. *JAMA Intern Med.* 2017;177:808–809.

Tiebosch AT, Frederick PM, van Breda Vriesman PJ, et al. Thin-basement-membrane nephropathy in adults with persistent hematuria. *N Engl J Med.* 1989;320:14–18.

Topham PS, Harper SJ, Furnss PN, et al. Glomerular disease as a cause of isolated microscopic hematuria. *Q J Med.* 1994;87:329–335.

Van der Molen AJ, Hovius MC. Hematuria: a problem based imaging algorithm illustrating the recent Dutch guidelines on hematuria. *AJR Am J Roentgenol.* 2012;198:1256–1265.

Vivante A, Afek A, Frenkel-Nir Y, et al. Persistent asymptomatic isolated microscopic hematuria in Israeli adolescents and young adults and the risk for end-stage renal disease. *JAMA.* 2011;306:729–736.

Wallis CJD, Juvet T, Lee Y, et al. Association between use of antithrombotic medication and hematuria-related complications. *JAMA.* 2017;318:1260–1271.

Wollin T, Laroche B, Psooy K. Canadian guidelines for the management of asymptomatic microscopic hematuria in adults. *Can Urol Assoc J.* 2009;30:77–80.

Zhou J, Chen X, Xie Y, et al. A differential diagnostic model of diabetic nephropathy and non-diabetic renal diseases. *Nephrol Dial Transplant.* 2008;23:1940–1945.

20 Nephrotic Range Proteinuria

Jeroen K.J. Deegens and
Jack F.M. Wetzels

Nephrotic range proteinuria is defined as a protein excretion >3 to 3.5 g/day or a spot urine protein-to-creatinine ratio of >3 to 3.5 g protein/g creatinine (g protein/10-mmol creatinine). Several glomerular diseases can cause nephrotic range proteinuria (Table 20.1). These glomerular diseases can be either idiopathic (unknown cause) or secondary to systemic diseases such as diabetes mellitus and systemic lupus erythematosus (SLE), or to drugs, infections, or tumors. Currently, diabetic nephropathy is the most common cause of nephrotic range proteinuria in adults. In nondiabetic adults, focal segmental glomerulosclerosis (FSGS) and membranous nephropathy (MN) account for the majority of cases.

CLINICAL PRESENTATION

Patients with nephrotic range proteinuria usually present with nephrotic syndrome, a constellation of symptoms characterized by heavy proteinuria, peripheral edema, hypoalbuminemia (<3.0 g/dL [30 g/L]), and hyperlipidemia. In addition, patients may present with symptoms related to the underlying cause (Table 20.1) or related to complications of nephrotic syndrome. Not all patients with nephrotic range proteinuria develop nephrotic syndrome. Nephrotic range proteinuria with normal or slightly decreased serum albumin levels is characteristic for FSGS secondary to maladaptive responses. Often these patients are asymptomatic and usually come to medical attention after a routine examination or because of symptoms related to chronic kidney failure.

COMPLICATIONS OF NEPHROTIC RANGE PROTEINURIA

Complications of nephrotic range proteinuria result primarily from metabolic changes related to nephrotic syndrome.

Peripheral Edema

Typically, peripheral edema is located around the eyes in the morning and in the legs and feet during the day and evening. In more severe forms, the edema can become generalized, accompanied by pleural effusion and/or ascites. Classically, formation of nephrotic edema has been considered to be the result of increased kidney sodium retention secondary to intravascular volume depletion that is due to hypoalbuminemia and a low plasma oncotic pressure. However, this "underfilling edema" seems to be limited to patients with acute-onset minimal

| **TABLE 20.1** | Common Glomerular Diseases Associated With Nephrotic Range Proteinuria |

Diabetic Nephropathy

Focal segmental glomerulosclerosis
  Idiopathic
  Secondary
    Familial/genetic (mutations in podocyte/slit diaphragm proteins)
    Virus associated (parvovirus B19, HIV)
    Drug induced (pamidronate/alendronate, lithium, heroin, interferon)
    Maladaptive responses following loss of functioning nephrons (obesity, hypertension, unilateral kidney agenesis, reflux nephropathy, kidney dysplasia)
    Malignancy (lymphoma)
    Kidney scarring that is due to other glomerular diseases (membranous nephropathy, IgA nephropathy, diabetic nephropathy)

Membranous nephropathy
  Primary
  Secondary
    Malignancy (carcinoma of lung, breast, colon)
    Infections (hepatitis B and C, syphilis)
    Drugs and toxic agents (gold, penicillamine, captopril)
    Autoimmune disease (SLE, Sjögren syndrome, diabetes mellitus)

Minimal change disease
  Idiopathic
  Secondary
    Malignancy (lymphoma, leukemia)
    Drugs (NSAIDs)
    Atopy (fungi, pollen, house dust, poison ivy, bee stings)
    Infections (syphilis, HIV, *Mycoplasma pneumoniae*)

IgA nephropathy
  Idiopathic
  Secondary
    Henoch–Schonlein disease
    Infectious (HIV, hepatitis B)
    Gastrointestinal diseases (celiac disease)
    Autoimmune disease (sarcoidosis, rheumatoid arthritis, Reiter disease, spondylitis, dermatitis herpetiformis)

Membranoproliferative glomerulonephritis
  With deposition of immunoglobulin and C3
    Infections (hepatitis B and C, endocarditis)
    Mixed cryoglobulinemia
    Autoimmune disease (SLE, Sjögren syndrome)
    Malignancy (lymphoma, chronic lymphocytic leukemia, kidney cell carcinoma, paraprotein related)
  With dominant C3 deposition
    C3 glomerulopathy
    Autoantibodies (C3 or C4 nephritic factor; anti-factor H or anti-factor B antibodies)
    Monoclonal gammopathy
    Genetic mutations (C3, CFH, CFI, CFB, CFHR5)
    Postinfectious glomerulonephritis

Renal amyloidosis
  AL amyloidosis
  AA amyloidosis
    Chronic infections
    Inflammatory disease (rheumatoid arthritis, ankylosing spondylitis, psoriatic arthritis, Crohn disease, cystic fibrosis, and familial Mediterranean fever)

Lupus nephritis

Note: The secondary causes reported in this list are illustrative and not meant to be exhaustive.
CFB, complement factor B; CFH, complement factor H; CFI, complement factor I; CFHR5, complement factor H–related protein; HIV, human immunodeficiency virus; SLE, systemic lupus erythematosus; NSAIDs, nonsteroidal anti-inflammatory drugs; IgA, immunoglobulin A.

change disease (MCD) and patients with a very low serum albumin (<1.0 g/dL [10 g/L]). Blood volume is normal or even increased in the majority of adult nephrotic patients, and in these patients primary kidney sodium retention contributes to edema formation.

Cardiovascular Complications

Abnormal lipid metabolism is almost always present in patients with nephrotic syndrome. Both increased hepatic production of lipoproteins and decreased lipid catabolism play a role. Most prominent are an increased low-density lipoprotein (LDL) cholesterol level, hypertriglyceridemia, and an increased lipoprotein(a) level. This combination is highly atherogenic and carries a five- to sixfold increased risk for myocardial infarction and a two- to threefold increased risk of coronary death.

Thromboembolic Events

Patients with nephrotic syndrome are at increased risk for venous and arterial thrombotic events, especially in the first 6 to 48 months after presentation. Venous thrombotic events include deep and kidney vein thrombosis as well as pulmonary embolism. Estimates of risk for developing thrombosis vary from 1.5% to values as high as 45% when including patients with a clinically silent venous thrombotic event such as kidney vein thrombosis. At highest risk are patients with MN with a serum albumin <2.5 g/dL (25 g/L). The increased risk is caused by an imbalance between pro- and antithrombotic proteins, enhanced platelet aggregation, and impaired thrombolytic activity.

Protein Malnutrition

Urinary losses of proteins, kidney protein degradation, and poor intake all contribute to a negative nitrogen balance, which can result in a significant reduction of lean body mass.

Infections

Before the introduction of antibiotics, infections were an important cause of mortality in patients with nephrotic syndrome. The susceptibility to bacterial infections has been attributed to urinary losses of immunoglobulin G (IgG) and complement and to reduced cell-mediated immunity. Patients are especially susceptible to infections with encapsulated bacteria, such as *Streptococcus* and *Haemophilus*.

Acute Kidney Injury

Acute kidney injury (AKI) is a frequent complication of nephrotic syndrome due to MCD, and is observed in 40% of patients. AKI typically develops in elderly male patients and is associated with more severe proteinuria. AKI is attributed to a reduced glomerular permeability that is due to damaged podocyte foot processes, ischemic kidney injury (as a result of decreased effective arterial volume, especially in older patients with atherosclerosis and hypertension), or intrarenal edema with tubular collapse. Although at follow-up, estimated glomerular filtration rate (eGFR) is lower in patients with AKI, this is mostly related to the higher age and few patients have persistent chronic kidney disease (Maas, 2017; Waldman, 2007).

In patients with nephrotic syndrome, AKI more often results from the use of drugs such as nonsteroidal anti-inflammatory drugs (NSAIDs), angiotensin-converting enzyme inhibitors (ACEIs), and diuretics. In this setting AKI usually is the consequence of volume depletion and interference with kidney autoregulation. Rarer causes of AKI are drug-induced tubulointerstitial nephritis, bilateral kidney vein thrombosis, and extracapillary glomerulonephritis superimposed on MN or immunoglobulin A (IgA) nephropathy. In IgA nephropathy, heavy glomerular hematuria can lead to AKI as a result of hemoglobin-induced acute tubular necrosis or occlusion of the tubules by red cells.

Disorders in Calcium Metabolism and Bone Lesions

Serum levels of 25-hydroxyvitamin D are reduced in nephrotic syndrome because of urinary loss of vitamin D–binding protein. However, if kidney function is not impaired, then free serum calcitriol levels usually are normal. Only a small fraction of nephrotic patients with normal kidney function has low serum calcitriol levels resulting in hypocalcemia (low ionized serum calcium or low total serum calcium corrected for albumin concentration). If left untreated, these metabolic disturbances can lead to secondary hyperparathyroidism and bone lesions, such as osteomalacia and osteitis fibrosa. In some patients, bone lesions may develop without alterations in calcium and vitamin D metabolism. The underlying mechanism remains elusive, but patients with a prolonged duration of nephrotic syndrome and high levels of proteinuria appear to be at highest risk. Chronic kidney insufficiency and treatment with corticosteroids are other causes of bone lesions in nephrotic patients.

PROGNOSIS AND PREDICTIVE FACTORS

Proteinuria is an important risk factor and the best predictor of progression to end-stage kidney disease (ESKD) in both diabetic and nondiabetic nephropathy. Risk increases for every g/L increase of proteinuria. Other predictors of risk of ESKD are baseline kidney function and blood pressure. The single best predictor of a favorable outcome is attainment of a complete (<0.2 g/day) remission of proteinuria. Thus, the main goal of treatment is maximal lowering of proteinuria, which often can be achieved by non–disease-specific measures. Additional disease-specific treatment may be required to attain a remission. Therefore, patients with nephrotic range proteinuria must be thoroughly evaluated to determine the underlying cause.

INITIAL EVALUATION

The initial evaluation of patients with nephrotic range proteinuria should include quantification of proteinuria, assessment for the presence of complications, and establishing the underlying cause of nephrotic range proteinuria.

Quantification of Proteinuria

If proteinuria is suspected, screening can be performed using a dip-stick. If positive, proteinuria should be quantified. Daily proteinuria can be estimated by calculating total protein-to-creatinine ratio in a first morning or random spot urine. Protein-to-creatinine ratio (expressed as mg/g or g/10 mmol) is calculated by dividing urinary protein concentration (in mg/dL [g/L]) by urinary creatinine concentration (in mg/dL [or mmol/L]). This is a simple and convenient method. In most patients, total protein-to-creatinine ratio correlates very well with daily protein excretion. However, this method may over-estimate proteinuria in patients with a low creatinine excretion that is due to reduced muscle mass (e.g., malnourished or elderly nephrotic patients and women, whose creatinine excretion on average is 15% to 25% lower compared with men) and underestimate proteinuria in muscular patients. Therefore, some consider 24-hour urine testing as best practice. We believe that for the follow-up of patients, quantitation of proteinuria in spot urine samples is sufficient, although we advise confirming results of spot urinalysis once in each patient by collecting a 24-hour urine sample. This 24-hour urine sample will provide additional useful information on total creatinine excretion and thus relative muscle mass, and is helpful in the assessment of the sodium intake as well as protein intake if urine urea excretion is analyzed.

Assessment of Complications

A detailed history, physical examination, and baseline laboratory studies should be performed to assess whether complications are present (Table 20.2). Most complications are readily identifiable. Screening for asymptomatic kidney vein thrombosis is not recommended because of the absence of evidence of benefit. However, signs of acute kidney vein thrombosis (flank pain, gross hematuria, or significant elevation of serum lactate dehydrogenase [LDH]) warrant further diagnostic evaluation with spiral computed tomographic (CT) angiography. Magnetic resonance imaging (MRI) is a suitable alternative, although reported sensitivity and specificity of MRI are lower than CT angiography. The choice also depends on local radiologic expertise. Of note, these radiologic imaging techniques are not without risk in patients with kidney insufficiency. Iodinated radiocontrast agents are associated with nephrotoxicity, whereas especially linear gadolinium-containing contrast agents carry the risk of nephrogenic systemic fibrosis. The reader is advised to carefully balance the risk and benefits of either technique. CT angiography is indicated for suspected pulmonary embolism.

Establishing an Underlying Cause

In patients with insulin-dependent diabetes mellitus, proteinuria is most likely the consequence of diabetic nephropathy. Diabetic nephropathy typically develops more than 10 years after the onset of type 1 diabetes. In type 2 diabetes, in which onset usually is not specifically known, nephropathy may appear to occur earlier. Onset of nephrotic range proteinuria is preceded by a period of many

TABLE 20.2	Evaluation of Patients With Nephrotic Range Proteinuria
History	Edema, flank pain, hematuria, dyspnea, fever, medication, infections, diabetes, signs of malignancy, skin lesions, family history, kidney disease, urologic procedures, or hypertension in past medical history
Physical examination	Edema, blood pressure, weight, length, skin, joints, breasts, lymph nodes, digital rectal examination of prostate

Basic laboratory tests

Blood	Full blood count, serum creatinine, blood urea nitrogen, serum electrolytes (sodium, potassium, calcium), serum albumin, liver functions, glucose, and fasting lipid profile
Urine	Spot urine protein-to-creatinine ratio, protein selectivity index, protein and creatinine in 24-hour urine, examination of urine sediment for red cell casts
Chest x-ray	Check for malignancies, pleural effusion
Ultrasonography kidneys	Check for kidney size, two kidneys present, hydronephrosis, obstruction
Kidney biopsy	Consult with nephrologists
CT angiography	In case of suspected kidney vein thrombosis or pulmonary embolism

Additional tests depending on underlying glomerular disease[a]

FSGS	HIV test, chest x-ray
Membranous nephropathy	Anti-PLA2R antibodies, hepatitis B and C, prostate specific antigen in men >50 years, antinuclear antibodies (if positive, anti–double-stranded DNA and C3/C4 should be measured), fecal occult blood test, chest x-ray, mammography in women >40 years
	Patients with AKI: antiglomerular antibodies and consider repeat kidney biopsy if AKI developed after first biopsy; urinary excretion of α_1- or β_2-microglobulin (optional to determine prognosis in primary MN; Fig. 20.2)
Minimal change disease	HIV (in case of clinical suspicion), chest x-ray
IgA nephropathy	HIV (in case of clinical suspicion).
	Patients with AKI not preceded by gross hematuria, repeat kidney biopsy if ARF developed after first kidney biopsy. ARF developing shortly after gross macroscopic hematuria usually resolves within 1 week. If no improvement after 1 week, consider repeat kidney biopsy.
MPGN	Hepatitis B and C, cryoglobulins, C3 and C4, serum and urine protein electrophoresis, anti–double-stranded DNA
Lupus nephritis	Antinuclear antibody, anti–double-stranded DNA, C3 and C4
AL amyloidosis	Serum and urine protein electrophoresis
AA amyloidosis	C-reactive protein

[a]More tests may be necessary depending on the history and physical examination.

CT, computed tomography; FSGS, focal segmental glomerulosclerosis; HIV, human immunodeficiency virus; AKI, acute kidney injury; MN, membranous nephropathy; IgA, immunoglobulin A; MPGN, membranoproliferative glomerulonephritis.

years with microalbuminuria. Patients with established diabetic nephropathy almost always have diabetic retinopathy. Thus, in diabetic patients who fulfill these criteria, a kidney biopsy usually will not be performed.

In patients without diabetes, nephrotic range proteinuria without hypoalbuminemia is mostly the consequence of secondary FSGS. This diagnosis can be suspected by the finding of hypoplastic kidneys, kidney scarring, long-standing hypertension, or morbid obesity. In these patients, a kidney biopsy may be postponed and effects of supportive treatment may be awaited.

The recent discovery of antibodies against the phospholipase A_2 receptor (anti-PLA2R) in more than 70% of patients with MN will change the diagnostic algorithm in patients with nephrotic syndrome. The specificity for diagnosing MN exceeds 95%. Therefore, in the presence of these antibodies a diagnosis of MN can be made without the need for a kidney biopsy (De Vriese, 2017). In the absence of anti-PLA2R, a kidney biopsy is necessary to verify the diagnosis, because the specificity of the clinical history and radiologic and laboratory studies are not high enough to warrant the use of aggressive disease-specific treatment. A kidney biopsy should only be performed after consultation with a nephrologist. Once a specific glomerular disease is diagnosed, an additional search for an underlying secondary cause may be needed (Table 20.2).

SYMPTOMATIC TREATMENT OF NEPHROTIC RANGE PROTEINURIA

Symptomatic or non–disease-specific treatment is aimed at reducing proteinuria to prevent or slow progression to ESKD and at reducing symptoms and complications of nephrotic syndrome (Table 20.3).

Edema

Edema results from kidney sodium retention. Therefore, patients with edema should restrict dietary sodium intake to 50 mmol/day (1.15 g/day). Treatment with diuretics is indicated in the case of severe edema or mild edema unresponsive to sodium restriction. Edema should be reversed slowly to prevent acute hypovolemia or AKI. Higher doses of loop diuretics often are required to achieve effective kidney sodium excretion because of excessive tubular sodium retention, hypoalbuminemia, which results in an impaired delivery of albumin-bound diuretics to the kidney and binding to albumin within the tubular fluid rendering the diuretic inactive.

The initial treatment consists of a loop diuretic once daily (Fig. 20.1). Patients should weigh themselves daily, and dosage is adjusted to achieve weight loss of 0.5 to 1 kg/day. The absence of a significant diuresis following ingestion of a loop diuretic usually is an indication of low tubular diuretic concentrations. Increasing the dose is indicated. Loop diuretics have a short half-life, and the initial natriuresis may be counterbalanced by avid sodium restriction during the rest of the day. Therefore, if weight loss is insufficient in patients who respond with initially appropriate diuresis, dosing twice daily will be

Treatment	Which Patients?	Treatment Target
Diuretics	Patients with edema	Resolution of edema (see Fig. 20.1).
ACEI	Patients with nephrotic range proteinuria	Proteinuria <0.5 g/day.
		Blood pressure ≤130/80 mm Hg.
Sodium restriction	Patients with nephrotic syndrome	60–80 mmol/day (1.5–2 g) sodium per day.
	Patients treated with ACEI/ARB and persistent high blood pressure or persistent proteinuria ≥1 g/day	
Protein restriction	Patients with nephrotic syndrome	0.8 g/kg per day.
	Patients with eGFR <60 mL/min per 1.73 m²	
Statin	≥50 years	Existing evidence does not support a specific LDL target.
	18–49 years with an additional risk factor: MI or coronary revascularization, diabetes mellitus, prior ischemic stroke, or an estimated 10-year incidence of coronary death or nonfatal MI >10%	Adjusting the statin dose based on LDL levels is not required.
Prophylactic anticoagulation	Patients with membranous nephropathy and serum albumin <2.5 g/dL	INR 2.0–3.0 with warfarin treatment.
	Patients with serum albumin <2 g/dL and additional risk factor for thrombosis[a]	
	Patients with membranous nephropathy and serum albumin <3.2 g/dL not eligible for treatment with warfarin and a calculated risk of ATE >20/1,000 person-years	Aspirin.
Vitamin D treatment	Patients with nephrotic syndrome, hypocalcemia, and low serum 25-hydroxyvitamin D	Normal serum calcium and 25-hydroxyvitamin D levels.
Bisphosphonate	Women not of childbearing potential[b] and men <40 years treated with glucocorticoids at moderate or high risk for osteoporotic fractures and	Reduction of bone disease and fractures.

(continued)

Treatment	Which Patients?	Treatment Target
	■ a prior osteoporotic fracture	
	■ a Z-score <−3 or rapid bone loss ≥10% at the hip or spine over 1 year and continuing glucocorticoid treatment ≥7.5 mg/day for >6 months	
	■ 30 years and initial prednisone (or equivalent) dose ≥30 mg/day and a cumulative dose of >5 g in the past year	
	Women not of childbearing potential[b] and men ≥40 years treated with glucocorticoids at moderate or high risk for osteoporotic fracture:	
	Moderate risk:	
	■ FRAX 10-year risk for major osteoporotic fracture 10–20%[c] *or* for hip fracture >1–3%[c]	
	High risk irrespective of the prednisone dose and treatment duration:	
	■ FRAX 10-year risk for major osteoporotic fracture ≥20%[c] *or* for hip fracture ≥3%[c]	
	■ men ≥50 years and postmenopausal women with a BMD T-score at the hip or spine ≤−2.5	
	■ initial prednisone (or equivalent) dose ≥30 mg/day and a cumulative dose of >5 g in the past year	

[a]Previous thromboembolic event, prolonged bed rest or immobility, congestive heart failure.
[b]Consider treatment in women of childbearing potential who do not plan to become pregnant within the period of bisphosphonate treatment and are using effective birth control or are not sexually active.
[c]Increase the risk generated with FRAX by 1.15 for major osteoporotic fracture and 1.2 for hip fracture if glucocorticoid treatment is >7.5 mg/day (e.g., if hip fracture risk is 2.0%, increase to 2.4%).
ACEI, angiotensin-converting enzyme inhibitor; ARB, angiotensin receptor blocker; INR, international normalized ratio; ATE, arterial thrombotic events; eGFR, estimated glomerular filtration rate; LDL, low-density lipoprotein; MI, myocardial infarction.

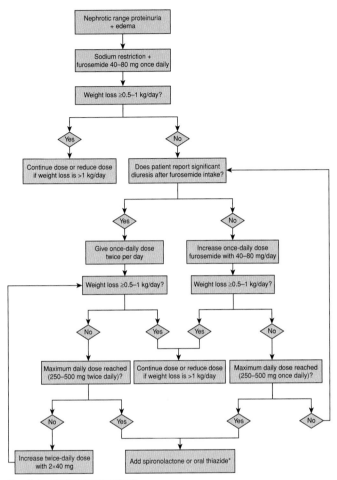

FIGURE 20.1 Treatment of edema in patients with nephrotic range proteinuria.

more effective. The total daily dose may be as high as 500 to 1,000 mg for furosemide.

In patients with severe nephrotic syndrome, treatment with a loop diuretic may be insufficient because of avid sodium retention in other parts of the nephron. Activation of the epithelial sodium channel by proteases in nephrotic urine appears to play an important role in sodium retention. Therefore, if serum potassium levels are normal, amiloride or triamterene may be added. Other options include addition of a thiazide diuretic or spironolactone. It is important to realize that the simultaneous use of diuretics from different classes increases the risk of volume contraction and potassium disturbances. Serum electrolytes, blood urea nitrogen (BUN), creatinine, body weight, and blood pressure should be measured within 1 week of starting dual diuretic treatment and monitored closely thereafter.

Patients who do not respond to oral treatment may benefit from intravenous administration of loop diuretics. Some authors even suggest using a mixture of furosemide and salt-poor albumin if severe generalized edema persists in patients with hypoalbuminemia. However, this strategy has not been proven to be effective.

Proteinuria

A decrease in proteinuria can prevent progression to kidney failure and reduce complications associated with nephrotic syndrome, such as hypoalbuminemia, hyperlipidemia, and edema. Strict blood pressure control is the most important measure to reduce proteinuria. ACEI or, in case of side effects, angiotensin receptor blockers (ARBs) are the preferred agents, as they reduce proteinuria and slow progression of kidney disease more effectively than other antihypertensive agents. ACEI and ARBs act by reducing the intraglomerular pressure and by improving the size-selective properties of the glomerular capillary wall, both of which contribute to reducing protein excretion.

The antiproteinuric and antihypertensive effects of ACEI and ARBs are strongly dependent on the degree of sodium depletion. Therefore, it is necessary to restrict sodium intake to 60 to 80 mmol/day (1.5 to 2 g/day). ACEI and ARBs should not be started at the same time as the loop diuretic, because the combined effects of intravascular volume depletion and impairment of autoregulation increase the risk of AKI. Low-dose ACEI and ARBs can be introduced once a stable dose of the loop diuretic is reached. ACEI and ARBs are titrated upward slowly while monitoring blood pressure, kidney function, and serum potassium. Treatment should be discontinued in case of an increase in serum creatinine >30%. Mild hyperkalemia can first be treated with a low-potassium diet and potassium-binding resins before considering discontinuation of ACEI or ARBs.

We recommend to aim for a blood pressure ≤130/80 mm Hg and to adjust antihypertensive treatment based on the response in terms of proteinuria (KDIGO, 2012). Even if proteinuria is not at target, systolic blood pressures <110 mm Hg and diastolic blood pressures <70 mm Hg should be avoided in patients with diabetes or cardiovascular disease because of an increase in (cardiovascular) death (Bohm, 2017). A systolic blood pressure target of ≤130 may not be appropriate for patients with high pulse pressures. High systolic blood pressure may prevail over too low diastolic blood pressures, for example, in a patient with a blood pressure of 190/70 mm Hg it is wise to try and reach values of 160/60 mm Hg. Proteinuria should be reduced to <0.5 g/day, although this target often is difficult to reach in patients with nephrotic syndrome.

If the goals for blood pressure and proteinuria are not reached with ACEI or ARBs, a diuretic should be added in patients who are not already being treated with a loop diuretic. If blood pressure or proteinuria is not on target, additional treatment modalities include adding a calcium channel blocker, spironolactone, or a β-blocker.

The choice in the individual patient must be tailored and depends on clinical and laboratory parameters, such as prior vascular morbidity, potassium levels, or evidence of hyperaldosteronism.

The combination of ACEI and ARB should be used with care (see Chapter 14). Use of dual blockade may cause complications, such as hypotension and syncope. It has been suggested that nondihydropyridine calcium antagonists, but not dihydropyridine calcium antagonists, lower proteinuria. However, the antiproteinuric effect of nondihydropyridine calcium channel blockers has been questioned (Ruggenenti, 2005). Monotherapy with dihydropyridine calcium antagonists should be avoided in patients with proteinuria. However, they can be used safely in patients who are using ACEI.

Other options to reduce proteinuria include treatment with NSAIDs. However, NSAIDs can have severe side effects, such as hyperkalemia, sodium retention, AKI, and gastrointestinal bleeding. Therefore, we are very reluctant to use NSAIDs in these patients.

Hyperlipidemia

Patients with nephrotic range proteinuria, with or without nephrotic syndrome, are at risk for development of cardiovascular disease. Lipid-lowering treatment with an HMG-CoA reductase inhibitor (statin) is indicated if proteinuria is expected to persist for at least several months in adults aged ≥50 years and in adults aged 18 to 49 years with one or more of the following risk factors: known coronary disease (MI or coronary revascularization), diabetes mellitus, prior ischemic stroke, or an estimated 10-year incidence of coronary death or nonfatal MI >10% (Tonelli and Wanner, 2014).

Thromboembolic Complications

Nephrotic syndrome carries a high risk for the development of thromboembolic complications. Patients with MN are at the highest risk for venous thrombotic complications. Current guidelines advise to consider prophylactic anticoagulation in patients with MN and serum albumin <2.5 g/dL (KDIGO, 2012). Physicians can balance the risk and benefits of such treatment using a web-based calculator put together by the University of North Carolina and the University of Toronto (http://www.med.unc.edu/gntools/). Regardless of the underlying cause, prophylactic anticoagulation also seems appropriate in patients with severe hypoalbuminemia and other risk factors for thrombosis, such as a previous thromboembolic event, congestive heart failure, prolonged bed rest, or immobilization.

Initial prophylactic treatment consists of a combination of warfarin and unfractionated or low–molecular-weight heparin (LMWH) in sufficient dosage to obtain prolongation of the clotting time. Treatment with unfractionated heparin/LMWH can be discontinued if the international normalized ratio (INR) has been on target (2.0 to 3.0) for two consecutive measurements. Prophylactic treatment is continued until serum albumin concentration is >3.0 g/dL (30 g/L) or as long as the additional risk factor is present.

Recent data also provide evidence for an increased risk of arterial thrombotic events, particularly in patients with MN and a serum albumin <3.2 g/dL. In these patients, we start treatment with aspirin if they are not eligible for treatment with prophylactic anticoagulation with warfarin and the calculated risk of arterial thrombotic events exceeds 20/1,000 person-years (Hofstra and Wetzels, 2016).

Therapeutic anticoagulation with heparin/LMWH and warfarin is indicated in patients with deep vein thrombosis, pulmonary embolism, and kidney vein thrombosis. Treatment with warfarin is continued as long as nephrotic syndrome persists, with a minimum duration of 6 to 12 months.

Although evidence is limited, in the absence of contraindications, thrombolytic therapy with or without thrombectomy should be considered in patients with kidney vein thrombosis with evidence of extension of the thrombus into the inferior vena cava, AKI, thrombosis of the contralateral kidney vein, recurrent pulmonary embolisms, or severe flank pain.

Dietary Protein Intake

A high dietary protein intake should be avoided in patients with nephrotic syndrome as this can increase the rate of protein catabolism and urine protein excretion. In contrast, protein restriction has been shown to slow kidney function deterioration in patients with diabetic and nondiabetic kidney diseases. However, the optimal level of protein intake is unclear, and care must be taken to avoid malnutrition. Therefore, in patients with nephrotic syndrome or nephrotic range proteinuria with chronic kidney insufficiency, a moderate protein restriction of 0.8 g/kg body weight per day is advised while maintaining a normal caloric intake. For optimal treatment, referral to a dietitian is strongly recommended.

Infection

Although nephrotic syndrome is well known to be a predisposing factor to bacterial infection, data on the effectiveness of preventive measures are limited. Pneumococcal and influenza vaccination are recommended for all patients with nephrotic syndrome. Although strong evidence for the effectiveness of pneumococcal vaccination is lacking, a small case-control study showed similar antibody response to pneumococcal vaccination in nephrotic children on high-dose corticosteroids versus children in complete remission and no increase in relapse rate (Ulinski, 2008). In patients with recurrent bacterial infections (erysipelas, pneumonia, peritonitis), total serum IgG levels should be measured. If serum IgG is <6 g/L, prophylactic IgG may be useful. Alternatively, patients with recurrent skin infections may benefit from intermittent intramuscular benzylpenicillin. Still, the best advice is to remain alert for signs and symptoms of infection in patients with nephrotic syndrome to allow early treatment with antibiotic therapy.

Acute Kidney Injury

If AKI does occur, then drugs that can cause AKI (e.g., NSAIDs, ACEI, ARBs) should be discontinued. Diuretics should be discontinued in patients with signs of hypovolemia. Most important, however, is specific treatment of the underlying glomerular disease to induce a remission of proteinuria. Obviously, patients with AKI resulting from bilateral deep vein thrombosis or extracapillary proliferative glomerulonephritis should be treated accordingly.

Disorders in Vitamin D and Calcium Metabolism

Treatment of abnormalities in calcium and vitamin D homeostasis is aimed at preventing development of secondary hyperparathyroidism and bone diseases such as osteomalacia, osteitis fibrosa, and osteoporosis. Unfortunately, there are few data available to guide treatment. In patients with nephrotic syndrome and normal kidney function, treatment with 1,000 IU/day vitamin D (cholecalciferol or ergocalciferol) seems reasonable if 25-hydroxyvitamin D deficiency causes low-ionized or corrected total serum calcium levels. Depending on the response, higher doses may be necessary. Other causes of hypocalcemia, such as hypomagnesemia, hypoparathyroidism, and use of calcium-lowering drugs (bisphosphonates, cinacalcet), should be excluded before initiating treatment. Serum levels of calcium and 25-hydroxyvitamin D should be followed.

Provision of vitamin D supplements usually is insufficient to prevent bone disease in patients with nephrotic range proteinuria (with or without nephrotic syndrome) and chronic kidney insufficiency. Phosphate retention, which may develop with loss of kidney function, interferes with the conversion of 25-hydroxyvitamin D to calcitriol by the kidneys. As a result, secondary hyperparathyroidism develops. Treatment consists of dietary phosphate restriction and calcitriol as discussed in Chapter 8.

Glucocorticoid-Induced Osteoporosis

Patients with nephrotic syndrome often require prolonged treatment with corticosteroids to induce a remission of proteinuria. Use of corticosteroids for 3 months is complicated by substantial loss of trabecular bone and an increased risk for fractures of the spine and hips. Fractures occur at higher bone mineral density (BMD) in comparison with postmenopausal osteoporosis. Prevention and treatment of glucocorticoid-induced osteoporosis should be started early, as bone loss is most pronounced in the first 6 to 12 months of treatment. To oppose the negative calcium balance induced by corticosteroids, it is recommended that all patients maintain a calcium intake of 1,000 to 1,500 mg/day and a vitamin D intake of 800 IU/day. If dietary intake is too low, supplements should be prescribed. Adequate calcium and vitamin D intake is not sufficient to prevent bone loss in patients at high risk of glucocorticoid-induced osteoporosis and bisphosphonates are recommended in these patients.

The 2017 American College of Rheumatology guidelines for the treatment of glucocorticoid-induced osteoporosis are summarized in Table 20.3 (Buckley, 2017). The recommendations, taking into account the predicted risk of a fracture using the FRAX tool (www.sheffield.ac.uk/FRAX/) with adjustment for low or higher than usual steroid dose, are mainly based on studies that included postmenopausal women, patients with rheumatoid arthritis or other inflammatory diseases (causing bone loss themselves) and used the change in BMD as the main outcome measure. Therefore, and in view of the role of steroids in bisphosphonate-induced osteonecrosis, we use prophylactic treatment more cautiously. Bisphosphonates are not recommended for patients with an eGFR <30 mL/min per 1.73 m², because their safety and efficacy in this patient group are unknown. Bisphosphonates should be used with caution in premenopausal women who are at risk of becoming pregnant, because these drugs can accumulate in the fetal bone. Premenopausal women started on bisphosphonates should be counseled regarding the use of appropriate contraception.

SPECIALIZED LABORATORY TESTS

Depending on the underlying glomerular disease, additional studies may be needed to assess secondary causes (Table 20.2). It may also be useful to perform additional studies to guide treatment at start and during follow-up.

Urinary Biomarkers

Both urinary IgG (a marker of glomerular size selectivity) and β_2-microglobulin (marker of tubulointerstitial damage) have been proven to be valuable markers in predicting prognosis. In patients with idiopathic MN and normal kidney function, a high excretion of α_1- or β_2-microglobulin (Fig. 20.2) has been shown to be associated with a high risk for developing ESKD (van den Brand, 2011). Other urinary biomarkers for the early identification of AKI have been described, including kidney injury molecule 1 and neutrophil gelatinase–associated lipocalin. These biomarkers also show strong correlation with clinical disease activity in glomerular diseases. However, their predictive value in proteinuric kidney disease remains to be determined (Maas, 2016; Peters, 2011).

Selectivity Index

Proteinuria selectivity index (SI) can be used to assess changes in the glomerular permeability for proteins. Urinary protein loss can be selective (resulting in loss of small–molecular-weight proteins, such as albumin) or nonselective (with loss of larger–molecular-weight proteins, such as immunoglobulins). A selective proteinuria (SI <0.2) is primarily seen in patients with MCD and some patients with FSGS and MN. In patients with idiopathic FSGS, a selective proteinuria predicts a high spontaneous remission rate (Fig. 20.3) (Deegens, 2005). SI is calculated by dividing the clearance of IgG by the clearance of transferrin (or albumin):

$$SI = \frac{\text{urinary IgG} \times \text{serum transferrin}}{\text{serum IgG} \times \text{urinary transferrin}}$$

Other Tests

In patients with MN, treatment response can be guided by repeated measurement of antibodies in PLA2R positive patients. In AL amyloidosis,

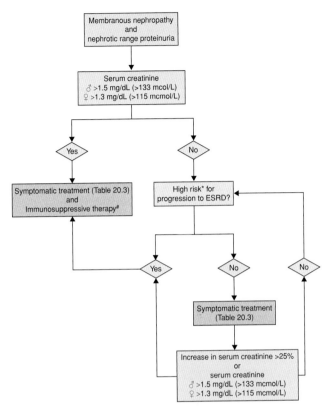

*If low, repeat measurement after 6 months.
#Initial therapy 6 months of treatment with steroids and cyclophosphamide.
Alternative 6 months of calcineurin inhibitor with low dose steroids.

FIGURE 20.2 Flowchart of diagnosis and treatment in membranous nephropathy. (Adapted from Hofstra JM, Fervenza FC, Wetzels JF. Treatment of idiopathic membranous nephropathy. *Nat Rev Nephrol.* 2013;9:443–458.)

response to treatment can be monitored by measurement of paraproteins and light chains; in AA amyloidosis, C-reactive protein can be monitored as an index of inflammation; and in lupus nephritis, anti–double-stranded DNA (anti-dsDNA) antibody levels and levels of complement C3 reflect disease activity.

TREATMENT OF IDIOPATHIC GLOMERULAR DISEASES

All patients with nephrotic range proteinuria should receive anti-proteinuric and symptomatic treatment, irrespective of the underlying cause, to control the complications of nephrotic syndrome. In patients with idiopathic glomerular diseases, spontaneous remissions do occur and sometimes can be awaited. On the other hand, there is little evidence that symptomatic treatment induces a remission of nephrotic range proteinuria in patients with idiopathic glomerular

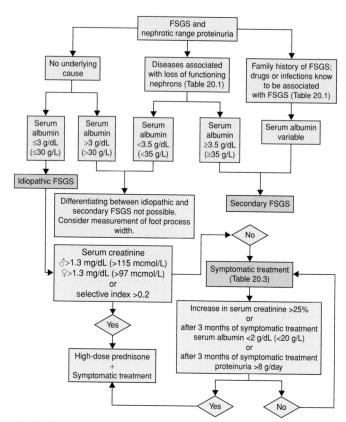

FIGURE 20.3 Flowchart of diagnosis and treatment in idiopathic focal segmental glomerulosclerosis. (Adapted from Deegens JK, Steenbergen EJ, Wetzels JF. Review on diagnosis and treatment of focal segmental glomerulosclerosis. *Neth J Med*. 2008;66:3–12.)

diseases and prevents development of ESKD. In high-risk patients, disease-specific therapies—usually a combination of immunosuppressive drugs—are necessary to induce a remission of proteinuria.

Membranous Nephropathy

Histologically, MN is characterized by the formation of subepithelial immune deposits and thickening of glomerular capillary loops. MN can be idiopathic or secondary to other underlying diseases (Table 20.1). The discovery of antibodies against podocyte antigens in the serum of patients with MN has confirmed that MN is a kidney-limited autoimmune disease. Recognized antigens are PLA2R and thrombospondin type-1 domain-containing 7A (Beck, 2009; Tomas, 2014).

The natural history of MN is variable. Outcome in patients who never have had nephrotic range proteinuria is good, with 10-year kidney survival rates approximating 100%. In contrast, nearly half of the patients with MN and nephrotic range proteinuria develop kidney failure. About 30% to 40% of patients spontaneously enter a remission. A smaller percentage will continue to have nephrotic range proteinuria without progression to kidney failure.

Immunosuppressive treatment should be reserved for patients with idiopathic MN who are at highest risk for ESKD: patients with established kidney insufficiency (not caused by diuretics/ACEI), patients with long-standing and severe proteinuria, and patients with high levels of urinary β_2-microglobulin or α_1-microglobulin (Fig. 20.2). Patients with high levels of PLA2R antibodies are also less likely to develop a spontaneous remission. Prednisone given alone is not effective. Although treatment with cyclophosphamide has proven to be effective, the side effects lead many physicians and patients to consider alternative therapies. Calcineurin inhibitors (CNIs) and rituximab may be suitable alternatives, although their efficacy is unproven, especially in patients with high antibody titers (van de Logt, 2018).

Focal Segmental Glomerulosclerosis

FSGS is a histologic diagnosis characterized by scarring lesions in portions (segments) of some (focal) but not all glomeruli. In addition to the classical form (FSGS not otherwise specified), four other histologic variants (FSGS tip lesion, collapsing FSGS, perihilar FSGS, and cellular FSGS) have been defined based on the character and glomerular distribution of the lesions. Although these variants correlate to some degree with outcome, they cannot be used to guide treatment (Deegens, 2008b).

Generally, the distinction between idiopathic and secondary FSGS can be made from the history, additional laboratory tests, and radiologic studies (Table 20.2). Serum albumin levels are very informative and often allow differentiating between idiopathic FSGS, where serum albumin tends to be low, and FSGS secondary to maladaptive responses, where serum albumin tends to be closer to normal. When in doubt, measurement of podocyte foot process width on electron microscopic examination can be helpful (Deegens, 2008a). Secondary causes also include mutations in proteins involved in maintaining podocyte and glomerular basement membrane function. Underlying genetic mutations should be considered in patients with a family history of kidney disease and in young adults with steroid-resistant FSGS.

Spontaneous remissions do occur in patients with idiopathic FSGS who present with normal kidney function and selective proteinuria. In patients whose nephrotic syndrome can be controlled with symptomatic treatment, we advise to wait at least 3 months before starting immunosuppressive treatment (Fig. 20.3) (Deegens, 2008b; De Vriese, 2018). Initial immunosuppressive treatment consists of prednisone 1 mg/kg per day (up to 80 mg/day). Complete remission rates range from 30% to 60%. In patients with steroid-dependent or frequently relapsing idiopathic FSGS, cyclophosphamide for 2 to 3 months in combination with prednisone results in more stable remissions. A CNI with low-dose prednisone is effective in patients unresponsive to corticosteroids. If a remission occurs, CNI therapy is continued for 1 year and then slowly tapered off to prevent a relapse. In the absence of a remission, CNI therapy should be stopped after 6 months. Because of the increased risk of complications, such as nephrotoxicity, we caution against the use of CNI in patients with moderate to severe kidney insufficiency.

Minimal Change Disease

MCD is defined by the absence of histologic glomerular abnormalities other than epithelial foot process effacement on electron microscopic examination. Most cases are idiopathic. Idiopathic MCD (iMCD) is considered a relatively benign disease. Indeed, progression to ESKD is extremely rare. Onset of progressive kidney failure usually is associated with the development of FSGS lesions, and in these cases it is uncertain if FSGS lesions reflect progression of iMCD or if FSGS was missed on previous biopsies because of a sampling error. It has been suggested that in untreated adults, the spontaneous remission rate may be as high as 70%, although this may take up to 3 years to manifest. These data likely are biased, because many patients need treatment to manage nephrotic syndrome. Still, in patients with preserved kidney function whose nephrotic syndrome can be controlled with symptomatic treatment, we advise to wait at least 3 months before starting immunosuppressive treatment.

Treatment with prednisone 1 mg/kg per day (up to 80 mg/day) is advised if serum albumin does not progressively increase to ≥3.0 g/dL (30 g/L), complications of nephrotic syndrome develop, or kidney function deteriorates (KDIGO, 2012). The initial dose should be given for a minimum of 4 weeks and can be slowly tapered over a period of 24 weeks once a complete remission is attained.

Relapses occur in approximately 50% of patients (Maas, 2017). A first relapse can be treated with a new course of prednisone. In steroid-dependent or frequently relapsing patients, an 8- to 12-week course of cyclophosphamide and prednisone can induce more stable remissions. A CNI with low-dose prednisone is advised for patients relapsing after cyclophosphamide treatment, or for patients with contraindications to cyclophosphamide. Relapses are frequent after cessation of a CNI, and many patients need continuous treatment with CNI to maintain a remission (Kyrieleis, 2009). Although limited data are available, mycophenolate mofetil (MMF) may be a less nephrotoxic alternative to treatment with CNI if dosed adequately (area under the curve >50 mcg/mL) (Gellermann, 2013).

In children, MCD generally has been considered a benign disorder with cessation of relapses after puberty. However, a significant number of children continue to relapse into adulthood. These patients frequently suffer from side effects of long-term immunosuppressive treatment, and balancing between achieving a remission and adverse treatment effects can be difficult. Therefore, we recommend referring patients with iMCD that persists into adulthood to a specialized center. In these children with severe side effects, treatment with rituximab, a chimeric anti-CD20 monoclonal antibody, can be considered to achieve a drug-free remission (Ravani, 2016).

Immunoglobulin A Nephropathy

IgA nephropathy is characterized by deposits of IgA in the glomerular mesangium. The majority of patients present with hematuria (macroscopic or microscopic) or nonnephrotic proteinuria. Nephrotic range proteinuria is a less common presentation. A subgroup of patients with IgA nephropathy who present with acute-onset nephrotic syndrome and preserved kidney function have minimal glomerular changes on kidney biopsy. These patients probably have two coinciding glomerular diseases (i.e., MCD with IgA deposits of questionable significance). These patients should be treated as patients with MCD.

Most patients with IgA nephropathy and nephrotic range proteinuria have significant structural glomerular damage on kidney biopsy and progressive kidney dysfunction. Supportive treatment, including ACEI or ARB, can effectively reduce proteinuria and slow progression to ESKD. Proteinuria <0.5 to 1 g/day during follow-up invariably predicts a good outcome (Berthoux, 2011).

In patients with eGFR >50 mL/min per 1.73 m^2 and persistent proteinuria >1 g/day despite maximal symptomatic treatment, a 6-month course of steroids can be offered (KDIGO, 2012). This approach has been challenged by results from the STOP IgAN Trial, which showed that addition of immunosuppressive therapy to intensive supportive care in patients with persistent proteinuria ≥0.75 g/day did not change the rate of decrease in eGFR, even though complete remissions were significantly higher after immunosuppressive treatment (Rauen, 2015). However, the study pooled results from two different immunosuppressive regimens and was not powered to detect a beneficial effect on eGFR in the subgroup of patients with eGFR >60 mL/min per 1.73 m^2 treated with high-dose steroid monotherapy. In fact, in this subgroup proteinuria decreased to <1 g/day in the majority of patients and complete remission rate was much higher compared to the pooled results. Therefore, we feel that steroid treatment, as recommended by KDIGO, is still an acceptable option.

A novel formulation of budesonide (a type of corticosteroid) specifically targeting intestinal mucosal immunity was evaluated (Fellstrom, 2017). Nine-month treatment with budesonide significantly reduced proteinuria and stabilized eGFR compared to placebo, albeit with more corticosteroid-related side effects. Further studies are needed to evaluate the efficacy and side effects of targeted-release budesonide in comparison to prednisone. Data from one prospective study suggest that patients with more advanced disease (serum creatinine 1.5 to 2.8 g/dL; 133 to 250 mcmol/L), nephrotic range proteinuria, and a rapid deterioration of kidney function (>15% increase in serum creatinine in 1 year) may benefit from treatment with prednisone and cyclophosphamide followed by azathioprine (Ballardie, 2002). The role of fish oil in IgA nephropathy is uncertain. It may reduce kidney inflammation and slow kidney function decline, but evidence is weak.

TREATMENT OF SECONDARY GLOMERULAR DISEASES

Secondary glomerular diseases are conditions in which an underlying cause can be established. Treatment should be primarily directed at the underlying cause (Table 20.1). In all patients antiproteinuric treatment is important to slow progression of kidney disease.

Diabetes mellitus is the most common secondary cause of nephrotic range proteinuria. Strict blood glucose control, reduction of proteinuria, and lowering blood pressure are the mainstay of treatment in diabetic nephropathy, as reviewed in Chapter 13.

Obesity

In many patients, FSGS is secondary to hyperfiltration in remnant nephrons, with typical examples including hypoplastic kidney, reflux nephropathy, and long-standing hypertension. Obesity (body mass index [BMI] >30 kg/m^2) is a risk factor for progression to ESKD in patients with pre-existing kidney disease or reduced kidney mass. Moreover, patients with obesity are at increased risk for developing obesity-related glomerulopathy, where on kidney biopsy the glomeruli are enlarged, often with FSGS lesions. The pathophysiology is unclear but may include hyperfiltration and increased kidney venous pressure.

Nephrotic range proteinuria is common in obesity-related glomerulopathy but, as in other causes of FSGS secondary to maladaptive responses, serum albumin is relatively normal and edema is absent. The reduction in proteinuria shows a significant correlation with the percentage of weight reduction, and modest weight losses of 5% or less can already induce a decrease in proteinuria ≥30% (Morales, 2003). However, maintaining weight loss often is difficult, and many patients relapse. Approaches to weight loss and results of bariatric surgery are described in Chapter 4.

Lupus Nephritis

SLE is a chronic inflammatory disease that can affect many organs. The majority of patients are women of childbearing age. The kidney is involved in up to 60% of patients. Kidney involvement may occur at any time in the course but is more likely to occur in the first year after diagnosis. Based on the findings on kidney biopsy, lupus nephritis is divided into six classes. Nephrotic range proteinuria can be present in patients with focal proliferative lupus nephritis (class III), diffuse proliferative lupus nephritis (class IV), and membranous lupus nephritis (class V).

Patients with nephrotic range proteinuria and active lupus nephritis class III, IV, or V should receive immunosuppressive treatment. Induction therapy consists of a combination of prednisone with oral MMF or intravenous cyclophosphamide. For maintenance therapy MMF or azathioprine are used. In African-American patients MMF is superior to azathioprine. Cyclophosphamide should not be used as maintenance therapy as treatment duration >3 months is associated with an increased infertility risk.

Prednisone monotherapy may be sufficient in patients with a pure MN pathology of SLE without a proliferative component. However, many patients need additional immunosuppressive treatment (e.g., azathioprine or cyclophosphamide added to prednisone), either to induce a remission or to allow use of a lower dose of prednisone.

Hydroxychloroquine should be given to patients with SLE during the whole course of the disease, irrespective of disease severity and should be continued during pregnancy. Hydroxychloroquine may prevent lupus flares, increases long-term survival of patients with SLE, and may help protect against irreversible organ damage, thrombosis, and bone mass loss (Ruiz-Irastorza, 2010). Patients should be checked for hydroxychloroquine-related ophthalmologic toxicity. It is recommended that all patients receive a baseline eye examination within the first year of use followed by annual screening after 5 years. Earlier screening is indicated in case of a daily dose >6.5 mg/kg or a cumulative dose >1,000 g and in patients with known retinal disease, kidney insufficiency or liver disease.

Amyloidosis

Nephrotic syndrome is a common manifestation of renal amyloidosis. Renal amyloidosis is characterized by pathologic deposition of fibrillary proteins in the kidney. In AL amyloidosis, a single clone of malignant plasma cells produces monoclonal immunoglobulin light chains that accumulate in the glomerulus. Although multiple myeloma may be present, the plasma cell clone often is undetectable by bone marrow examination. Treatment is aimed at suppressing or eliminating the plasma cell clone. Myeloablative therapy with stem cell rescue is used in selected patients. Persistent disease often results in a rapid progression to ESKD. AA amyloidosis is a complication of chronic infections and chronic inflammation. AA amyloid is built from serum amyloid A protein, an acute-phase reactant produced by the liver. Treatment of the underlying inflammatory process is the most effective measure to induce a remission of proteinuria. Eprodisate, an agent directed at preventing fibril formation, was not effective in slowing renal functional decline in AA amyloidosis (Merlini, 2016).

THE ELDERLY PATIENT WITH NEPHROTIC RANGE PROTEINURIA

Diabetic nephropathy and MN are the most common causes of nephrotic range proteinuria in elderly patients (≥65 years). The clinical presentation of nephrotic syndrome is not different from that in younger patients. However, edema often is mistakenly attributed to heart failure or venous insufficiency of the lower limbs. Therefore, elderly patients with edema should be screened for proteinuria. Malignancies are an important cause of glomerular diseases in older patients. An underlying malignancy is present in 20% to 25% of elderly patients with MN (Deegens and Wetzels, 2007). Remission of proteinuria can be attained after successful treatment of the tumor. It may take up to 18 months before resolution of proteinuria is seen. Symptomatic treatment is also indicated in elderly patients with nephrotic range proteinuria. Thromboembolic complications appear to be more common in elderly patients with MN and nephrotic syndrome than in younger patients. Symptomatic treatment should be monitored closely, as elderly patients are more prone to side effects of antihypertensive drugs and diuretics. Immunosuppressive drugs are effective in elderly patients, although adverse effects are more common. Therefore, immunosuppressive treatment should be tailored to the individual patient, taking into consideration comorbidity, life expectancy, and activities of daily living.

CASE STUDY
A 53-year-old man came to his primary care physician reporting nausea, vomiting, and dizziness. Past medical history was unremarkable, except for high blood pressure and proteinuria at a routine examination 5 years earlier. However, he had not received antihypertensive treatment. On physical examination, blood pressure was markedly elevated at 200/110 mm Hg, height was 170 cm, weight was 90 kg (BMI = 31.1 kg/m^2). There was no peripheral edema. Laboratory investigation showed normal serum electrolytes, creatinine 1.4 mg/dL (124 mcmol/L), albumin 4.0 g/dL (40 g/L), LDL cholesterol 263 mg/dL (6.8 mmol/L), and SI 0.25. Proteinuria was 4.1 g/g creatinine, and eGFR was 56 mL/min per 1.73 m^2. An ultrasound showed two normal-sized kidneys.

The absence of hypoalbuminemia and edema in spite of nephrotic range proteinuria strongly suggested a diagnosis of FSGS secondary to hypertension and/or obesity, and a kidney biopsy was postponed to await the effect of symptomatic treatment. Blood pressure remained high despite treatment with an ACEI and salt restriction. A 24-hour urine collection showed poor compliance with the sodium-restricted diet (urinary sodium excretion was 200 mmol [4.6 g]/day). Therefore, a thiazide diuretic was added, which resulted in a significant decline in blood pressure. Because blood pressure and proteinuria were not at target, a calcium channel blocker was added. Over the next year, proteinuria decreased to <0.2 g/day. Kidney function has remained stable during a follow-up of more than 6 years.

CASE STUDY
A 45-year-old woman came to her doctor's office because she had been tired for 3 weeks and had noticed progressive edema of the lower legs. She had a past history of hypertension that had been effectively treated with a β-blocker. The family history was significant in that a sister had SLE. On physical examination blood pressure was 180/100 mm Hg, weight 67 kg, and height 160 cm (BMI was 26.2 kg/m^2). There was bilateral 2+ pitting edema of the legs, but no skin lesions. Laboratory investigation showed normal serum electrolytes, creatinine 0.9 mg/dL (80 mcmol/L), BUN 10 mg/dL (3.6 mmol/L), albumin 1.8 g/dL (18 g/L), and LDL cholesterol 275 mg/dL (7.12 mmol/L). Urine analysis showed that proteinuria was 10.8 g/g of creatinine. Anti-PLA2R antibodies were positive. Additional studies for secondary disease—including hepatitis B and C, antinuclear antibody, chest x-ray—were all negative. Therefore a kidney biopsy was not performed and a diagnosis of MN was made. The patient was started on diuretics and a low-sodium and low-protein diet.

To assess the risk of progression to kidney failure, urinary excretion of β_2-microglobulin (0.36 mg/10 mmol) was measured. This value is indicative of a low risk of progression, and symptomatic treatment with an ACEI, a statin, and prophylactic anticoagulation was started. Because blood pressure and proteinuria were not at target, a calcium channel blocker was added. Urinary β_2-microglobulin excretion remained low after 6 months of treatment. Over the next 1.5 years, serum albumin progressively increased and proteinuria started to decrease. Two years after presentation, a complete spontaneous remission was attained.

References and Suggested Readings

Ballardie FW, Roberts IS. Controlled prospective trial of prednisolone and cytotoxics in progressive IgA nephropathy. *J Am Soc Nephrol*. 2002;13:142–148.

Beck LH Jr, Bonegio RG, Lambeau G, et al. M-type phospholipase A2 receptor as target antigen in idiopathic membranous nephropathy. *N Engl J Med*. 2009;361:11–21.

Berthoux F, Mohey H, Laurent B, et al. Predicting the risk for dialysis or death in IgA nephropathy. *J Am Soc Nephrol*. 2011;22:752–761.

Bohm M, Schumacher H, Teo KK, et al. Achieved blood pressure and cardiovascular outcomes in high-risk patients: results from ONTARGET and TRANSCEND trials. *Lancet*. 2017;389:2226–2237.

Briot K, Cortet B, Roux C, et al; Bone Section of the French Society for Rheumatology (SFR) and Osteoporosis Research and Information Group (GRIO). 2014 update of recommendations on the prevention and treatment of glucocorticoid-induced osteoporosis. *Joint Bone Spine*. 2014;81:493–501.

Buckley L, Guyatt G, Fink HA, et al. 2017 American College of Rheumatology Guideline for the prevention and treatment of glucocorticoid-induced osteoporosis. *Arthritis Rheumatol*. 2017;69:1521–1537.

Deegens JK, Assmann KJ, Steenbergen EJ, et al. Idiopathic focal segmental glomerulosclerosis: a favourable prognosis in untreated patients? *Neth J Med*. 2005;63:393–398.

Deegens JK, Dijkman HB, Borm GF, et al. Podocyte foot process effacement as a diagnostic tool in focal segmental glomerulosclerosis. *Kidney Int*. 2008a;74:1568–1576.

Deegens JK, Steenbergen EJ, Wetzels JF. Review on diagnosis and treatment of focal segmental glomerulosclerosis. *Neth J Med*. 2008b;66:3–12.

Deegens JK, Wetzels JF. Membranous nephropathy in the older adult: epidemiology, diagnosis and management. *Drugs Aging*. 2007;24:717–732.

De Vriese AS, Glassock RJ, Nath KA, et al. A proposal for a serology-based approach to membranous nephropathy. *J Am Soc Nephrol*. 2017;28:421–430.

De Vriese AS, Sethi S, Nath KA, et al. Differentiating primary, genetic, and secondary FSGS in adults: a clinicopathologic approach. *J Am Soc Nephrol*. 2018;29:759–774.

Fellstrom BC, Barratt J, Cook H, et al. Targeted-release budesonide versus placebo in patients with IgA nephropathy (NEFIGAN): a double-blind, randomised, placebo-controlled phase 2b trial. *Lancet*. 2017;389:2117–2127.

Gellermann J, Weber L, Pape L, et al; Gesellschaft für Pädiatrische Nephrologie (GPN). Mycophenolate mofetil versus cyclosporin A in children with frequently relapsing nephrotic syndrome. *J Am Soc Nephrol*. 2013;24:1689–1697.

Hofstra JM, Wetzels JF. Should aspirin be used for primary prevention of thrombotic events in patients with membranous nephropathy? *Kidney Int*. 2016;89:981–983.

Kidney Disease: Improving Global Outcomes (KDIGO) Glomerulonephritis Work Group. KDIGO clinical practice guideline for glomerulonephritis. *Kidney Int Suppl*. 2012;2:139–274.

Kyrieleis HA, Lowik MM, Pronk I, et al. Long-term outcome of biopsy-proven, frequently relapsing minimal-change nephrotic syndrome in children. *Clin J Am Soc Nephrol*. 2009;4:1593–1600.

Maas RJ, Deegens JK, Beukhof JR, et al. The clinical course of minimal change nephrotic syndrome with onset in adulthood or late adolescence: a case series. *Am J Kidney Dis*. 2017;69:637–646.

Maas RJ, van den Brand JA, Waanders F, et al. Kidney injury molecule-1 and neutrophil gelatinase-associated lipocalin as prognostic markers in idiopathic membranous nephropathy. *Ann Clin Biochem.* 2016;53:51–57.

Merlini G. *Phase 3 KIACTA Results, 15th International Symposium on Amyloidosis.* Uppsala, Sweden, July 3–7. 2016. Available from http://www.raredr.com/news/5-year-aa-amyloidosis. Accessed June 3, 2018.

Morales E, Valero MA, Leon M, et al. Beneficial effects of weight loss in overweight patients with chronic proteinuric nephropathies. *Am J Kidney Dis.* 2003;41:319–327.

Peters HP, Waanders F, Meijer E, et al. High urinary excretion of kidney injury molecule-1 is an independent predictor of end-stage renal disease in patients with IgA nephropathy. *Nephrol Dial Transplant.* 2011;26:3581–3588.

Rauen T, Eitner F, Fitzner C, et al; STOP-IgAN Investigators. Intensive supportive care plus immunosuppression in IgA nephropathy. *N Engl J Med.* 2015;373:2225–2236.

Ravani P, Bonanni A, Rossi R, et al. Anti-CD20 antibodies for idiopathic nephrotic syndrome in children. *Clin J Am Soc Nephrol.* 2016;11:710–720.

Ruggenenti P, Perna A, Loriga G, et al; REIN-2 Study Group. Blood-pressure control for renoprotection in patients with non-diabetic chronic renal disease (REIN-2): multicentre, randomised controlled trial. *Lancet.* 2005;365:939–946.

Ruiz-Irastorza G, Ramos-Casals M, Brito-Zeron P, et al. Clinical efficacy and side effects of antimalarials in systemic lupus erythematosus: a systematic review. *Ann Rheum Dis.* 2010;69:20–28.

Tomas NM, Beck LH Jr, Meyer-Schwesinger C, et al. Thrombospondin type-1 domain-containing 7A in idiopathic membranous nephropathy. *N Engl J Med.* 2014;371:2277–2287.

Tonelli M, Wanner C; Kidney Disease: Improving Global Outcomes Lipid Guideline Development Work Group Members. Lipid management in chronic kidney disease: synopsis of the Kidney Disease: Improving Global Outcomes 2013 clinical practice guideline. *Ann Intern Med.* 2014;160:182.

Ulinski T, Leroy S, Dubrel M, et al. High serological response to pneumococcal vaccine in nephrotic children at disease onset on high-dose prednisone. *Pediatr Nephrol.* 2008;23:1107–1113.

van den Brand JA, Hofstra JM, Wetzels JF. Low-molecular-weight proteins as prognostic markers in idiopathic membranous nephropathy. *Clin J Am Soc Nephrol.* 2011;6:2846–2853.

van de Logt AE, Dahan K, Rousseau A, et al. Immunological remission in PLA2R-antibody-associated membranous nephropathy: cyclophosphamide versus rituximab. *Kidney Int.* 2018;93:1016–1017.

Waldman M, Crew RJ, Valeri A, et al. Adult minimal-change disease: clinical characteristics, treatment, and outcomes. *Clin J Am Soc Nephrol.* 2007;2:445–453.

21 | Acute Kidney Injury

Michael Heung and Lenar Yessayan

Acute kidney injury (AKI) is a syndrome characterized by an abrupt decline in kidney function, which can range from mild to severe. A variety of definitions for AKI (previously referred to as acute renal failure) have been used in the literature, but recent efforts have resulted in the development of a consensus definition and staging system (Table 21.1) (KDIGO, 2012).

AKI and CKD are now well-recognized as intertwined syndromes. On the one hand, AKI—even with apparent renal recovery—is associated with increased risk for future CKD and end-stage renal disease (ESRD). On the other hand, CKD is a major predisposing factor for AKI (Chawla, 2014). Clinicians need to be aware of this bidirectional relationship when managing patients with CKD.

AKI is a common and potentially devastating complication, occurring in about 20% of hospitalized adult patients and with overall hospital mortality rates approaching nearly 25% (Susantitaphong, 2013).

APPROACH TO DIFFERENTIAL DIAGNOSIS OF AKI

An important first step in management of AKI is to identify underlying causes, which may in turn define management. Causes of AKI can be divided into prerenal, intrinsic, and postrenal etiologies. Prerenal AKI results from decreased renal perfusion (Table 21.2). Intrinsic AKI may be caused by a variety of conditions that affect the glomeruli, renal tubules, interstitium, or blood vessels (Table 21.3). Postrenal AKI results from obstruction to urine flow at the level of the ureters, bladder outlet or urethra. Key investigations in AKI are summarized in Table 21.4. Here we will discuss some of the more commonly encountered AKI scenarios.

Acute Tubular Necrosis

Acute tubular necrosis (ATN) is characterized by acute tubular cell injury and dysfunction and is the most common form of intrinsic AKI in hospitalized patients. It may be secondary to ischemic injury (e.g., hypotension or shock, postcardiac bypass, or aorta surgery), nephrotoxic injury, or septic injury (with or without overt hypotension). Exogenous nephrotoxins commonly associated with the development of ATN include aminoglycosides, amphotericin B, cisplatinum, and radiocontrast media. Endogenous nephrotoxins include pigments such as hemoglobin and myoglobin (hemolysis and rhabdomyolysis) and light chains (myeloma cast nephropathy). In ATN,

TABLE 21.1   Kidney Disease Improving Global Outcomes (KDIGO) Staging of Acute Kidney Injury (AKI)

Stage	Serum Creatinine	Urine Output
1	≥0.3 mg/dL (≥26.5 µmol/L) increase, *or* 1.5–1.9 times baseline	<0.5 mL/kg per hour for 6–12 hours
2	2.0–2.9 times baseline	<0.5 mL/kg per hour for ≥12 hours
3	≥3.0 times baseline, *or* Increase to ≥4.0 mg/dL (≥353.6 µmol/L), *or* Initiation of renal replacement therapy, *or* In patients <18 years, decrease in eGFR to <35 mL/min per 1.73 m²	<0.3 mL/kg per hour for ≥24 hours or Anuria for ≥12 hours

TABLE 21.2   Prerenal Causes of Acute Kidney Injury

Hypovolemia
Renal losses
Gastrointestinal losses
Cutaneous losses
Blood loss
Fluid loss to the third space
  ■ Tissue damage (e.g., pancreatitis)
  ■ Hypoalbuminemia (e.g., the nephrotic syndrome)

Decreased Cardiac Output
Heart failure
Pulmonary embolism
Myocardial infarction
Abdominal compartment syndrome

Systemic Vasodilation
Sepsis
Anaphylaxis
Anesthetics
Vasodilators

Local Hypoperfusion
Bilateral renal artery obstruction (stenosis, embolism, thrombosis, dissection)
Bilateral renal vein thrombosis

Afferent Arteriolar Vasoconstriction
Hypercalcemia
Drugs (NSAIDs, calcineurin inhibitors, radiocontrast agents, norepinephrine, amphotericin B)
Hepatorenal syndrome

Efferent Arteriolar Vasodilation
Drugs (angiotensin-converting enzyme inhibitors, angiotensin receptor blockers)

NSAIDs, nonsteroidal anti-inflammatory drugs.

TABLE 21.3 Intrinsic Causes of Acute Kidney Injury

Glomerular
ANCA-associated GN
Anti-GBM GN
Immune complex GN
Lupus nephritis
Lupus-like nephritis (drugs: quinidine, methyldopa, hydralazine, procainamide)
Postinfectious GN
Cryoglobulinemic GN
Membranoproliferative GN
Henoch–Schönlein purpura
Minimal change disease (drugs: NSAIDs, interferon, pamidronate)
Focal segmental glomerulosclerosis (drugs: interferon, pamidronate)

Vascular
Atheroembolic disease
Thrombotic microangiopathy
- TTP, HUS, DIC, HELLP syndrome, scleroderma renal crisis, malignant hypertension
- Drugs: Anti-angiogenesis agents (bevacizumab), calcineurin inhibitors, chemotherapeutics (interferon, gemcitabine, mitomycin C), platelet aggregation inhibitors (ticlopidine, clopidogrel), interferon, quinine
Vasculitis
- ANCA-associated GN
- Anti-GBM GN
- Drugs (+/– ANCA): cocaine (levamisole), hydralazine, infliximab, propylthiouracil

Tubular
Ischemic
Other
- Heme pigment (rhabdomyolysis, intravascular hemolysis)
- Crystals (uric acid, atazanavir, acyclovir, sulfonamides, quinolone, methotrexate, ascorbic acid, orlistat, triamterene, sodium phosphate purgatives)
- Drugs (vancomycin, aminoglycosides, polymyxins, tenofovir, amphotericin B, cisplatin, ifosfamide, radiocontrast agents), synthetic cannabinoid use

Interstitial
Drugs (proton pump inhibitors, penicillins, cephalosporins, NSAIDs, allopurinol, rifampin, mesalamine, sulfonamides)
Infection (pyelonephritis, viral infection)
Systemic disease (Sjögren syndrome, sarcoidosis, SLE, lymphoma, leukemia)

ANCA, antineutrophil cytoplasmic antibody; GN, glomerulonephritis; GBM, glomerular basement membrane; NSAIDs, nonsteroidal anti-inflammatory drugs; TTP, thrombotic thrombocytopenic purpura; HUS, hemolytic uremic syndrome; DIC, disseminated intravascular coagulation; HELLP, hemolysis, elevated liver function tests, low platelets.

urine output may vary from <500 mL/day to normal values. Common diagnostic findings are urine specific gravity <1.015, urine osmolality <450 mOsm/kg (usually <350), and muddy brown granular casts and tubular epithelial cells on urine sediment examination. In oliguric patients one can calculate a **fractional excretion of sodium** (FE_{Na}):

$$\left(FE_{Na} = \left[\frac{(UrineNa \times PlasmaCr)}{(PlasmaNa \times UrineCr)} \right] \times 100\% \right)$$

21.4 Key Investigations Pointing Toward Specific Causes of AKI

Laboratory Finding	Possible Cause for AKI
Urine dipstick: positive blood or protein	Renal inflammatory process
Proteinuria and dipstick negative for protein	Myeloma cast nephropathy
Urinary dysmorphic red blood cells or casts	Glomerulonephritis, TMA
Urinary WBC or WBC cell casts	AIN
Urinary granular casts or renal epithelial cells	ATN
Crystalluria	Uric acid, drugs (see Tables 21.3 and 23.3)
Anemia	Hemorrhage, hemolysis
Anemia with rouleaux formation	Plasma cell dyscrasia
Eosinophilia	AIN, cholesterol emboli, vasculitis
Microangiopathic hemolytic anemia + thrombocytopenia	TTP, HUS, DIC
Coagulopathy	Liver disease, DIC, antiphospholipid antibody syndrome
Hypercalcemia	Malignancy, myeloma cast nephropathy, hyperparathyroidism, granulomatous disease
Hyperphosphatemia	Rhabdomyolysis and TLS; may be elevated in other causes of AKI if duration is prolonged
Elevated creatinine phosphokinase	Rhabdomyolysis
Elevated uric acid	TLS, acute uric acid nephropathy
Elevated serum anion, osmolal gap, or both	Ethylene glycol or methanol intoxication
Monoclonal increase in serum immunoglobulins or free light chains	Myeloma, plasma cell dyscrasias
Antinuclear antibody (ANA)	Autoimmune diseases
Anti–double-stranded antibodies anti-dsDNA Ab)	Autoimmune diseases, more specific than ANA for SLE
Anti-Smith (anti-Sm) antibodies	Highly specific for SLE
Antineutrophil cytoplasmic antibody (ANCA)	C-ANCA and anti-PR3 antibodies in GPA granulomatosis, P-ANCA and anti-MPO in microscopic polyangiitis
Elevated anti-glomerular basement membrane antibodies (anti-GBM Ab)	Good pasture syndrome
Low complement	SLE, post-infectious glomerulonephritis, cryoglobulinemia
Elevated cryoglobulins	Hepatitis C, lymphoproliferative disorders

TMA, thrombotic microangiopathy; AIN, allergic interstitial nephritis; ATN, acute tubular necrosis; TTP, thrombotic thrombocytopenic purpura; HUS, hemolytic uremic syndrome; DIC, disseminated intravascular coagulation; TLS, tumor lysis syndrome; GPA, granulomatosis with polyangiitis; SLE, systemic lupus erythematosus; PR3, proteinase 3; MPO, myeloperoxidase.

FE_{Na} is typically >1% and may help differentiate ATN from prerenal azotemia where FE_{Na} is <1%. FE_{Na} may be falsely low in ATN secondary to contrast-induced nephropathy and pigment nephropathy (rhabdomyolysis, hemolysis) or when severe renal hypoperfusion coexists. High FE_{Na} is not specific to ATN and may be seen in diuretic-induced prerenal azotemia or in patients with CKD. Fractional excretion of urea (FE_{urea} = [(UrineUr × PlasmaCr) / (PlasmaUr × UrineCr)] × 100%) is more useful than FE_{Na} during diuretic therapy. FE_{urea} <35% suggests prerenal AKI; FE_{urea} >50% indicates ATN.

Treatment is etiology specific and primarily supportive. Hemodynamic abnormalities should be corrected and potentially nephrotoxic agents discontinued. In severe cases, dialysis may be required until renal function is restored. Kidney function typically recovers within 1 to 3 weeks from onset. However, some may remain dialysis dependent for up to 3 months or indefinitely.

Acute Interstitial Nephritis

Acute interstitial nephritis (AIN) is characterized by leukocyte infiltration of the renal interstitium. It is seen in at least 10% of kidney biopsies with AKI and therefore its prevalence is likely underestimated. It is most often associated with medication use and typically develops 10 to 14 days after exposure to the medication (earlier if patient was previously exposed). Other causes include infections, malignancy, and immune disorders. The most common culprit medications include β-lactams, sulfonamides, rifampin, fluoroquinolones, H_2 antagonists, proton pump inhibitors, allopurinol, and NSAIDs.

Diagnosis is often made by finding a temporal association between AKI onset and use of known culprit drug, or resolution with discontinuation of a drug. Signs and symptoms are nonspecific. The classic triad of fever, rash, and eosinophilia is observed in only 5% of cases. Eosinophiluria is neither sensitive nor specific for AIN and should not be used to diagnose or rule out AIN. Urinalysis and urine sediment analysis may show proteinuria (rarely exceeding 2 g/day), glucosuria, white blood cells (WBCs), WBC casts, and red blood cells. Nonsteroidal anti-inflammatory drug (NSAID)–induced AIN may present with nephrotic range proteinuria. Biopsy may be considered when the diagnosis is not clear or when withdrawal of a potential culprit drug may affect patient care.

The benefit of corticosteroid therapy is controversial. It may be considered in those who have not responded to drug withdrawal alone. The duration of treatment should be short, and steroids should be tapered and discontinued if no response is observed after 4 weeks of therapy (Raghavan and Eknoyan, 2014).

Hepatorenal Syndrome

Hepatorenal syndrome (HRS) is a functional cause of AKI that occurs in patients with acute liver disease (acute hepatitis, fulminant hepatic failure) or in patients with advanced cirrhosis and portal hypertension. HRS is associated with a poor prognosis: untreated, type 1 (characterized by rapid renal function decline) is associated with >90% mortality at 3 months; and type 2 (characterized by refractory ascites and slower renal function decline) is associated with 30% mortality at 3 months and 60% at 1 year.

The pathophysiology of HRS is characterized by splanchnic vasodilation that results in decreased total vascular resistance in spite of peripheral vasoconstriction, activation of renin–angiotensin and sympathetic nervous systems, and rise in cardiac output. Intense renal vasoconstriction results in GFR reduction. Precipitating triggers include bacterial infections, gastrointestinal hemorrhage, or large volume paracentesis. Occasionally, no clear precipitating factor is identified.

HRS is a diagnosis of exclusion. HRS is associated with oliguria and bland urine sediment. However, nonoliguric state or active urine sediment (blood and/or protein) does not exclude the diagnosis of HRS. The diagnostic criteria for HRS have recently been revised to include the KDIGO definitions of AKI and removal of a fixed cutoff value of serum creatinine (Table 21.5).

Liver transplantation is the ideal treatment for HRS. Medical therapy should include albumin (1 g/kg per day), intravenous vasopressors (norepinephrine or vasopressin) in critically ill patients, and either terlipressin (not available in the United States) or combination of midodrine and octreotide in noncritically ill patients. In patients with severe renal impairment who are liver transplant candidates or expected to survive from acute liver injury, dialysis should be considered.

Abdominal Compartment Syndrome

Abdominal compartment syndrome (ACS) is characterized by a sustained increase in intra-abdominal pressure of >20 mm Hg with new

TABLE 21.5	Diagnostic Criteria of Hepatorenal Syndrome (HRS) Type of Acute Kidney Injury (AKI) in Patients With Cirrhosis According to Revised Consensus Recommendations of the International Club of Ascites

- Diagnosis of cirrhosis and ascites
- Diagnosis of AKI according to ICA-AKI criteria:
  Increase in serum creatinine ≥0.3 mg/dL (≥26.5 µmol/L) within 48 hours; or,
  Percentage increase serum creatinine ≥50% from baseline which is known, or presumed, to have occurred within the prior 7 days
- No response after 2 consecutive days of diuretic withdrawal and plasma volume expansion with albumin 1 g/kg of body weight
- Absence of shock
- No current or recent use of nephrotoxic drugs (NSAIDs, aminoglycosides, iodinated contrast media, etc.)
- No macroscopic signs of structural kidney injury, defined as:
  Absence of proteinuria (>500 mg/day)
  Absence of microhematuria (>50 RBCs per high-power field)
  Normal findings on renal ultrasonography

ICA, International Club of Ascites; NSAIDs, nonsteroidal anti-inflammatory drugs; RBCs, red blood cells.

organ dysfunction. AKI results from decreased renal perfusion pressure as a result of increased renal venous pressure and congestion, diminished cardiac output, and renal vasoconstriction. Common causes of ACS include intra-abdominal or retroperitoneal hemorrhage, pancreatitis, massive fluid resuscitation, laparoscopy and pneumoperitoneum, and ileus. In critically ill patients, the incidence of ACS may be as high as 12%. Common early signs include tense abdomen, oliguria, elevated airway pressures, and difficulty ventilating.

Intra-abdominal pressure can be estimated by a variety of approaches. Bladder pressure, using an indwelling catheter, is the most common method used. The measurement is obtained with the patient in supine position, at end expiration, and in the absence of abdominal contractions. Similar to other states with kidney hypoperfusion, FE_{Na} is low in ACS.

Management is supportive and includes surgical decompression when appropriate. Gastrointestinal decompression is required if ACS is due to intestinal distention. Paracentesis may be needed in patients with tense ascites. Sedation and chemical paralysis (in mechanically ventilated patients) may be required to relax abdominal muscles and maintain adequate ventilation.

Urinary Tract Obstruction

Urinary flow obstruction may occur at any level of the urinary tract. It may be secondary to bladder outlet obstruction (prostatic enlargement, urethral fibrosis), bilateral ureteral obstruction (stones, bladder masses, retroperitoneal fibrosis), or unilateral ureteral obstruction in patients with solitary functioning kidney. Obstruction may also be precipitated by functional bladder impairment from medications (e.g., narcotics or anticholinergic agents).

Ultrasonography is the most commonly used imaging technique to diagnose obstructive nephropathy. Findings include dilatation of ureters and pelvicalyceal systems. False-positive results may be seen in conditions associated with chronic pelvicalyceal dilatation. The presence of periodic ureteral urinary jets on Doppler imaging of the bladder suggests nonobstructive dilatation of these systems (false positives). False-negative results may be seen in cases of acute obstruction (<24 hours), low urine flow rates (severe volume depletion or renal failure), or when ureters are encased by masses or fibrous tissue. The sensitivity of ultrasound for diagnosis of obstruction can be improved by measuring the resistive index with color Doppler ultrasound. A resistive index above 0.7 reflects increased vascular resistance present in obstruction and effectively discriminates between obstructed and nonobstructed kidneys.

Lower urinary tract obstruction (bladder outlet) is treated by inserting a urethral catheter and if this cannot be passed, by placing a suprapubic catheter. Upper urinary tract obstruction is treated by placement of nephrostomy tubes or placement of ureteral stents during cystoscopy. Percutaneous nephrostomy is generally the appropriate emergency treatment of upper urinary tract obstruction in the setting of AKI. After relief of the obstruction, the exact site and the cause of the obstructing lesion will determine the approach to a more definitive therapy.

PROGNOSTIC INFORMATION

Once AKI has been recognized, it is important to gauge the renal prognosis. Will the AKI be quickly reversible, or will it get progressively worse? Several factors can help inform this question:

Staging Criteria and Clinical Setting

The severity of AKI, as defined by staging criteria, correlates with short and long term mortality. In one prospective multicenter study, the 90-day mortality risk stratified by KDIGO stage was 17% in those without AKI, 29% for stage 1, 34% for stage 2, and 39% for stage 3 AKI (Nisula, 2013). Other adverse impacts of AKI include increased risk of readmission (Bedford, 2014), developing CKD (7 times the risk) (Rimes-Stigare, 2015; Thakar, 2011) and progression to ESRD (22 times the risk) (Ishani, 2009; Rimes-Stigare, 2015). In critically ill patients (intensive care setting), the mortality rate for patients with severe AKI requiring acute dialysis is approximately 50% (Hoste and Schurgers, 2008).

Oliguria

Oliguria has been used as a biomarker of renal injury for centuries (Heberden, 1818). Urine output measurement has been incorporated in the recent consensus definitions of AKI (Table 21.1). In the KDIGO definition, a urine output of less than 0.5 mL/kg per hour for a period of at least 6 hours is an alternative to creatinine rise in defining the earliest stage of AKI. Oliguria does not always indicate kidney tissue damage. It may be secondary to reduced GFR (with or without tubular damage), increased tubular reabsorption (osmotic and nonosmotic release of ADH), or obstruction. Profound oliguria (< 0.3 mL/kg per hour) indicates reduction in GFR unless the cause is urinary obstruction.

Oliguria in the presence of biochemical markers of kidney injury usually indicates a more severe form of AKI. In observational studies of ATN, higher peak serum creatinine concentration (Anderson, 1977), and higher risks of dialysis and mortality (Mandelbaum, 2013; Oh, 2013; Wald, 2006) are reported in oliguric than nonoliguric ATN.

Furosemide Challenge Test

Furosemide, a loop diuretic, reaches the urinary space through active secretion in the proximal tubule. Thus, the urinary output in response to furosemide challenge may be used to distinguish between impaired tubular function and functional AKI occurring in response to osmotic or hemodynamic stimuli. In patients with early AKI, a urine volume of <200 mL in the first 2 hours after

1.0 to 1.5 mg/kg furosemide administration has been shown to predict progression to KDIGO stage 3 AKI with a sensitivity of 87% and a specificity of 84% (Chawla, 2013). In a secondary analysis of the study, furosemide challenge test outperformed biomarkers of renal tubular injury in predicting progression of AKI, need for renal replacement therapy, and inpatient mortality (Koyner, 2015).

TIMING OF INITIATION OF RENAL REPLACEMENT THERAPY

As discussed earlier, a first step in AKI management is to identify and treat potential contributing factors. Beyond this, there are no proven medical therapies to reverse established AKI, and care of these patients is primarily supportive. In severe cases, this can include acute initiation of dialysis. The decision to initiate dialysis in AKI is unambiguous when life-threatening complications are present, such as severe hyperkalemia, acidemia, pulmonary edema, or uremic complications. The optimal timing of dialysis for AKI is less clear when these factors are not present or are not severe.

Several single-center nonrandomized controlled studies in cardiac surgery patients and observational cohort studies in the ICU have suggested a mortality benefit with "early" dialysis. These studies vary widely in their definition of "early" dialysis and often include arbitrary cutoffs for serum creatinine, urea, urine output, time from ICU admission, and duration of AKI when defining "early" dialysis.

Two prospective randomized controlled trials examined the impact of early dialysis initiation but differed in their conclusions. A single center study, the early vs late initiation of renal replacement therapy in critically Ill patients with acute kidney injury (ELAIN) trial (Zarbock, 2016), showed greater survival over the first 90 days in those undergoing early dialysis, while the multicenter artificial kidney initiation in kidney injury (AKIKI) study (Gaudry, 2016) did not show survival benefit for early dialysis. Importantly, the two studies significantly differed in their definitions of "early" and "delayed" dialysis (Table 21.6). Also, in both studies a substantial proportion of patients randomized to late dialysis did not end up requiring dialysis (9% in the ELAIN trial and 49% in the AKIKI trial). At present, there is inadequate evidence to recommend early initiation of dialysis for AKI. Results from ongoing randomized clinical trials addressing this issue will hopefully provide data to resolve this debate.

PREVENTION OF AKI AND AKI-RELATED COMPLICATIONS

Given the lack of effective therapies for established nonimmunologic AKI (i.e., ATN), an important focus must be placed on prevention. In primary prevention, interventions are designed to prevent AKI occurrence. For secondary prevention, among patients who already have AKI, goals include preventing AKI worsening, avoiding later complications or AKI, and preventing AKI recurrence. Importantly, iatrogenic insults can play a major role in development or worsening

	21.6 Comparison Between ELAIN and AKIKI Randomized Clinical Trials Examining Timing of Renal Replacement Therapy in Patients With Acute Kidney Injury	
	ELAIN Trial ($N = 231$) (Zarbock, 2016)	AKIKI Trial ($N = 620$) (Gaudry, 2016)
Centers	1	31
Inclusion Criteria		
AKI stage	KDIGO stage 2	KDIGO stage 3
Other Criteria	At least 1 of: ■ Severe sepsis ■ On vasopressors ■ Refractory fluid overload ■ SOFA score ≥2	At least 1 of: ■ Mechanically ventilated ■ On vasopressors
Biomarker	Serum NGAL >150 ng/mL	None
Dialysis Triggers		
Early Group Definition	Within 8 hours of KDIGO stage 2	Within 6 hours of KDIGO stage 3
Delayed Group Definition	12 hours after progressing to KDIGO stage 3 AKI *or* any of the following dialysis triggers: ■ BUN >100 mg/dL ■ K >6 mEq/L (or ECG changes) ■ Mg >4 mmol/L ■ Urine <200 mL/24 hours ■ Organ edema despite diuretics	Any of the following dialysis triggers: ■ BUN >112 mg/dL ■ K >6 mEq/L (or 5.5 with treatment) ■ pH <7.15 (pure metabolic or mixed) ■ Pulmonary edema with FiO_2 >0.5 or O_2 >5 L/min *or* oligo/anuria >72 hours
Outcomes		
90-day mortality (early vs. delayed)	39.3% vs. 54.7% ($p = 0.03$)	48.5% vs. 49.7% ($p = 0.79$)
% Patients Needing Dialysis in Delayed Group	90.8%	51.0%

NGAL, neutrophil gelatinase–associated lipocalin; KDIGO, Kidney Disease: Improving Global Outcomes; SOFA, sequential organ failure assessment; BUN, blood urea nitrogen; K, potassium; Mg, magnesium.

of AKI, and studies have suggested that a significant proportion (as much as 20% to 40%) of hospital-acquired AKI cases might have been preventable (Aitken, 2013; Fuhrman and Kellum, 2017).

Identifying patients at high risk for AKI is important to guide preventative measures as well as to educate patients and obtain fully informed consent. Risk prediction scores for AKI have been developed for a variety of different clinical situations, although these have had limited external validation and have therefore not been widely adopted. Nonetheless, there are several well-established risk factors for AKI that clinicians should be aware of (Table 21.7). In addition, there are some common and specific clinical scenarios that are particularly amenable to preventative measures.

TABLE 21.7	Established Patient Risk Factors for Acute Kidney Injury

Pre-existing chronic kidney disease
Older age
Congestive heart failure
Diabetes mellitus
Proteinuria
Emergent (compared to elective) surgery
Prior history of AKI

Cardiac Surgery

This is one of the most studied settings in AKI prevention research. AKI complicates about 24% of cardiac surgery cases and is a significant negative prognostic factor (Fuhrman and Kellum, 2017). The pathophysiology of cardiac surgery–related AKI includes ischemia related to cardiopulmonary bypass, and this is influenced both by blood oxygen saturation and oxygen-carrying capacity (i.e., hemoglobin and hemodilution). Additional factors include presence of endogenous nephrotoxins such as hemoglobinuria from hemolysis and myoglobinuria from rhabdomyolysis, and atheroemboli that can be dislodged during vascular manipulation. Inflammation is increasingly recognized as a pathogenic factor, and this may develop from exposure to the cardiopulmonary bypass machine or transfusions.

Despite significant research, at present there remain no proven pharmacologic therapies for prevention of cardiac surgery–related AKI. Clinical trials have evaluated a variety of agents including dopamine, loop diuretics, N-acetylcysteine, fenoldopam, and atrial natriuretic peptide. In addition, off-pump cardiac surgery has been compared to the traditional on-pump approach. Unfortunately, none of these interventions have proven beneficial in decreasing the risk of AKI.

Protocol-driven approaches have been found beneficial in reducing risk of cardiac surgery–related AKI (Meersch, 2017). Interestingly, studies suggest that having a protocolized (vs. nonprotocolized) approach appears beneficial irrespective of the specific protocol targets (Brienza, 2009). Such protocols generally focus on the following elements:

Hemodynamic Optimization

It is generally recommended that blood pressure be maintained for adequate renal perfusion. While there is a lack of strong evidence basis in this area, a typical target is mean arterial pressure >65 mm Hg. Vasopressor use may be required.

Intravascular Volume Optimization

Both volume depletion (i.e., prerenal state) and volume overload (e.g., decompensated congestive heart failure) can increase the risk of AKI in the perioperative setting. Postoperative fluid overload has also been implicated in renal venous congestion and risk of AKI.

Decreasing Preoperative Kidney Injury Risk

Cardiac surgery patients will typically require a preoperative cardiac catheterization with nephrotoxic contrast dye exposure. Allowing time between contrast exposure and surgery (>48 hours) is advised whenever possible. Other considerations include holding angiotensin-converting enzyme inhibitors and angiotensin receptor blockers preoperatively.

Limiting Postoperative Nephrotoxic Exposures

Examples include routine use of NSAIDs for postoperative pain management; prophylactic administration of nephrotoxic antibiotics such as aminoglycosides; and iodinated contrast with CT imaging.

Close Observation

Monitoring of urine output in the intra- and postoperative periods can help to identify patients developing AKI before routine lab testing, and help guide interventions at an earlier stage.

Iodinated Contrast Exposure (CT Scan or Angiography)

As with cardiac surgery, much research effort has gone into trying to prevent contrast-related AKI. Overall, the AKI risk appears to have decreased with the transition from hyperosmolar to more iso-osmolar contrast agents, and recent studies suggest that the risk of contrast-related AKI is quite low in patients with normal to moderately decreased renal function (eGFR >30 mL/min).

The most proven approach to decreasing risk of contrast-related AKI is fluid administration, which presumably speeds up contrast transit through the nephron and thus decreases tubular cell toxicity. However, there remains controversy in this area, as a recent trial did not demonstrate benefit from prophylactic fluid administration (Nijssen, 2017). Care must be taken when prescribing rapid fluid administration to patients with congestive heart failure or existing fluid overload. There are no consensus hydration regimens, but guidelines generally suggest giving an isotonic fluid at least 1 hour before exposure and continuing 3 to 6 hours post exposure (KDIGO, 2012).

Another effective approach is to minimize the amount of contrast used. For cardiac catheterization, this can be accomplished by foregoing a left ventriculogram, using biplane imaging, and doing selective catheterization only. For CT imaging, in high-risk patients there should be a discussion with radiology to determine how necessary contrast is to answer the clinical question. Importantly, the presence of CKD should not automatically preclude a necessary procedure involving contrast. For example, cardiovascular disease is the leading cause of death in patients with CKD, and this population appears to benefit from percutaneous coronary interventions. Yet studies have found that CKD patients presenting with an acute coronary syndrome are less likely to undergo intervention compared to patients without CKD.

Secondary Prevention

In some situations, primary prevention may not be possible, for example, in those patients presenting with community-acquired AKI. However, in these cases there may be a role for secondary prevention of worsening AKI and AKI complications. An important step in limiting the extent of AKI is a careful review of medications with the goal of limiting the extent of potential nephrotoxic exposures, as well as to properly dose adjust medications in the setting of evolving renal function impairment. Additional measures include close monitoring of renal function (serum creatinine and urine output), hemodynamic and volume status optimization, and avoidance of hyperglycemia. Studies have demonstrated that implementation of these "bundled" measures can be effective in preventing more severe AKI (Meersch, 2017).

Patients surviving an episode of AKI remain at high risk for complications. One study found that, among patients who recovered from dialysis-requiring AKI, early nephrology follow-up post hospitalization was associated with lower all-cause mortality (Harel, 2013). While this finding needs to be confirmed, patients with AKI are clearly at risk for adverse renal outcomes, such as the development of CKD and even ESRD. Careful follow-up of these patients is therefore important to monitor renal function and implement appropriate therapies to delay CKD progression (Silver, 2015). In addition, survivors of AKI appear to be at higher risk for cardiovascular complications (Go, 2018).

NEPHROLOGY CONSULTATION

As mentioned above, AKI is a very common occurrence among hospitalized patients. The majority of patients will have mild (stage 1) AKI, with common etiologies being volume depletion (prerenal) and toxin-mediated injury (e.g., intravenous iodinated contrast, medications, myoglobin from rhabdomyolysis). In most of these cases, patients will respond to supportive measures and not require additional workup. However, clinicians should also be cognizant of scenarios where additional evaluation, including nephrology consultation, may be needed.

Uncertain Etiology of AKI

In the absence of a clear cause for AKI, or if obvious causes have been ruled out (e.g., lack of response to fluid challenge), further evaluation is warranted, especially if renal function continues to decline. Initial workup should include a urinalysis and renal ultrasound. Findings on the urinalysis, as outlined earlier in this chapter, play a major role in delineating the relevant differential diagnoses and directing subsequent workup. Renal ultrasound can help assess for chronicity of the renal insufficiency if unknown, and also rule out an obstructive process. Nephrology consultation can assist with completing the workup based on these initial tests, including cases in which a kidney biopsy may be indicated.

Suspected Glomerulonephritis

The presence of the hallmarks of the acute nephritic syndrome (hypertension, hematuria and proteinuria, AKI) should prompt urgent nephrology consultation for expedited workup. In severe cases (i.e., the syndrome of rapidly progressive glomerulonephritis), early intervention can be organ preserving and even lifesaving. While serologic testing (e.g., for systemic lupus erythematosus, ANCA-associated vasculitis, or anti-glomerular basement membrane disease) can be informative, the diagnostic gold standard is kidney biopsy which provides additional important information such as severity of the disease and renal prognosis (e.g., degree of scarring observed).

Moderate to Severe AKI

Consideration for nephrology consultation should also be given for patients who present with stage 2 or 3 AKI. In these situations, a careful review of potential contributing factors is warranted in order to limit any further kidney damage and ideally facilitate kidney function recovery before the need for renal replacement therapy. In patients who are at high risk for progressing to needing renal replacement therapy, earlier consultation can allow appropriate patient education and counseling, as well as avoid having to start acute dialysis in an emergent situation.

Preventive Measures

This is perhaps the most underutilized form of consultation, yet arguably the most effective. Nephrologists are often consulted after the development of AKI, when interventions to halt evolution of the disease are much more limited. In situations with high risk of anticipated nephrotoxic insult, consultation may help inform optimal measures to prevent AKI. Examples include patients with advanced CKD undergoing cardiac catheterization or elective cardiovascular surgery. At a minimum, pre-AKI consultation can help provide full informed consent for patients and prepare them for potential complications.

PATIENT/FAMILY EDUCATION

Considering how frequently AKI occurs and how serious its consequences can be, clinicians must be comfortable counseling patients and their family members on expectations with this syndrome. Here we discuss some of the questions most commonly asked by patients with severe AKI who may require acute dialysis:

What Does Dialysis Do? Does Dialysis Help the Kidneys?

Dialysis, also referred to as renal replacement therapy, helps to perform some of the key functions of the kidneys, namely solute clearance, electrolyte and acid–base homeostasis, and volume balance. However, dialysis (hemodialysis or peritoneal dialysis) does not directly promote kidney recovery (except perhaps by improving vascular congestion through fluid removal). As such, dialysis should be considered as supportive care.

Will the Patient Need to Be on Dialysis Permanently? What Is the Likelihood of Recovery?

In general, the expectation with initiation of acute dialysis should be eventual recovery of kidney function and the vast majority of AKI patients with normal baseline kidney function will be able to come off dialysis. However, there are a number of factors to consider. Worse baseline CKD is associated with lower likelihood of recovery. Recovery is lower with advanced age, presumably also because of lower kidney function reserve. Longer duration of AKI correlates with lower likelihood of recovery. Nevertheless, recovery can occur weeks to months after the initial insult and even after discharge from the hospital (Pajewski, 2018). The likelihood of recovery may be lower in the presence of some comorbidities, in particular congestive heart failure and liver failure with portal hypertension.

Is There Anything That Can Be Done to Promote Kidney Recovery?

Unfortunately, there are no proven medical therapies to reverse established severe AKI.

What Are the Risks of Dialysis? Does It Hurt?

Dialysis catheter insertion is mildly uncomfortable and carries the risk of damage to internal organs and bleeding, as well as subsequent risk of infection. Dialysis itself is typically not associated with severe symptoms. Complications of dialysis include hemodynamic instability such as hypotension and less commonly cardiac arrhythmias.

What Will Happen if the Patient Chooses Not to Pursue Dialysis? Or to Stop Dialysis at a Later Point?

If kidney function recovery does not occur, patients with severe AKI will have progressive uremia and other biochemical abnormalities (e.g., hyperkalemia, metabolic acidosis) which will eventually be fatal. If a comfort care approach is chosen, symptoms (such as pain, nausea, and even shortness of breath) can typically be managed medically. Involvement of a palliative care team is beneficial in this setting.

References and Suggested Readings

Aitken E, Carruthers C, Gall L, et al. Acute kidney injury: outcomes and quality of care. *QJM.* 2013;106:323–332.

Anderson RJ, Linas SL, Berns AS, et al. Nonoliguric acute renal failure. *N Engl J Med.* 1977;296:1134–1138.

Bedford M, Stevens PE, Wheeler TW, et al. What is the real impact of acute kidney injury? *BMC Nephrol.* 2014;15:95.

Brienza N, Giglio MT, Marucci M, et al. Does perioperative hemodynamic optimization protect renal function in surgical patients? A meta-analytic study. *Crit Care Med.* 2009;37:2079–2090.

Chawla LS, Davison DL, Brasha-Mitchell E, et al. Development and standardization of a furosemide stress test to predict the severity of acute kidney injury. *Crit Care.* 2013;17:R207.

Chawla LS, Eggers PW, Star RA, et al. Acute kidney injury and chronic kidney disease as interconnected syndromes. *N Engl J Med.* 2014;371:58–66.

Fuhrman DY, Kellum JA. Epidemiology and pathophysiology of cardiac surgery-associated acute kidney injury. *Curr Opin Anaesthesiol.* 2017;30:60–65.

Gaudry S, Hajage D, Schortgen F, et al; AKIKI Study Group. Initiation strategies for renal-replacement therapy in the intensive care unit. *N Engl J Med.* 2016;375:122–133.

Go AS, Hsu CY, Yang J, et al. Acute kidney injury and risk of heart failure and atherosclerotic events. *Clin J Am Soc Nephrol* 2018; May 17 (epub).

Harel Z, Wald R, Bargman JM, et al. Nephrologist follow-up improves all-cause mortality of severe acute kidney injury survivors. *Kidney Int.* 2013;83:901–908.

Heberden W. Commentaries on the History and Cure of Diseases. Boston, MA: Wells and Lilly; 1818.

Hoste EA, Schurgers M. Epidemiology of acute kidney injury: how big is the problem? *Crit Care Med.* 2008;36:S146–S151.

Ishani A, Xue JL, Himmelfarb J, et al. Acute kidney injury increases risk of ESRD among elderly. *J Am Soc Nephrol.* 2009;20:223–228.

Kidney Disease: Improving Global Outcomes (KDIGO) Acute Kidney Injury Workgroup. KDIGO clinical practice guideline for acute kidney injury. *Kidney Int Suppl.* 2012;2:1–138.

Koyner JL, Davison DL, Brasha-Mitchell E, et al. Furosemide stress test and biomarkers for the prediction of AKI severity. *J Am Soc Nephrol.* 2015;26:2023–2031.

Mandelbaum T, Lee J, Scott DJ, et al. Empirical relationships among oliguria, creatinine, mortality, and renal replacement therapy in the critically ill. *Intensive Care Med.* 2013;39:414–419.

Meersch M, Schmidt C, Hoffmeier A, et al. Prevention of cardiac surgery-associated AKI by implementing the KDIGO guidelines in high risk patients identified by biomarkers: the PrevAKI randomized controlled trial. *Intensive Care Med.* 2017;43:1551–1561.

Nijssen EC, Rennenberg RJ, Nelemans PJ, et al. Prophylactic hydration to protect renal function from intravascular iodinated contrast material in patients at high risk of contrast-induced nephropathy (AMACING): a prospective, randomised, phase 3, controlled, open-label, non-inferiority trial. *Lancet.* 2017;389:1312–1322.

Nisula S, Vaara ST, Kaukonen KM, et al; FINNAKI-QOL Study Group. Six-month survival and quality of life of intensive care patients with acute kidney injury. *Crit Care.* 2013;17:R250.

Oh HJ, Shin DH, Lee MJ, et al. Urine output is associated with prognosis in patients with acute kidney injury requiring continuous renal replacement therapy. *J Crit Care.* 2013;28:379–388.

Pajewski R, Gipson P, Heung M. Predictors of post-hospitalization recovery of renal function among patients with acute kidney injury requiring dialysis. *Hemodialysis Int.* 2018;22:66–73.

Raghavan R, Eknoyan G. Acute interstitial nephritis—a reappraisal and update. *Clin Nephrol.* 2014;82:149–162.

Rimes-Stigare C, Frumento P, Bottai M, et al. Evolution of chronic renal impairment and long-term mortality after de novo acute kidney injury in the critically ill; a Swedish multi-centre cohort study. *Crit Care.* 2015;19:221.

Silver SA, Goldstein SL, Harel Z, et al. Ambulatory care after acute kidney injury: an opportunity to improve patient outcomes. *Can J Kidney Health Dis.* 2015;2:36.

Stewart J, Findlay G, Smith N, et al. Adding insult to injury: a review of the care of patients who died in hospital with a primary diagnosis of acute kidney injury (acute renal failure). A report by the National Confidential Enquiry into Patient Outcome and Death, London. 2009. Available from http://www.ncepod.org.uk/2009aki.html. Accessed June 1, 2018.

Susantitaphong P, Cruz DN, Cerda J, et al; Acute Kidney Injury Advisory Group of the American Society of Nephrology. World incidence of AKI: a meta-analysis. *Clin J Am Soc Nephrol.* 2013;8:1482–1493.

Thakar CV, Christianson A, Himmelfarb J, et al. Acute kidney injury episodes and chronic kidney disease risk in diabetes mellitus. *Clin J Am Soc Nephrol.* 2011;6:2567–2572.

Wald R, Deshpande R, Bell CM, et al. Survival to discharge among patients treated with continuous renal replacement therapy. *Hemodial Int.* 2006;10:82–87.

Zarbock A, Kellum JA, Schmidt C, et al. Effect of early vs delayed initiation of renal replacement therapy on mortality in critically ill patients with acute kidney injury: The ELAIN randomized clinical trial. *JAMA.* 2016;315:2190–2199.

22 Anemia

Iain C. Macdougall

Anemia is a common complication of chronic kidney disease (CKD), generally worsening as renal function declines and being particularly prevalent in CKD stages 3 to 5. The most important cause is an inappropriately low secretion of erythropoietin (EPO) from the diseased kidneys, but iron deficiency, inflammation, hyperparathyroidism, and other etiologies also play an important role.

PATHOPHYSIOLOGY

Erythropoietin

EPO is the key regulator of erythropoiesis. In adults, the kidney is the major site of EPO production, with the liver making a small contribution. Within the kidney, peritubular interstitial fibroblasts are the predominant cells involved in EPO synthesis. EPO acts in the bone marrow to increase the red cell mass, predominantly by preventing death of erythroid progenitor cells by apoptosis.

Hypoxia-Inducible Factor

Hypoxia is the major stimulus for EPO production. The pivotal link between the two is the molecule hypoxia-inducible factor (HIF). HIF stimulates EPO gene transcription. Normally, HIF is turned off because in the presence of adequate tissue oxygen, HIF is continuously being inactivated by an enzyme called prolyl hydroxylase. If hypoxia occurs, however, prolyl hydroxylase is inhibited, suppression of HIF ceases, and the increased HIF activity then upregulates EPO production.

Hepcidin and Ferroportin

Hepcidin is a critical mediator of the anemia of inflammation. Hepcidin acts to stop iron efflux from gut epithelial cells (enterocytes), liver cells, and reticuloendothelial cells (macrophages). Hepcidin does this by causing internalization and eventual degradation of **ferroportin**, a membrane-based iron exporter present on these cells. Thus, when hepcidin levels are high, which occurs in response to high serum iron levels or to inflammation, iron is poorly absorbed, as it is not released from enterocytes. Hepcidin also prevents release of iron into the circulation from liver and reticuloendothelial storage sites.

Iron

Iron is a critical mineral for red blood cell (RBC) production, being incorporated into heme at the erythroblast stage of red cell development. Many CKD patients are in negative iron balance because of increased iron losses and/or reduced iron absorption. Anorexia with reduced intake may exacerbate iron deficiency, but reduced gut absorption of iron that is due to inflammation-induced increases in hepcidin may also play a major role.

Inflammation

CKD is a state of chronic inflammation. Proinflammatory cytokines reduce erythropoiesis in several ways: They are potent stimulators of hepcidin production, they directly inhibit EPO production, and they antagonize the antiapoptotic action of EPO on RBC progenitor cells.

PREVALENCE OF ANEMIA IN CHRONIC KIDNEY DISEASE

The prevalence of anemia in CKD depends on what definition of anemia is used. A commonly used classification, now quite old, is based on a World Health Organization Report from 1968 which defined anemia as a hemoglobin (Hb) <13 g/dL in men and <12 in women. In one study (Levin, 1996), CKD patients were categorized into four groups based on their creatinine clearance (>50 mL/min, 35 to 49, 25 to 34, and <25). The prevalence of anemia according to the above definition increased from around 25% in patients with early renal insufficiency to more than 80% for the group with a creatinine clearance of <25 mL/min. Data from the Third National Health and Nutrition Examination Survey (Hsu, 2002) showed a statistically significant decrease in Hb among men that began when creatinine clearance was <70 mL/min, and among women when creatinine clearance was <50. In men with a creatinine clearance between 20 and 30, the Hb was 1.4 g/dL lower than in men with a normal creatinine clearance, whereas the decrement in women was 1.0 g/dL.

POTENTIAL BENEFITS OF CORRECTING ANEMIA

Moderately Severe Anemia

For the correction of severe anemia (Hb in the range of 6.0 to 9.0 g/dL, which often was seen in dialysis patients before the availability of EPO), the benefits of anemia correction are not in dispute. Correction of anemia markedly reduces the need for blood transfusions with the attendant risks of viral infection and immune sensitization (which might compromise eligibility and outcomes of a future kidney transplant). Exercise tolerance, quality of life, and cognitive function are markedly improved, as is cardiac status. Also, there is an increased risk of bleeding that is due to prolongation of the bleeding time when Hb is <10 g/dL. Correction of Hb can reduce the bleeding time toward normal. The improvement is presumably due to improved functional platelet localization to the periphery of blood vessels at higher Hb levels and also to increased fibrinogen and factor VIII levels.

Correction of Mild Anemia

After erythropoiesis-stimulating agents (ESAs) corrected severe anemia in dialysis patients, attention focused on the potential benefits of correcting mild anemia (in the range of 9 to 11 g/dL) to normal or almost normal levels (in the range of 12 to 14). Here the results are not so clear-cut, and evidence of increased risk became apparent in several important and much-publicized randomized controlled trials.

Cardiovascular End-Point Results

For the so-called hard outcome measures—including mortality, hospitalizations, and cardiovascular events—there is a discrepancy between the observational data and that obtained from randomized controlled trials. A large amount of observational data suggested that mortality and cardiovascular complications are reduced at high Hb concentrations, and this trend continues up through relatively high Hb levels (e.g., 13 g/dL). This, however, is in contrast to results from randomized controlled trials, which all show a similar pattern. The first large trial in predialysis patients, CREATE (Drueke, 2006), showed no difference in the primary end point (a composite of eight cardiovascular events) in patients randomized to a hemoglobin of 13 to 15 g/dL versus a hemoglobin of 10.5 to 11.5. The second study, CHOIR (Singh, 2006), indicated a significantly worse primary end point (a composite of four cardiovascular end points) in patients randomized to a hemoglobin of 13.5 g/dL versus those randomized to a hemoglobin of 11.3. In a third large trial, the TREAT study (Pfeffer, 2009), predialysis diabetic CKD patients were given either an EPO-like drug (darbepoetin alfa) or placebo to a target Hb level of 13 g/dL. The rates of occurrence of cardiovascular end points were not different between the two Hb groups. Transfusions in the darbepoetin alfa group were 44% lower compared to placebo ($p < 0.001$), and there was a modest reduction in patient fatigue, but the price was a statistically significant increase in stroke and venous thromboembolism.

Improved Quality of Life

Observational data suggest that quality of life increases in a relatively linear fashion up to normal Hb concentrations, and the CREATE randomized controlled study showed significantly improved quality of life at a hemoglobin of around 14 g/dL versus a hemoglobin of around 10 to 11. Most other controlled studies have shown similar findings, the one exception being the CHOIR study, in which the increment in Hb between the two groups was probably too small to be able to detect a significant difference. In the TREAT trial, fatigue was reduced in the darbepoetin-treated group targeting a hemoglobin level of 13 g/dL compared with controls.

Regression of Left Ventricular Hypertrophy

Observational studies in which left ventricular hypertrophy and Hb are measured show a significant inverse association between the two, even up to Hb values in the near-normal range (Cerasola, 2011). However, in the Canadian randomized trial (Levin, 2005), administration of ESAs failed to show any effect on left ventricular mass index over a 24-month period compared with a control group in which ESAs were not given. The Hb levels in the two groups at the end of the Canadian trial were 12.7 versus 11.5 g/dL, respectively; these were not very different, possibly accounting for the negative results. In agreement with observational studies, in those patients in whom Hb levels fell, the left ventricular mass index did increase.

Transfusion Avoidance

When treating mild anemia, a transfusion benefit still occurs, but to a much lesser extent than when correcting severe anemia, because usually there is no need for transfusion when the Hb is >10 g/dL. The situation in which a transfusion reduction may occur after correction of mild anemia, for example, is when the patient suffers bleeding or another event that acutely lowers Hb by, for example, 3 g/dL. Because the patient is now starting at a higher Hb baseline, the postevent Hb does not diminish to a value at which transfusion is deemed necessary.

APPROACH TO ANEMIA IN CHRONIC KIDNEY DISEASE

Many detailed guidelines have been published on the approach to the anemic CKD patient. All of these are consistent with the author's simplified three-step approach to managing this condition: (a) exclude another cause for anemia, (b) correct iron deficiency if present, and (c) treat with ESA if Hb is still not within the desired target range.

Determining the Cause for Anemia

The first step is to exclude another cause for anemia. This is relevant for all stages of CKD but is particularly important for patients in CKD stages 1 to 3, in whom it is much less likely that EPO deficiency alone is the cause of the anemia. Thus, a minimum workup for anemia should include investigation for gastrointestinal blood loss (essential if iron deficiency is present) and measurement of factors related to RBC production, namely serum ferritin (reflecting iron status), serum vitamin B_{12}, and folate levels. The C-reactive protein (CRP) level may be helpful in screening for an underlying inflammatory condition. Low levels of 25 vitamin D (see Chapter 8) have been associated with an increased risk of anemia in CKD patients even after adjusting for levels of parathyroid hormone (Patel, 2010); although it is reasonable to recommend that low 25-D levels should be sought and corrected if found, there is no evidence from interventional trials that this helps to correct anemia. Hyperparathyroidism can cause anemia because of its secondary fibrotic actions on the bone marrow; serum parathyroid hormone levels should be determined and corrected to the extent possible as described in Chapter 8. Investigation for hemolysis and primary bone marrow disorders may be indicated in individual cases. In certain geographical areas and ethnic groups, a hemoglobinopathy screen may be helpful to exclude thalassemia or sickle cell disease. In patients who have renal impairment and anemia in whom the cause of the kidney disease has not been ascertained, serum immunoglobulins and protein electrophoresis should be performed to exclude myeloma as a cause for both conditions.

Diagnosis of Iron Deficiency

The gold standard measure of iron stores relevant to erythropoiesis is a biopsy core of the bone marrow that has been stained for iron. This is rarely done, and several laboratory tests of the blood are used to assess whether a patient has iron deficiency.

Ferritin

Ferritin is a ubiquitously present protein that is used to store iron in a nontoxic form. Free iron is toxic to cells, because it acts as a catalyst to form free radicals. Within cells, iron is safely bound to ferritin. Ferritin can be thought of as a barrel for iron, and in fact it is structured as a large hollow sphere pierced by channels through which iron can enter. Ferritin is a storage molecule and not an iron transporter. However, some ferritin leaks out of cells and is found in the serum, such that serum ferritin levels normally reflect total-body iron stores. Serum ferritin is normally cleared by the liver, and in the case of liver dysfunction, this clearance mechanism falters, and serum ferritin levels can be markedly increased without any iron overload. Ferritin also is an acute phase reactant, and serum ferritin levels increase markedly in certain cancers, in malnutrition, and with inflammation. Recognizing iron deficiency is easy if the absolute ferritin level is <50 mcg/L, but ferritin levels well in excess of 100 mcg/L still may coexist with iron deficiency if there is concomitant inflammation (the CRP level may give a clue).

Transferrin, Serum Iron, and Transferrin Saturation

The main transporter of iron in the blood is **transferrin**, a glycoprotein made mostly in the liver. Each transferrin molecule has the capacity to carry two iron molecules. When a transferrin molecule loaded with iron encounters a cell with a transferrin receptor, it docks, and the molecule is taken into the cell by endocytosis via a vesicle that forms around it. Once inside the cell, the transferrin molecule releases its iron, and then the empty molecule is extruded.

All of the iron in the blood that is not bound to Hb is present in the serum bound to transferrin. Normal serum iron values range from 60 to 175 mcg/dL (11 to 31 mcmol/L). As a surrogate for serum transferrin, the **total iron binding capacity (TIBC)** is usually measured; this test measures the maximum amount of iron that the serum can carry. In effect, TIBC reflects transferrin, because after loading the serum sample with iron, the measurable iron is proportional to the now fully loaded transferrin concentration in the serum, but the units are in terms of iron. Normal values for TIBC are 240 to 450 mcg/dL (43.0 to 80.6 mcmol/L). The **percent transferrin saturation** (TSAT) is calculated by dividing the serum iron by the TIBC, and is usually about 30% (range 20% to 50%).

In the case of **true (or absolute) iron deficiency**, the serum iron level will be low, and transferrin levels are elevated (a compensatory response), leading to a low TSAT, <20%. Serum ferritin levels also will be low. In the case of **functional iron deficiency**, a condition in which total-body iron stores are normal or even increased, but there is a failure to deliver iron to the bone marrow rapidly enough to meet the demand, ferritin levels are normal or high, while TSAT is low. This may occur either with excessively enhanced erythropoiesis, or alternatively in the presence of inflammation, when **reticuloendothelial blockade** occurs. In the latter condition, hepcidin levels are high, lowering the density of ferroportin on reticuloendothelial cells and enterocytes. The low ferroportin density severely inhibits iron entry into the blood from the gut (via enterocytes) and from recycling (via the reticuloendothelial cells). Serum iron in such a case will also be low. TSAT may not be much reduced, as inflammation can suppress synthesis of transferrin, so TIBC, the denominator of TSAT, is reduced as well as serum iron, the numerator. With inflammation, ferritin levels may be normal or high, even when total-body iron stores are actually depleted. Thus, **malnutrition or inflammation** will increase serum ferritin, leading to a reduction of its sensitivity as a marker of iron deficiency, and inflammation will lower serum transferrin, raising the TSAT for any given level of serum iron and potentially masking iron deficiency.

The associations of TSAT and ferritin with mortality were studied in 461 male patients evaluated for nondialysis CKD at a U.S. veterans hospital (Kovesdy, 2009). Mortality was lowest when TSAT was 20% to 30% and increased markedly at lower values. Mortality increased when ferritin was >300, probably reflecting inflammation. The lowest mortality was when ferritin was >100 and TSAT was >15%.

Reticulocyte Hemoglobin Content

The reticulocyte hemoglobin content is a readily available test on the standard automated complete blood count. It measures the amount of Hb in reticulocytes, which are newly produced RBCs. As such, it is a measure of the recent availability of iron for erythropoiesis. This test is less affected by inflammation than either ferritin or transferrin saturation. Normal values are 24.5 to 31.8 pg. Iron deficiency is indicated by values of 26 pg or lower, with values of 28 pg or lower being suggestive of this condition.

NONHEMATOLOGIC EFFECTS OF IRON

Iron has a number of physiologic functions beyond red cell development, including nerve and muscle function (myoglobin), mitochondrial function, and energy generation. Correction of iron deficiency has been shown to have a number of effects on the body that do not seem to be related to changes in Hb level. These include improvements in physical performance and cognitive function, restoration of ability to maintain core body temperature in response to cold stress, amelioration of restless legs syndrome, and improvement of neutrophil and macrophage function. On the other hand, a number of bacteria require iron for growth, and supplementation of iron to malnourished children can increase their rates of death from infectious causes (Sazawal, 2006).

REPLACING IRON

Patients not yet on dialysis are different from those undergoing hemodialysis in that their maintenance iron needs are lower. Iron replacement can be implemented either orally or using one of several intravenous (IV) iron preparations that are available. In more advanced stages of CKD, partly because of hepcidin-induced reduction of gut iron absorption and partly because of increased gastrointestinal blood loss, regular IV iron administration often is required. In those patients also requiring an ESA, use of IV iron is required because of enhanced iron needs for stimulated erythropoiesis. Oral iron may be sufficient to maintain iron stores in some CKD patients, although a number of studies have found that the rate of increase of Hb, as well as the final increase in Hb, often is lower with oral iron than if IV iron is used.

Oral Iron

This has traditionally been given as ferrous sulfate, fumarate, or gluconate, with a usual dosage of 200 mg/day. Absorption is higher if the iron is given on an empty stomach; however, side effects, particularly dyspepsia and bloating, may then be worse. Other problems with oral iron include constipation and diarrhea, and, of course, the stools will become black in color. Because the absorption of iron is increased at low gastric pH, absorption of oral iron is lower when drugs used to increase gastric pH such as antacids or histamine-2 antagonists or proton pump inhibitors are used concomitantly. Delayed-release preparations of iron are available, which minimize release of iron in the stomach with the goal of decreasing dyspepsia. In recent times, several newer preparations of oral iron have become available, such as iron polysaccharide complexes (Niferex-150, Nu-Iron 150), heme iron polypeptide, and ferric citrate. The most promising of these is ferric citrate, which was originally developed as a phosphate binder, but which was found to be absorbed more readily than ferrous iron salts, and which could evoke an increase in serum ferritin and transferrin saturation even in hemodialysis patients.

Intravenous Iron Preparations

IV iron compounds have been available for several decades. When parenteral administration of iron salts was found to be toxic in the 1930s, strategies were developed to complex the iron salts with a carbohydrate polymer to allow slow release of iron from the iron–carbohydrate complex, at a rate at which it could be bound to transferrin. The prototype compound was iron dextran, and other iron–carbohydrate complexes such as iron sucrose and sodium ferric gluconate followed. Newer iron preparations include ferric carboxymaltose, iron isomaltoside-1000, and ferumoxytol. These latter compounds allow larger quantities of iron to be given IV as a single administration, and may be particularly useful in patients who are needle-phobic, those with poor venous access, and those living far from the hospital.

Potential Risks of Intravenous Iron

Potential risks of IV iron include very rare, but sometimes life-threatening, hypersensitivity reactions. Fatal anaphylactic reactions were previously seen with a high molecular weight iron dextran which was subsequently withdrawn from the market. Other concerns about IV iron include its potential to exacerbate oxidative stress and infections. More recently, some, but not all, IV iron preparations have been associated with the development of hypophosphatemia, possibly exacerbating osteomalacia.

Hypersensitivity Reactions to IV Iron. All IV iron preparations have the potential to induce hypersensitivity reactions. Most of these are mild and self-limiting, but occasionally more severe reactions are seen. The anaphylactic reactions previously seen with iron dextran were believed to be mediated via immunoglobulin, whereas the pathogenesis of the milder reactions seen nowadays seems to be due to free iron in circulation, or alternatively complement activation–related pseudoallergy (CARPA). One of the major factors in the development of IV iron reactions is the speed of iron administration, and reducing the dose and rate of administration may be helpful.

Infection. Iron is a key nutrient that many pathogenic bacteria, including *Staphylococci*, thrive on. Iron also may interfere with phagocytic ability of white blood cells. Data from large observational studies have been conflicting as far as an association between IV iron and infections is concerned, with some studies suggesting an association and others showing no such association. Randomized controlled data are lacking and are much needed. In the meantime, IV iron should not be given during episodes of acute bacterial or fungal infection.

Oxidation and Kidney Damage. Some iron invariably escapes from the infused carrier, and in vitro studies have shown increased serum markers of oxidation after IV iron infusion. Of some concern is a study by Agarwal (2004), in which an infusion of IV iron resulted not only in blood markers of oxidative damage but also transient proteinuria and excretion in the urine of markers of kidney injury. However, two recent randomized controlled trials have failed to show any adverse effect of IV iron on progression of renal impairment (Agarwal, 2015; Macdougall, 2014).

Intravenous Iron Administration Strategies

In managing outpatients, the need to administer an appropriate amount of IV iron conveniently is a challenge. There is the need for IV access, the potential risk of damaging veins that may be needed in the future for vascular access, and the need to schedule sometimes repeated outpatient appointments. The older iron preparations have a maximum recommended infusion amount per sitting of 125 to 200 mg of iron, which may be satisfactory for use in hemodialysis patients. For nondialysis patients, however, the ability to forego multiple injections is a distinct advantage. The newer IV iron preparations, such as ferumoxytol and ferric carboxymaltose, allow larger doses of iron to be given more rapidly at a single sitting.

Calculating the Initial Iron Deficit

Formulae have been devised in an attempt to calculate the body's iron deficits (e.g., Ganzoni), and therefore the dose of iron required. Unfortunately, these are somewhat flawed, since they take into account the hemoglobin and the ferritin deficits, but no consideration is given to iron losses from the body. Their utility in routine clinical practice remains questionable.

Intravenous Iron Administration

For each IV iron product, there is a maximum amount of iron that can safely be given at one time, and the amount also depends on whether the iron product is given as a slow IV push or an IV infusion. The practitioner should refer to product safety labeling information for these limits. For **iron sucrose**, current (always check the most recently updated labeling) U.S.-approved infusion guidelines are 200 mg given IV push over 2 to 5 minutes. For **ferric gluconate**, 125 mg can be given over 10 minutes. For **ferumoxytol**, a 30-mL vial containing 510 mg of elemental iron can be infused over 30 minutes. With **ferric carboxymaltose**, up to 1,000 mg dissolved in normal saline can be given over 15 minutes as a single infusion. With ferumoxytol and ferric carboxymaltose, the number of sessions of treatment can be reduced, as larger doses can be given at a single sitting.

Therapeutic Trial of Intravenous Iron

In anemic nondialysis CKD patients, there is controversy over whether oral iron should be tried first or whether IV iron may be more effective. Many physicians will try oral iron, and if there is lack of efficacy or gastrointestinal intolerance (which can occur in up to 30% of patients), then IV iron may be used. The FIND-CKD trial (Macdougall, 2014) showed that IV iron, targeting a higher ferritin level of 400 to 600 mcg/L, achieves a larger and faster increment in hemoglobin than oral iron. Availability of services to deliver IV iron will also significantly impact on whether IV iron may be used.

ERYTHROPOIESIS-STIMULATING AGENT THERAPY

The final stepwise approach to managing CKD anemia is the introduction of ESA therapy. Many agents are now available worldwide, and these can be divided into short-, medium-, and long-acting agents. The original agents **(epoetin alfa or beta)** were short acting, and were preparations of human EPO manufactured using recombinant DNA technology. The main disadvantage of epoetin was the need for twice- or thrice-weekly administration, and so strategies were developed to prolong the duration of action of the molecule.

A medium-acting preparation with extra carbohydrate side chains (**darbepoetin alfa; Aranesp**) was introduced in 2002, and 5 years later a pegylated form of epoetin was released (**methoxy polyethylene glycol epoetin beta or continuous erythropoietin receptor activator [CERA; Mircera]**). Since then, following expiry of the patent for epoetin, several "biosimilar" preparations of epoetin have been available in Europe since 2009, and subsequently have become available in the United States. In clinical practice, epoetin usually is given two to three times a week IV (hemodialysis patients) or subcutaneously, darbepoetin once weekly or every 2 weeks, and CERA once a month in the maintenance phase.

Risks of Erythropoiesis-Stimulating Agent Therapy

The interaction between ESA and a higher Hb concentration to increase the risk of cardiovascular disease (CHOIR study) and stroke (TREAT study) has been discussed above. It still is not clear if a higher Hb per se is harmful, or if driving the Hb up to higher levels using ESA therapy may be responsible for these adverse effects. The exact mechanisms by which ESA therapy may be harmful are not well understood.

Iron Deficiency, Stroke Risk, Erythropoiesis-Stimulating Agent Therapy, and Thrombocytosis

Iron deficiency is known to increase platelet count and risk of thrombotic events (Keung and Owen, 2004). In some reports, thrombosis risk was noted to be high with iron deficiency, independent of the platelet count. These two factors may play a role in the increased mortality seen with ESA treatment in randomized trials, in which mortality could be related to a higher ESA dose (Szczech, 2008). High ESA doses may increase the platelet count, given that EPO and thrombopoietin, the hormone that stimulates platelet generation, are closely related. Also, high ESA doses may increase the platelet count by creating a state of functional iron deficiency (Besarab, 2009). In one observational study of a large number of dialysis patients, those in whom Hb levels were >13 g/dL showed an increased risk of mortality if there was coexisting thrombocytosis (Streja, 2008). The clinical implications of these concepts are not completely clear.

Other Risks of Erythropoiesis-Stimulating Agent Treatment

Worsening of hypertension and, uncommonly, associated encephalopathy and seizures are known adverse effects of ESA treatment and are more likely to occur when the rise in Hb is very rapid. Also, there is an increased risk of venous thrombosis according to reports in which ESAs were given in a perisurgical setting. There has been controversy for many years as to whether ESA therapy exacerbates tumor growth or is harmful in patients with malignancy; the latest evidence suggests that as long as the guidelines are followed, particularly in relation to target hemoglobin, then this risk is probably small.

Target Hemoglobin Levels

The current target Hb levels for anemia in predialysis CKD patients vary slightly between various guideline bodies, but are generally in the range of 10 to 12 g/dL. In the United States, the Food and Drug Administration (FDA) has insisted that all EPO-like drugs (known as ESAs) carry a "black box warning" informing the care provider as well as the patient about the risks of targeting a high Hb value with ESA therapy. In recent times, the target hemoglobin range has become stricter in the United States than in Europe and the rest of the world, with many U.S. physicians aiming for a target hemoglobin of between 10 and 11 g/dL, compared to physicians in the rest of the world, who aim for a target hemoglobin of 10 to 12 g/dL.

Erythropoiesis-Stimulating Agent Dosing Recommendations

ESA treatment should not be started if there is evidence of iron deficiency. Once iron stores are replete, initial ESA therapy can be introduced. The dosing frequency depends on the product used (Table 22.1). If epoetin therapy is used, then starting doses in the range of 2,000 IU twice or thrice weekly are appropriate (sometimes epoetin is dosed weekly). For darbepoetin alfa, a reasonable starting dose would be 20 to 30 mcg/wk (or 40 to 60 mcg every alternate week). CERA may be commenced at a dose of 30 to 50 mcg every 2 weeks, or alternatively 75 to 50 mcg/mo. Doses calculated per kg body weight are not usually required, although often this is recommended in the product literature and summary of product characteristics for the ESAs.

Adjusting the Dose and Monitoring

It is important to recheck the Hb 2 to 4 weeks after starting ESA therapy so that the increment in Hb can be assessed and the ESA

	Stepwise Approach to the Management of Chronic Kidney Disease Anemia

Exclude other causes of anemia, especially if eGFR >60 mL/min

Exclude and treat iron deficiency with a trial of IV iron, if necessary

If Hb still <10 g/dL AND eGFR <60 mL/min AND not iron deficient, then consider starting ESA therapy
- *Epoetin 2,000 units 2–3x/week or 6,000 units once weekly*
- *Darbepoetin alfa 30 mcg/wk or 60–75 mcg every 2 weeks*
- *CERA 30–50 mcg every 2 weeks or 75 mcg every month*

Monitor Hb every 2–4 weeks

If Hb response <1 g/dL in first 4 weeks, and Hb still below target, then increase the dose of ESA by 50%

If no response after 2 months, then look for causes of EPO resistance, and consider algorithm shown in Figure 22.1

Monitor iron status (ferritin, TSAT) every 3 months or so, and supplement as necessary

eGFR, estimated glomerular filtration rate normalized to 1.73 m² body surface area; IV, intravenous; Hb, hemoglobin; ESA, erythropoiesis-stimulating agent; CERA, continuous erythropoietin receptor activator; TSAT, transferrin saturation.

Poor response to ESAs - investigation

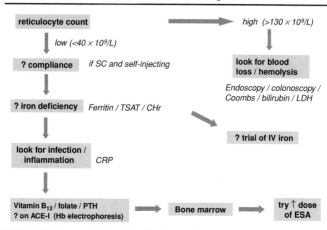

FIGURE 22.1 Suggested clinical algorithm for managing a poor response to erythropoiesis-stimulating agent therapy. SC, subcutaneously injected; CHr, reticulocyte hemoglobin content; CRP, C-reactive protein; LDH, lactate dehydrogenase.

dose adjusted as required. The U.S. FDA in the ESA package insert warns that the rate of Hb rise should not exceed 1 g/dL in any 2-week period. The Hb should continue to be monitored at 2 to 4 weekly intervals until the level stabilizes, realizing that this will not occur at a given ESA dose until 60 to 100 days. The dose of ESA should not be increased by more than once in a given month, and not at all in the first month; even if the Hb has not increased much in the first 2 weeks, the long delay in ESA effect may be responsible for the apparent lack of response. If the Hb exceeds 12 g/dL, the ESA dose should be reduced, probably by around 25%, and the dose should be held if the Hb exceeds 13 g/dL, restarting at a lower level once Hb decreases to ≤12 g/dL. The blood pressure should be monitored regularly; a sustained increase in blood pressure of 10/5 systolic/diastolic should be reported immediately and prompt an evaluation of the Hb level and the ESA dose. Whereas current guidelines do not call for monitoring of platelets, in patients with higher platelet counts, particular caution should be exercised in giving higher doses of ESAs, and consideration should be given to ensuring that iron stores have been fully repleted.

Causes of Erythropoiesis-Stimulating Agent Resistance

Causes of ESA resistance include iron insufficiency, inflammation and infection, covert or occult bleeding, and sometimes previously undetected malignancy. Hyperparathyroidism, severe enough to reduce erythropoiesis, occurs much less commonly in nondialysis CKD patients compared with those on dialysis.

Erythropoiesis-Stimulating Agent Resistance

Because the ESA dose response curve does tend to plateau, and because high ESA doses have, for whatever reason, been associated with a poor outcome in randomized trials such as the CHOIR study (Szczech, 2008), one should avoid the temptation to markedly increase the ESA dose. Attention should focus on making sure that iron stores are repleted, perhaps giving a trial of IV iron and looking for sources of occult bleeding, inflammation, or malignancy.

Pure Red Cell Aplasia and Antierythropoietin Antibodies

A very rare complication of ESA therapy is the induction of antierythropoietin antibodies, causing severe transfusion-dependent pure red cell aplasia. This was a major problem a few years ago with one of the epoetin alfa preparations marketed outside the United States (Eprex; Erypo in Germany), although it was subsequently reported to occur with epoetin beta and darbepoetin alfa, also. Experimental evidence suggested that this may be due to the combination of a number of factors, including the generation of immune adjuvants caused by rubber leachates in the syringes used for administration of this agent, a break in the cold storage chain, and possible breakdown or aggregation of the protein by other factors. The single most important factor was the removal of human serum albumin from the formulation, as mandated by the European Union following concerns about Creutzfeldt–Jakob disease in the late 1990s.

Replacement of the rubber plungers in the Eprex syringes with Teflon stoppers seems to have reduced the incidence of this condition, but the exact triggering mechanism for this condition is still not clear. It does seem to be related to the formulation of the ESA and also the storage conditions, and it is particularly a concern with cheaper "copy" epoetin products from less developed parts of the world. It is likely that in the future non–protein-based ESAs will become available, and these may be less immunogenic, avoiding this complication altogether.

Peginesatide (Hematide)

Peginesatide (Hematide) was a peptide-based ESA manufactured using cheaper synthetic chemistry techniques rather than the more expensive recombinant DNA technology. Following successful completion of a phase 3 program, this product was licensed as Omontys in the United States for use in dialysis patients. Unfortunately, within 1 year of launch, several life-threatening and fatal anaphylactic reactions were seen, and the product was voluntarily withdrawn from the market. One of the major advantages of this ESA was that it did not produce antibodies that cross-reacted with either endogenous or recombinant EPO, and therefore should never cause pure red cell aplasia. Indeed, peginesatide was used successfully to treat patients who had developed antibody-mediated pure red cell aplasia induced by other ESAs (Macdougall, 2009).

HIF Stabilizers (Prolyl Hydroxylase Inhibitors)

A new strategy for stimulating erythropoiesis involves an orally active molecule that mimics hypoxia by causing stabilization of hypoxia-inducible factor-alfa (HIF-alfa), the major transcription factor for the EPO gene. Thus, administration of a HIF stabilizer will increase the endogenous production of EPO, even in dialysis-dependent CKD, and is effective in correcting anemia (Koury and Haase, 2015; Maxwell and Eckardt, 2016). Four such agents completed their phase 2 program (roxadustat, daprodustat, vadadustat, and molidustat), and three of these are currently in phase 3 trials. Apart from being orally active, one of the major advantages of this new class of drugs is their ability to improve iron availability, probably via an effect on iron regulatory genes and an indirect effect on hepcidin. Although the studies to date have not raised any concerns, potentially these agents can upregulate several hundred other genes, and their long-term safety will have to be proven (Tanaka and Eckardt, 2018).

References and Suggested Readings

Agarwal R. Nonhematological benefits of iron. *Am J Nephrol.* 2007;27:565–571.

Agarwal R. Individualizing decision-making—resurrecting the doctor-patient relationship in the anemia debate. *Clin J Am Soc Nephrol.* 2010;5:1340–1346.

Agarwal R, Kusek JW, Pappas MK. A randomized trial of intravenous and oral iron in chronic kidney disease. *Kidney Int.* 2015;88:905–914.

Agarwal R, Vasavada N, Sachs NG, et al. Oxidative stress and renal injury with intravenous iron in patients with chronic kidney disease. *Kidney Int.* 2004;65:2279–2289.

Barraclough KA, Noble E, Leary D, et al. Rationale and design of the oral HEMe iron polypeptide Against Treatment with Oral Controlled Release Iron Tablets trial for the correction of anaemia in peritoneal dialysis patients (HEMATOCRIT trial). *BMC Nephrol.* 2009;10:20.

Besarab A, Hörl WH, Silverberg D. Iron metabolism, iron deficiency, thrombocytosis, and the cardiorenal anemia syndrome. *Oncologist.* 2009;14:22–33.

Cerasola G, Nardi E, Palermo A, et al. Epidemiology and pathophysiology of left ventricular abnormalities in chronic kidney disease: a review. *J Nephrol.* 2011;24:1–10.

Devine BJ. Gentamicin therapy. *Drug Intell Clin Pharm.* 1974;8:650–655.

Drueke TB, Locatelli F, Clyne N, et al. Normalization of hemoglobin level in patients with chronic kidney disease and anemia. *N Engl J Med.* 2006;355:2071–2084.

Fliser D, Haller H. Erythropoietin and treatment of non-anemic conditions—cardiovascular protection. *Semin Hematol.* 2007;44:212–217.

Hsu CY, McCulloch CE, Curhan GC. Epidemiology of anemia associated with chronic renal insufficiency among adults in the United States: results from the Third National Health and Nutrition Examination Survey. *J Am Soc Nephrol.* 2002;13:504–510.

Kalicki RM, Uehlinger DE. Red cell survival in relation to changes in the hematocrit: more important than you think. *Blood Purif.* 2008;26:355–360.

Keung YK, Owen J. Iron deficiency and thrombosis: literature review. *Clin Appl Thromb Hemost.* 2004;10:387–391.

Koury MJ, Haase VH. Anaemia in kidney disease: harnessing hypoxia responses for therapy. *Nat Rev Nephrol.* 2015;11:394–410.

Kovesdy CP, Estrada W, Ahmadzadeh S, et al. Association of markers of iron stores with outcomes in patients with nondialysis-dependent chronic kidney disease. *Clin J Am Soc Nephrol.* 2009;4:435–441.

Kruse A, Thijssen S, Kotanko P, et al. Relationship between red blood cell lifespan and inflammation. *J Am Soc Nephrol.* 2009;20:173A (Abstract).

Levin A, Djurdjev O, Thompson C, et al. Canadian randomized trial of hemoglobin maintenance to prevent or delay left ventricular mass growth in patients with CKD. *Am J Kidney Dis.* 2005;46:799–811.

Levin A, Singer J, Thompson CR, et al. Prevalent left ventricular hypertrophy in the predialysis population: identifying opportunities for intervention. *Am J Kidney Dis.* 1996;27:347–354.

Macdougall IC, Bock AH, Carrera F, et al; FIND-CKD Study Investigators. FIND-CKD: a randomized trial of intravenous ferric carboxymaltose versus oral iron in patients with chronic kidney disease and iron deficiency anaemia. *Nephrol Dial Transplant.* 2014;29:2075–2084.

Macdougall IC, Rossert J, Casadevall N, et al. A peptide-based erythropoietin-receptor agonist for pure red-cell aplasia. *N Engl J Med.* 2009;361:1848–1855.

Maxwell PH, Eckardt KU. HIF prolyl hydroxylase inhibitors for the treatment of renal anaemia and beyond. *Nat Rev Nephrol.* 2016;12:157–168.

McMahon LP, Kent AB, Kerr PG, et al. Maintenance of elevated versus physiological iron indices in non-anaemic patients with chronic kidney disease: a randomized controlled trial. *Nephrol Dial Transplant.* 2010;25:920–926.

Patel NM, Gutiérrez OM, Andress DL, et al. Vitamin D deficiency and anemia in early chronic kidney disease. *Kidney Int.* 2010;77:715–720.

Peters HP, Laarakkers CM, Swinkels DW, et al. Serum hepcidin-25 levels in patients with chronic kidney disease are independent of glomerular filtration rate. *Nephrol Dial Transplant.* 2010;25:848–853.

Pfeffer MA, Burdmann EA, Chen CY, et al; TREAT Investigators. A trial of darbepoetin alfa in type 2 diabetes and chronic kidney disease. *N Engl J Med.* 2009;361:2019–2032.

Sazawal S, Black RE, Ramsan M, et al. Effects of routine prophylactic supplementation with iron and folic acid on admission to hospital and mortality in preschool children in a high malaria transmission setting: community-based, randomised, placebo-controlled trial. *Lancet.* 2006;367:133–143.

Singh AK, Szczech L, Tang KL, et al. Correction of anemia with epoetin alfa in chronic kidney disease. *N Engl J Med.* 2006;355:2085–2098.

Stancu S, Bârsan L, Stanciu A, et al. Can the response to iron therapy be predicted in anemic nondialysis patients with chronic kidney disease? *Clin J Am Soc Nephrol.* 2010;5:409–416.

Streja E, Kovesdy CP, Greenland S, et al. Erythropoietin, iron depletion, and relative thrombocytosis: a possible explanation for hemoglobin-survival paradox in hemodialysis. *Am J Kidney Dis.* 2008;52:727–736.

Szczech LA, Barnhart HX, Inrig JK, et al. Secondary analysis of the CHOIR trial epoetin-alpha dose and achieved hemoglobin outcomes. *Kidney Int.* 2008;74:791–798.

Tanaka T, Eckardt KU. HIF activation against CVD in CKD: novel treatment opportunities. *Semin Nephrol.* 2018;38:267–276.

World Health Organization Technical Report Series. No. 405. Nutritional Anaemias: Report of a WHO scientific group, Geneva, 1968. Available from http://apps.who.int/iris/handle/10665/40707. Accessed June 6, 2018.

23

Drug Dosing in Chronic Kidney Disease

Gregory J. Roberti, Joseph B. Lockridge, and Ali J. Olyaei

INTRODUCTION

Impaired renal function changes the metabolism and elimination of many pharmacologic agents. The pharmacokinetics of some hepatically metabolized medications can be affected as well. Many of these drugs have pharmacologically active metabolites that are renally excreted. Additionally, chronic kidney disease (CKD) may nonspecifically inhibit hepatic cytochrome P450 (CYP)-based metabolism of medications. For a select group of medications, inactivation by enzymes within kidney cells plays an important role in their metabolism. For these reasons, to avoid drug toxicity and ensure therapeutic efficacy in CKD, dosage adjustment of many medications is required. In this chapter the pharmacologic parameters that are altered by renal dysfunction are summarized, and an approach to dosage adjustment is described.

ALTERED PHARMACOKINETIC PRINCIPLES IN RENAL FAILURE

A given drug may reach several different compartments in the body before being eliminated (Fig. 23.1). Alterations in renal function may affect bioavailability, volume of distribution, protein binding, biotransformation, or elimination.

Bioavailability

The bioavailability of a drug refers to the fraction of a dose which reaches systemic circulation. It is reported as a percentage. The rate and route of administration determine bioavailability. A medication given intravenously generally has 100% bioavailability because the entire dose by definition reaches the systemic circulation. When a dose is given by an oral, intramuscular, or subcutaneous route, a smaller percentage of the dose reaches the systemic circulation. For example, furosemide has 100% bioavailability when given intravenously but only 50% when taken orally. This fact explains the common practice of doubling the dose of furosemide when a patient is transitioned from intravenous to oral dosing. In patients with CKD, the bioavailability of oral furosemide ranges from 10% to 50%.

Medication absorption may be altered in patients with kidney disease for various reasons. For instance, uremia-induced vomiting or gastroparesis caused by neuropathic changes associated with concomitant diabetes mellitus or aging may impair oral absorption.

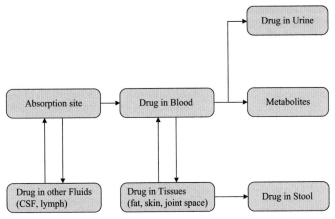

FIGURE 23.1 Factors that may alter the pharmacokinetics and pharmacodynamics.

Patients with CKD and heart failure or nephrotic syndrome commonly have bowel wall edema, which can diminish absorption. Concomitant administration of phosphate- or lipid-binding resins may result in the formation of insoluble complexes with the administered medication that limit drug absorption and slow gut motility. Absorption of medications such as the fluoroquinolones is impaired by the concurrent administration of iron and this may increase the risk of therapeutic failure.

Volume of Distribution
The volume of distribution (Vd) of a medication can be used to calculate the dose required to achieve a desired systemic drug level. The Vd does not refer to a specific anatomic compartment but is a hypothetical volume: It is a proportionality constant that relates the total amount of drug in the body to its serum concentration. As a general rule, there is an inverse correlation between the serum concentration and the Vd. By virtue of increasing total body water, edema and ascites tend to increase the Vd of water-soluble agents, resulting in lower serum concentrations. Conversely, both digoxin and insulin have been shown to have a markedly decreased Vd in end-stage renal disease (ESRD) patients, with relatively increased serum concentrations for a given dose.

Protein Binding
Although compounds circulate in both protein-bound and unbound forms, it is only the unbound form that is distributed and biologically active. The portion of a given agent that is bound to plasma proteins can be thought of as a storage pool. Renal dysfunction decreases protein binding for most medications because organic waste products block the binding sites on carrier proteins and thus displace the drug. Consequently, a larger proportion of the medication circulates

in its unbound, active form. For instance, acidosis and urea decrease binding of mycophenolate to albumin, which leads to an increase in mycophenolate free fraction. This, in turn, can increase mycophenolate clearance, causing lower total concentrations. Because standard drug assays often measure the total drug concentrations (i.e., both bound and unbound drug), it may be prudent to specifically monitor unbound drug levels. This is particularly important for medications with a narrow therapeutic window (e.g., phenytoin). Most acidic medications bind to albumin and most basic medications bind to nonalbumin proteins. There is one offsetting factor to reduced protein binding in CKD: most nonalbumin proteins are acute phase reactants, and in patients with CKD plasma levels of these, are often elevated. This results in increased protein binding of some alkaline medications such as propranolol and vancomycin.

Biotransformation

The liver and kidney are set up in series as a waste-processing system. Biotransformation of medications occurs mainly in the liver, although cells in the intestine, lungs, and kidney also can contain the enzymes that produce these reactions. These metabolic reactions have been divided into two phases. Phase 1 reactions, which are predominantly executed by the CYP system, detoxify medications and naturally occurring substances by reactions that primarily include oxidation, reduction, and hydrolysis. Phase 2 biotransformation reactions act to transform a parent medication or metabolite of a phase 1 reaction into a water-soluble compound that can be easily excreted in the urine or bile (Yeung, 2014).

It is a common misconception that in the CKD population, it is unnecessary to adjust the dosage for medications exclusively cleared by hepatic metabolism and transport. Reduction of CYP activity in CKD may increase medication accumulation and cause potential drug toxicity, even of medications that normally are not renally excreted (Nolin, 2015). Patients with CKD experience globally reduced activity of phase 1 biotransformation reactions by the CYP system due to both nonspecific inhibition of the liver enzymes and decreased activity of CYP reactions which, to a limited extent, occur in renal tissues. Reductions of CYP3A4 activity of up to 28% have been demonstrated in patients with ESRD (Dowling, 2003). The phase 2 hepatic conjugation reactions such as glucuronidation and acetylation are significantly reduced in CKD as well (Yeung, 2014).

Despite the known alterations in CYP drug metabolism due to CKD, it is difficult to predict which medications and under what clinical situations, significant variation in metabolic clearance warrants dosage adjustment. Several groups of clinically important CYP enzymes are presented in Table 23.1. When a second medication is given that is metabolized by the same CYP enzyme group as the first medication, the CYP biotransformation of the first medication is reduced, and its blood levels may increase. An example is the antiarrhythmic amiodarone in a patient taking cyclosporine: both are

TABLE 23.1 Drugs Metabolized by the P450 CYP3A4/5, CYP2C9/19, and CYP2D6 Enzyme Systems

CYP3A4/5	CYP2C9/19	CYP2D6
Amiodarone	Amiodarone	Carvedilol
Amlodipine	Amitriptyline	Desipramine
Azithromycin	Azole antifungals	Nortriptyline
Cannabinoids	Chloramphenicol	Propranolol
Clarithromycin	Celecoxib	Metoprolol
Cyclosporine	Cimetidine	Timolol
Danazol	Diclofenac	
Delavirdine	Fluoxetine	
Diltiazem	Fluvastatin	
Erythromycin	Fluvoxamine	
Fluconazole	Glipizide	
Fluoxetine	Glyburide	
Fluvoxamine	Ibuprofen	
Grapefruit juice	Irbesartan	
Indinavir	Losartan	
Itraconazole	Metronidazole	
Ketoconazole	Omeprazole	
Metronidazole	Phenytoin	
Mibefradil	Ritonavir	
Miconazole	Rosiglitazone	
Nefazodone	Rosuvastatin	
Nelfinavir	Tolbutamide	
Norfloxacin	Warfarin	
Omeprazole		
Propoxyphene		
Quinine		
Ritonavir		
Saquinavir		
Sertraline		
Troleandomycin		
Verapamil		
Zafirlukast		

CYP, cytochrome P.

metabolized by CYP3A, and as a result of inhibition of CYP3A by amiodarone, the plasma cyclosporine levels can increase substantially.

Biotransformation reactions most often result in inactive metabolites, but notable exceptions exist that may have untoward effects in the CKD patient. The antidiabetic agent glyburide has pharmacologically active metabolites that depend partially on renal elimination; these accumulate in CKD, increasing the risk of hypoglycemia. The narcotic meperidine is metabolized to normeperidine, which requires renal elimination. Although normeperidine has little narcotic effect, it is a central nervous system irritant and can accumulate in patients with impaired renal function, lowering the seizure threshold. Morphine sulfate undergoes phase 2 metabolism to produce morphine-3-glucuronide (M3G) and morphine-6-glucuronide (M6G). Both metabolites may accumulate in CKD, with M3G decreasing the seizure threshold and M6G causing respiratory depression. Clinicians should be aware of renally cleared medications with active metabolites and the consequences of their accumulation in CKD.

In addition to the phase 1 and phase 2 biotransformation reactions discussed, the kidney itself can play a role in drug metabolism. The topic of insulin metabolism by the kidney is discussed in Chapter 13. Insulin is filtered at the glomerulus and metabolized in the proximal tubule. With CKD, this process is inhibited and as a result insulin can have a prolonged duration of action. The antibiotic imipenem is metabolized by renal enzymes called peptidases, and so its half-life will be substantially altered in CKD. For a more complete discussion of this topic, see Knights (2013).

Pharmacogenomics

Genome-based differences in drug metabolism and nephrotoxicity may be an important factor for optimal drug dosing and identifying patient subgroups that may be particularly resistant or sensitive to a given drug. For example, genetic variation in expression of *N*-acetyltransferase can result in significant drug toxicities in patients on antituberculosis (INH), antihypertensive (hydralazine), and antiarrhythmic agents (procainamide). Genetic variants are called "snips," or single-nucleotide polymorphisms (SNPs). The variability of the genome at these various SNPs is termed *polymorphism*. For example, significant polymorphism in P-glycoprotein and cytochrome P450 has been observed in different individuals. Polymorphisms of cytochrome P isoenzymes and P-glycoproteins may directly and/or indirectly influence adverse drug reactions and drug–drug interactions.

As another example, significant heterogeneity is present in the expression of angiotensin-converting enzyme (ACE). Insertion or deletion polymorphisms in genes controlling ACE expression may affect the clinical outcome after attempted pharmacologic blockade of the renin–angiotensin–aldosterone system (RAAS). For immunosuppressive agents, African-American and Hispanic patients require higher oral doses of some drugs than other ethnic groups to achieve the same target blood concentrations. These differences can be partly related to different polymorphism-related expression of intestinal P-glycoprotein (the product of the multiple drug resistance gene MDR-1) and of cytochrome P450-IIIA.

The U.S. Food and Drug Administration has approved pharmacogenomic testing of cytochrome P450 2C9 for individualizing warfarin therapy. Patients with low or high expression of CYP450 2C9 are at greater risk of bleeding or thrombosis, respectively. Knowledge of which gene variant is present can highlight those patients in whom lower or higher warfarin doses are likely to be necessary. In patients with CKD, studies of microarrays have shown a modulation of gene expression at different stages of kidney disease; however, it is not yet clear how useful many of these gene markers will be in clinical practice.

Age-Related Effect on Kidney Function and Drug Dosing

Aging processes may affect muscle mass, protein binding, hepatic and renal function, and relative amounts of intracellular mass versus body fat and thereby volume of distribution. These changes alter the pharmacokinetics and pharmacodynamics of most drugs. Age-related deterioration in kidney function occurs in the absence of any pathologic disorders. In the kidney, there is a 0.5- to 1-cm decrease in kidney length and a 20% to 30% reduction in kidney mass between the ages of 30 and 80 years with corresponding loss of renal function. On kidney biopsy, one finds increased fibrosis, tubular atrophy, and arteriosclerosis, as well as microvascular disease and reduced vascular responsiveness. Similar changes take place with age in the liver; liver size as well as blood flow decrease, slowing the rate of both phase 1 and phase 2 biotransformation reactions and prolonging the half-life of pharmacologic agents. Thus, when adjusting the dose of drugs in the elderly, more than just estimated glomerular filtration rate (eGFR) needs to be considered.

Neurocognitive disorders are common in the elderly. The cause is multifactorial, but often medications contribute significantly. Benzodiazepines and other sedative–hypnotic agents are often used for the management of anxiety or sleep disorders. Approximately 15% of patients with kidney disease use these agents, with significantly higher use among women, smokers, and patients with chronic obstructive pulmonary disease. The use of benzodiazepines has been associated with acute or chronic confusion. In most patients, drug-induced confusion and delirium are dose dependent. Aging and CKD prolong the plasma half-life of these and other drugs and extend exposure to these agents. In the assessment of cognitive disorders in the elderly, particularly patients with CKD, it is important to review all medications.

Many different pharmacologic agents may cause confusion; for example, lithium, digoxin, theophylline, steroids (prednisone), H_2 blockers (cimetidine), benzodiazepines, antidepressants (tricyclic), dopamine agonists (levodopa), narcotics (morphine, meperidine), β-blockers, and diuretics are well known to increase the risk of drug-induced confusion. Drugs that can precipitate fluid and electrolyte abnormalities may impair neurotransmission and have been implicated in the pathogenesis of confusion and delirium in patients with CKD. Pharmacologic agents that cause electrolyte abnormalities are listed in Table 23.2.

Among geriatric patients, falls are the leading cause of injury and death. Approximately 50% of nursing home and hospitalized patients over age 65 will experience a fall every year. Polypharmacy (four prescriptions or more) increases risk of falls. Use of sedative–hypnotics

TABLE 23.2	Drugs That Alter Electrolyte and Mineral Values	
Abnormality	**Medication**	**Mechanism**
Hyponatremia	Thiazide diuretics	Impair urinary diluting capacity of collecting duct
	ACE inhibitors	Stimulate thirst via conversion of angiotensin I or II
	Trimethoprim-sulfamethoxazole	Block amiloride-sensitive Na channels in the collecting duct
	NSAIDs	Inhibition of prostaglandins and potentiation of vasopressin's effect on the tubule
	Proton pump inhibitors, cyclophosphamide, morphine, barbiturates, vincristine, carbamazepine, acetaminophen, ACE inhibitors, NSAIDs, antipsychotics, desmopressin, oxytocin, antidepressants (SSRIs, TCAs)	Syndrome of inappropriate antidiuretic hormone secretion
	Mannitol	Volume expansion secondary to increased osmolality
Hypernatremia	Loop diuretics	Increase renal clearance of water
	Mannitol	Volume depletion
	Amphotericin B, dexamethasone, dopamine, lithium, ofloxacin, orlistat, foscarnet	Nephrogenic diabetes insipidus
	Hypertonic (3%) saline or normal (0.9%) saline, hypertonic sodium bicarbonate, antibiotics containing sodium (piperacillin, erythromycin)	Exogenous sodium load
	Osmotic cathartic agents (lactulose, sorbitol)	Gastrointestinal loss
Hypokalemia	Loop and thiazide diuretics	Increase sodium delivery to distal nephron where it can stimulate potassium excretion
	Sympathomimetics (epinephrine, terbutaline, albuterol), insulin, dobutamine, theophylline, aminophylline	Stimulate Na^+/K^+ ATPase pump, thereby causing potassium entry into cells
	Osmotic diuretics	Increased sodium delivery to distal nephron
	Carbonic anhydrase inhibitors	Block proximal sodium absorption so more goes to distal nephron
	Glucocorticoids/ mineralocorticoids	Enhance resorption of sodium at the renal distal tubule

(*continued*)

TABLE 23.2   Drugs That Alter Electrolyte and Mineral Values (*Continued*)

Abnormality	Medication	Mechanism
	Penicillins, aminopenicillins, penicillinase-resistant penicillins	Promote potassium excretion via increased sodium delivery to the distal nephron
	Aminoglycosides (gentamicin, tobramycin, amikacin), foscarnet, cisplatin	Renal potassium wasting by inducing magnesium depletion
	Amphotericin B	Inhibits secretion of hydrogen ions by collecting duct
	Cation-exchange resin (sodium polystyrene sulfonate)	Exchanges sodium for potassium within lumen of intestine
Hyperkalemia	Potassium citrate, penicillin G, enteral and parenteral nutrition	Excess potassium administration
	Spironolactone/amiloride, triamterene, trimethoprim	Inhibit aldosterone/inhibit potassium secretion
	Metoprolol, propranolol, labetalol, digoxin	Inhibit Na^+/K^+ ATPase pump; shift K out of cells
	ACE inhibitor, ARB, NSAIDs, heparin	Reduce aldosterone synthesis and secretion
	Succinylcholine	Shifts K out of cells
Hypocalcemia	Chemotherapeutic agents (cisplatin, 5-FU, cyclophosphamide, doxorubicin), fluoride poisoning, bisphosphonates, calcitonin, amphotericin B, cimetidine, ethanol	Decreased bone resorption
	Foscarnet, phosphate, citrate, albumin, lipid emulsion, heparin	Calcium chelation
	Phenytoin, phenobarbital, rifampin, isoniazid, ketoconazole, primidone	Vitamin D deficiency
	Aspirin, estrogen, magnesium sulfate, colchicine, propylthiouracil	Reduced PTH secretion/action
	Aminoglycosides (gentamicin, tobramycin, amikacin, neomycin)	Hypomagnesemia
	Loop diuretics	Increased urinary calcium excretion
Hypercalcemia	Vitamin D, vitamin A	Increased calcium absorption
	Estrogen, tamoxifen, thiazide diuretics	Miscellaneous
	Lithium	Inhibits calcium transport through cellular membranes

(continued)

TABLE 23.2	Drugs That Alter Electrolyte and Mineral Values (*Continued*)	
Abnormality	**Medication**	**Mechanism**
Hypophosphatemia	Antacids, sucralfate, phosphate binders	Reduce gut absorption
	Aspirin (overdose), albuterol, epinephrine, dopamine, insulin (exogenous), sodium bicarbonate	Shift phosphate into cells
	Acetaminophen (overdose), diuretics (thiazide, loop, osmotic, carbonic anhydrase inhibitors), corticosteroids, theophylline, chemotherapeutic agents	Urinary excretion
Hyperphosphatemia	Phosphate-containing enema/laxative, phosphate (exogenous oral or intravenous)	Excess phosphate administration
Hypomagnesemia	Aminoglycosides, amphotericin B, cisplatin, cyclosporine, digoxin, diuretics, foscarnet, methotrexate, pentamidine, polymyxin B, ticarcillin	Increased renal excretion
Hypermagnesemia	Lithium	Decreased renal excretion
	Magnesium-containing enema/laxative/antacid, magnesium (exogenous oral or intravenous)	Excess magnesium administration

ACE, angiotensin-converting enzyme; ARB, angiotensin receptor blocker; K, potassium; Na, sodium; NSAIDs, nonsteroidal anti-inflammatory drugs; PTH, parathyroid hormone; SSRIs, selective serotonin reuptake inhibitors; TCAs, tricyclic antidepressants; 5-FU, 5-fluorouracil.

has been the strongest risk factor for falls in the elderly. Health care providers should identify patients at risk for falls, in particular those with a history of previous falls. Overaggressive fluid removal, polypharmacy, drugs that affect the sensorium, as well as drugs with the potential of electrolyte disturbances should be used with caution.

Drugs That Can Alter Renal Function or Cause Renal Injury

Drugs known to markedly alter renal function or induce kidney injury are listed in Table 23.3. In most circumstances, the mechanism of injury is multifactorial, and interactions among drugs, disease, and a number of risk factors contribute to kidney injury. A number of drugs can injure the kidney by virtue of causing renal vasoconstriction, thereby reducing blood flow to the "deep" part of the kidney termed the *renal medulla*. When such drugs are given to patients who already have an additional hemodynamic cause for renal vasoconstriction, glomerular filtration rate (GFR) can be decreased and blood urea nitrogen and creatinine can become markedly elevated.

TABLE 23.3

Drug-Induced Kidney Injury

Drug	Risk Factor	Pathophysiology	Prevention	Management
NSAIDs	Chronic kidney disease, heart failure, dehydration, and diuretic	Hemodynamically induced acute renal failure that is due to vasoconstriction by decreased prostaglandin production and acute and chronic tubulointerstitial nephropathy Chronic interstitial nephritis and papillary necrosis, Na retention, hyperkalemia, hypertension, and edema	Avoid diuretic use at the same time. Limit use when SCr >1.5 mg/dL (130 mcmol/L). Use NSAIDs with short half-life	Discontinue medication Consider alternative pain-reducing agents.
Aminoglycoside (neomycin, gentamicin, tobramycin, amikacin, streptomycin)	Excessive peak and/or trough levels; duration (>7 days), concurrent nephrotoxins	Aminoglycoside accumulates within PCT and induces acute tubular necrosis, nonoliguric kidney injury; magnesium wasting	Maintain therapeutic range Give once-daily dose if necessary	Reduce the dose, decrease frequency and duration of therapy. Oral magnesium supplement if there is magnesium wasting.
Acyclovir	High dose, IV bolus dose	Crystal nephropathy	Avoid rapid bolus infusion Adjust for dosage for CKD, prior hydration (with the urine output maintained >75 mL/h), and slow drug infusion over 1–2 hours	Discontinue medication if possible, hydration, and stop loop diuretic.

(continued)

TABLE 23.3 Drug-Induced Kidney Injury (*Continued*)

Drug	Risk Factor	Pathophysiology	Prevention	Management
Adefovir dipivoxil	≥30 mg/day Renal impairment Pre-existing tubular dysfunction Duration of therapy	Depletion of mitochondrial DNA, acute tubular degeneration	Dosage adjustment for CKD	Discontinue medication if possible.
Cidofovir	Dose and duration, mild renal dysfunction	Induced apoptosis in PCT, diabetes insipidus, renal failure, and Fanconi syndrome	Hydration and probenecid In BK nephropathy, use only 0.25 mg/kg per week	Hydration and discontinue medication if possible.
Tenofovir	Dose and duration, mild renal dysfunction, use of ACE inhibitor, ritonavir and low body weight, genetic polymorphisms	Renal toxicity is mediated by proximal tubule epithelial cells, Fanconi syndrome	Hydration and dosage adjustment	Hydration and discontinue medication if possible.
Indinavir	Bolus dose	Crystal neuropathy, nephrolithiasis, obstructive ARF	Hydration Establish high urine flow Avoid bolus dose	Discontinue medication. It takes 6–8 weeks before normalization of renal function.
Foscarnet	Dose and duration, mild renal dysfunction	Crystal neuropathy, direct tubular toxicity, acute tubular necrosis, nephrogenic diabetes insipidus	0.5–1 L NS infusion before each dose, adjust for stage of CKD	Dose reduction.

Interferon		Prerenal acute renal failure, tubulointerstitial nephritis, thrombotic microangiopathy, membranoproliferative glomerular nephropathy	Discontinuation.
IVIG	Sucrose-containing product, dehydration	Accumulation of sucrose in PCT forms vesicle, ↑ osmolarity and vacuolization	Avoid radiocontrast concomitantly Avoid sucrose-containing product	Hydration Discontinue sucrose-containing product.
Lithium	Renal impairment, dehydration from fever, vomiting, exposure, hyponatremia, diuretics—especially thiazides	Tubular dysfunction, chronic tubulointerstitial nephropathy (tubular atrophy and interstitial fibrosis), and progressive glomerulosclerosis	Therapeutic range (0.6–1.2 mEq/L) Prevent dehydration Avoid low Na diet Avoid thiazide and nephrotoxic drug	Amiloride for nephrogenic diabetes insipidus Fluid restoration Hemodialysis (Rebound can occur if stopped too early).
CsA/tacrolimus	Dose, age, CKD	Calcineurin inhibitor nephrotoxicity, decreased prostaglandin, vasoconstriction, reduced GFR, ischemic collapse or scarring of the glomeruli, focal areas of tubular atrophy and interstitial fibrosis (striped fibrosis)	Maintain in therapeutic range Avoid drugs that raise levels (CYP3A4 inhibitor)	Dose reduction
Oral sodium phosphate	Dose, repeated dose, age, ARB and ACE inhibitor, and CKD	Tubular and interstitial calcium phosphate deposits	Avoid if possible; aggressive hydration, minimizing the dose of oral sodium phosphate	Discontinuation Hydration

(continued)

		Drug-Induced Kidney Injury (*Continued*)		

TABLE 23.3 Drug-Induced Kidney Injury (*Continued*)

Drug	Risk Factor	Pathophysiology	Prevention	Management
ACE inhibitors	Concomitant diuretic therapy; NSAIDs	Dilate efferent arteriole, reducing GFR; injury mechanism unknown	Avoid in bilateral renal artery stenosis	Discontinuation
Methotrexate	Acidic urine High dose	Precipitates in the urine and induces tubular injury	Prior hydration, alkalinize urine to pH >7.0 (3L of dextrose in water + 44–66 mEq of NaHCO$_3$/day)	Loop diuretic Leucovorin rescue
Ifosfamide	Use cisplatin at the same time	Direct tubular injury and mito-chondrial damage, Fanconi syndrome, nephrogenic diabetes insipidus, hypokalemia	Use of mesna	Discontinuation
Cisplatin	Low chloride High dose used for bone marrow ablation	Acute tubular necrosis, nephrogenic diabetes insipidus, hypomagnesemia	Vigorous hydration with forced diuresis: 2,500 mL NS/h before and several hours after administration Mannitol or furosemide used Amifostine (thiophosphate) Thiosulfate	Discontinue; give magnesium supplementation as needed
Sulfonamide (sulfadiazine and sulfamethoxazole)	High dose during the treatment of toxoplasmosis in patients w/ AIDS, Urine pH <5.5	Crystal neuropathy, nephrolithiasis	Fluid intake >3 L/day, monitor urine for crystals; if crystals are seen, alkalinization of urine to pH >7.15	Hydration

Radiocontrast	Dose and frequency, osmolarity of contrast media	High osmolarity and medullary vasoconstriction	Hydration before and after the administration Acetylcysteine or NaHCO$_3$ before and after administration	Hydration
Aristolochia acid (Chinese herbal neuropathy and endemic Balkan nephropathy)	Use of vasoconstrictors such as fenfluramine/diethylpropion at the same time Batch-to-batch variability in toxin content Female sex Dose Genetic predisposition	Chronic tubulointerstitial nephritis; uroepithelial tumors	Avoid! Be wary of herbal medicines that may contain Aristolochia	Discontinue Corticosteroids
Amphotericin B	Dose and duration, other nephrotoxic agent	Afferent vasoconstriction, decreases renal blood flow, distal tubular injury, hypokalemia, hypomagnesemia, metabolic acidosis due to tubular acidosis, polyuria due to nephrogenic diabetes insipidus	Use liposomal formulation (does not contain deoxycholate) Sodium loading (500–1,000 mL of NS 30 min before administration) Regularly monitor K, Mg, and Na serum concentrations	Hydration Dose reduction

Note: All of the above medications should be dosed based on renal function. Avoid concomitant use of nephrotoxic medications and diuretics. Patient-related risk factors for all the above drugs are age, previous renal insufficiency, dehydration and volume depletion, concurrent use of nephrotoxic drugs, chronic renal failure, diabetic neuropathy, severe congestive heart failure. Adequate hydration before therapy and during the treatment of acute renal failure because of volume depletion is one of the most important risk factors. Obtain baseline blood urea nitrogen, serum creatinine, and electrolytes, and closely monitor renal function during the treatments.

AIDS, acquired immunodeficiency syndrome; ARF, acute renal failure; CKD, chronic kidney disease; CsA, cyclosporine; CYP, cytochrome P; GFR, glomerular filtration rate; IV, intravenous; IVIG, intravenous immunoglobulin; K, potassium; Mg, magnesium; Na, sodium; NS, normal saline; NSAIDs, nonsteroidal anti-inflammatory drugs; PCT, proximal convoluted tubule; SCr, serum creatinine.

Although usually reversible, permanent, ischemic damage can result. Renal vasoconstriction also affects the ability of the kidney to excrete free water, because it decreases sodium delivery to the distal nephron. This in turn may result in hyponatremia, which in the elderly has been related to an increased risk of gait instability, falls, and fractures. Also, decreased distal sodium delivery impedes excretion of acid and potassium.

Drugs notable for causing renal injury by vasoconstriction are the **nonsteroidal anti-inflammatory drugs** (NSAIDs) and **iodinated contrast agents**, although both can sometimes cause renal damage by other mechanisms as well. The ACE inhibitors and angiotensin receptor blockers (ARBs) can reversibly impair kidney function because they dilate the efferent arteriole. This causes reduced intraglomerular pressure, and the plasma entering the glomerulus tends to just pass on through with less ultrafiltrate entering the renal tubule. For this reason, a decrease in the GFR is commonly observed in patients with CKD who are placed on one of these medications.

Cyclosporine and **tacrolimus** may cause serious dose-independent and irreversible nephrotoxicity. Kidney biopsy in nonrenal transplant patients with cyclosporine and tacrolimus nephrotoxicity suggests damage to the blood vessels, especially the afferent arteriole, as well as damage to the renal tubules and interstitium. **Aminoglycosides, amphotericin B, antiviral agents, cisplatin,** and **zoledronate** are believed to induce acute kidney injury through direct tubular injury. Many antimicrobial agents and proton pump inhibitors cause injury by way of inducing inflammatory damage to the tubules and surrounding tissue, so-called interstitial nephritis. Another mechanism of drug-induced kidney injury is due to precipitation of drug or metabolite crystals within the renal tubules. This not only causes obstruction to tubular fluid outflow but can damage the renal tubular cells as well. **Acyclovir, methotrexate, foscarnet,** and several other antiviral agents are associated with such injury.

DOSAGE ADJUSTMENT IN CHRONIC KIDNEY DISEASE

The following five steps provide a framework for dosage adjustments in patients with CKD. It must be emphasized that this stepwise approach is only a starting point from which dosage adjustments must be closely monitored and modified on a patient-by-patient basis.

Step 1: Obtain Past Medical History and Perform Physical Examination

The first steps in determining the need for dosage adjustment in any patient are eliciting a complete and detailed past medical history and performing a physical examination. Renal dysfunction should be characterized as acute or chronic, and, if possible, the cause of the dysfunction should be ascertained. History of prior drug intolerance, allergy, or nephrotoxicity needs to be obtained. Medication history should include past and current medications, episodes of drug allergy, and use of over-the-counter medications, vitamins, health foods, and herbal supplements (see Chapter 10). Adherence to prescribed medication therapy should be reviewed and noted.

In patients with acute kidney insufficiency, the patient's volume status may change substantially from day to day, and therefore volume status should be assessed carefully because the Vd of a drug can be altered by large changes in the amount of extracellular fluid volume. Finally, the clinician should determine whether the patient has hepatic dysfunction in addition to renal impairment, because concomitant hepatic dysfunction may necessitate even greater drug dosage adjustments affecting a larger range of medications.

Step 2: Assess Renal Function

Methods of assessing kidney function are discussed in Chapter 1 and will not be repeated here. Several important principles can be emphasized, however.

1. Before applying the corrections for reduced renal function described here, the dose should be preoptimized for body size, because the method recommended adjusts for the amount of kidney function normalized to body surface area (BSA). The pharmacokinetics of most drugs in markedly obese patients has not been well studied (Martin, 2012). In the absence of better information, for drugs that are not fat soluble, the adjusted body weight (Appendix 2) can be used to compute initial dose (before dose reduction for renal function) to limit the risk of overdosage because of very large patient size.

2. GFR generally is slightly less than creatinine clearance (CrCl), because the latter also includes tubular secretion of creatinine. The extent to which GFR/CrCl is <1.0 depends on race (lower in African Americans) and also the degree of GFR. GFR/CrCl is about 0.80 in patients with moderate renal impairment.

3. For an adult (middle-aged) healthy person, the expected normal value of either GFR or creatinine depends on BSA and averages about 100 mL/min per 1.73 m^2 for GFR and about 120 mL/min per 1.73 m^2 for CrCl (Peralta, 2011). In young adults (subjects ages 20 to 29), the expected normal values for eGFR and estimated CrCl (eCrCl) are slightly higher, about 116 and 130 mL/min per 1.73 m^2, respectively.

4. The eGFR/1.73 m^2 values calculated by the Modification of Diet in Renal Disease (MDRD) or Chronic Kidney Disease Epidemiology Collaboration (CKD-EPI) equations are already normalized to 1.73 m^2 BSA. The Cockcroft–Gault (CG) and Ix equations described in Chapter 1 give a "raw" CrCl, which is not normalized to body size. This raw CrCl can be multiplied

by the ratio of actual BSA to 1.73 to calculate CrCl/1.73 m², similar to eGFR/1.73 m².

5. In morbidly obese patients, the CG and Ix equations will overestimate raw CrCl. These equations predict 24-hour creatinine excretion based on weight, but creatinine excretion is better predicted by lean body mass (LBM) than by body weight. Equations to compute LBM are given in Appendix 2. Because LBM/W differs by body mass index, age, and sex, one would need to use a modified CG or Ix equation with different age, sex, and mass coefficients tailored to LBM. Such an equation has not yet been validated. Until such an equation is available, eCrCl can be computed using the Salazar–Corcoran equation described in Appendix 1. One can estimate raw GFR in obese patients by using the MDRD equation. The true GFR/1.73 m² in patients with obesity tends to be increased because of obesity-associated glomerular hyperfiltration (Levey and Kramer, 2010).

Step 3: Determine Loading Dose

Steady-state drug concentrations are achieved after approximately five half-lives. CKD may significantly prolong a drug's half-life, and if no loading dose is given, achievement of steady-state levels and therapeutic efficacy may be significantly delayed. In general, the standard loading dose that is given to patients with normal renal function should also be given to those with renal insufficiency in order to rapidly reach therapeutic drug levels. Digoxin is a major exception to this rule: Only 50% to 75% of the usual loading dose of digoxin should be administered to patients with renal failure because of a marked reduction of digoxin Vd in this setting. The loading dose can be calculated by the following formula, in which the Vd is in L/kg and Cp is the desired plasma concentration in mg/L:

$$\text{Loading dose} = \text{Vd} \times \text{Cp}$$

Step 4: Determine Maintenance Dose

Two methods can be used to adjust the maintenance dose in patients with CKD. One is to lengthen the dosing interval while keeping the dose constant, and the second is to reduce the dose while leaving the dosage interval unchanged.

For many drugs, the maintenance doses are recommended in the product labeling. For patients with normal renal function, the recommended maintenance dose may or may not be adjusted for body size. For example, a dose of an antibiotic may simply be given as 250 mg twice a day, with 500 mg twice a day for serious infections. Then the product labeling, particularly of older drugs, may recommend dose reduction when CrCl or GFR is <30 mL/min.

In such a case, it may be wise to compute an estimate of CrCl or raw eGFR directly to see if it is close to 30 mL/min. For a normal-size patient, use of the MDRD/1.73 m^2 equation usually is sufficient, because 30 mL/min per 1.73 m^2 will ordinarily be close to 30 mL/min as long as BSA is within 10% to 15% of 1.73 m^2. However, in a small patient with a BSA of 1.4 m^2, a GFR of 30 would be equal to an eGFR/1.73 m^2 of 37 mL/min. So, dose reduction should begin at a slightly higher level of eGFR/1.73 m^2. In contrast, for a large patient with BSA of 2.3, for example, a raw GFR of 30 corresponds to a GFR/1.73 m^2 of $30 \times 1.73/2.30 = 26$, and so the recommended dose adjustment should not be made until eGFR/1.73 m^2 has fallen to about 26 mL/min. Basing dose adjustments on raw—as opposed to normalized—GFR values is recommended by the U.S. National Kidney Education Program (NKDEP, 2009), although the recommendation is opinion based.

For some drugs that are excreted almost wholly by the kidney, a logical step is to either reduce the dosing interval by 50% or to double the dosing interval when eGFR/1.73 m^2 has decreased to 50% of the value in a healthy adult. For this method of dosing reduction, one computes eGFR/1.73 m^2 and applies the adjustment if it is <50 mL/min. A more severe adjustment may also be applied if eGFR/1.73 m^2 is <25 mL/min. However, for this method to work without size bias, it is important that the maintenance dose be preoptimized to body size *before* applying the dose adjustment due to renal function. Such a method is most applicable to cases in which the drug dose is given in terms of mg/kg or mg/m^2.

Finally, in extremely obese patients, computation of both the loading dose and maintenance dose is fraught with potential error, and there is little clinical information to guide the clinician. For drugs distributed in the total body water, LBM estimates such as those by Janmahasatian (see Appendix 2) can be used. One would calculate LBM for the obese patient using this equation and compare this to LBM for a patient at ideal or standard body weight, and increase the dose proportionately. For drugs that are distributed in body fat, proportionately higher amounts may need to be given to the obese. As detailed in Chapter 1 and Appendix 1, the Ix and CG equations underestimate CrCl in markedly obese patients. This is an area of active investigation, but until validated equations are available, the Salazar–Corcoran estimate of CrCl can be used. Alternatively, the MDRD and CKD-EPI equations perform reasonably well in obesity, and eGFR/1.73 m^2 value can be converted to raw GFR by multiplying by BSA as described above (see also Pai, 2010).

There continues to be controversy about whether a CrCl should be used for drug dosing estimates (Khanal, 2017) or if the MDRD equation as described above can be used (Stevens and Levey, 2009). Some of the arguments in favor of using the CG equation relate to the steep age-related decline in eCrCl predicted by the CG equation, which seemed to coincide better with the markedly decreased clearance of some renally excreted drugs such as gentamicin in the elderly (Spruill, 2009). However, the steep age-related slope in the CG equation was not confirmed in a more recent equation predicting 24-hour creatinine excretion (Ix, 2011). Whatever correction method is used, caution must be used, especially in the elderly, in whom both renal function and other mechanisms for drug metabolism may be reduced, as well as in obese patients, in whom there is a risk of underdosing based on either an inadequate compensation for massive body size or to errors in estimation of the degree of renal function.

Step 5: Monitor Drug Levels

For drugs with narrow therapeutic windows, adjusting the dose or dosing interval may not be sufficient to avoid toxicity and ensure therapeutic efficacy. Therapeutic drug monitoring refers to adjustment of drug dosage according to measured plasma concentrations. Therapeutic drug monitoring can be performed after an appropriate loading dose or after three to four maintenance doses have been administered to ensure that steady-state concentrations have been reached. Peak levels reflect the highest drug concentration achieved after an initial rapid distribution phase and tend to correlate with drug efficacy. Trough levels are generally obtained immediately before the next dose is given to ascertain the lowest concentration of drug in the body and, thus, systemic clearance (Table 23.4).

Drug Dosing Adjustment Tables

Dose adjustment recommendations are listed in organ-system and clinical problem-focused tables (Tables 23.5 to 23.17). An extensive review of current medical literature was utilized in deriving these dosing recommendations, but studies in this area are often conflicting or were done in limited populations; dosage adjustment recommendations are almost never based on prospective controlled trials. Thus, the prescribing health care provider must not rely solely on the tables provided here, but rather should use them as a starting point only. Patient-specific comorbid conditions, age, and weight, as well as risk of drug interactions, also must be considered, and the most recent product prescribing information should be carefully read and heeded. FDA-compliant U.S. package inserts can be conveniently downloaded from a National Library of Medicine website, dailymed.nlm.nih.gov.

(*Text Continued on Page 438*)

TABLE 23.4 Therapeutic Drug Monitoring in Chronic Kidney Disease

Drug Name	When to Draw Sample	Therapeutic Range	How Often to Draw Levels
Aminoglycosides (conventional dosing): gentamicin, tobramycin, amikacin	Trough: immediately before dose Peak: 30 min after a 30–45-min infusion	*Gentamicin and tobramycin:* Trough: <2 mg/L Peak: 5–8 mg/L *Amikacin:* Peak: 20–30 mg/L Trough: <5–10 mg/L	Check peak and trough with 3rd dose. For therapy <72 hours, levels not necessary. Repeat drug levels weekly or if renal function changes.
Aminoglycosides (24-hr dosing): gentamicin, tobramycin, amikacin	Obtain random drug level 12 hours after dose	0.5–3 mg/L	After initial dose. Repeat drug level in 1 week or if renal function changes.
Carbamazepine	Trough: Immediately before dosing	4–12 mcg/mL	Check 2–4 days after first dose or change in dose.
Cyclosporine	Trough: Immediately before dosing	150–400 ng/mL	Daily for first week, then weekly.
Digoxin	12 hours after maintenance dose	0.8–2.0 ng/mL	5–7 days after first dose for patients with normal renal and hepatic function; 15–20 days in anephric patients.
Enoxaparin	4 hours after 2nd or 3rd dose	0.7–1.1 anti-Xa IU/mL	Weekly and as needed.
Lidocaine	8 hours after intravenous infusion started or changed	1–5 mcg/mL	As needed.
Lithium	Trough: before am dose at least 12 hours since last dose	Acute: 0.8–1.2 mmol/L Chronic: 0.6–0.8 mmol/L	As needed.
Phenobarbital	Trough: immediately before dosing	15–40 mcg/mL	Check 2 weeks after first dose or change in dose. Follow up level in 1–2 months.

(continued)

399

TABLE 23.4 Therapeutic Drug Monitoring in Chronic Kidney Disease (*Continued*)

Drug Name	When to Draw Sample	Therapeutic Range	How Often to Draw Levels
Phenytoin: free phenytoin	Trough: immediately before dosing	10–20 mcg/mL (total) 1–2 mcg/mL (free)	5–7 days after first dose or after change in dose.
Procainamide: NAPA (*N*-acetylprocainamide), a procainamide metabolite	Trough: immediately before next dose or 12–18 hours after starting or changing an infusion Draw with procainamide sample	4–10 mcg/mL Trough: 4 mcg/mL Peak: 8 mcg/mL	As needed. Procainamide + NAPA levels: 5–30 mcg/mL.
Sirolimus	Trough: immediately before next dose	10–20 ng/dL	Weekly for first month, then as needed.
Tacrolimus	Trough: immediately before next dose	5–10 ng/mL	Daily for first week, then weekly.
Valproic acid (divalproex sodium)	Trough: immediately before next dose	40–100 mcg/mL	Check 2–4 days after first dose or change in dose.
Vancomycin	Trough: immediately before dose Peak: 60 minutes after a 60-minute infusion	Trough: 10–20 mg/L Peak: 25–40 mg/L	With 3rd dose (when initially starting therapy, or after each dosage adjustment). For therapy <72 hours, levels not necessary. Repeat drug levels if renal function changes.

TABLE 23.5 Antimicrobial Agents Dosing in Chronic Kidney Disease

Drugs	Normal Dosage	% of Renal Excretion	Dosage Adjustment in CKD		Comments
			GFR30–60	GFR10–29	
Aminoglycoside Antibiotics					Nephrotoxic. Ototoxic. Toxicity worse when hyperbilirubinemic. Measure serum levels for efficacy and toxicity. Peritoneal absorption increases with presence of inflammation. Vd increases with edema, obesity, and ascites. For HD: dose after HD, check level before HD.
Gentamicin	1.5 mg/kg q8h	95%	100% q12–q24h	100% 24–q48h	Peak 5–8, trough <2 mg/L.
Tobramycin	1.5 mg/kg q8h	95%	100% q12–q24h	100% q24–q48h	Peak 5–8, trough <2 mg/L.
Netilmicin	2 mg/kg q8h	95%	100% q12–q24h	100% q24–q48h	May be less ototoxic than other members of class. Peak 5–8, trough <2 mg/L.
Amikacin	7.5 mg/kg q12h	95%	100% q12–q24h	100% q24–q48h	Monitor levels. Peak 20–30, trough <5–10 mg/L (<10 for severe infection).
Cephalosporins					Coagulation abnormalities, transitory elevation of BUN, rash, and serum sickness-like syndrome; seizures or confusion when giving higher IV doses in severe CKD.
Oral Cephalosporins					
Cefaclor	250–500 mg tid	70%	100%	50–100%	
Cefadroxil	500 mg–1 g bid	80%	100%	50–100%	
Cefixime	200–400 mg q12h	85%	100%	50–100%	
Cefpodoxime	200 mg q12h	30%	100%	50–100%	

(continued)

TABLE 23.5 Antimicrobial Agents Dosing in Chronic Kidney Disease (*Continued*)

Drugs	Normal Dosage	% of Renal Excretion	Dosage Adjustment in CKD			Comments
			GFR30–60	GFR10–29		
Ceftibuten	400 mg q24h	70%	100%	50–100%		
Cefuroxime axetil	250–500 mg bid	90%	100%	50–100%		Malabsorption in presence of H$_2$ blockers. Absorbed better with food.
Cephalexin	250–500 mg tid	95%	100%	50–100%		Rare allergic interstitial nephritis. May cause bleeding from impaired prothrombin biosynthesis.
Cephradine	250–500 mg tid	100%	100%	50–100%		Rare allergic interstitial nephritis. May cause bleeding from impaired prothrombin biosynthesis.
Cefdinir	300 mg po bid	20%	100%	50%		
IV Cephalosporins						
Cefamandole	1–2 g IV q6–q8h	100%	100%	50%		
Cefazolin	1–2 g IV q8h	80%	100%	50%		
Cefepime	1–2 g IV q8h	85%	100%	50%		
Cefmetazole	1–2 g IV q8h	85%	100%	50%		
Cefoperazone	1–2 g IV q12h	20%	100%	100%		Displaced from protein by bilirubin. Reduce dose by 50% for jaundice. May prolong prothrombin time.
Cefotaxime	1–2 g IV q6–q8h	60%	100%	50%		Active metabolite in ESRD. Reduce dose further for combined hepatic and renal failure.
Cefotetan	1–2 g IV q12h	75%	100%	50%		
Cefoxitin	1–2 g IV q6h	80%	100%	50%		
Ceftaroline						May produce false increase in serum creatinine by interference with assay.

Ceftolozane/tazobactam					
Ceftazidime-avibactam					
Ceftazidime	1–2 g IV q8h	70%	100%	25–50%	
Ceftriaxone	1–2 g IV q24h	50%	100%	100%	
Cefuroxime sodium	0.75–1.5 g IV q8h	90%	100%	50%	Rare allergic interstitial nephritis. May cause bleeding from impaired prothrombin biosynthesis.
Penicillins					Bleeding abnormalities, hypersensitivity. Seizures.
Oral Penicillin					
Amoxicillin	500 mg tid	60%	100%	50%	
Ampicillin	500 mg q6h	60%	100%	50%	
Dicloxacillin	250–500 mg q6h	50%	100%	50%	
Penicillin V	250–500 mg q6h	70%	100%	50%	
IV Penicillin					
Ampicillin	1–2 g IV q6h	60%	100%	50%	
Nafcillin	1–2 g IV q4h	35%	100%	100%	
Penicillin G	2–3 million units IV q4h	70%	100% q4–q6h	50%	Seizures. False-positive urine protein reactions. Six million units per day upper-limit dose in ESRD.
Piperacillin	3–4 g IV q4–q6h		100%	50%	Sodium content: 1.9 mmol/g.
Ticarcillin/clavulanate	3.1 g IV q4–q6h	85%	100%	50%	Sodium content: 5.2 mmol/g.
Piperacillin/tazobactam	3.375 g IV q6–q8h	75–90%	100%	50%	Sodium content: 1.9 mmol/g.
Quinolones					Increased renal toxicity with vancomycin.
Ciprofloxacin	200–400 mg IV q24h	60%	100%	50%	Photosensitivity; tendon rupture; food, tube feedings, and meds may decrease absorption. Use with caution with phosphate binders. Poorly absorbed with antacids, sucralfate, and phosphate binders. Decreases phenytoin levels.

(continued)

TABLE 23.5 Antimicrobial Agents Dosing in Chronic Kidney Disease (*Continued*)

Drugs	Normal Dosage	% of Renal Excretion	Dosage Adjustment in CKD		Comments
			GFR30–60	GFR10–29	
Levofloxacin	500 mg qd	70%	100%	50%	L-isomer of ofloxacin; appears to have similar pharmacokinetics and toxicities.
Moxifloxacin	400 mg qd	20%	100%	100%	Agents in this group are malabsorbed in the presence of magnesium, calcium, aluminum, and iron. Theophylline metabolism is impaired. Higher oral doses may be needed to treat CAPD peritonitis.
Nalidixic acid	1.0 g q6h	High	100%	Avoid	
Norfloxacin	400 mg q12h	30%	100%	100%	See above.
Ofloxacin	200–400 mg q12h	70%	100%	50%	See above.
Miscellaneous Agents					
Azithromycin	250–1,000 mg qd	6%	100%	100%	No drug–drug interaction with CsA/tacrolimus.
Colistin IV	2.5 mg/kg tid	100%	50%	25%	
Clarithromycin	500 mg bid	20%	100%	100%	
Clindamycin	150–450 mg tid	10%	100%	100%	Increases risk of *Clostridium difficile* infection.
Fosfomycin			100%	100%	
Erythromycin	250–500 mg qid	15–20%	100%	100%	Increases CsA/tacrolimus level.
Dalbavancin	1,500 mg ×1	33%	100%	50%	
Telavancin	10 mg/kg q24h	72%	75%	50%	

Drug	Dose				Comments
Imipenem/cilastatin	250–500 mg IV q6h	50%	100%	50%	Seizures in ESRD. Nonrenal clearance in acute renal failure is less than in chronic renal failure. Administered with cilastatin to prevent nephrotoxicity of renal metabolite.
Meropenem	1 g IV q8h	65%	100%	50%	
Ertapenem	1 g IV q24h	80%	100%	50%	
Doripenem	500 mg IV q8h	71%	50%	25%	
Metronidazole	500 mg IV q6h	20%	100%	100%	Peripheral neuropathy, increase LFTs, disulfiram reaction with alcoholic beverages.
Pentamidine	4 mg/kg per day	5%	100%	50%	Inhalation may cause bronchospasm, IV administration may cause hypotension, hypoglycemia, and nephrotoxicity.
Trimethoprim/sulfamethoxazole	800/160 mg bid	70%	100%	25–50%	Increases serum creatinine. Can cause hyperkalemia.
Vancomycin	1 g IV q12h	90%	75–100%	50%	Nephrotoxic; ototoxic; may prolong the neuromuscular blockade effect of muscle relaxants. Peak 30, trough 5–10.
Vancomycin oral	125–250 mg qid	0%	100%	100%	Oral vancomycin is indicated only for the treatment of *C. difficile.*
Daptomycin	6–8 mg/kg q24h	50%	100%	50%	Myalgia, arthralgia, fatigue.
Linezolid	600 mg po/IV q12h	1%	100%	100%	
Quinupristin/dalfopristin	7.5 mg/kg	10%	100%	100%	Gastrointestinal adverse reactions.
Tigecycline	50 mg IV q12h	22%	100%	100%	
Doxycycline	100 mg IV/po q12h	20%	100%	100%	Avoid in children.
Minocycline	100 mg po q12h	10%	100%	100%	
Antituberculosis Antibiotics					
Rifampin	300–600 mg qd	20%	100%	100%	Decreases CsA/tacrolimus level. Many drug interactions.
Antifungal Agents					
Amphotericin B	0.5 mg–1.5 mg/kg per day	<1%	100%	100%	Nephrotoxic, infusion-related reactions; give 250 cc NS before each dose.
Amphotec	4–6 mg/kg per day	<1%	100%	100%	

(continued)

405

TABLE 23.5 Antimicrobial Agents Dosing in Chronic Kidney Disease (*Continued*)

Drugs	Normal Dosage	% of Renal Excretion	Dosage Adjustment in CKD			Comments
			GFR30–60	GFR10–29		
Abelcet	5 mg/kg per day	<1%	100%	100%		
AmBisome	3–5 mg/kg per day	<1%	100%	100%		
Fluconazole	200–800 mg IV qd/bid	70%	100%	75–100%		Hepatic dysfunction. Marrow suppression more common in azotemic patients.
Flucytosine	37.5 mg/kg	90%	q12h	50%		
Azoles and Other Antifungals						
Griseofulvin	125–250 mg q6h	1%	100%	100%		Increase CsA/tacrolimus level, QT interval prolongation, many drug interactions.
Itraconazole	200 mg q12h	35%	100%	100%		Poor oral absorption.
Ketoconazole	200–400 mg qd	15%	100%	100%		Hepatotoxic.
Miconazole	1,200–3,600 mg/day	1%	100%	100%		
Terbinafine	250 mg qd	>1%	100%	50%		May cause congestive heart failure.
Voriconazole	4 mg/kg q12h	<2%	100%	100%		Avoid IV formulation when GFR <50; nephrotoxicity and risk of tubular damage; accumulation of solvent in severe CKD.
Posaconazole	300 mg po daily	13%	100%	Avoid IV formulation		
Isavuconazole	372 mg (isavuconazole 200 mg) once daily.	1%	100%	100%		

Drug	Dose				Comments
Micafungin	100 mg	1%	100%	100%	Hepatotoxicity.
Caspofungin	70 mg	1%	100%	100%	Disulfiram reactions.
Anidulafungin	100 mg	10%	100%	100%	
Antiviral Agents					
Abacavir	300–600 mg/day	<2%	100%	100%	
Acyclovir	200–800 mg 5×/day	50%	100%	25–50% (15% for IV)	Poor absorption. Neurotoxicity in severe CKD. Intravenous preparation can cause renal failure if injected rapidly.
Adefovir dipivoxil	10 mg daily	45%	50%	25%	For eGFR <10 mL/min; every 72 hours.
Amantadine	100–200 mg q12h	90%	50%	25%	Avoid in severe CKD.
Cidofovir	5 mg/kg weekly ×2 (induction); 5 mg/kg every 2 weeks	90%	Avoid	Avoid	Dose-limiting nephrotoxicity with proteinuria, glycosuria, renal insufficiency; nephrotoxicity and renal clearance reduced with coadministration of probenecid.
Delavirdine	400 mg q8h	5%	No data: 100%	No data	
Didanosine	200 mg q12h (125 mg if <60 kg)	40–69%	100%	200 q72h	Pancreatitis.
Efavirenz	600 mg/day	<1%	100%	100%	
Emtricitabine	200 mg/day	100%	200 q48h	200 q72h	For eGFR <10 mL/min; every 72 hours.
Entecavir	0.5 mg daily	70%	50%	25%	VZV: 500 mg po tid; HSV: 250 po bid. Metabolized to active compound penciclovir.
Famciclovir	250–500 mg po bid-tid	60%	100%	50%	
Foscarnet	40–80 mg IV q8h	85%	50%	25%	Nephrotoxic, neurotoxic, hypocalcemia, hypophosphatemia, hypomagnesemia, and hypokalemia.
Ganciclovir IV	5 mg/kg q12h	95%	100%	25–50%	Granulocytopenia and thrombocytopenia.
Ganciclovir po	1,000 mg po tid	95%	100%	50%	Oral ganciclovir should be used ONLY for prevention of CMV infection. Always use IV ganciclovir or valganciclovir for the treatment of CMV infection.

(continued)

TABLE 23.5 Antimicrobial Agents Dosing in Chronic Kidney Disease (*Continued*)

Drugs	Normal Dosage	% of Renal Excretion	Dosage Adjustment in CKD			Comments
			GFR30–60	GFR10–29		
Harvoni/(ledipasvir/ sofosbuvir)	Ledipasvir 90 mg/ sofosbuvir 400 mg once daily.	<1%	100%	No data		
Interferons						Peginterferon alfa-2a (Pegasys). Peginterferon alfa-2b (PegIntron, Sylatron). Interferon alfa-2b (Intron A).
Lamivudine	150 mg bid	80%	75–100%	50%		For hepatitis B.
Nelfinavir	750 mg q8h	No data	No data	No data		
Nevirapine	200 mg q24h × 14 days	<3	No data: 100%	No data		
Raltegravir	400 mg bid	7–14%	100%	100%		
Ribavirin	800 mg daily	60%	50%	25%		Hemolytic uremic syndrome.
Rifabutin	300 mg q24h	5–10%	100%	100%		
Rimantadine	100 mg bid	25%	100%	100%		
Ritonavir	600 mg q12h	3.50%	100%	100%		Many drug interactions.
Saquinavir	600 mg q8h	<4%	100%	100%		
Simeprevir	150 mg daily	<1%	100%	100%		
Sofosbuvir (Sovaldi)	400 mg once daily.	<1%	100%	No data		
Stavudine	30–40 mg q12h	35–40%	100%	100%		

Telbivudine	600 mg daily	42%	50%	25%	For eGFR <10 mL/min; every 72 hours. Consider alternative agents when GFR <50.
Tenofovir	300 mg/day	100%	300 q48h	300 q72–q96h	May cause acute renal failure or Fanconi syndrome. Use alafenamide formulation for CKD patients. Thrombotic thrombocytopenic purpura/hemolytic uremic syndrome.
Valacyclovir	500–1,000 mg q8h	50%	100%	50%	
Dasabuvir, ombitasvir, paritaprevir, and ritonavir (Viekira pak)		<1%	100%	100%	
Glecaprevir/pibrentasvir (Mavyret)		<1%	100%	100%	Drug of the choice in HD in CKD stages 4 and 5.
Sofosbuvir/velpatasvir (Epclusa)		<1%	100%	No data	
Sofosbuvir/velpatasvir/voxilaprevir (Vosevi)		<1%	100%	No data	
Elbasvir and grazoprevir (Zepatier)	Elbasvir 50 mg/grazoprevir 100 mg	<1%	100%	100%	
Valganciclovir	450–900 mg po bid	95%	75%	25–50%	
Vidarabine	15 mg/kg infusion q24h	50%	100%	100%	
Zalcitabine	0.75 mg q8h	75%	100%	q12h	
Zanamivir	2 puffs bid × 5 days	1%	100%	100%	Bioavailability from inhalation and systemic exposure to drug is low.
Zidovudine	200 mg q8h, 300 mg q12h	8–25%	100%	75%	Enormous interpatient variation. Metabolite renally excreted.

bid, twice daily; BUN, blood urea nitrogen; CAPD, continuous ambulatory peritoneal dialysis; CHF, congestive heart failure; CMV, cytomegalovirus; CrCl, creatinine clearance; CsA, cyclosporine; FK, tacrolimus; GFR, glomerular filtration rate; HSV, herpes simplex virus; IV, intravenous; LFT, liver function test; NS, normal saline; po, by mouth; qd, every day; tid, three times daily; Vd, volume of distribution; VZV, varicella zoster virus.

TABLE 23.6 Analgesic Dosing in Chronic Kidney Disease

Analgesics	Normal Dosage	% of Renal Excretion	Dosage Adjustment in CKD		Comments
			GFR 30–60	GFR 10–29	
Narcotics and Narcotic Antagonists					
Alfentanil	Anesthetic induction 8–40 g/kg	<1%	100%	100%	Titrate the dose regimen.
Butorphanol	2 mg q3–q4h	<1%	100%	75%	
Codeine	30–60 mg q4–q6h	<1%	100%	75%	
Fentanyl	Anesthetic induction (individualized)	<1%	100%	75%	
Meperidine	50–100 mg q3–q4h	<1%	100%	Avoid	Normeperidine, an active metabolite, accumulates in severe CKD and may cause seizures. Protein binding is reduced in severe CKD. Avoid when GFR <20.
Methadone	2.5–5 mg q6–q8h	<1%	100%	100%	
Morphine	20–25 mg q4h	<1%	100%	75%	Increased sensitivity to drug effect in severe CKD. Active metabolite.
Naloxone	2 mg IV	<1%	100%	100%	
Pentazocine	50 mg q4h	<1%	100%	75%	
Sufentanil	Anesthetic induction	<1%	100%	100%	
Nonnarcotics					
Acetaminophen	650 mg q4h	<1%	100%	100%	Overdose may be nephrotoxic. Drug is major metabolite of phenacetin.
Acetylsalicylic acid	650 mg q4h	<1%	100%	100%	Nephrotoxic in high doses. May decrease GFR when renal blood flow is prostaglandin dependent. May add to uremic GI and hematologic symptoms. Protein binding reduced in severe CKD.

GFR, glomerular filtration rate; GI, gastrointestinal; IV, intravenous.

TABLE 23.7 Antihypertensive and Cardiovascular Drugs Dosing in Chronic Kidney Disease

Antihypertensive and Cardiovascular Agents	Normal Dosage	% of Renal Excretion	Dosage Adjustment in CKD GFR 30–60	Dosage Adjustment in CKD GFR 10–29	Comments
ACE Inhibitors					
Benazepril	10 mg qd	20%	100%	75%	Hyperkalemia, acute renal failure, angioedema, rash, cough, anemia, and liver toxicity. 2% cross-risk of angioedema with ARB.
Captopril	6.25–25 mg tid	35%	100%	75%	Rare proteinuria, nephrotic syndrome, dysgeusia, granulocytopenia. Increases serum digoxin levels.
Enalapril	5 mg qd	45%	100%	75%	Enalaprilat, the active moiety formed in liver.
Fosinopril	10 mg bid	20%	100%	100%	Fosinoprilat, the active moiety formed in liver. Drug less likely than other ACE inhibitors to accumulate in renal failure.
Lisinopril	2.5 mg qd	80%	100%	50–75%	Lysine analog of a pharmacologically active enalapril metabolite.
Pentopril	125 mg q24h	80–90%	100%	50–75%	
Perindopril	2 mg q24h	<10%	100%	75%	Active metabolite is perindoprilat. The clearance of perindoprilat and its metabolites is almost exclusively renal. Approximately 60% of circulating perindopril is bound to plasma proteins, and only 10–20% of perindoprilat is bound.
Quinapril	10 mg qd	30%	100%	75–100%	Active metabolite is quinaprilat. 96% of quinaprilat is excreted renally.
Ramipril	2.5 mg qd	15%	100%	50–75%	Active metabolite is ramiprilat. Data are for ramiprilat.

(continued)

411

TABLE 23.7 Antihypertensive and Cardiovascular Drugs Dosing in Chronic Kidney Disease (*Continued*)

Antihypertensive and Cardiovascular Agents	Normal Dosage	% of Renal Excretion	Dosage Adjustment in CKD			Comments
			GFR 30–60	GFR 10–29		
Trandolapril	1–2 mg qd	33%	100%	50–100%		Hyperkalemia, angioedema (less common than with ACE inhibitors), 2% risk of cross-angioedema with ARB.
Angiotensin II receptor blockers						
Candesartan	16 mg qd	33%	100%	100%		Candesartan cilexetil is rapidly and completely bioactivated by ester hydrolysis during absorption from the gastrointestinal tract to candesartan.
Eprosartan	600 mg qd	25%	100%	100%		Eprosartan pharmacokinetics more variable in severe CKD. Decreased protein binding in uremia.
Irbesartan	150 mg qd	20%	100%	100%		
Losartan	50 mg qd	13%	100%	100%		
Valsartan	80 mg qd	7%	100%	100%		
Telmisartan	20–80 mg qd	<5%	100%	100%		
β-Blockers						Decrease HDL. Mask symptoms of hypoglycemia, bronchospasm, fatigue, insomnia, depression, and sexual dysfunction.
Acebutolol	400 mg q24h or bid	55%	100%	50%		Active metabolites with long half-lives.
Atenolol	25 mg qd	90%	100%	50–75%		Accumulates in severe CKD.
Betaxolol	20 mg q24h	100%	100%	50%		
Bopindolol	1 mg q24h	<10%	100%	100%		
Carteolol	0.5 mg q24h	<50%	100%	50%		

Normal Dosage (second group):
- Trandolapril Angiotensin II receptor blockers: —
- Candesartan: 32 mg qd
- Eprosartan: 400–800 mg qd
- Irbesartan: 300 mg qd
- Losartan: 100 mg qd
- Valsartan: 160 mg bid
- Acebutolol: 600 mg q24h or bid
- Atenolol: 100 mg qd
- Betaxolol: 80–90%
- Bopindolol: 4 mg q24h
- Carteolol: 10 mg q24h

Carvedilol	3.125 mg tid	25 mg tid	2%	100%	100%	Kinetics is dose dependent. Plasma concentrations of carvedilol reported to be increased in patients with renal impairment.
Celiprolol	200 mg q24h	10%	100%	100%	
Dilevalol	200 mg bid	400 mg bid	<5%	100%	100%	
Esmolol (IV only)	50 mcg/kg per minute	300 mcg/kg per minute	10%	100%	100%	Active metabolite retained in renal failure. For IV use: 20 mg slow IV injection over a 2-min period. Additional injections of 40 or 80 mg can be given at 10-min intervals until a total of 300 mg or continuous infusion of 2 mg/min.
Labetalol	50 mg po bid	400 mg bid	5%	100%	100%	
Metoprolol	50 mg bid	100 mg bid	<5%	100%	100%	
Nadolol	80 mg qd	160 mg bid	90%	100%	25–50%	Start with prolonged interval and titrate.
Penbutolol	10 mg q24h	40 mg q24h	<10	100%	100%	
Pindolol	10 mg bid	40 mg bid	40%	100%	100%	
Propranolol	40–160 mg tid	320 mg/day	<5%	100%	100%	Bioavailability may increase in ESRD. Metabolites may cause increased bilirubin by assay interference in ESRD. Hypoglycemia reported in ESRD.
Sotalol	80 bid	160 mg bid	70%	100%	25–50%	Avoid in severe CKD due to risk of arrhythmia.
Timolol	10 mg bid	20 mg bid	15%	100%	100%	
Calcium Channel Blockers						Dihydropyridine: headache, ankle edema, gingival hyperplasia and flushing. Nondihydropyridine: bradycardia, constipation, gingival hyperplasia, and AV block.
Amlodipine	2.5 qd	10 mg qd	10%	100%	100%	May increase digoxin and cyclosporine levels. Weak vasodilator and antihypertensive.
Bepridil	No data	<1%	No data	No data	No data	Acute renal dysfunction. May exacerbate hyperkalemia.
Diltiazem	30 mg tid	90 mg tid	10%	100%	100%	May increase digoxin and cyclosporine levels.

(continued)

413

TABLE 23.7 Antihypertensive and Cardiovascular Drugs Dosing in Chronic Kidney Disease (*Continued*)

Antihypertensive and Cardiovascular Agents	Normal Dosage	% of Renal Excretion	Dosage Adjustment in CKD		Comments
			GFR 30–60	GFR 10–29	
Felodipine	5 mg bid	1%	100%	100%	May increase digoxin levels.
Isradipine	5 mg bid	<5%	100%	100%	May increase digoxin levels.
Nicardipine	20 mg tid	<1%	100%	100%	Uremia inhibits hepatic metabolism. May increase digoxin levels.
Nifedipine XL or CC	30 mg qd	10%	100%	100%	Avoid short-acting nifedipine formulation.
Nimodipine	30 mg q8h	10%	100%	100%	May lower blood pressure.
Nisoldipine	20 mg qd	10%	100%	100%	May increase digoxin levels.
Verapamil	40 mg tid	10%	100%	100%	Acute renal dysfunction. Active metabolites accumulate particularly with sustained-release forms.
Diuretics					Hypokalemia/hyperkalemia (potassium-sparing agents), hyperuricemia, hyperglycemia, hypomagnesemia, increase serum cholesterol.
Acetazolamide	125 mg tid	90%	100%	50%	May potentiate acidosis. Ineffective as diuretic in severe CKD. May cause neurologic side effects in severe CKD.
Amiloride	5 mg qd	50%	100%	100%	Hyperkalemia with GFR <30 mL/min, especially in diabetic patients. Hyperchloremic metabolic acidosis.
Bumetanide	1–2 mg qd	35%	100%	100%	Ototoxicity increased in ESRD in combination with aminoglycosides. High doses effective in severe CKD. Muscle pain, gynecomastia.

Chlorthalidone	25 mg q24h	50%	100%	Much better agent for CKD patients with HTN; less effective when GFR <30.
Ethacrynic acid	50 mg qd	20%	100%	Ototoxicity increased in severe CKD in combination with aminoglycosides.
Furosemide	40–80 mg qd	70%	100%	Ototoxicity increased in severe CKD, especially in combination with aminoglycosides. High doses effective in severe CKD.
Indapamide	2.5 mg q24h	<5%	100%	Not believed effective when GFR <30.
Metolazone	2.5 mg qd	70%	100%	High doses effective in severe CKD. Gynecomastia, impotence.
Piretanide	6 mg q24h	40–60%	100%	High doses effective in severe CKD. Ototoxicity.
Spironolactone	100 mg qd	25%	100%	Active metabolites with long half-life. Hyperkalemia common when GFR <30, especially in diabetic patients. Gynecomastia, hyperchloremic acidosis. Increases serum by immunoassay interference.
Thiazides	25 mg qd	>95%	Avoid	Not effective when GFR <30.
Torosemide	5 mg bid	25%	100%	High doses effective in ESRD. Ototoxicity.
Triamterene	25 mg bid	5–10%	100%	Hyperkalemia common when GFR <30, especially in diabetic patients. Active metabolite with long half-life in severe CKD. Folic acid antagonist. Urolithiasis. Crystalluria in acid urine. May cause acute renal failure.
Miscellaneous Agents				
Amrinone	5 mg/kg per minute daily dose <10 mg/kg	10 mg/kg per minute daily dose <10 mg/kg	10–40%	100%	Thrombocytopenia. Nausea, vomiting in ESRD.
Clonidine	0.1 bid/tid	1.2 mg/day	45%	100%	Sexual dysfunction, dizziness, portal hypotension.

(continued)

415

TABLE 23.7 Antihypertensive and Cardiovascular Drugs Dosing in Chronic Kidney Disease (*Continued*)

Antihypertensive and Cardiovascular Agents	Normal Dosage	% of Renal Excretion	Dosage Adjustment in CKD			Comments
			GFR 30–60	GFR 10–29		
Digoxin	0.125 mg qod/qd	0.25 mg qd	25%	100%	100%	Decrease loading dose by 50% in severe CKD. Radioimmunoassay may overestimate serum levels in uremia. Clearance decreased by amiodarone, spironolactone, quinidine, and verapamil. Hypokalemia and hypomagnesemia enhance toxicity. Vd and total body clearance decreased in severe CKD. Serum level 12 hours after dose is best guide in severe CKD. Digoxin immune antibodies can treat severe toxicity.
Hydralazine	10 mg qid	100 mg qid	25%	100%	100%	Lupus-like reaction.
Midodrine	No data	No data	75–80%	5–10 mg q8h	5–10 mg q8h	Increased blood pressure.
Minoxidil	2.5 mg bid	10 mg bid	20%	100%	100%	Pericardial effusion, fluid retention, hypertrichosis, and tachycardia.
Nitroprusside	1 mcg/kg per minute	10 mcg/kg per minute	<10%	100%	100%	Cyanide toxicity, avoid prolonged use (more than 2–3 days).
Dobutamine	2.5 mcg/kg per minute	15 mcg/kg per minute	10%	100%	100%	
Milrinone	0.375 mcg/kg per minute	0.75 mcg/kg per minute	10%	100%	100%	Hypotension, long half-life, start low in CKD patients.

ACE, angiotensin-converting enzyme; ARB, angiotensin receptor blocker; AV, atrioventricular; bid, twice daily; CKD, chronic kidney disease; GFR, glomerular filtration rate; HDL, high-density lipoprotein; HTN, hypertension; IV, intravenous; po, by mouth; qd, every day; qid, four times daily; qod, every other day; tid, three times daily; Vd, volume of distribution.

TABLE 23.8 Endocrine and Metabolic Dosing in Chronic Kidney Disease

Hypoglycemic Agents	Normal Dosage	% of Renal Excretion	Dosage Adjustment in CKD GFR>30–60	GFR10–29	Comments
Acarbose	25 mg tid	35%	100%	50%	Avoid all oral hypoglycemic agents on CRRT. Abdominal pain, nausea, and flatulence.
Acetohexamide	250 mg q24h	None	Avoid	Avoid	Diuretic effect. May falsely elevate serum creatinine. Active metabolite has T½ of 5–8 hours in healthy subjects and is eliminated by the kidney. Prolonged hypoglycemia in azotemic patients.
Alogliptin	25 mg qd	70%	50%	25%	Pharyngitis, headache.
Canagliflozine	100 mg qd	40%	50%	Avoid	Fungal UTI infections, dehydration and AKI.
Chlorpropamide	100 mg q24h	47%	50%	Avoid	Impairs water excretion. Prolonged hypoglycemia in azotemic patients.
Dapagliflozin	10 mg qd	<2%	50%	Avoid	Fungal UTI infections, dehydration and AKI.
Exenatide	5 mcg subq q12h	1%	100%	Avoid	N/V and diarrhea.
Glibornuride	12.5 mg q24h	No data	No data	No data	
Gliclazide	80 mg q24h	<20%	50–100%	Avoid	
Glipizide	5 mg qd	5%	100%	50%	
Glyburide	2.5 mg qd	50%	100%	Avoid	Active metabolite.
Linagliptin	5 mg qd	5%	100%	100%	Pharyngitis, headache.
Liraglutide	0.6 mg qd	1%	100%	100%	N/V and diarrhea.

(continued)

TABLE 23.8 Endocrine and Metabolic Dosing in Chronic Kidney Disease (*Continued*)

Hypoglycemic Agents	Normal Dosage	% of Renal Excretion	Dosage Adjustment in CKD		Comments
			GFR>30–60	GFR10–29	
Metformin	500 mg bid	95%	100%	Avoid	Lactic acidosis, should be avoided in patients with SCr >1.5 mg/dL (130 mcmol/L).
Pioglitazone	2,550 mg/day (bid or tid)				
	15 mg qd	10%	100%	100%	Increased risk of bladder cancer.
Repaglinide	30 mg qd				
Rosiglitazone	0.5–1 mg	1%	100%	100%	Increased risk of nonfatal heart attack.
	4 mg tid				
Saxagliptin	8 mg qd	75%	50%	25%	Pharyngitis, headache.
Sitagliptin	2.5 mg qd	80%	50%	25%	Pharyngitis, headache.
Tolazamide	5 mg qd	7%	100%	100%	Diuretic effects.
Tolbutamide	100 mg qd	<1%	100%	100%	May impair water excretion.
	250 mg q24h				
	1 g q24h				
Parenteral Agent					
Insulin	Variable	Renally metabolized	100%	75%	Dosage guided by blood glucose levels. Renal metabolism of insulin decreases with azotemia.
Antilipidemic Agents					
Atorvastatin	10 mg/day	<2%	100%	100%	Liver dysfunction, myalgia, and rhabdomyolysis with CsA/tacrolimus.
	80 mg/day				
Bezafibrate	200 mg bid–qid	50%	50–100%	25–50%	
	400 mg SR q24h				

Cholestyramine	4 g bid	24 g/day	<1%	100%	100%	No data.
Clofibrate	500 mg bid	1,000 mg bid	40–70%	q6–q12h	q12–q18h	No data.
Colestipol	5 g bid	30 g/day	<1%	100%	100%	No data.
Fluvastatin	20 mg daily	80 mg/day	<1%	100%	100%	No data.
Gemfibrozil	600 mg bid	600 mg bid	<1%	100%	100%	No data.
Lovastatin	5 mg daily	20 mg/day	<1%	100%	100%	No data.
Nicotinic acid	1 g tid	2 g tid	<1%	100%	50%	No data.
Pravastatin	10–40 mg daily	80 mg/day	<10%	100%	100%	No data.
Probucol	500 mg bid		<2%	100%	100%	
Rosuvastatin	5 mg daily	40 mg/day	10%	100%	100%	5 mg qd; maintenance not to exceed 10 mg qd.
Simvastatin	5 mg qd	20 mg qd	13%	100%	100%	No data.
Thyroid and Antithyroid Agents						
Methimazole	5–20 mg tid		7	100%	100%	
Propylthiouracil	100 mg tid		<10	100%	100%	

bid, twice daily; CsA, cyclosporine; qd, every day; SCr, serum creatinine; SR, sustained release; tid, three times daily.

TABLE 23.9 Gastrointestinal Dosing in Chronic Kidney Disease

Gastrointestinal Agents	Normal Doses		% of Renal Excretion	Dosage Adjustment in CKD			Comments
	Starting Dose	Maximum Dose		GFR 30–60	GFR 10–29	GFR 10–29	

Gastrointestinal Agents	Starting Dose	Maximum Dose	% of Renal Excretion	GFR 30–60	GFR 10–29	Comments
Antiulcer Agents						
Cimetidine	300 mg tid	800 mg bid	60%	100%	25–50%	Multiple drug–drug interactions: β-blockers, sulfonylurea, theophylline, warfarin; may raise serum creatinine.
Famotidine	20 mg bid	40 mg bid	70%	100%	25–50%	Headache, fatigue, thrombocytopenia, alopecia.
Lansoprazole	15 mg qd	30 mg bid	<1%	100%	100%	Headache, diarrhea.
Nizatidine	150 mg bid	300 mg bid	20%	100%	75%	Headache, fatigue, thrombocytopenia, alopecia.
Omeprazole	20 mg qd	40 mg bid	<1%	100%	100%	Headache, diarrhea.
Rabeprazole	20 mg qd	40 mg bid	<1%	100%	100%	Headache, diarrhea.
Pantoprazole	40 mg qd	80 mg bid	<1%	100%	100%	Headache, diarrhea.
Ranitidine	150 mg bid	300 mg bid	80%	100%	50–75%	Headache, fatigue, thrombocytopenia, alopecia.
Cisapride	10 mg tid	20 mg qid	5%	100%	100%	Avoid with azole antifungals, macrolide antibiotics, and other P450 3A4 inhibitors. Prolongs the QT interval.
Metoclopramide	10 mg tid	30 mg qid<1%	15%	100%	100%	Increases cyclosporine/tacrolimus level. Neurotoxic.
Misoprostol	100 mcg bid	200 mcg qid	<1%	100%	100%	Diarrhea, nausea, vomiting. Abortifacient agent.
Sucralfate	1 g qid	1 g qid	<1%	100%	100%	Constipation, decreased absorption of MMF.

bid, twice daily; MMF, mycophenolate mofetil; qd, every day; qid, four times daily; tid, three times daily.

| | | | | | TABLE 23.10 | | Neurologic/Anticonvulsant Dosing in Chronic Kidney Disease |

Anticonvulsants	Normal Dosage	% of Renal Excretion	Dosage Adjustment in CKD			Comments
			GFR 30–60	GFR 10–29	GFR 10–29	
Carbamazepine	2–8 mg/kg per day; adjust for side effects and TDM	2%	100%	100%		Plasma concentration: 4–12 mcg/mL Double vision, fluid retention, myelosuppression.
Clonazepam	2 mg tid	1%	100%	100%		Although no dose reduction is recommended, the drug has not been studied in patients with renal impairment. Recommendations are based on known drug characteristics, not clinical trials data.
Ethosuximide	5 mg/kg per day; adjust for side effects and TDM	20%	100%	100%		Plasma concentration: 40–100 mcg/mL Headache.
Felbamate	400 mg/tid	90%	100%	50%		Anorexia, vomiting, insomnia, nausea.
Gabapentin	150 mg tid	77%	100%	50%		Fewer CNS side effects compared with other agents.
Lamotrigine	25–50 mg/day	1%	100%	100%		Autoinduction, major drug–drug interaction with valproate.
Levetiracetam	500 mg bid	66%	100%	50%		
Oxcarbazepine	300 mg bid	1%	100%	100%		Less effect on P450 compared with carbamazepine.
Phenobarbital	20 mg/kg per day; adjust for side effects and TDM	1%	100%	100%		Plasma concentration: 15–40 mcg/mL Insomnia.
Phenytoin	20 mg/kg per day; adjust for side effects and TDM	1%	100%	100%		Plasma concentration: 10–20 mcg/mL Nystagmus Check free phenytoin level.

(continued)

421

TABLE 23.10 Neurologic/Anticonvulsant Dosing in Chronic Kidney Disease (*Continued*)

Anticonvulsants	Normal Dosage	% of Renal Excretion	Dosage Adjustment in CKD			Comments
			GFR 30–60	GFR 10–29		
Primidone	50 mg	1%	100%	100%		Plasma concentration: 5–12 mcg/mL.
Sodium valproate	7.5–15 mg/kg per day; adjust for side effects and TDM	1%	100%	100%		Plasma concentration: 50–150 mcg/mL Weight gain, hepatitis Check free valproate level.
Tiagabine	4 mg qd, increase 4 mg/day, titrate weekly	2%	100%	100%		Total daily dose may be increased by 4–8 mg at weekly intervals until clinical response is achieved or up to 32 mg/day. The total daily dose should be given in divided doses two to four times daily.
Topiramate	50 mg/day	70%	100%	50%		
Trimethadione	300 mg tid–qid	<1%	q8h	q8–q12h		Active metabolites with long half-life in ESRD. Nephrotic syndrome.
Vigabatrin	1 g bid	70%	100%	50%		Encephalopathy with drug accumulation.
Zonisamide	100 mg qd	30%	100%	75%		Manufacturer recommends that zonisamide should not be used in patients with renal failure (estimated GFR <50 mL/min), as there has been insufficient experience concerning drug dosing and toxicity. The initial dose should be 100 mg daily.

bid, twice daily; CNS, central nervous system; GFR, glomerular filtration rate; qd, every day; qid, four times daily; TDM, therapeutic drug monitoring; tid, three times daily.

TABLE 23.11 Rheumatologic Dosing in Chronic Kidney Disease

Arthritis and Gout Agents	Normal Dosage	% of Renal Excretion	Dosage Adjustment in CKD			Comments
			GFR 30–60	GFR 10–29		
Allopurinol	300 mg q24h	30%	75%	50%		Interstitial nephritis. Rare xanthine stones. Renal excretion of active metabolite with T½ of 25 hours in normal renal function; T½ 1 week in patients with severe CKD. Exfoliative dermatitis.
Auranofin	6 mg q24h	50%	50%	Avoid		Proteinuria and nephritic syndrome.
Colchicine	Acute: 2 mg then 0.5 mg q6h Chronic: 0.5–1.0 mg q24h	5–17%	100%	50–100%		Avoid prolonged use if GFR <50 mL/min.
Gold sodium	25–50 mg	60–90%	50%	Avoid		Thiomalate proteinuria, nephritic syndrome, membranous nephritis.
Penicillamine	250–1,000 mg q24h	40%	100%	Avoid		Nephrotic syndrome.
Probenecid	500 mg bid	<2%	100%	Avoid		Ineffective at decreased GFR.
Nonsteroidal Anti-Inflammatory Drugs						Decrease renal function and platelet aggregation, nephrotic syndrome, interstitial nephritis, hyperkalemia, sodium retention, and increased risk of CVD, MI, and stroke.
Diclofenac	25–75 mg bid	<1%	50–100%	Avoid		
Diflunisal	250–500 mg bid	<3%	100%	Avoid		
Etodolac	200 mg bid	<1%	100%	Avoid		
Fenoprofen	300–600 mg qid	30%	100%	Avoid		
Flurbiprofen	100 mg bid–tid	20%	100%	Avoid		
Ibuprofen	800 mg tid	1%	100%	Avoid		

(continued)

TABLE 23.11 Rheumatologic Dosing in Chronic Kidney Disease (*Continued*)

Arthritis and Gout Agents	Normal Dosage	% of Renal Excretion	Dosage Adjustment in CKD		Comments
			GFR 30–60	GFR 10–29	
Indomethacin	25–50 mg tid	30%	100%	Avoid	
Ketoprofen	25–75 mg tid	<1%	100%	Avoid	
Ketorolac	30–60-mg load then 15–30 mg q6h	30–60%	100%	Avoid	Acute hearing loss in severe CKD.
Meclofenamic acid	50–100 tid–qid	2–4%	100%	Avoid	
Mefenamic acid	250 mg qid	<6%	100%	Avoid	
Nabumetone	1.0–2.0 g q24h	<1%	100%	Avoid	
Naproxen	500 mg bid	<1%	100%	Avoid	
Oxaprozin	1,200 mg q24h	<1%	100%	Avoid	
Phenylbutazone	100 mg tid–qid	1%	100%	Avoid	
Piroxicam	20 mg q24h	10%	100%	Avoid	
Sulindac	200 mg bid	7%	100%	Avoid	Active sulfide metabolite in severe CKD.
Tolmetin	400 mg tid	15%	100%	Avoid	

bid, twice daily; CVD, cardiovascular disease; GFR, glomerular filtration rate; MI, myocardial infarction; qid, four times daily; tid, three times daily.

TABLE 23.12

Rheumatologic (Biologic) Dosing in Chronic Kidney Disease

Biologic Agents	Normal Dosage	% of Renal Excretion	Dosage Adjustment in CKD		Comments
			GFR 30–60	GFR 10–29	
Etanercept	50 mg SC weekly	<1%	100%	100%	Increased risk of TB and other infections.
Infliximab	3 mg/kg IV at 0, 2, and 6 weeks, then q 8 weeks, + methotrexate	<1%	100%	100%	Increased risk of TB and other infections.
Adalimumab	40 mg SC every other week	<1%	100%	100%	May be continued during therapy; may increase to 40 mg SC q week in patients not receiving concomitant methotrexate. May cause glomerulonephritis.
Anakinra	100 mg/day SC	25%	100%	25%	Anakinra elimination is reduced significantly in patients with GFR less than 30 ml/min.
Rituximab	375 mg/m² every other week	<1%	100%	100%	Increased risk of TB and other infections.

CrCl, creatinine clearance; GFR, glomerular filtration rate; IV, intravenous; SC, subcutaneous; TB, tuberculosis.

TABLE 23.13 Sedative Dosing in Chronic Kidney Disease

Sedatives	Normal Dosage	% of Renal Excretion	Dosage Adjustment in CKD		Comments
			GFR 30–60	GFR 10–29	
Barbiturates					
Pentobarbital	30 mg q6–q8h	<1%	100%	100%	May cause excessive sedation. Increased osteomalacia in severe CKD. Charcoal hemoperfusion and hemodialysis more effective than peritoneal dialysis for poisoning.
Phenobarbital	50–100 mg q8–q12h	<1%	100%	100%	Up to 50% unchanged drug excreted with urine with alkaline diuresis.
Secobarbital	30–50 mg q6–q8h	<1%	100%	100%	
Thiopental	Anesthesia induction (individualized)	<1%	100%	100%	
Benzodiazepines					
Alprazolam	0.25–5.0 mg q8h	<1%	100%	100%	May cause excessive sedation and encephalopathy in severe CKD.
Clorazepate	15–60 mg q24h	<1%	100%	100%	
Chlordiazepoxide	15–100 mg q24h	<1%	100%	100%	
Clonazepam	1.5 mg q24h	<1%	100%	100%	Although no dose reduction is foreseen from pharmacokinetics, the drug has not been studied in patients with severe renal impairment.
Diazepam	5–40 mg q24h	<1%	100%	100%	Active metabolites, desmethyldiazepam, and oxazepam may accumulate in renal failure. Dose should be reduced if given longer than a few days. Protein binding decreases in uremia.
Estazolam	1 mg qhs	<1%	100%	100%	
Flurazepam	15–30 mg qhs	<1%	100%	100%	

Drug	Dose				Comments
Lorazepam	1–2 mg q8–q12h	<1%	100%	100%	
Midazolam	Individualized	<1%	100%	100%	
Oxazepam	30–120 mg q24h	<1%	100%	100%	
Quazepam	15 mg qhs	<1%	100%	100%	
Temazepam	30 mg qhs	<1%	100%	100%	
Triazolam	0.25–0.50 mg qhs	<1%	100%	100%	May cause excessive sedation and encephalopathy in severe CKD.
Benzodiazepines: Benzodiazepine Antagonist					
Flumazenil	0.2 mg IV over 15 seconds	<1%	100%	100%	
Miscellaneous Sedative Agents					
Buspirone	5 mg q8h	<1%	100%	100%	Removed by hemoperfusion. Excessive sedation.
Ethchlorvynol	500 mg qhs	<1%	100%	Avoid	Hypertension, excessive sedation.
Haloperidol	1–2 mg q8–q12h	<1%	100%	100%	Nephrotoxic. Nephrogenic diabetes insipidus. Nephrotic syndrome.
Lithium carbonate	0.9–1.2 g q24h	100%	100%	<50%, follow levels	Renal tubular acidosis. Interstitial fibrosis. Acute toxicity when serum levels >1.2 mEq/L. Serum levels should be measured periodically 12 hours after dose. T½ does not reflect extensive tissue accumulation. Plasma levels rebound after dialysis. Toxicity enhanced by volume depletion, NSAIDs, and diuretics.
Meprobamate	1.2–1.6 g q24h	25%	100%	50%	Excessive sedation. Excretion enhanced by forced diuresis.

GFR, glomerular filtration rate; IV, intravenous; NSAIDs, nonsteroidal anti-inflammatory drugs; qhs, at bedtime.

TABLE 23.14 Antiparkinson Dosing in Chronic Kidney Disease

Antiparkinson Agents	Normal Dosage	% of Renal Excretion	Dosage Adjustment in CKD		Comments
			GFR 30–60	GFR 10–29	
Carbidopa	1–2 tab tid/qid (30–200 mg qd)	30%	100%	100%	Require careful titration of dose according to clinical response.
Levodopa	1–2 tab tid/qid (300–2,000 mg qd)	<1%	100%	50–100%	Active and inactive metabolites excreted in urine. Active metabolites with long T½ in severe CKD.
Rasagiline (MAO-B inhibitor)	1 mg qd	<1%	100%	100%	

MAO-B, monamine oxidase B; qd, every day; qid, four times daily; tid, three times daily.

TABLE
23.15

Antipsychotic Dosing in Chronic Kidney Disease

Antipsychotics	Normal Dosage	% of Renal Excretion	Dosage Adjustment in CKD		Comments
			GFR 30–60	GFR 10–29	
Phenothiazines					
Chlorpromazine	300–800 mg q24h	<1%	100%	100%	Orthostatic hypotension, extrapyramidal symptoms, and confusion can occur.
Promethazine	20–100 mg q24h	<1%	100%	100%	Excessive sedation may occur in severe CKD.
Thioridazine	50–100 mg po tid. Increase gradually. Maximum of 800 mg/day.	<1%	100%	100%	
Trifluoperazine	1–2 mg bid. Increase to no more than 6 mg.	<1%	100%	100%	
Perphenazine	8–16 mg po bid, tid, or qid. Increase to 64 mg daily.	<1%	100%	100%	
Thiothixene	2 mg po tid. Increase gradually to 15 mg daily.	<1%	100%	100%	
Haloperidol	1–2 mg q8–q12h	<1%	100%	100%	Hypotension, excessive sedation
Loxapine	12.5–50 mg IM q4–q6h	<1%	100%	100%	Do not administer drug IV.
Clozapine	12.5 mg po. 25–50 mg daily to 300–450 mg by end of 2 weeks. Maximum: 900 mg daily.	<1%	100%	100%	
Risperidone	1 mg po bid. Increase to 3 mg bid.	<1%	100%	100%	
Olanzapine	5–10 mg	<1%	100%	100%	Potential hypotensive effects
Quetiapine	25 mg po bid. Increase in increments of 25–50 bid or tid. 300–400 mg daily by day 4.	<1%	100%	100%	
Ziprasidone	20–100 mg q12h	<1%	100%	100%	

bid, twice daily; GFR, glomerular filtration rate; IM, intramuscularly; IV, intravenously; po, by mouth; qid, four times daily; tid, three times daily.

TABLE 23.16 Anticoagulation in Chronic Kidney Disease

Anticoagulants	Normal Dosage	% of Renal Excretion	Dosage Adjustment in CKD			Comments
			GFR 30–60	GFR 10–29		
Alteplase	60 mg over 1 hour, then 20 mg/h for 2 hours	<1%	100%	100%		Tissue-type plasminogen activator (tPA)
Anistreplase	30 U over 2–5 min	<1%	100%	100%		
Apixaban	5 mg po bid	25%	100%	50%		
Aspirin	81–325 mg/day	10%	100%	100%		GI irritation and bleeding tendency
Clopidogrel	75 mg/day	50%	100%	100%		GI irritation and bleeding tendency
Dabigatran	150 mg po bid	80%	100%	Avoid		
Dalteparin	100 U/kg	No data	100%	Avoid		Check anti-factor Xa activity 4 hours after 2nd dose in patients with renal dysfunction.
Dipyridamole	50 mg tid	No data	100%	100%		
Enoxaparin	1 mg/kg q12h	8%	100%	75–50%		1 mg/kg q12h for treatment of DVT. Check anti-factor Xa activity 4 hours after 2nd dose in patients with renal dysfunction. Some evidence of drug accumulation in renal failure.
Fondaparinux	2.5–10 mg subq	<1%	100%	Avoid		Half-life increases with renal failure. Should be used for patients with HIT only.
Heparin	75 U/kg load then 15 U/kg per hour	<1%	100%	100%		Half-life increases with dose.
Iloprost	0.5–2.0 ng/kg per minute for 5–12 hours	<1%	100%	100%		
Prasugrel	10 mg	<1%	100%	100%		GI irritation and bleeding tendency. Higher risk of bleeding than clopidogrel.

430

Drug	Dose				Comments
Rivaroxaban	20 mg daily	80%	100%	Avoid	Acute renal failure. Uricosuric effect at low GFR.
Streptokinase	250,000-U load, then 100,000 U/h	<1%	100%	100%	Decrease CsA level. May cause severe neutropenia and thrombocytopenia.
Sulfinpyrazone	200 mg bid	25–50%	100%	100%	
Ticlopidine	250 mg bid	2%	100%	100%	
Tinzaparin	175 U/kg	No data	100%	Avoid	175 U/kg for treatment of DVT. Check anti-factor Xa activity 4 hours after 2nd dose in patients with renal dysfunction. Some evidence of drug accumulation in renal failure.
Tranexamic acid	25 mg/kg tid–qid	90%	50%	25%	
Urokinase	4,400-U/kg load, then 4,400 U/kg/h	<1%	100%	100%	
Warfarin	5 mg/day then adjust per INR	<1%	100%	50–100%	Monitor INR very closely. Start at 5 mg/day. 1 mg vitamin K IV over 30 min or 2.5–5 mg po can be used to normalize INR.

bid, twice daily; CsA, cyclosporine; DVT, deep vein thrombosis; GFR, glomerular filtration rate; GI, gastrointestinal; HIT, heparin-induced thrombocytopenia; INR, international normalized ratio; IV, intravenous; po, by mouth; qid, four times daily; subq, subcutaneous; tid, three times daily.

TABLE 23.17 Oncologic Agents in Chronic Kidney Disease

Oncologic Drugs	Normal Dosage	Dosage Adjustment in CKD			Comments
		GFR 30–60	GFR 10–29		
Bleomycin	No adjustment needed	40–50 mL/min, reduce dose by 30% 30–40 mL/min, reduce dose by 40%	20–30 mL/min, reduce dose by 45% 10–20 mL/min, reduce dose by 55%		Because pulmonary toxicity is a dose limiting toxicity, repeat pulmonary function tests prior to each administration
Capecitabine (Xeloda)	No dose reduction	25% dose reduction	Contraindicated *Note:* has been used at 50–80% dose reduction (Aymanns, 2010; Cockcroft and Gault, 1976)		
Carboplatin	No adjustment needed	Reduce dose by 50%	Reduce dose by 50%		Nephrotoxicity often appears as hypomagnesemia (reversible tubular injury), and is most common in patients previously treated with cisplatin
Carfilzomib (Kyprolis)	Reduced initial dose 15 mg/m² daily on cycle 1, 20 mg/m² on cycle 2, and 27 mg/m² on cycles 3 and beyond	Reduced initial dose 15 mg/m² daily on cycle 1, 20 mg/m² on cycle 2, and 27 mg/m² on cycles 3 and beyond	Reduced initial dose 15 mg/m² daily on cycle 1, 20 mg/m² on cycle 2, and 27 mg/m² on cycles 3 and beyond		

Drug				Comments
Carmustine (BiCNU)	Insufficient data	Insufficient data	Avoid	Progressive azotemia, increased serum creatinine, and renal failure reported during and after discontinuation of prolonged therapy
Cetuximab	No adjustment needed	No adjustment needed	No adjustment needed	Nephrotoxicity often appears as hypomagnesemia (tubular injury)
Chlorambucil (Leukeran) (Nolin, 2015)	No dose adjustment	No dose adjustment	No dose adjustment	
Cisplatin	Reduce dose by 25%	Reduce dose by 50%	Reduce dose by 50% or consider use of alternate agent	Per manufacturer recommendation cisplatin should not be administered to any patient with pre-existing renal impairment. Nephrotoxicity often appears as renal failure, renal tubular acidosis, and hypomagnesemia (tubulointerstitial injury).
Cladribine	No adjustment needed	Reduce dose by 25%	Reduce dose by 25%	
Clofarabine (Clolar)	50% dose reduction	50% dose reduction	Insufficient data	Hematuria or rapid-onset acute renal failure with proteinuria.
Crizotinib	No adjustment needed	No adjustment needed	Administer 250 mg qd	
Cyclophosphamide	No adjustment needed	No adjustment needed	50% of the dose	Nephrotoxicity often appears as hyponatremia (SIADH and increased N/V) and hemorrhagic cystitis.
Cytarabine (high dose 1–3 g/m²)	Reduce dose by 40%	Reduce dose by 50%	Consider alternative agent or dose 100–200 mg/m² per day CIV	Renal adjustments are only required in high doses (1–3 g/m²) possibly for >500 mg/m²
Dacarbazine (DTIC)	Insufficient data	Insufficient data	Insufficient data	Mild to moderate azotemia without permanent damage

(continued)

TABLE 23.17 Oncologic Agents in Chronic Kidney Disease (*Continued*)

Oncologic Drugs	Normal Dosage	Dosage Adjustment in CKD			Comments
		GFR 30–60	GFR 10–29		
Daunorubicin	No adjustment needed	No adjustment needed	No adjustment needed		Mainly excreted through the bile; however, per FDA recommendations, at 50% dose reduction is recommended in patients with a SCr >3
Epirubicin	No adjustment needed	No adjustment needed	No adjustment needed		Mainly excreted through the bile; however, per FDA recommendations, at 50% dose reduction is recommended in patients with a SCr >5
Eribulin	Reduce to 1.1 mg/m² per dose	Reduce to 1.1 mg/m² per dose	No data		
Erlotinib (Tarceva) (Wagner, 2015)	Insufficient data	Insufficient data *Note:* hold if CrCl <30 due to treatment	Insufficient data *Note:* hold if CrCl <30 due to treatment		
Etoposide	Reduce dose by 15%	Reduce dose by 20%	Reduce dose by 25%		About 50% of every dose is excreted through urine
Fludarabine	Reduce dose to 20 mg/m²	Reduce dose to 20 mg/m²	Avoid use		No reports of nephrotoxicity *Note:* <4% renal elimination
Gefitinib (Iressa) (Walker, 2009)	No dose adjustment	No dose adjustment	No dose adjustment *Note:* use caution		Nephrotoxicity often appears as hemolytic uremic syndrome (microangiopathic lesions)
Gemcitabine	No adjustment needed	No adjustment needed	No adjustment needed		

Drug				Comments
Hydroxyurea (Droxia) (Yeung, 2014)	50% dose reduction 7.5 mg/kg daily	50% dose reduction 7.5 mg/kg daily	50% dose reduction 7.5 mg/kg daily	Temporarily impaired tubular function with elevated serum uric acid, BUN, and creatinine.
Ibrutinib (Imbruvica) (Zhang, 2009)	No dose adjustment MCL: 560 mg po daily	No dose adjustment MCL: 560 mg po daily	Insufficient data	Renal failure preceded by increases in creatinine of 1.5–3 times the upper limit of normal. *Note:* <1% excreted renally
Ifosfamide	Reduce dose by 20%	Reduce dose by 25%	Reduce dose by 30%	Nephrotoxicity often appears as Fanconi syndrome, renal tubular acidosis, nephrogenic diabetes insipidus, and hemorrhagic cystitis. 18% of the drug is excreted through urine
Imatinib	No adjustment needed	CrCl 59–40 mL/min max recommended dose of 600 mg	CrCl 39–20 mL/min reduce starting dose by 50%, increase as tolerated. Max recommended dose 400 mg	
Interferons	No adjustment needed	No adjustment needed	No adjustment needed	Nephrotoxicity often appears as proteinuria, (minimal change, and acute tubular necrosis)
Interleukin-2	No adjustment needed	No adjustment needed	No adjustment needed	Nephrotoxicity often appears as prerenal azotemia from renal hypoperfusion (capillary leak syndrome). Use with caution.
Irinotecan	No adjustment needed	No adjustment needed	No adjustment needed	Patients with multiple myeloma frequently have renal insufficiency. T½ and AUC increase as creatinine clearance decreases.
Lenalidomide	MCL: dose 10 mg daily MDS: dose 5 mg daily MM: dose 10 mg daily	MCL: dose 10 mg daily MDS: dose 5 mg daily MM: dose 10 mg daily	MCL: dose 15 mg q48h MDS: dose 2.5 mg daily MM: dose 15 mg q48h	

(continued)

TABLE
23.17

Oncologic Agents in Chronic Kidney Disease (*Continued*)

Oncologic Drugs	Normal Dosage	Dosage Adjustment in CKD		Comments
		GFR 30–60	GFR 10–29	
Lomustine	Reduce dose by 25%	Reduce dose by 30%	Avoid use	Nephrotoxicity often appears as a slowly progressive, chronic interstitial nephritis, which is generally irreversible and can be induced by prolonged therapy time.
Melphalan	Reduce dose by 15%	Reduce dose by 25%	Reduce dose by 30%	Nephrotoxicity often appears as SIADH. Have patients maintain adequate hydration during therapy.
Methotrexate	Reduce dose by 35%	Reduce dose by 50%	Avoid use	Nephrotoxicity often appears as nonoliguric renal failure (intratubular deposition of methotrexate). Avoid nephrotoxicity with aggressive hydration with NS, urine alkalinization, and forced diuresis (3 L/day)
Mitomycin	Limited data	Limited data	CrCl <10 mL/min, reduce dose by 25%	HUS and TTP
Oxaliplatin	No adjustment needed	No adjustment needed	Reduce dose from 85–65 mg/m^2	Nephrotoxicity rarely appears as acute tubular necrosis; however, the significance is much less than the previous generation platins (cisplatin and carboplatin)

Drug				
Paclitaxel (Taxol)	No dose adjustment (NKDEP, 2009) 135 or 175 mg/m²	No dose adjustment (NKDEP, 2009) 135 or 175 mg/m²	No dose adjustment (NKDEP, 2009) 135 or 175 mg/m²	Mild to severe elevations in serum creatinine
Panitumumab	No adjustment needed	No adjustment needed	No adjustment needed	Nephrotoxicity often appears as hypomagnesemia
Pemetrexed	No adjustment needed	No adjustment needed	Limited data; avoid use	ATN
Pentostatin	Reduce dose by 30%	Reduce dose by 40%	Consider an alternative agent	
Rituximab	No adjustment needed	No adjustment needed	No adjustment needed	HUS and TTP
Sorafenib	Reduce dose to 400 mg bid	Reduce dose to 200 mg bid	Limited data	Nephrotoxicity may be delayed as long as several years after discontinuation.
Streptozocin	No adjustment needed	Reduce dose by 25%	CrCl <10 mL/min, reduce dose by 50%	Proteinuria, and nephrotic syndrome (renal thrombotic microangiopathy)
Sunitinib	No adjustment needed	No adjustment needed	No adjustment needed	
Temozolomide (Temodar)	Insufficient data; Note: pharmacokinetics equivalent for CrCl 36–130 mL/min	Insufficient data	Insufficient data	
Topotecan	Reduce dose by 20%	Reduce dose by 25%	Reduce dose by 30%	
Vandetanib	Reduce initial dose to 200 mg daily	Reduce initial dose to 200 mg daily	Reduce initial dose to 200 mg daily	Increased SCr, and proteinuria
Vemurafenib (Zelboraf)	No dose adjustment; 960 mg po every 12 hours; Note: clearance similar to patients with normal renal function	No dose adjustment; 960 mg po every 12 hours; Note: clearance similar to patients with normal renal function	Insufficient data	
Vinca alkaloids	No adjustment needed	No adjustment needed	No adjustment needed	Hypernatremia secondary to SIADH. Maintain adequate hydration during treatment

ATN, acute tubular necrosis; AUC, area under the curve; CrCl, creatinine clearance; g, gram; GFR, glomerular filtration rate; HUS, hemolytic uremic syndrome; MCL, mantle-cell lymphoma; MDS, myelodysplastic syndromes; MM, multiple myeloma; NS, normal saline; N/V, nausea and vomiting; qd, daily; SCr, serum creatinine; SIADH, syndrome of inappropriate antidiuretic hormone; T1/2, half-life; TTP, thrombotic thrombocytopenic purpura; U/Kg/h, units/kg/h.

References and Suggested Readings

Aronoff GR, Bennett WM, Berns JS, et al. Drug Prescribing in Renal Failure: Dosing Guidelines for Adults and Children. 5th ed. Philadelphia, PA: American College of Physicians-American Society of Internal Medicine; 2007.

Aymanns C, Keller F, Maus S, et al. Review on pharmacokinetics and pharmacodynamics and the aging kidney. *Clin J Am Soc Nephrol.* 2010;5:314–327.

Cockcroft DW, Gault MH. Prediction of creatinine clearance from serum creatinine. *Nephron.* 1976;16:31–41.

Corsonello A, Onder G, Bustacchini S, et al. Estimating renal function to reduce the risk of adverse drug reactions. *Drug Saf.* 2012;35:47–54.

Dowling TC, Briglia AE, Fink JC, et al. Characterization of hepatic cytochrome P450 3A activity in patients with end-stage renal disease. *Clin Pharmacol Ther.* 2003;73: 427–434.

Hart RG, Eikelboom JW, Ingram AJ, et al. Anticoagulants in atrial fibrillation patients with chronic kidney disease. *Nat Rev Nephrol.* 2012;8:569–578.

Hudson JQ, Nyman HA. Use of estimated glomerular filtration rate for drug dosing in the chronic kidney disease patient. *Curr Opin Nephrol Hypertens.* 2011;20: 482–491.

Ix JH, Wassel CL, Stevens LA, et al. Equations to estimate creatinine excretion rate: the CKD epidemiology collaboration. *Clin J Am Soc Nephrol.* 2011;6:184–191.

Khanal A, Peterson GM, Jose MD, et al. Comparison of equations for dosing of medications in renal impairment. *Nephrology (Carlton).* 2017;22:470–477.

Knights KM, Rowland A, Miners JO. Renal drug metabolism in humans: the potential for drug-endobiotic interactions involving cytochrome P450 (CYP) and UDP-glucuronosyltransferase (UGT). *Br J Clin Pharmacol.* 2013;76:587–602.

Levey AS, Kramer H. Obesity, glomerular hyperfiltration, and the surface area correction. *Am J Kidney Dis.* 2010;56:255–258.

Lindeman RD, Tobin J, Shock NW. Longitudinal studies on the rate of decline in renal function with age. *J Am Geriatr Soc.* 1985;33:278–285.

Martin JH, Saleem M, Looke D. Therapeutic drug monitoring to adjust dosing in morbid obesity—a new use for an old methodology. *Br J Clin Pharmacol.* 2012;73: 685–690.

National Kidney Disease Education Program. NKDEP's suggested approach to drug dosing, 2009. Available from https://www.niddk.nih.gov/health-information/professionals/clinical-tools-patient-education-outreach/ckd-drug-dosing-providers. Accessed June 6, 2018.

Nolin TD. A synopsis of clinical pharmacokinetic alterations in advanced CKD. *Semin Dial.* 2015;28:325–329.

Olyaei AJ, Bennett WM. Drug dosing in the elderly patients with chronic kidney disease. *Clin Geriatr Med.* 2009;25:459–527. Review.

Pai MP. Estimating the glomerular filtration rate in obese adult patients for drug dosing. *Adv Chronic Kidney Dis.* 2010;17:e53–e62.

Peralta CA, Shlipak MG, Judd S, et al. Detection of chronic kidney disease with creatinine, cystatin C, and urine albumin-to-creatinine ratio and association with progression to end-stage renal disease and mortality. *JAMA.* 2011;305:1545–1552.

Salazar DE, Corcoran GB. Predicting creatinine clearance and renal drug clearance in obese patients from estimated fat-free body mass. *Am J Med.* 1988;84:1053–1060.

Spruill WJ, Wade WE, Cobb HH 3rd. Continuing the use of the Cockcroft–Gault equation for drug dosing in patients with impaired renal function. *Clin Pharmacol Ther.* 2009;86:468–470.

Stevens LA, Levey AS. Use of the MDRD equation to estimate kidney function for drug dosing. *Clin Pharmacol Ther.* 2009;86:465–467.

Stevens LA, Nolin TD, Richardson MM, et al. Comparison of drug dosing recommendations based on measured GFR and kidney function estimating equations. *Am J Kidney Dis.* 2009;54:33–42.

Tawfic QA, Bellingham G. Postoperative pain management in patients with chronic kidney disease. *J Anaesthesiol Clin Pharmacol.* 2015;31:6–13.

Wagner LA, Tata AL, Fink JC. Patient safety issues in CKD: core curriculum 2015. *Am J Kidney Dis.* 2015;66:159–169.

Walker DB, Walker TJ, Jacobson TA. Chronic kidney disease and statins: improving cardiovascular outcomes. *Curr Atheroscler Rep*. 2009;11:301–308.

Yeung CK, Shen DD, Thummel KE, et al. Effects of chronic kidney disease and uremia on hepatic drug metabolism and transport. *Kidney Int*. 2014;85:522–528.

Zhang Y, Zhang L, Abraham S, et al. Assessment of the impact of renal impairment on systemic exposure of new molecular entities: evaluation of recent new drug applications. *Clin Pharmacol Ther*. 2009;85:305–311.

24 Chronic Kidney Disease in Children

Agnes Trautmann and Franz Schaefer

Children with chronic kidney disease (CKD) differ from the adult population with respect to the demographics of the disorder, the spectrum of underlying diseases, the associated comorbidities, and the nature and severity of complications. Psychosocial and ethical aspects related to coping with CKD as well as its treatment also have unique aspects in children.

DEMOGRAPHICS AND ETIOLOGY

The prevalence of end-stage renal disease (ESRD) and renal replacement therapy (RRT) in children and adolescents across the world ranges from 18 to 100 per million population. The median annual incidence is 9 patients per million similarly aged children. Variations in incidence may reflect variations in the incidence of CKD, differences in pre-ESRD care, differences in the propensity to treat patients with ESRD, or in the timing of RRT commencement. In many countries, the prevalence is rising due to the combination of a fairly steady incidence and improved patient survival on RRT (Harambat, 2012).

The pediatric incidence is only 10% of that observed in young adults and <2% of that observed in the elderly. Most of the available epidemiologic data come from ESRD registries, and information on the demographics of mild to moderate CKD in children is limited but likely to be in similar proportion to the adult population. In countries with a high prevalence of consanguineous marriage, the prevalence of CKD in children is estimated to be several fold higher than in Western countries.

The spectrum of kidney disorders underlying pediatric CKD differs greatly from the distribution of nephropathies in adults. Approximately 60% to 70% of affected children were born with congenital abnormalities of the kidneys and/or urinary tract with a reduced number of functioning nephrons because of variable degrees of renal hypo/dysplasia. Obstructive uropathies (posterior urethral valves, pelvicoureteric or distal ureteric stenosis) usually are detected in the neonatal period and relieved surgically if functionally relevant. In these cases, the emergence of CKD depends on the degree of renal hypo/dysplasia present at birth. Approximately 50% of boys born with urethral valves ultimately will develop ESRD in later life.

Inherited monogenic kidney disorders constitute another major cause of pediatric CKD, accounting cumulatively for another 15% to

20% of cases. Nephronophthisis, polycystic kidney disease, oxalosis, cystinosis, and Alport syndrome are caused by identifiable genetic defects; genetic defects are also responsible for a large proportion of children presenting with focal segmental glomerulosclerosis and atypical hemolytic uremic syndrome.

Other causes include kidney injury following ischemic insults that has become chronic (most importantly perinatal asphyxia and septicemia). In contrast, even large pediatric patient registries have not reported significant numbers of children with diabetic or hypertensive nephropathy, the two most common causes of CKD in adult populations. Acquired glomerulopathies, causing 5% of CKD, usually affect primarily older children and are limited to rare cases of Immunoglobulin A (IgA) nephropathy or Henoch–Schönlein nephritis, and systemic vasculitis such as systemic lupus erythematosus and granulomatosis with polyangiitis.

ASSOCIATED COMORBIDITIES

Because of the predominantly genetic origin of pediatric nephropathies, CKD in children frequently is associated with a variety of extrarenal abnormalities. The prevalence of severe, associated comorbidities appears to have increased in recent years as a growing number of children with severe syndromal disease is accepted to CKD and ESRD management programs. In the Registry of the International Pediatric PD Network, 13% of children with CKD starting dialysis suffered from a defined syndrome with one or several extrarenal manifestations. Impaired neurocognitive development was observed in 16%, cardiac anomalies in 15%, ocular abnormalities in 13%, and hearing abnormalities in 5% of patients.

Impaired neurodevelopment and sensory dysfunctions are among the most disabling general handicaps interfering with psychosocial adjustment and integration. Twenty to 25% of infants undergoing appropriate neurodevelopmental testing show moderate to severe developmental delays, which usually remain unchanged after successful kidney transplantation. IQ testing at school age usually reveals an IQ distribution that is shifted downward with respect to total verbal and performance compared with healthy controls, but testing may be biased in a substantial proportion of patients because of associated sensory disorders such as hearing loss or visual impairment. Whereas the deficits usually are most striking in the ESRD population, significant neurocognitive deficits concerning memory, attention and executive function have been demonstrated in children with stages 2 to 4 CKD, also. These concerning findings clearly define a need for regular assessment of neurodevelopment and/or neurocognitive function in all children with significant glomerular filtration rate (GFR) impairment and the development of interventional programs, including individualized plans to optimize developmental and educational outcomes.

ASSESSMENT OF KIDNEY FUNCTION IN CHILDREN

Glomerular Filtration Rate

Several issues need to be considered when assessing and interpreting kidney function in children. Childhood is the final extrauterine period of growth and maturation. During this phase, the metabolic needs of the organism on the one hand and the functional capacity of the kidneys on the other undergo profound, synchronized changes. From birth to adulthood, body weight increases 20-fold, body length three-to fourfold, and body surface area (BSA) (the closest correlate of basal metabolic rate) eightfold. By convention, the GFR is normalized to the BSA of an average-size adult (i.e., 1.73 m^2).

Although nephron formation is complete by the 30th gestational week, nephrons continue to grow in size and functional capacity after birth. In early postnatal life, nephron size and capacity increase not only in absolute terms but also relative to BSA, resulting in a significant physiologic gain in normalized global renal function. The average GFR/1.73 m^2 in the neonate is 20 to 30 mL/min, increasing rapidly in the first few months of life (Table 24.1). From age 18 months onward, the absolute increase of GFR precisely matches the growth in BSA, resulting in a constant normal range of BSA-indexed GFR throughout childhood and adolescence. After 2 years of age, the conventional CKD staging system (see Chapter 1), which assigns stages of CKD according to estimated GFR (eGFR)/1.73 m^2 in multiples of 15 and 30 mL/min, can be used.

Regular assessments of GFR are crucial in the staging and monitoring of renal function in children with CKD. The direct measurement of GFR is a challenging task in children. Although inulin clearance is still considered the gold standard, inulin is unavailable in many countries,

TABLE 24.1	Normal Glomerular Filtration Rate by Postnatal Age in Term and Preterm Neonates, Children, and Adolescents
Age	**GFR/1.73 m^2 mean ± SD (mL/min)**
1 week, preterm (29–34 weeks GA)	15±6
2–8 weeks, preterm (29–34 weeks GA)	29±14
>8 weeks, preterm (29–34 weeks GA)	51
1 week, born at term	41±15
2–8 weeks, born at term	66±25
>8 weeks, born at term	96±22
2–12 years	133±27
13–21 years, males	140±30
13–21 years, females	126±22

GFR, glomerular filtration rate; SD, standard deviation; GA, gestational age.
Source: Adapted from Schwartz GJ, Brion LP, Spitzer A. The use of plasma creatinine concentration for estimating glomerular filtration rate in infants, children, and adolescents. *Pediatr Clin North Am.* 1987;34:571–590; Hogg RJ, Furth S, Lemley KV, et al. National Kidney Foundation's Kidney Disease Outcomes Quality Initiative clinical practice guidelines for chronic kidney disease in children and adolescents: evaluation, classification, and stratification. *Pediatrics.* 2003;111:1416–1421.

and formal steady-state inulin clearance studies are difficult to perform in the pediatric setting, because of both technical and ethical aspects. Radioisotope single-injection dilution studies (e.g., using ^{51}Cr-EDTA chromium or ^{99}Tc-DTPA) have been largely abandoned because of significant radiation exposure. A simplified single-injection clearance protocol utilizing the radiocontrast agent iohexol has been validated in children with CKD. However, even iohexol carries a small but definite risk of toxicity, and injection and timed blood collection protocols are not trivial to establish and perform regularly in busy clinical programs. Therefore, utilization of such protocols will depend on the availability of valid, non-invasive alternatives.

Creatinine-Based Estimates of Glomerular Filtration Rate

The most commonly used direct GFR measurement in children is the endogenous creatinine clearance, measured and normalized to 1.73 m^2 BSA as described in Chapter 1. Creatinine clearance measurements require that children be able to control their voiding. Shortened protocols with timed urine collections over 3 to 6 hours in outpatient settings are a valid alternative to 24-hour sampling. Creatinine clearance accurately reflects GFR in patients with normal or mildly impaired renal function. As GFR declines, tubular creatinine secretion increases, resulting in an overestimation of true GFR. In advanced CKD (GFR/1.73 m^2 <20 mL/min), the mean of creatinine and urea clearances is a well-established equivalent of GFR.

The need for simple and rapid GFR assessment in clinical practice has led to the development of prediction equations that allow eGFR from levels of serum markers. The most widely used eGFR markers are creatinine, a product of muscle metabolism; and cystatin C, a low–molecular-weight protein (13 kDa), which happens to be a cysteine protease inhibitor.

Creatinine generation, and consequently the steady-state serum creatinine level, depends strongly on the relative amount of muscle mass, which in turn depends on age and sex. Mean serum creatinine levels gradually increase during childhood from 0.3 to 0.4 mg/dL (26 to 35 mcmol/L) in early infancy to 1.0 mg/dL in female and 1.3 mg/dL in male adolescents (88 and 115 mcmol/L, respectively).

Schwartz devised a formula to estimate GFR from serum creatinine accounting for developmental changes in creatinine generation. According to this formula, eGFR equals the ratio of height over serum creatinine times a constant k (Schwartz, 1987). In the original Schwartz equation, k was age and sex specific. The Schwartz formula, because of its simplicity and ready availability, has found wide acceptance in the field of pediatrics, but validation studies have demonstrated poor precision and accuracy of the original equation. True GFR tends to be overestimated by 10% to 15%, and the average 95% confidence intervals typically range from −40% to +50%.

Because the relationship of serum creatinine with GFR is exponential, with very little change in serum creatinine down to a GFR of 50 to 60, serum creatinine–based prediction equations are particularly insensitive in detecting GFR changes in CKD stage 2. Another problem arises from changes in laboratory methodology. The original values for the constant k term in the Schwartz equation were validated using the Jaffe method to measure creatinine. Most laboratories today use enzymatic assays; and more recently, an isotope-dilution mass spectrometry assay has been introduced to which creatinine assays should now all be calibrated. Both enzymatic assays and isotope-dilution mass spectrometry-calibrated assays yield systematically lower serum creatinine values than those obtained using the legacy Jaffe technique, and this results in GFR overestimations by 5% to 10% when using the original k values in the Schwartz GFR estimating equation. To address this issue, Schwartz (2009) subsequently validated a new equation adapted for use with enzymatic creatinine measurements. The new Schwartz formula uses a uniform k value for both sexes and is valid in children from 1 to 16 years:

Estimated GFR = height (cm) × 0.413/serum creatinine (mg/dL)

Cystatin-Based Estimates of Glomerular Filtration Rate

In recent years, cystatin C has been advocated as a serum marker of GFR. Cystatin C is produced by all nucleated cells at a relatively stable rate. The principal mode of excretion of cystatin C is renal: Cystatin C is freely filtered by the glomerulus and is then metabolized after being reabsorbed in the proximal tubule. Because of this, serum cystatin C levels increase in a predictable fashion as GFR falls. Cystatin C–based eGFR may be particularly advantageous in children as its production rate, after correcting for BSA, is much less influenced by age than is serum creatinine, and serum cystatin levels are independent of sex and muscle mass. After a decrease by approximately 50% in the first year of life, cystatin C plasma levels remain stable until about age 50 years. For these reasons, cystatin C appears to be a more sensitive and reliable marker of GFR than serum creatinine, with an earlier increase of serum levels in patients with CKD (Table 24.2). Filler and Lepage (2003) derived an equation to predict GFR from serum cystatin C in a pediatric validation study using ^{99}Tc-DTPA single-injection clearance as the standard. The sensitivity of detecting children with CKD stage 2 was 74% for serum cystatin C as compared to 46% for serum

TABLE 24.2	Reference Ranges for Serum Cystatin C
	Reference Interval (mg/L)
Preterm infants	1.34–2.57
Full-term infants	1.36–2.23
>8 days–1 year	0.75–1.87
>1–3 years	0.68–1.90
>3–16 years	0.51–1.31

Source: From Filler G, Lepage N. Should the Schwartz formula for estimation of GFR be replaced by cystatin C formula? *Pediatr Nephrol.* 2003;18:981–985.

creatinine. Confidence intervals were consistently narrower for cystatin C than for creatinine-based eGFR. In children with CKD stages 3 to 5, the intrapatient coefficient of variation of cystatin C was significantly lower than that of serum creatinine, suggesting that cystatin C is a better tool for longitudinal monitoring of patients with advanced CKD.

In their recent study, Schwartz (2009) derived a best-fitting GFR prediction equation based on height, serum creatinine, cystatin C, blood urea nitrogen (BUN), and sex. Validated against iohexol clearance in North American children, this refined formula promises improved precision and accuracy of GFR estimation:

$$\text{Estimated GFR (mL/min/1.73 m}^2) = 39.1 \, [\text{height (m)/Scr (mg/dL)}]^{0.516}$$
$$\times [1.8/\text{cystatin C (mg/L)}]^{0.294}$$
$$\times [39/\text{BUN (mg/dL)}]^{0.169} \times [1.099]^{\text{male}}$$
$$\times [\text{height (m)}/1.4]^{0.188}$$

The new formula is claimed to be useful in the range of GFR/1.73 m^2 from 15 to 75 mL/min but awaits validation outside this range of kidney function and in non-U.S. cohorts.

Assessment of Proteinuria

Proteinuria is a common laboratory finding in children. A rapid semiquantitative assessment of proteinuria can be made using dipstick staining. The most precise quantitation is obtained by measuring protein excretion in 12- or 24-hour samples using the Coomassie blue method. However, precise urine collections usually are difficult to perform in infants and young children. If timed urine collections are not possible, assessment of the protein/creatinine ratio (UPr/Cr) and/or albumin/creatinine ratio (UA/Cr) as markers for glomerular proteinuria in random urine samples is a valid alternative. Markers of tubular proteinuria are α_1-microglobulin/creatinine ratio, β_2-microglobulin/creatinine ratio, and retinol-binding protein measured in a random urine sample.

Most healthy children excrete small amounts of protein in their urine. Physiologic proteinuria varies with age and the size of the child: When corrected for BSA, the upper normal limit of protein excretion is 300 mg/m^2 per day at age 1 month in full-term babies, 250 mg at 1 year, 200 mg at 10 years, and 150 mg in late adolescence. Any protein excretion in excess of 1.0 g/m^2 per day is termed "gross" or "nephrotic" proteinuria.

The upper limit of normal for the UPr/Cr (as mg protein/mg creatinine) is 0.5 at age younger than 2 years, and 0.2 in older children and adolescents (Hogg, 2003). A UPr/Cr >2.0 is consistent with nephrotic-range proteinuria.

Isolated asymptomatic proteinuria in children can occur either as a transient phenomenon (e.g., caused by fever, strenuous exercise, extreme cold exposure, epinephrine administration, emotional stress, congestive heart failure, abdominal surgery, or seizures) or as a persistent abnormality. It can represent a benign condition (e.g., orthostatic proteinuria) or a serious CKD.

Estimates of the prevalence of isolated asymptomatic proteinuria in children range between 0.6% and 6%. Orthostatic proteinuria accounts for up to 60% of all cases of asymptomatic proteinuria reported in children, with an even higher incidence in adolescents. Children with orthostatic proteinuria usually excrete <1 g of protein per day (UPr/Cr <1.0). Although patients with orthostatic proteinuria have an excellent prognosis, the long-term prognosis for children with isolated fixed proteinuria remains unknown (Loghman-Adham, 1999).

HYPERTENSION

Prevalence, Etiology, and Mechanisms

In contrast to adults, the majority of hypertensive children suffer from a specific underlying disease and secondary forms of hypertension (National Heart, Lung and Blood Institute, 2005) and are at greater risk of long-term target-organ damage. However, the investigation of pediatric hypertension poses numerous practical and scientific problems in three main areas: measuring blood pressure, defining hypertension, and deciding about the extent of further investigations in the hypertensive patient. The changing cardiovascular physiology, pathology, and body dimensions in childhood add complexity in each of these areas.

Renal parenchymal disease accounts for at least 75% of pediatric cases, and renovascular disease for an additional 10%. Coarctation of the aorta, endocrine disease, and monogenetic inherited forms of hypertension are less common causes. The proportion of essential hypertension varies from 2% to 75% depending on region and age. As nearly all prepubertal children have an identifiable underlying cause, age is a much more reliable clue toward essential hypertension than overweight (Hadtstein and Schaefer, 2007).

Arterial hypertension is very common in children at all stages of CKD. The prevalence of hypertension is around 25% to 50% in children with CKD stages 2 to 4, and approaches 90% by the time ESRD is reached (Schaefer, 2017). Left ventricular hypertrophy (LVH) is present in one-third of the CKD patients, increased carotid intima–media–thickness (IMT) in 42%. Because blood pressure is associated with target-organ damage in childhood and is closely related to the rate of renal failure progression, early detection and consequent management of arterial hypertension can contribute to better long-term renal survival and a decreased risk of cardiovascular complications (Mitsnefes, 2003).

CKD-associated hypertension develops by a variety of pathophysiologic mechanisms (Hadtstein and Schaefer, 2008). Fluid overload and activation of the renin–angiotensin system are certainly crucial in this process, and sympathetic hyperactivation, endothelial dysfunction, and chronic hyperparathyroidism are likely to contribute to pediatric nephropathies as they do to adult kidney disorders. Drugs such as erythropoietin, glucocorticoids, and cyclosporin A can also cause blood pressure elevation in a dose-dependent manner.

Definition of Hypertension in Childhood

The definition of arterial hypertension in the pediatric population is a challenging issue. Because of the low mortality and the long time lag to cardiovascular complications, hard clinical outcome criteria are not available to define critical cutoff blood pressure values in children. Moreover, blood pressure undergoes a marked physiologic increase with age and body size during childhood and adolescence. Therefore, childhood hypertension is defined by the distribution of blood pressure in the age- and sex-matched general population. Because blood pressure is closely correlated with body height independent of age, blood pressure percentiles are related to both age and relative height.

Specific pediatric hypertension guidelines have been published in the United States (Flynn, 2017) and Europe (Lurbe, 2016). Hypertension is defined as a systolic and/or diastolic blood pressure that on at least three occasions is greater than or equal to the 95th percentile for age, sex, and height. Systolic and/or diastolic blood pressure levels exceeding the 90th but not the 95th percentile are designated as persistently elevated blood pressure (formerly termed prehypertension). In analogy to adult definitions, any blood pressure levels ≥120/80 mm Hg, even if below the 90th percentile for age and height, should also be considered elevated. Persistently elevated blood pressure is considered a treatment indication for children and adolescents at high risk for end-organ damage, including the CKD population (Flynn, 2017; National High Blood Pressure Education Program Working Group on High Blood Pressure in Children and Adolescents, 2004). Blood pressure values >12 mm Hg above the 95th percentile define stage 2 hypertension. The hypertension cutoff values currently recommended for children and adolescents growing at the 50th height percentile are given in Tables 24.3 and 24.4 (a detailed chart is available on the home page of the International Pediatric Hypertension Association, http://www.iphapediatrichypertension. org). Data on normative blood pressure for infants below 1 year are limited. Oscillometric normal ranges are available for infants 0 to 5 years of age (Park, 2005) and newborns (Dionne, 2012; Dionne and Flynn, 2017), given in Table 24.5.

Children may be hypertensive at absolute blood pressure values that may not seem high by adult criteria. For example, 120/75 mm Hg constitutes severe stage 2 hypertension in a 2 year old, stage 1 hypertension in a 7 year old, and prehypertension in an 11 year old of average height. In addition to age, stature plays an important role in what constitutes normal blood pressure. Figure 24.1A,B gives the upper normal limit of casual systolic blood pressure (95th percentile) for boys and girls, respectively, by age and height percentile.

Measurement of Blood Pressure in Children

Blood pressure measurements that are taken intermittently in the clinical setting usually are referred to as "casual," "clinic," or "office" measurements. Casual blood pressure percentiles have been calculated

	Blood Pressure Limits (mm Hg) for Boys Growing Along the 50th Height Percentile (Based on Normal-Weight Children)		
24.3			
Age (year[s]) (Boys)	Elevated Blood Pressure ≥90th Percentile	Stage 1 Hypertension ≥95th Percentile	Stage 2 Hypertension >95th Percentile +12 mm Hg
1	100/53	103/55	115/67
2	102/56	106/59	118/71
3	103/59	107/62	119/74
4	105/62	108/66	120/78
5	106/65	109/69	121/81
6	107/68	111/71	123/83
7	109/70	112/73	124/85
8	110/71	114/74	126/86
9	110/73	115/76	127/88
10	112/74	116/77	128/89
11	114/75	118/78	130/90
12	117/75	121/78	133/90
13	121/75[a]	125/75[b]	137/90[c]
14	126/77[a]	130/81[b]	142/93[c]
15	128/79[a]	132/83[b]	144/95[c]
16	129/80[a]	134/84[b]	146/96[c]
17	131/81[a]	135/85[b]	147/97[c]

[a]Any blood pressure >120 systolic and 80 diastolic should be considered elevated in adolescents ≥13 years of age with chronic kidney disease.
[b]Stage 1 hypertension: Blood pressure 130/80–139/89 mm Hg in adolescents ≥13 years of age (in parallel to the forthcoming American Heart Association and American College of Cardiology adult BP guidelines).
[c]Stage 2 hypertension: Blood pressure ≥140/90 mm Hg in adolescents ≥13 years of age.
Source: From Flynn JT, Kaelber DC, Baker-Smith CM, et al; Subcommittee on Screening and Management of High Blood Pressure in Children. Clinical practice guideline for screening and management of high blood pressure in children and adolescents. *Pediatrics.* 2017;140:pii:e20171904.

according to sex, age, and height (available on www.nhlbi.nih.gov). However, casual blood pressure measurements have rather poor reproducibility.

Physiologic day-to-day variation of blood pressure, reading and device inaccuracies, and insufficient standardization of measurement compromise the reproducibility of blood pressure readings. Different cuff sizes are available for pediatric use; the cuff width should be 40% and the cuff length 80% to 100% of the upper-arm length. Most importantly, however, pediatric patients are prone to a marked "white-coat" effect. This alerting response to the medical setting occurs to a variable extent in up to 60% of children. White-coat hypertension can be differentiated from permanently elevated blood pressure by 24-hour ambulatory blood pressure monitoring (ABPM). ABPM is feasible in most children from 3 years of age. Normal ranges for daytime, nighttime, and 24-hour blood pressure are available for the age range 6 to 18 years (Wühl, 2002).

In contrast to adults, children have higher daytime ABPM values than clinic blood pressures because of their greater physical activity during the day (Hadtstein and Schaefer, 2008).

TABLE 24.4	Blood Pressure Limits (mm Hg) for Girls Growing Along the 50th Height Percentile (Based on Normal-Weight Children)		
Age (year[s]) (Girls)	Elevated Blood Pressure ≥90th Percentile	Stage 1 Hypertension ≥95th Percentile	Stage 2 Hypertension >95th Percentile +12 mm Hg
1	100/56	103/60	115/72
2	103/60	106/64	118/76
3	102/62	108/68	120/78
4	106/65	109/69	121/81
5	107/67	110/71	122/83
6	108/69	111/72	123/84
7	109/70	112/73	124/85
8	110/72	113/74	125/86
9	111/73	114/75	126/87
10	112/73	116/76	128/88
11	114/74	118/77	130/89
12	118/75	122/78	134/90
13	121/76[a]	124/79[b]	136/91[c]
14	122/76[a]	125/80[b]	137/92[c]
15	122/77[a]	126/81[b]	138/93[c]
16	123/77[a]	127/81[b]	139/93[c]
17	124/77[a]	127/81[b]	139/93[c]

[a]Any blood pressure >120 systolic and 80 diastolic should be considered elevated in adolescents with chronic kidney disease.
[b]Stage 1 hypertension: Blood pressure 130/80–139/89 mm Hg in adolescents ≥13 years of age (in parallel to the forthcoming American Heart Association and American College of Cardiology adult BP guidelines).
[c]Stage 2 hypertension: Blood pressure ≥140/90 mm Hg in adolescents ≥13 years of age.
Source: From Flynn JT, Kaelber DC, Baker-Smith CM, et al; Subcommittee on Screening and Management of High Blood Pressure in Children. Clinical practice guideline for screening and management of high blood pressure in children and adolescents. *Pediatrics.* 2017;140:pii:e20171904.

TABLE 24.5	Blood Pressure Limits (mm Hg) for Infants After 2 Weeks of Life by Postmenstrual Age (Systolic BP/Diastolic BP [Mean Arterial Pressure])		
Postmenstrual Age (weeks)	50th Percentile	95th Percentile	99th Percentile
44	88/50 (63)	105/68 (80)	110/73 (85)
42	85/50 (62)	98/65 (76)	102/70 (81)
40	80/50 (62)	95/65 (75)	100/70 (80)
38	77/50 (59)	92/65 (74)	97/70 (79)
36	72/50 (57)	87/65 (72)	92/70 (77)
34	70/40 (50)	85/55 (65)	90/60 (70)
32	68/40 (49)	83/55 (64)	88/60 (69)
30	65/40 (48)	80/55 (63)	85/60 (68)
28	60/38 (45)	75/50 (58)	80/54 (63)
26	55/30 (38)	72/50 (57)	77/56 (63)

Source: From Dionne JM, Abitbol CL, Flynn JT. Hypertension in infancy: diagnosis, management and outcome. *Pediatr Nephrol.* 2012;27:17–32.

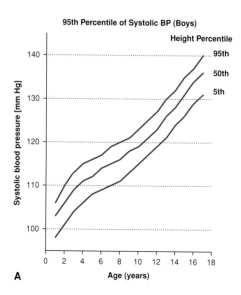

A

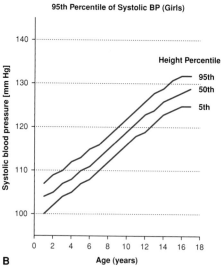

B

FIGURE 24.1   A: Upper normal limit (95th percentile) of systolic casual blood pressure **in boys** according to relative height as expressed by 5th, 50th, and 95th height percentiles. Blood pressure physiologically increases by 30 mm Hg from age 1 to 17 years and differs based on height percentile at any given age by up to 10 mm Hg. **B:** Upper normal limit (95th percentile) of systolic casual blood pressure **in girls** according to relative height as expressed by 5th, 50th, and 95th height percentiles.

The physiologic nocturnal decrease of blood pressure (dipping phenomenon) develops along with normal sleeping patterns in early infancy; loss of nocturnal dipping is common in children with CKD and is assumed to be an independent cardiovascular risk factor in children as it is in adult patients. Altered day–night blood pressure patterns as described in adult CKD patients can also be detected in children (Wühl, 2005). These children frequently have isolated night-time hypertension with normal daytime blood pressure. An elevated ambulatory blood pressure despite normal clinic blood pressure is observed in approximately 10% of children with CKD; this condition, termed *masked hypertension,* appears to be of clinical importance as evidenced by the LVH frequently observed in these patients (Lurbe, 2005). As a result of its superior diagnostic sensitivity, ABPM has become a standard tool in the diagnostics and management of hypertension in centers specializing in pediatric CKD.

End-Organ Damage From Childhood Hypertension

A common assumption in cardiovascular medicine is that high blood pressure and other risk factors identified in adult populations affect only the elderly. However, increasing evidence suggests that CKD-associated cardiovascular disease is present already in childhood and manifests relatively early in the course of CKD (Schaefer, 2017). Although cardiovascular disease is encountered rarely in the general pediatric population, morbidity and mortality from cardiovascular causes has a significant incidence in pediatric ESRD. In those patients with ESRD younger than age 19 years, cardiac disease is responsible for 22 deaths/1,000 patient-years, accounting for 16% of all deaths in whites and 26% in blacks. This represents an up to 1,000-fold increase in risk when compared with the general population. Hypertension may be a major contributor to this risk, as 80% to 90% of children entering ESRD are hypertensive and/or on antihypertensive medication.

Hypertension has been linked to a number of important markers of cardiovascular disease in children. LVH and increased carotid IMT have been demonstrated not only in hypertensive children with advanced CKD, in whom alterations of mineral metabolism and volume overload are important superimposed risk factors, but also in children with early essential hypertension and even in children with masked hypertension. With increasing evidence of clinical relevance of IMT, assessment of IMT should become part of the routine hypertension workup. Recently, pediatric normative data were established (Doyon, 2013).

It should be noted that because of infrequent screening for blood pressure and renal disease in the general pediatric population, severe complications from hypertension at first presentation (e.g., congestive heart failure, encephalopathy) are common. Approximately, 50% of hypertensive children suffer from hypertensive retinopathy at the time of diagnosis. Severe hypertension is particularly common in infants with renoparenchymal disease.

Management of Hypertension in Children
With Chronic Kidney Disease

Blood pressure should be screened regularly in all children with CKD. In addition to clinic measurements, ABPM should be performed at least once a year and within 1 to 2 months of modification of therapy in patients receiving antihypertensive medication. As in current treatment recommendations for adults, children with CKD should be considered at increased risk for cardiovascular complications, and therapeutic interventions should be initiated when blood pressure rises to the prehypertensive range (exceeding the 90th percentile for age and height). The Effect of Strict Blood Pressure Control and ACE Inhibition on Progression of Chronic Renal Failure in Pediatric Patients (ESCAPE) trial demonstrated that in children with CKD, intensified blood pressure control, that is, targeting 24-hour mean arterial blood pressure levels below the 50th percentile, provides substantial renoprotection (Wühl, 2009). Interventions should aim at achieving a blood pressure well below the 75th percentile.

Lifestyle changes such as increased physical activity, avoidance of salty foods, and reduction of weight in obese patients are recommended also for children with CKD but are rarely effective as sole measures (Hadtstein and Schaefer, 2008). Angiotensin-converting enzyme inhibitors (ACEIs) and angiotensin receptor blockers (ARBs) should be the first choice for antihypertensive medications (see "Progression" section below) and, if given at appropriate doses (e.g., ramipril 6 mg/m^2 per day (Wühl, 2004) or candesartan 0.2 to 0.4 mg/kg per day (Schaefer, 2010)), will normalize blood pressure in the majority of patients. If the blood pressure–lowering effect is insufficient, a loop diuretic should be added (e.g., furosemide 2 to 4 mg/kg per day), followed by a calcium channel antagonist (e.g., amlodipine 0.2 mg/kg per day). The timing of drug intake should be adapted to achieve optimal blood pressure control throughout 24 hours as verified by ABPM.

THE HEART IN PEDIATRIC CHRONIC KIDNEY DISEASE

LVH is the most common identifiable cardiac alteration in CKD and the most important indicator of cardiovascular risk both in the general population (Groothoff, 2002) and in adult patients with ESRD (McDonald and Craig, 2004; Parekh, 2002; Silberberg, 1989). LVH is believed to contribute to the high risk of sudden cardiac death in children with CKD as a result of lethal arrhythmias brought about by myocardial fibrosis and cellular hypertrophy. A cross-sectional analysis of more than 130 children revealed that LVH was present in one-third of patients with CKD stages 2 to 4 (Matteucci, 2006).

Left ventricular mass seems to increase with stage of CKD. The Cardiovascular Comorbidity in Children With CKD (4C) study confirmed an increasing prevalence of LVH with each CKD stage from 11% in CKD stage 3a to 48% in CKD stage 5 (Schaefer, 2017). The International Pediatric Peritoneal Dialysis Network (IPPN) observed a

48% prevalence of LVH among more than 500 children on chronic PD (Bakkaloglu, 2011; Borzych, 2011). Children on hemodialysis appear to have an even higher LVH prevalence (82%) than children on peritoneal dialysis (68%) (Mitsnefes, 2000), possibly due to poorer blood pressure control on hemodialysis.

In mild to moderate CKD, the geometry of LVH is eccentric in two-thirds of cases, indicating that volume overload may be common even in children with mild to moderate CKD, and that volume overload may be more relevant to causing cardiac pathology than concomitant hypertension (Schaefer, 2008). An increase in circulating volume early in CKD might be brought about by hyperactivation of the renin–angiotensin–aldosterone and sympathetic nervous systems. Moreover, the uremic state is known to affect left ventricular growth through nonhemodynamic mechanisms, including upregulation of inflammatory cytokines and other autocrine and paracrine pathways. Finally, male sex and a high body mass have been identified as independent risk factors for cardiac hypertrophy (Borzych, 2011).

In addition to these morphologic changes, a subclinical impairment of left ventricular systolic function was found in some 25% of children with mild to moderate CKD (Chinali, 2007). Systolic dysfunction was most common in patients with concentric LVH and associated with low GFR and anemia. A high prevalence of systolic dysfunction, characterized by reduced radial and transmural circumferential strain of the left ventricle paired with a mild cardiac systolic dyssynchrony, was recently documented with the speckle-tracking technology in children with CKD. Remarkably, these subclinical abnormalities in LV mechanics were observed in the presence of a normal ejection fraction (Chinali, 2015).

PROGRESSION OF CHRONIC KIDNEY DISEASE IN CHILDREN

The natural course of renal function in pediatric CKD is mainly determined by the age and degree of renal failure at the time of first disease manifestation. In children born with renal hypoplasia, the physiologic early increase in GFR is typically extended to the first 3 to 4 years of life, potentially reflecting an adaptive hypertrophy of the reduced number of functioning nephrons. In approximately 50% of children, this early incremental phase is followed by a period of stable or very slowly deteriorating renal function, which usually lasts for 5 to 8 years (Wingen, 1997; Wühl, 2009, 2013). Around the onset of puberty, the GFR loss tends to accelerate, typically leading to ESRD in late adolescence or early adulthood (Gonzalez Celedon, 2007).

The reasons for this nonlinear renal failure progression are incompletely understood and may include an insufficient capacity of the nephrons to adapt to the rapidly growing metabolic needs during the pubertal growth spurt, adverse renal effects of puberty-related increases in sex steroid production, and/or an accelerated sclerotic degeneration by a diminishing number of remnant, hyperfiltering nephrons.

In children with very severe renal hypoplasia, the early increase in GFR may be blunted, and early progression to ESRD may occur instead. Around 20% of renal hypoplasia patients maintain stable GFR even beyond puberty. Follow-up studies have shown that in these patients with mild bilateral renal hypoplasia, progressive deterioration of GFR frequently ensues in the third decade of life.

Among the numerous factors predicting progressive renal failure in adult populations and in animal models, hypertension and proteinuria have been documented as the most important modifiable risk factors, also in children. Hypertension is prevalent in 20% to 80% of children with CKD, depending on the degree of renal dysfunction and underlying kidney disorder. In the European Study for Nutritional Treatment of Chronic Renal Failure in Childhood, systolic blood pressure >120 mm Hg was associated with a significantly faster decline of GFR (Wingen, 1997). Recently, the randomized prospective ESCAPE trial demonstrated that in children with CKD resulting from various disorders, intensified antihypertensive treatment, forcing blood pressure to the low normal range (<50th percentile for age), is associated with improved long-term renal survival (Wühl, 2009).

Proteinuria is predictive of CKD progression in children as it is in adult populations. Proteinuria predicts renal disease progression in children with renal hypo/dysplasia, and even in children with normal kidney function, persistent nephrotic-range proteinuria is a risk factor for progressive renal injury. In the children receiving fixed-dose ACE inhibition in the ESCAPE trial, residual proteinuria proved predictive of CKD progression despite treatment. These findings provide a strong rationale for the early and consistent application of renin–angiotensin system antagonist treatment protocols (Wühl, 2009).

Both ACEIs and ARBs have been shown to be safe and effective in children with CKD. Ramipril, administered at a dose of 6 mg/m^2 per day, normalized blood pressure and lowered proteinuria by approximately 50% in the patients participating in the ESCAPE trial (Wühl, 2004). Similar results have been reported with the ARBs losartan (Ellis, 2004), valsartan (Flynn, 2008), or candesartan (Schaefer, 2010); randomized trials with other ARBs are in progress.

The goal of antiproteinuric treatment is to reduce proteinuria as much as possible, ideally to <300 mg/m^2 per day. This degree of proteinuria reduction appears to be associated with the maximal renoprotective effect in adult studies (Jafar, 2001; Ruggenenti, 1999).

It should be noted that the renoprotective superiority of renin–angiotensin system antagonists over other antihypertensive agents has not been formally demonstrated in pediatric CKD. Data from the ItalKid Registry did not show significant modification of CKD progression by ACEI treatment in children with hypo/dysplastic kidney disease compared with matched untreated subjects (Ardissino, 2007). However, no information with respect to the type and dosage of ACEIs used and the prevailing degree of proteinuria was available, and the baseline progression rate was very slow in that retrospective study. A recent analysis from the CKiD study cohort showed an association between ACEI use and slowing of progression of CKD to ESRD (Abraham, 2017).

Another important observation in the ESCAPE trial was a gradual return of proteinuria despite ongoing ACEI treatment. This effect was dissociated from persistently excellent blood pressure control and might limit the long-term renoprotective efficacy of ACEI monotherapy in pediatric CKD (Wühl, 2009).

In a post hoc analysis of the ESCAPE trial, vitamin D deficiency was associated with proteinuria and more rapid progression of CKD (Shroff, 2016). A recent analysis of the 4C study cohort found that severe metabolic acidosis (serum bicarbonate <18 mmol/L) was associated with poor renal survival (Harambat, 2017). These observations suggest a potential causative role of easily correctable metabolic and endocrine abnormalities in CKD progression.

The application of diets with reduced protein content has been extensively tested for a potential renal protective effect both in adults and in children with CKD. A randomized controlled trial in 200 children with CKD did not show any significant beneficial effect of a low-protein diet (Wingen, 1997). Whereas CKD progression does not appear to be influenced favorably by protein restriction, limiting protein intake may still be useful to postpone the need for RRT in CKD stage 5 by lowering the nitrogenous waste product load.

RENAL OSTEODYSTROPHY

Consequences of Altered Bone and Mineral Metabolism in Children

Adequate control of bone and mineral metabolism is one of the major clinical challenges in the management of children with CKD. Long-term follow-up studies have clearly demonstrated that renal osteodystrophy beginning in childhood may cause permanent bone disease in adult life. Among children, CKD-related bone disease may manifest by bone pain, deformities, epiphyseal slipping, and an increased risk of fractures, including microfractures.

In a population-based Dutch study in young adults with childhood-onset ESRD, severe growth retardation was found in 61%, persistent symptomatic bone disease in 37%, limb deformities in 25%, and disabling bone disease in 18%, of young adult survivors of pediatric ESRD (Groothoff, 2003).

Increasing evidence suggests that the alteration of mineral metabolism and its treatment affects not only bone and mineral metabolism, but also contributes to the development of calcifying uremic vasculopathy as a consequence of a redistribution of mineral salts from the skeleton to the large arteries and soft-tissue compartments.

Vascular calcification in the coronary arteries is found in individual adolescent patients on dialysis (Civilibal, 2006; Goodman, 2000) and already in more than 90% of young adults with childhood-onset CKD (Oh, 2002). Early signs of vasculopathy, such as an increased IMT and stiffness of the carotid artery, can be detected as early as in the second decade of life (Litwin, 2005; Oh, 2002; Shroff, 2007). Both morphologic and functional alterations are progressive over time and most marked in adolescents on dialysis, but they also may be seen in children with moderate CKD. IMT and stiffness of the carotid artery correlate with the degree of hyperparathyroidism, the serum calcium × phosphorus ion product, the cumulative dose of calcium-containing phosphate binders, and with plasma parathyroid hormone (PTH) levels (Oh, 2002; Shroff, 2007). Increasing evidence suggests that CKD-associated vasculopathy is a major cause of the excessive morbidity and mortality both during childhood and in early adult life.

Markers of Bone and Mineral Metabolism in Children

Some specific pediatric features need to be considered in the assessment and interpretation of markers of mineral metabolism in children. The serum phosphate concentration is age dependent, and the renal phosphate threshold varies markedly during childhood. The upper limit of normal serum phosphate concentration is 2.7 mmol/L in neonates, 2.4 mmol/L in small infants, 2.1 and 1.9 mmol/L in preschool- and schoolchildren, and 1.4 to 1.9 mmol/L in adolescents (for English measurements, the upper limit values are 8.4 mg/dL in neonates, 7.45 mg/dL in small infants, 6.5 and 5.9 in preschool- and schoolchildren, and 4.35 to 5.9 mg/dL in adolescents).

Age-specific ranges must also be considered for serum calcium, with slightly higher levels in neonates and young infants. Serum calcium usually is normal or low in untreated patients with advanced CKD, with the maintenance of calcium homeostasis being exerted mainly by a compensatory increase in PTH. Once treatment with active vitamin D and calcium-containing phosphate binders is initiated, serum calcium levels increase, but significant hypercalcemia remains rare in growing children with stage 4 CKD, even on calcitriol therapy (Schmitt, 2003).

Likewise, the upper normal limit for the serum calcium × phosphorus ion product is age dependent. The recommended upper normal limit in adults is also applicable in adolescents ($55 \text{ mg}^2/\text{dL}^2$), whereas the upper normal limit is higher in children younger than 12 years of age ($65 \text{ mg}^2/\text{dL}^2$) and even higher in small infants.

Plasma PTH levels are independent of age. However, the usefulness of plasma-intact PTH measurements in predicting bone histopathology is as limited in children as in adult patients (Gal-Moscovici and Popvtzer, 2005). The optimal range of plasma PTH levels which allows for normal bone turnover and growth at minimal vascular calcification risk is a matter of controversy. European consensus guidelines suggest to maintain PTH within the normal range in all children with CKD before dialysis (Klaus, 2006), but North American (KDOQI) guidelines (discussed in Chapter 8) argue in favor of permissive mild hyperparathyroidism as GFR declines to prevent low-turnover bone disease.

A study of the IPPN found a markedly increased risk of symptomatic bone disease with PTH exceeding 300 pg/mL and impaired longitudinal growth at mean PTH concentrations above 500 pg/mL, whereas the risk of hypercalcemia increased at levels below 100 pg/mL (Borzych, 2010). PTH levels exceeding 200 pg/mL were also associated with an increased risk of LVH in the IPPN cohort (Bakkaloglu, 2011). In another study, children with PTH levels within twice the upper limit of normal had less vascular calcification compared to those with PTH levels above their threshold (Shroff, 2007). PTH levels were also found positively associated with fracture risk in children with CKD (Denburg, 2016). Considering all these pieces of evidence from large observational studies, 100 to 200 pg/mL may be the most appropriate PTH target range (Haffner and Schaefer, 2013).

Serum levels of 25-hydroxyvitamin D (25D) give an estimate of vitamin D body stores and should be >30 to 40 ng/mL (75 to 100 nmol/L). The upper range of normal serum 25D levels in healthy children is 70 ng/mL (175 nmol/L), but this has not been validated for patients with CKD. The serum levels of 25D should be measured if serum PTH increases above the target range and routinely at least twice a year. Serum half-life of 25D is 3 weeks.

Measurements of bone biomarkers can be helpful in assessing bone turnover in conjunction with PTH. Alkaline phosphatase is a classical marker of osteoblast activity. Normal values depend strongly on skeletal age, chronologic age, and pubertal stage, with higher activity present during periods of rapid growth. Bone-specific alkaline phosphatase (BAP) may improve the reflection of bone turnover. In children with CKD, both markers of bone formation (BAP) and bone resorption (TRAP5b) are increased, whereas sclerostin, an inhibitor of bone formation, was found decreased compared to healthy controls (Doyon, 2015). Growth hormone (GH) treatment and catch-up growth are associated with higher BAP and lower TRAP5b levels, reflecting an osteoanabolic state.

Therapeutic Options

CKD-MBD management in children needs to focus on three key areas. First, to maintain normal calcium–phosphate homeostasis so as to obtain acceptable bone quality and cardiovascular status, secondly to provide optimal growth in order to maximize the final height, and thirdly, to correct all metabolic and clinical abnormalities that can worsen bone disease, growth, and cardiovascular disease, that is, 25-hydroxy vitamin D deficiency, metabolic acidosis, and malnutrition.

Optimal control of serum phosphorus is probably the key element of preventive management of bone and mineral metabolism. To prevent hyperphosphatemia, regular dietary counseling by experienced pediatric dieticians should be performed and pharmacologic therapy should be initiated early in the course of CKD. Phosphorus intake can be optimized efficiently in young infants by controlled administration of formula nutrition specifically adapted to CKD needs (KDOQI Work Group, 2009). Enteral feeding via a nasogastric tube or percutaneous gastrostomy usually is introduced in young infants to ensure optimal nutrition. In contrast, schoolchildren and adolescents, with their common preference for processed foods, typically have major difficulties in maintaining an adequate diet, and hyperphosphatemia is frequently seen in CKD stage 4. Advanced educational programs using age-appropriate materials and even software are used in specialized pediatric CKD clinics to optimize dietary behaviors and utilization of phosphate binders. Still, adherence to dietary restrictions remains a challenging issue in children beyond infancy.

Serum calcium should be maintained in the normal range, taking care to maintain a normal serum calcium phosphorus ion product. In CKD stage 5, even serum calcium levels in the upper normal range should be avoided to limit the risk of vascular calcifications (KDOQI Work Group, 2009).

Most schoolchildren and adolescents require regular intake of phosphate binders. Calcium-based phosphate binders (calcium carbonate, calcium acetate) are still first choice in most pediatric units. While in hypocalcemic and rapidly growing children the additional calcium load is beneficial, prolonged administration increases the risk of developing hypercalcemia. Because of their contributions to calcium–phosphate ion product elevations and association with uremic vasculopathy, calcium-free alternatives are increasingly considered. Sevelamer is effective in lowering serum calcium, reduces the incidence of hypercalcemic episodes, and improves bone turnover relative to calcium carbonate in children (Salusky, 2005). Sevelamer carbonate is available as a powder, which facilitates its administration in tube-fed infants and children who are unable to swallow large capsules. Iron-based phosphate binders reduce serum phosphate and fibroblast growth factor (FGF)-23 concentrations while simultaneously increasing serum iron stores (Yokoyama, 2014), but pediatric experience is still lacking. Their use in children may be limited by GI side effects (Floege, 2014). The administration of lanthanum carbonate is currently not recommended in children due to the possible risk of accumulation of lanthanum in serum and tissue.

Oral treatment with ergocalciferol or cholecalciferol is recommended in all children with CKD. This is particularly relevant in infants who have higher metabolic needs. In children with normal kidney function, the recommended upper limit of daily vitamin D intake is 1,000 IU in the first year of life and 2,000 IU for all other ages. A daily dose of 1,000 to 2,000 units of cholecalciferol should be given to children with CKD to prevent 25D deficiency (KDOQI Work Group, 2009). The specific dosing of ergocalciferol or cholecalciferol in children with vitamin D deficiency or insufficiency should be guided by serum 25D levels. In severe vitamin D deficiency (25D concentration <5 ng/mL), 8,000 IU/day should be administered for 4 weeks, followed by 4,000 IU/day over 2 months. Alternatively, intermittent high-dose therapy is possible: 50,000 IU once per week for 4 weeks, then twice per month for another 2 months. Whereas mild vitamin D deficiency (5 to 15 ng/mL or 12 to 37 nmol/L) should be treated with a dose of 4,000 IU/day for 3 months or 50,000 IU every other week, 2,000 IU/day or 50,000 IU every week for 3 months is recommended to treat vitamin D insufficiency (16 to 30 ng/mL or 38 to 75 nmol/L). In children younger than 1 year, smaller doses of vitamin D are probably sufficient.

If plasma PTH levels remain elevated despite normal serum 25D and phosphate levels, treatment with calcitriol or analogues is required. Calcitriol or 1-α hydroxyvitamin D_2 is used in most children with CKD stages 4 and 5 to compensate for reduced renal 1-α hydroxylase activity and to prevent and control secondary hyperparathyroidism. 1-α hydroxyvitamin D_2 is almost the same molecule as calcitriol; 1-α hydroxyvitamin D_2 is the yeast-based ergocalciferol (D_2) backbone molecule that has been hydroxylated at the 25- and 1-positions and so is fully active, whereas calcitriol is the animal-based cholecalciferol (D_3) backbone molecule hydroxylated at these same positions. The dose of calcitriol depends on initial PTH, calcium, and phosphate values. An initial dose of 5 to 10 ng/kg per day is effective and safe in most children. The frequency of calcium, phosphate, and PTH monitoring should be adapted to the dose of vitamin D administered. Liquid formulations of calcitriol and 1-α hydroxyvitamin D_2 are available that can be given orally. Because these oily solutions are adsorbed to plastic materials, they should not be given via feeding tubes. Calcitriol use is often limited by aggravated hyperphosphatemia and hypercalcemia.

Synthetic vitamin D analogues have been developed to reduce intestinal calcium and phosphate absorption at equipotent PTH suppressive action. Three different sterols have been approved for use in various countries: 22-oxacalcitriol (maxacalcitol), 19-nor-1,25 dihydroxyvitamin D_2 (paricalcitol), and 1-α hydroxyvitamin D_2 (doxercalciferol). Only paricalcitol has been studied in children on hemodialysis (Greenbaum, 2007; Seeherunvong, 2006), but off-label use is common.

Cinacalcet, the first commercially available calcimimetic agent, has a unique profile of action that appears highly attractive for pediatric usage, and the early clinical experience in children with otherwise refractory hyperparathyroidism is promising (Muscheites, 2008). However, the use of cinacalcet in predialytic CKD patients is compromised by a high incidence of hypocalcemia. In children and adolescents, additional safety concerns are caused by the fact that the calcium-sensing receptor is abundantly expressed in epiphyseal growth plates, although animal studies do not suggest an impact on longitudinal growth. So far, off-label use is very common. Pediatric clinical trials focusing on the safety are currently underway. It remains to be seen whether cinacalcet will become established for treating secondary hyperparathyroidism in children with CKD (Alharthi, 2015).

Some children with CKD may develop severe treatment refractory hyperparathyroidism requiring parathyroidectomy but the incidence seems to be reduced with early treatment start. Of note, GH should not be given to patients with uncontrolled hyperparathyroidism, symptomatic high turnover bone disease or slipped epiphysis.

GROWTH, NUTRITION, AND DEVELOPMENT IN CHILDREN WITH CHRONIC KIDNEY DISEASE

Impaired statural growth and sexual development are among the most obvious and important complications of CKD in childhood. Growth retardation and delayed maturation can interfere markedly with psychosocial adjustment and are mentioned most consistently by young adult survivors of childhood-onset CKD as major factors compromising their social integration and subjective quality of life.

Patterns of Uremic Growth Failure

The impact of uremia and its sequelae on longitudinal growth largely depends on the age at first manifestation of CKD. Approximately one-third of total postnatal growth occurs during the first 2 years of life. Therefore, any circumstances affecting growth rates during the infancy period will cause rapid and severe growth retardation. Untreated uremia during the first year of life can result in a loss of up to 0.5 standard deviations (SDs) in relative height per month (Haffner and Nissel, 2008).

During the mid-childhood period, starting around 18 to 24 months of age and lasting until the onset of puberty, the growth inhibitory effect of CKD is more subtle, and relative height is lost gradually over periods of years rather than months. In general, growth patterns appear stable as long as GFR/1.73 m^2 remains >25 mL/min; if GFR falls below this level, then the growth rate decreases from percentile-predicted values. At 10 years of age, a mean cumulative loss of 6 cm of predicted final height was observed in children who had a mean GFR/1.73 m^2 <25 since early childhood (Schaefer, 1996). In children with CKD in whom height is increasing as expected along a given percentile line but in whom absolute height is reduced, successful kidney transplantation often results in prompt catch-up growth into the normal range as optimal growth conditions are restored.

The onset of clinical signs of puberty as well as the start of the pubertal growth spurt occurs with a delay of up to 2 years, depending on the degree of renal dysfunction (Schaefer, 1990). The height gain during the pubertal growth spurt is diminished by up to 50% (e.g., from 30, to 15 cm) in adolescents with ESRD. Final adult heights below the normal range are attained by 30% to 50% of children with CKD, although a trend of improving final heights has been noted during the past decade: The percentage of patients growing up to a subnormal height increases from 10% to 15% in CKD stage 3 to more than 50% in patients who reach ESRD during childhood. The duration of CKD, the presence of a congenital nephropathy, and male sex are among the most important predictors of a reduced final height (Haffner and Nissel, 2008).

Etiology of Growth Failure and Developmental Delay in Chronic Kidney Disease

During the infancy period, growth is largely dependent on nutritional and metabolic factors. Growth failure in infants with CKD usually is caused by inadequate spontaneous intake of nutrients because of anorexia and frequent vomiting. Reduced spontaneous energy intake resulting from uremic anorexia starts to impair growth rates when it falls below 80% of the recommended dietary allowance. The anorexia and wasting almost inevitably observed in infants with CKD may or may not also be related to a subclinical microinflammatory state similar to the one seen in adult patients (Bamgbola and Kaskel, 2003). Additional factors contributing to vomiting and anorexia include the accumulation of inadequately cleared circulating satiety factors and a general retardation of psychomotor development in the uremic state. Gastric emptying has been shown to be abnormally slow in infants with CKD. Fluid and electrolyte losses that are due to tubular dysfunction in dysplastic kidney disorders and catabolic episodes related to intercurrent infections may also play a role in worsening infantile growth.

Metabolic acidosis, which usually occurs when GFR is below 50% of normal, contributes to CKD-associated growth failure by various mechanisms. Increased protein breakdown has been observed in acidotic children with CKD. Moreover, spontaneous GH secretion, the expression of GH and insulin growth factor-1 (IGF-1) receptors in target tissues, and IGF-1 serum concentrations are all decreased in the acidotic state. Hence, metabolic acidosis in CKD induces a state of GH insufficiency and insensitivity (Haffner and Nissel, 2008).

Independent of metabolic acidosis, the somatotropic hormone axis shows a complex dysregulation in the uremic state. Circulating GH levels are normal or increased because of impaired metabolic clearance, but pituitary GH secretion rates are normal or diminished. GH-induced IGF-1 synthesis is impaired in uremia as a result of impaired activation of the GH-specific JAK2/STAT5 intracellular signaling pathway (Rabkin, 2005). In addition, accumulation of several IGF-1–binding proteins results in a molar excess of IGF-binding proteins relative to circulating IGFs, resulting in reduced IGF bioactivity. Finally, the normal or reduced GH secretion in the presence of markedly reduced IGF-1 bioactivity is compatible with an insufficient feedback activation of the somatotropic hormone axis at the hypothalamic and pituitary levels. In summary, these findings indicate multilevel homeostatic failure of the GH–IGF-1 system in uremia.

The gonadotropic hormone axis appears to be subject to a similarly impaired activation in CKD. Peripubertal patients with advanced and end-stage renal disease show normal or low sex-steroid levels in the presence of elevated circulating gonadotropins. However, the elevation of gonadotropins is entirely explained by impaired metabolic hormone clearance, whereas pituitary secretion rates are low, possibly because of impaired hypothalamic gonadotropin-releasing hormone (GnRH) secretion related to an increased local neurotransmitter tone. On top of this, there is deficient central nervous system activation, predominant secretion of less bioactive isoforms of the luteinizing hormone, and accumulation of circulating factors that inhibit GnRH release from the hypothalamus and testosterone release from Leydig cells. Finally, the cross talk between gonadotropic and somatotropic hormones during puberty appears to be impaired, as evidenced by a blunted surge of GH secretion in response to rising sex-steroid levels. Hence, uremia appears to cause a state of multiple endocrine resistance, effectively inhibiting both longitudinal growth and sexual development.

Among the other typical complications of CKD, renal anemia (Jabs, 1996) and secondary hyperparathyroidism do not appear to affect growth and puberty to a major extent.

Mild to moderate hyperparathyroidism and calcitriol treatment are not related to longitudinal growth rates, whereas severe hyperparathyroidism (PTH levels above 500 pg/mL) can cause growth failure (Borzych, 2010) and excessive hyperparathyroidism occasionally can result in a growth arrest by destroying the metaphyseal bone architecture (Klaus, 2006; Mehls, 1986).

Treatment of Uremic Growth Failure

In children with CKD, during the first 12 to 18 months of life, the most important measures for avoiding uremic growth failure are the provision of adequate energy intake, the correction of metabolic acidosis, and the maintenance of fluid and electrolyte balance. Supplementary feedings via nasogastric tube or gastrostomy frequently are required to achieve these targets.

Caloric intake should be targeted to provide 80% to 100% of the regular daily allowance (RDA) of healthy children. To account for the degree of growth retardation, the prescription should be related to the patient's height age rather than to chronologic age. Increasing caloric intake above 100% of the RDA does not induce further catch-up growth but rather results in obesity, with a potential adverse impact on long-term cardiovascular health.

Protein intake should be at least 100% of the RDA but should not exceed 140% RDA in patients with CKD stages 2 and 3 and 120% RDA in children with stages 4 and 5 CKD (KDOQI Work Group, 2009). It seems advisable to avoid excessive protein intake in advancing CKD to limit phosphorus and acid load in patients with failing kidney function. Restricted protein intake appears to be safe with respect to the preservation of growth and nutritional status; in a randomized trial in 200 children with CKD followed for 2 years, protein restriction to the lowest intake subjectively acceptable by the patients did not negatively affect growth or nutritional measures (Wingen, 1997).

Metabolic acidosis should be rigorously treated by oral alkaline supplementation. In addition, the supplementation of water and electrolytes is essential for children presenting with polyuria and/or salt-losing nephropathies. Water and electrolyte losses are very common and frequently underestimated in children with hypo- and dysplastic renal malformations.

The concept of early and consistent provision of supplementary nutrients, fluids, and electrolytes—when delivery has been ensured by enteral feeding via nasogastric tube or percutaneous gastrostomy when necessary—has dramatically improved the growth and development of children with CKD (Haffner and Nissel, 2008; Parekh, 2001; Rees, 2011). It has become possible to maintain height and weight within the normal range in the large majority of infants, even those with advanced or end-stage renal disease. Such measures also can largely abolish secondary complications of malnutrition and fluid, acid–base, and electrolyte imbalances.

In the postinfantile phase of childhood, nutrition as well as fluid and electrolyte balance continue to be permissive factors for adequate longitudinal growth, but catch-up growth can rarely be provided by dietary and supplementary measures alone. If height velocity is subnormal despite adequate provision of nutrients, salts, and fluids, and if growth failure is imminent or height is already subnormal, then treatment with recombinant growth hormone (rGH) is a viable option. The efficacy and safety of rGH has been demonstrated in numerous short- and long-term trials in children with CKD. The administration of rGH at pharmacologic doses (0.05 mcg/kg per day subcutaneously) overcomes endogenous GH resistance and markedly increases systemic and local IGF-1 production, with only a slight effect on IGF-binding proteins. This restores normal IGF-1 bioactivity and stimulates longitudinal growth. In children with predialytic CKD, height velocity typically doubles in the first treatment-year, and steady, albeit less, marked catch-up growth continues to be observed during subsequent years of therapy. After 5 to 6 treatment-years, standardized height (with −2, 0, and +2 representing the 5th, 50th and 97.5th percentiles of height distribution in the general pediatric population) had increased from −2.6 to −0.7 in one North American study, from −3.4 to −1.9 in a group of German children, and from −3.0 to −0.5 in one Dutch study.

The therapeutic response to rGH in CKD patients is superior to that observed in children on dialysis or after kidney transplantation, probably because of a more marked uremic GH resistance in ESRD and the growth suppressive effect of glucocorticoids in renal allograft recipients. In patients studied on rGH around age 9 to 10 years and followed through puberty until attainment of final height, catch-up growth was largely limited to the prepubertal period (Haffner, 2000). Final height was markedly improved in comparison with an untreated control group with an overall benefit attributable to rGH treatment of 10 to 15 cm. Total height gain was positively correlated with the duration of rGH therapy and negatively affected by the time spent on dialysis. These experiences permit one to conclude that rGH therapy should be initiated as early as possible in the predialytic CKD period, preferentially before severe growth retardation has occurred.

In addition to its excellent efficacy, long-term rGH therapy causes remarkably few adverse effects. These include hyperinsulinemia and an occasional slight aggravation of secondary hyperparathyroidism. Early reports suggesting an increased incidence of intracranial hypertension, a condition of high prevalence in CKD, have not been substantiated in controlled trials. Likewise, there is no clinical evidence of accelerated progression of renal failure secondary to sustained glomerular hyperfiltration induced by long-term rGH treatment.

WHEN SHOULD DIALYSIS BE INITIATED IN CHILDREN AND ADOLESCENTS WITH CHRONIC KIDNEY DISEASE?

The initiation of chronic dialysis in children with CKD is a dramatic event for the patient and family. In some patients, the urgent need for beginning dialysis is obvious because manifestations of renal failure cause significant morbidity and mortality. A variety of signs and symptoms are absolute indication for dialysis initiation. These include neurologic consequences of uremia (encephalopathy, confusion, seizure), refractory hypertension, pulmonary edema that is due to volume overload unresponsive to diuretics, uremic pericarditis, bleeding diathesis, refractory nausea and emesis, and anuria. More often than not, such absolute indications are lacking. In these cases, the decision to initiate dialysis requires consideration of various clinical parameters, laboratory data, and psychosocial issues. These include the occurrence of hyperkalemic episodes, hyperphosphatemia, uncontrolled hypertension due to fluid overload, malnutrition, and growth failure, but also of less dramatic sequelae of uremia, such as persistent fatigue, weakness, cognitive dysfunction, decreased school performance, pruritus, depression, nausea, emesis, anorexia, and altered sleeping patterns. Although dialysis usually becomes necessary when GFR (measured by the mean of creatinine and urea clearance) declines to 5 to 10 mL/min per 1.73 m^2, the decision usually is not based on a strict number but rather on overall patient well-being (Greenbaum and Schaefer, 2004).

Some measures can be taken to delay the need for dialysis. Metabolic acidosis, hyperkalemia, and hyperphosphatemia can temporarily be treated with dietary counseling and medications, but the approach is not always successful. In infants and young children, the institution of tube feeding facilitates adequate intake of critical nutrients (potassium, phosphorus, protein) and maintenance of adequate nutrition and fluid status. Often this allows postponement of dialysis initiation for some time. In contrast, adolescents usually are less compliant with medication and dietary restrictions, and may be better off with a timely start of dialysis. Anemia can be controlled well in advanced CKD by erythropoietin and oral or intravenous iron administration. Growth failure in children with CKD is treatable with rGH. The efficacy of GH largely depends on residual renal function, mandating a timely start of treatment. Nonresponsiveness to GH is considered only a relative argument for starting dialysis, because hemo- or peritoneal dialysis as conventionally prescribed do not improve growth rates substantially in the majority of children (Greenbaum and Schaefer, 2004).

References and Suggested Readings

Abraham AG, Betoko A, Fadrowski JJ, et al. Renin-angiotensin II-aldosterone system blockers and time to renal replacement therapy in children with CKD. *Pediatr Nephrol.* 2017;32:643–649.

Alharthi AA, Kamal NM, Abukhatwah MW, et al. Cinacalcet in pediatric and adolescent chronic kidney disease: a single-center experience. *Medicine* (Baltimore). 2015;94:e401.

Ardissino G, Viganò S, Testa S, et al; ItalKid Project. No clear evidence of ACEi efficacy on the progression of chronic kidney disease in children with hypodysplastic nephropathy–report from the ItalKid Project database. *Nephrol Dial Transplant.* 2007;22:2525–2530.

Bakkaloglu SA, Borzych D, Soo Ha I, et al. Cardiac geometry in children receiving chronic peritoneal dialysis: findings from the International Pediatric Peritoneal Dialysis Network (IPPN) registry. *Clin J Am Soc Nephrol.* 2011;6:1926–1933.

Bamgbola FO, Kaskel FJ. Uremic malnutrition-inflammation syndrome in chronic renal disease: a pathobiologic entity. *J Ren Nutr.* 2003;13:250–258.

Borzych D, Bakkaloglu SA, Zaritsky J, et al; International Pediatric Peritoneal Dialysis Network. Defining left ventricular hypertrophy in children on peritoneal dialysis. *Clin J Am Soc Nephrol.* 2011;6:1934–1943.

Borzych D, Rees L, Ha IS, et al; International Pediatric PD Network (IPPN). The bone and mineral disorder of children undergoing chronic peritoneal dialysis. *Kidney Int.* 2010;78:1295–1304.

Chinali M, de Simone G, Matteucci MC, et al; ESCAPE Trial Group. Reduced systolic myocardial function in children with chronic renal insufficiency. *J Am Soc Nephrol.* 2007;18:593–598.

Chinali M, Matteucci MC, Franceschini A, et al. Advanced parameters of cardiac mechanics in children with CKD: the 4C Study. *Clin J Am Soc Nephrol.* 2015;10: 1357–1363.

Civilibal M, Caliskan S, Adaletli I, et al. Coronary artery calcifications in children with end-stage renal disease. *Pediatr Nephrol.* 2006;21:1426–1433.

Denburg MR, Kumar J, Jemielita T, et al. Fracture burden and risk factors in childhood CKD: results from the CKiD Cohort Study. *J Am Soc Nephrol.* 2016;27:543–550.

Dionne JM, Abitbol CL, Flynn JT. Hypertension in infancy: diagnosis, management and outcome. *Pediatr Nephrol.* 2012;27:17–32.

Dionne JM, Flynn JT. Management of severe hypertension in the newborn. *Arch Dis Child.* 2017;102:1176–1179.

Doyon A, Fischer DC, Bayazit AK, et al; 4C Study Consortium. Markers of bone metabolism are affected by renal function and growth hormone therapy in children with chronic kidney disease. *PLoS One.* 2015;10:e0113482.

Doyon A, Kracht D, Bayazit AK, et al. Carotid artery intima-media thickness and distensibility in children and adolescents: reference values and role of body dimensions. *Hypertension.* 2013;62:550–556.

Ellis D, Moritz ML, Vats A, et al. Antihypertensive and renoprotective efficacy and safety of losartan: a long-term study in children with renal disorders. *Am J Hypertens.* 2004;17:928–935.

Filler G, Lepage N. Should the Schwartz formula for estimation of GFR be replaced by cystatin C formula? *Pediatr Nephrol.* 2003;18:981–985.

Floege J, Covic AC, Ketteler M, et al; PA21 Study Group. A phase III study of the efficacy and safety of a novel iron-based phosphate binder in dialysis patients. *Kidney Int.* 2014;86:638–647.

Flynn JT, Kaelber DC, Baker-Smith CM, et al; Subcommittee on Screening and Management of High Blood Pressure in Children. Clinical practice guideline for screening and management of high blood pressure in children and adolescents. *Pediatrics.* 2017;140:pii:e20171904.

Flynn JT, Meyers KEC, Neto JP, et al; Pediatric Valsartan Study Group. Efficacy and safety of the angiotensin receptor blocking agent valsartan in children with hypertension aged 1 to 5 years. *Hypertension.* 2008;52:222–228.

Gal-Moscovici A, Popvtzer MM. New worldwide trends in presentation of renal osteodystrophy and its relationship to parathyroid hormone levels. *Clin Nephrol.* 2005;63:284–289.

Gonzalez Celedon C, Bitsori M, Tullus K. Progression of chronic renal failure in children with dysplastic kidneys. *Pediatr Nephrol.* 2007;22:1014–1020.

Goodman WG, Goldin J, Kuizon BD, et al. Coronary-artery calcification in young adults with end-stage renal disease who are undergoing dialysis. *N Engl J Med.* 2000;342:1478–1483.

Greenbaum LA, Benador N, Goldstein SL, et al. Intravenous paricalcitol for treatment of secondary hyperparathyroidism in children on hemodialysis. *Am J Kidney Dis.* 2007;49:814–823.

Greenbaum L, Schaefer FS. The decision to initiate dialysis in children and adolescents. In: Warady BA, Schaefer FS, Fine RN, et al., eds. *Pediatric Dialysis.* Dordrecht: Kluwer Academic Publishers; 2004:177–196.

Groothoff JW, Gruppen MP, Offringa M, et al. Mortality and causes of death of end-stage renal disease in children: a Dutch cohort study. *Kidney Int.* 2002;61:621–629.

Groothoff JW, Offringa M, Van Eck-Smit BL, et al. Severe bone disease and low bone mineral density after juvenile renal failure. *Kidney Int.* 2003;63:266–275.

Hadtstein C, Schaefer F. What adult nephrologists should know about childhood pressure. *Nephrol Dial Transplant.* 2007;22:2119–2123.

Hadtstein C, Schaefer F. Hypertension in children with chronic kidney disease: pathophysiology and management. *Pediatr Nephrol.* 2008;23:363–371.

Haffner D, Nissel R. Growth and puberty in chronic kidney disease. In: Geary DF, Schaefer F, eds. *Comprehensive Pediatric Nephrology.* Philadelphia, PA: Mosby Elsevier; 2008:709–732.

Haffner D, Schaefer F. Searching the optimal PTH target range in children undergoing peritoneal dialysis: new insights from international cohort studies. *Pediatr Nephrol.* 2013;28:537–545.

Haffner D, Schaefer F, Nissel R, et al. Effect of growth hormone treatment on the adult height of children with chronic renal failure. German Study Group for growth hormone treatment in chronic renal failure. *N Engl J Med.* 2000;343:923–930.

Harambat J, Kunzmann K, Azukaitis K, et al; 4C Study Consortium. Metabolic acidosis is common and associates with disease progression in children with chronic kidney disease. *Kidney Int.* 2017;92:1507–1514.

Harambat J, van Stralen KJ, Kim JJ, et al. Epidemiology of chronic kidney disease in children. *Pediatr Nephrol.* 2012;27:363–373.

Hogg RJ, Furth S, Lemley KV, et al. National Kidney Foundation's Kidney Disease Outcomes Quality Initiative clinical practice guidelines for chronic kidney disease in children and adolescents: evaluation, classification, and stratification. *Pediatrics.* 2003;111:1416–1421.

Jabs K. The effects of recombinant human erythropoietin on growth and nutritional status. *Pediatr Nephrol.* 1996;10:324–327.

Jafar TH, Schmid CH, Landa M, et al. Angiotensin-converting enzyme inhibitors and progression of nondiabetic renal disease. A meta-analysis of patient-level data. *Ann Intern Med.* 2001;135: 73–87.

KDOQI Work Group. KDOQI Clinical Practice Guideline for Nutrition in children with CKD: 2008 update. Executive summary. *Am J Kidney Dis.* 2009;53: S11–S104.

Klaus G, Watson A, Edefonti A, et al; European Pediatric Dialysis Working Group (EPDWG). Prevention and treatment of renal osteodystrophy in children on chronic renal failure: European Guidelines. *Pediatr Nephrol.* 2006;21:151–159.

Litwin M, Wuhl E, Jourdan C, et al. Altered morphologic properties of large arteries in children with chronic renal failure and after renal transplantation. *J Am Soc Nephrol.* 2005;16:1494–1500.

Loghman-Adham M. Evaluating proteinuria in children. *Am Fam Physician.* 1998; 58:1145–1152,1158–1159.

Lurbe E, Agabiti-Rosei E, Cruickshank JK, et al. 2016 European Society of Hypertension guidelines for the management of high blood pressure in children and adolescents. *J Hypertens.* 2016;34:1887–1920.

Lurbe E, Torro I, Alvarez V, et al. Prevalence, persistence, and clinical significance of masked hypertension in youth. *Hypertension.* 2005;45:493–498.

Matteucci MC, Wühl E, Picca S, et al; ESCAPE Trial Group. Left ventricular geometry in children with mild to moderate chronic renal insufficiency. *J Am Soc Nephrol.* 2006;17:218–226.

McDonald SP, Craig JC; Australian and New Zealand Paediatric Nephrology Association. Long-term survival of children with end-stage renal disease. *N Engl J Med.* 2004;350:2654–2662.

Mehls O, Ritz E, Gilli G, et al. Role of hormonal disturbances in uremic growth failure. *Contrib Nephrol.* 1986;50:119–129.

Mitsnefes MM, Daniels SR, Schwartz SM, et al. Severe left ventricular hypertrophy in pediatric dialysis: prevalence and predictors. *Pediatr Nephrol.* 2000;14: 898–902.

Mitsnefes MM, Ho PL, McEnery PT. Hypertension and progression of chronic renal insufficiency in children: a report of the North American Pediatric Renal Transplant Cooperative Study (NAPRTCS). *J Am Soc Nephrol.* 2003;14:2618–2622.

Muscheites J, Wigger M, Drueckler E, et al. Cinacalcet for secondary hyperparathyroidism in children with end-stage renal disease. *Pediatr Nephrol.* 2008;23:1823–1829.

National Heart, Lung and Blood Institute. The fourth report on the diagnosis, evaluation, and treatment of high blood pressure in children and adolescents. Revised, 2005. Available from http://www.nhlbi.nih.gov/health/prof/heart/hbp/hbp_ped. pdf Accessed January 20, 2011.

National High Blood Pressure Education Program Working Group on High Blood Pressure in Children and Adolescents. The fourth report on the diagnosis, evaluation, and treatment of high blood pressure in children and adolescents. *Pediatrics.* 2004;114:555–576.

Oh J, Wunsch R, Turzer M, et al. Advanced coronary and carotid arteriopathy in young adults with childhood-onset chronic renal failure. *Circulation.* 2002;106:100–105.

Parekh RS, Carroll CE, Wolfe RA, et al. Cardiovascular mortality in children and young adults with end-stage kidney disease. *J Pediatr.* 2002;141:191–197.

Parekh RS, Flynn JT, Smoyer WE, et al. Improved growth in young children with severe chronic renal insufficiency who use specified nutritional therapy. *J Am Soc Nephrol.* 2001;12:2418–2426.

Park MK, Menard SW, Schoolfield J. Oscillometric blood pressure standards for children. *Pediatr Cardiol.* 2005;26:601–607.

Rabkin R, Sun DF, Chen Y, et al. Growth hormone resistance in uremia, a role for impaired JAK/STAT signaling. *Pediatr Nephrol.* 2005;20:313–318.

Rees L, Azocar M, Borzych D, et al; International Pediatric Peritoneal Dialysis Network (IPPN) registry. Growth in very young children undergoing chronic peritoneal dialysis. *J Am Soc Nephrol.* 2011;22:2303–2312.

Ruggenenti P, Perna A, Gherardi G, et al. Renoprotective properties of ACE-inhibition in non-diabetic nephropathies with non-nephrotic proteinuria. *Lancet.* 1999;354:359–364.

Salusky IB, Goodman WG, Sahney S, et al. Sevelamer controls parathyroid hormone-induced bone disease as efficiently as calcium carbonate without increasing serum calcium levels during therapy with active vitamin D sterols. *J Am Soc Nephrol.* 2005;16:2501–2508.

Schaefer F. Cardiac disease in children with mild-to-moderate chronic kidney disease. *Curr Opin Nephrol Hypertens.* 2008;17:292–297.

Schaefer F, Doyon A, Azukaitis K, et al; 4C Study Consortium. Cardiovascular phenotypes in children with CKD: the 4C Study. *Clin J Am Soc Nephrol.* 2017;12:19–28.

Schaefer F, Seidel C, Binding A, et al. Pubertal growth in chronic renal failure. *Pediatr Res.* 1990;28:5–10.

Schaefer F, van de Walle J, Zurowska A, et al; Candesartan in Children With Hypertension Investigators. Efficacy, safety and pharmacokinetics of candesartan cilexetil in hypertensive children from 1 to less than 6 years of age. *J Hypertens.* 2010;28:1083–1090.

Schaefer F, Wingen AM, Hennicke M, et al. Growth charts for prepubertal children with chronic renal failure due to congenital renal disorders. European Study Group for Nutritional Treatment of Chronic Renal Failure in Childhood. *Pediatr Nephrol.* 1996;10:288–293.

Schmitt CP, Ardissino G, Testa S, et al. Growth in children with chronic renal failure on intermittent versus daily calcitriol. *Pediatr Nephrol.* 2003;18:440–444.

Schwartz GJ, Brion LP, Spitzer A. The use of plasma creatinine concentration for estimating glomerular filtration rate in infants, children, and adolescents. *Pediatr Clin North Am.* 1987;34:571–590.

Schwartz GJ, Munoz A, Schneider MF, et al. New equations to estimate GFR in children with CKD. *J Am Soc Nephrol.* 2009;20:629–637.

Seeherunvong W, Nwobi O, Abitbol CL, et al. Paricalcitol versus calcitriol treatment for hyperparathyroidism in pediatric hemodialysis patients. *Pediatr Nephrol.* 2006;21:1434–1439.

Shroff R, Aitkenhead H, Costa N, et al; ESCAPE Trial Group. Normal 25-hydroxyvitamin D levels are associated with less proteinuria and attenuate renal failure progression in children with CKD. *J Am Soc Nephrol.* 2016;27:314–322.

Shroff RC, Donald AE, Hiorns MP, et al. Mineral metabolism and vascular damage in children on dialysis. *J Am Soc Nephrol.* 2007;18:2996–3003.

Silberberg JS, Barre PE, Prichard SS, et al. Impact of left ventricular hypertrophy on survival in end-stage renal disease. *Kidney Int.* 1989;36:286–290.

Wingen AM, Fabian-Bach C, Schaefer F, et al. Randomised multicentre study of a low-protein diet on the progression of chronic renal failure in children. European Study Group of Nutritional Treatment of Chronic Renal Failure in Childhood. *Lancet.* 1997;349:1117–1123.

Wühl E, Hadtstein C, Mehls O, et al; ESCAPE Trial Group. Ultradian but not circadian blood pressure rhythms correlate with renal dysfunction in children with chronic renal failure. *J Am Soc Nephrol.* 2005;16:746–754.

Wühl E, Mehls O, Schaefer F; ESCAPE Trial Group. Antihypertensive and antiproteinuric efficacy of ramipril in children with chronic renal failure. *Kidney Int.* 2004;66:768–776.

Wühl E, Trivelli A, Picca S, et al; ESCAPE Trial Group. Strict blood pressure control and renal failure progression in children. *N Engl J Med.* 2009;361:1639–1650.

Wühl E, van Stralen KJ, Verrina E, et al. Timing and outcome of renal replacement therapy in patients with congenital malformations of the kidney and urinary tract. *Clin J Am Soc Nephrol.* 2013;8:67–74.

Wühl E, Witte K, Soergel M, et al; German Working Group on Pediatric Hypertension. Distribution of 24-h ambulatory blood pressure in children: normalized reference values and role of body dimensions. *J Hypertens.* 2002;20:1995–2007.

Yokoyama K, Hirakata H, Akiba T, et al. Ferric citrate hydrate for the treatment of hyperphosphatemia in nondialysis-dependent CKD. *Clin J Am Soc Nephrol.* 2014;9:543–552.

25

Pregnancy in Chronic Kidney Disease

Kavitha Vellanki and Susan Hou

Pregnant women with chronic kidney disease (CKD) are at increased risk of hypertension, proteinuria, preeclampsia, premature labor, urinary tract infections, and thrombosis. Maladaptation to pregnancy predisposes pregnant women with moderate to severe CKD to the risk of progressive decline in renal function that may be irreversible. This occurs irrespective of the cause of the underlying renal disease, and the risk of rapid progression appears to increase dramatically once a critical degree of baseline renal insufficiency is present. Fertility rates decline with severity of renal failure and hence, conception is rare in dialysis-dependent women. Thus, only a small number of pregnant CKD women are cared for at any center and since pregnancy does not lend itself to randomization, most of the available evidence is from cross-sectional or observational studies.

RENAL CHANGES IN PREGNANCY

The kidney undergoes profound anatomical and physiologic changes during pregnancy, and major changes occur in both systemic and renal hemodynamics (Table 25.1). Glomerular filtration rate (GFR) and renal plasma flow (RPF) increase by approximately 50%. Increase in GFR is noted as early as 4 weeks of gestation, reaching peak level in the first half of pregnancy and exceeding nongravid GFR by 40% to 60% (Davison, 1983). Such changes are noted even in women with a single functional kidney, albeit to a lesser degree. There are no long-term effects on glomerular function or structure in women with normal renal function, even with repetitive pregnancies, as intraglomerular pressure remains normal despite drastic changes in GFR and RPF. While it is widely perceived that pregnancy-induced hemodynamic changes do not always occur in women with CKD, to what extent such maladaptation occurs is not known.

FERTILITY

Fertility is decreased in CKD, particularly in more advanced stages. Because there is no known estimate of the number of women with CKD who are trying to conceive, the precise stage of CKD at which fertility decreases is not known. However, it is rare to see women with a serum creatinine >1.5 mg/dL (130 mcmol/L) become pregnant. Disruption of hypothalamic–pituitary–gonadal axis at various levels leading to low estrogen levels is thought to be the major factor contributing to menstrual irregularities and infertility in advanced

TABLE 25.1	Normal "Adaptive" Changes During Pregnancy

Structural Changes in the Kidney
- Increase in kidney size by 1–1.5 cm (and up to 30% in volume)
- Dilatation of the collecting system, more prominent on the right

Systemic Hemodynamic Changes
- Increase in cardiac output and plasma volume by 40–50% of normal
- Drop in SBP by approx. 9 mm of Hg and DBP by 17 mm of Hg (prominent in second trimester)
- Hormonal changes: 10–20-fold increase in aldosterone, eightfold increase in renin, and fourfold increase in angiotensin
- Resistance to pressor effect of angiotensin
- Increased production of prostacyclin and nitric oxide

Renal Hemodynamic Changes
- Increase in GFR and RPF by 50% above normal
- Decrease in glomerular capillary oncotic pressure

Metabolic Changes
- Decrease in BUN (<13 mg/dL [4.6 mmol/L]) and serum creatinine (0.4–0.5 mg/dL [35–44 mcmol/L])
- Increase in proteinuria but generally <300 mg/day
- Increase in total body water by 6–8 L
- Net retention of approx. 900 mmol of sodium
- Decrease in plasma osmolality by 10 mOsm/L due to reset osmostat
- Decrease in serum sodium by 4–5 mmol/L
- Mild respiratory alkalosis with compensatory drop in bicarbonate (bicarb of 18–22 mmol/L)
- Decrease in serum uric acid levels (2.5–4 mg/dL; 150–240 mcmol/L)
- Increased glucose excretion leading to glucosuria irrespective of blood sugar levels

CKD. Hyperprolactinemia may play a role in decreased fertility, but prolactin increases occur fairly late unless the woman is taking drugs that increase prolactin.

Despite reduced fertility rates in CKD, pregnancy occurs often enough that birth control should be discussed even if they are on dialysis. Barrier methods of contraception, if used as directed, are safe and effective. The infection risks associated with intrauterine devices (IUDs) for contraception do not appear to differ in women with CKD or in women who have received a kidney transplant compared to healthy women. However, there may be decreased efficacy of IUDs in women taking immunosuppressive drugs (Zerner, 1981). Oral contraceptive pills are associated with risks of hypertension and thrombosis in the general population, and CKD patients are already at an increased risk of both. At present there are only scant data available on the use of oral contraceptives in CKD, the one exception being patients with lupus, in whom the complications of pregnancy are higher than the risk of using oral contraceptives. Low-dose estrogen pills can be used with relative safety in patients with lupus nephritis and CKD as long as there is no history of thrombosis or presence of anticardiolipin antibodies or poorly controlled hypertension.

Since pregnancy in women with moderate to severe renal insufficiency is fraught with hazard, few attempts have been made to reverse infertility, although some women have ovulated with hormone treatment and had children with the help of surrogate mothers.

ESTIMATION OF GLOMERULAR FILTRATION RATE IN PREGNANCY

The formulas most frequently used for GFR estimation are based on serum creatinine, and to date we do not have an accurate formula for calculating estimated GFR (eGFR) in pregnant patients. Modified MDRD underestimates GFR in normal pregnancy and Cockcroft–Gault formula overestimates GFR by 40 mL/min when compared to creatinine clearance. Studies have shown that even in pregnant CKD patients, the MDRD equation underestimated "true" GFR as measured by using inulin clearance by about 25 mL/min. Serum cystatin C does not fare any better (Saxena, 2012). Despite its inherent limitations, 24-hour urine creatinine clearance remains the most practical test to estimate GFR during pregnancy.

HYPERTENSION AND PREECLAMPSIA

Hypertension

Hypertension is the most common medical complication of pregnancy and the second leading cause of maternal mortality in United States, after pulmonary embolism, accounting for 1% of maternal deaths. Hypertension in pregnancy is defined as BP ≥140 mm Hg systolic or ≥90 mm Hg diastolic, measured on at least two separate occasions. The severity of hypertension during pregnancy is classified as mild (BP of 140 to 149/90 to 99 mm Hg), moderate (150 to 159/100 to 109 mm Hg), and severe (>160/110 mm Hg), with treatment considered only in severe hypertension in the absence of comorbid conditions.

Preeclampsia

Preeclampsia is a multisystem disease unique to human pregnancy. It is the most frequently encountered renal complication during pregnancy. The Task Force on Hypertension in Pregnancy modified the diagnostic criteria for preeclampsia and severe preeclampsia (American College of Obstetricians and Gynecologists, 2013). Dependence on proteinuria for the diagnosis of preeclampsia has been eliminated. Preeclampsia is now characterized by new onset of hypertension and either proteinuria or end-organ dysfunction, usually after 20 weeks of gestation in a previously normotensive woman (Table 25.2). Severe preeclampsia is characterized by any of the following: BP ≥160/110 mm Hg on two separate occasions, thrombocytopenia, elevated liver enzymes or severe persistent right upper quadrant or epigastric pain not accounted for by alternate diagnoses, progressive renal insufficiency, pulmonary edema, or new-onset cerebral or visual disturbances (Table 25.3). Eclampsia is defined as the occurrence of seizures in a woman with preeclampsia that cannot be attributed to other causes.

TABLE 25.2	2013 ACOG Criteria for Diagnosis of Preeclampsia
Blood pressure	SBP ≥140 mm Hg or DBP ≥90 mm Hg on two occasions at least 4 hours apart after 20 weeks of gestation in a previously normotensive patient. If SBP is ≥160 mm Hg or DBP is ≥110 mm Hg, confirmation within minutes is sufficient.
Proteinuria	Proteinuria ≥0.3 g in a 24-hour urine specimen or protein (mg/dL)/creatinine (mg/dL) ratio ≥0.3. Dipstick 1+ if a quantitative measurement is unavailable.

In patients with new-onset hypertension without proteinuria, the new onset of any of the following is diagnostic of preeclampsia:

Platelet count	<100,000/microliter
Serum creatinine	>1.1 mg/dL (>100 mcmol/L) or doubling of serum creatinine in the absence of other renal disease
Liver transaminases	At least twice the normal concentrations
Pulmonary edema	
Cerebral or visual symptoms	

ACOG, American College of Obstetricians and Gynecologists.

Pathophysiology. A placenta, but not a fetus, is required for the development of preeclampsia as it can occur in molar pregnancy, too. Placental ischemia is a universal finding. Personal or family history of preeclampsia, advanced maternal age, first pregnancy (or second pregnancy with a different father), more than one fetus, and underlying medical conditions such as hypertension, diabetes (usually with microalbuminuria), antiphospholipid antibodies, obesity, and CKD also predispose to preeclampsia. In predisposed pregnancies, impaired deep placentation is thought to cause placental ischemia; the injured placenta is then thought to release factors into maternal circulation that disrupt angiogenesis and induce preeclampsia.

TABLE 25.3	Clinical Features of Severe Preeclampsia (Any of These Findings)

SBP ≥160 mm Hg or DBP ≥110 mm Hg on two occasions at least 4 hours apart while the patient is on bed rest (unless antihypertensive medication has been initiated before this time).

Thrombocytopenia—platelet count <100,000/microliter.

Impaired liver function as indicated by abnormally elevated blood concentrations of liver enzymes (two times the normal limit), severe persistent right upper quadrant or epigastric pain unresponsive to medication and not accounted by alternative diagnoses or both.

Progressive renal insufficiency (serum creatinine >1.1 mg/dL (>100 mcmol/L) or doubling of serum creatinine in the absence of other renal disease).

Pulmonary edema.

New-onset cerebral or visual disturbances.

That preeclampsia results from the release of circulating factors by the placenta was first proposed in 1989. Accumulating evidence supports this hypothesis. An imbalance between angiogenic and antiangiogenic factors has emerged as the central pathogenic mechanism (Maynard and Karumanchi, 2011). Angiogenic factors include vascular endothelial growth factor (VEGF) and placental growth factor (PLGF) and antiangiogenic factors include soluble fms-like tyrosine kinase-1 (sFlt-1) and soluble endoglin (sEng).

Diagnosis and Prevention. Symptoms of preeclampsia include severe headache; problems with vision, such as blurring or flashing before the eyes; severe pain just below the ribs; vomiting; frothy urine; and sudden swelling of the face, hands, or feet. Pregnant women should be warned to seek immediate medical care when they develop any of the above. The degree of proteinuria and severity of maternal hypertension are highly variable, as is the gestational age at onset, with symptoms developing as early as 20 weeks of gestation and as late as during labor and, rarely, even postpartum. Edema is generally present, although most pregnant women have edema.

HELLP syndrome is characterized by microangiopathic hemolytic anemia, elevated liver enzymes (sometimes over 1,000 IU), and low platelets. HELLP syndrome occurs in 10% to 20% of patients with preeclampsia. Although it is thought to represent a severe form of preeclampsia, questions exist as to whether it could be a separate entity by itself as 15% to 20% do not have antecedent hypertension or proteinuria. Preeclampsia progresses to eclampsia (seizures) in 2 to 3% of cases.

There is no single cost-effective screening test for preeclampsia available at the current time. A wide variety of serologic markers have been proposed, but none of these tests are available for routine clinical practice now. The levels of angiogenic factors such as VEGF and PLGF decrease and those of antiangiogenic factors such as sFlt-1 and sEng increase in women who eventually develop preeclampsia (Chaiworapongsa, 2014). Similar changes were noted in pregnant women with CKD who developed preeclampsia but not in women with CKD alone (Masuyama, 2012). The sensitivity and specificity of the available tests are not robust enough to be used for routine screening of preeclampsia. Whether this sensitivity and specificity improve when only at-risk populations are evaluated is unknown. Women at high risk for preeclampsia should have baseline renal function, hemoglobin, platelet count, liver function tests, urinalysis, and urine quantification of protein done and repeated during the second and third trimesters. Once a diagnosis of preeclampsia has been made, monitoring of laboratory tests should be performed at least weekly.

Definitive management of preeclampsia is delivery of the fetus and placenta. When the fetus is mature enough to be delivered, the decision is easy. When the fetus is immature, close monitoring of both the fetus and mother with treatment of hypertension and prevention of maternal seizures are the key. Pilot studies exploring dextran sulfate apheresis and heparin-mediated extracorporeal LDL-precipitation (H.E.L.P.) apheresis have shown promising results in management of preeclampsia (Thadhani, 2016; Winkler, 2018). While some small studies reported improved outcomes with high-dose steroids for HELLP syndrome, a Cochrane analysis concluded that there is no clear-cut evidence for a benefit of steroid treatment on clinical outcomes. Continuous magnesium infusion to prevent eclampsia must be done with caution in CKD, with frequent monitoring of serum magnesium levels and reducing the maintenance dose to 1 g/h or less, depending on the renal function.

Low-dose aspirin (60 to 150 mg) decreases platelet thromboxane synthesis with no significant effect on prostacyclin synthesis in the blood vessels. Aspirin decreases the risk of preeclampsia in moderate to high-risk patients. Cochrane meta-analysis reported a 17% risk reduction of preeclampsia with antiplatelet agents, largely with low-dose aspirin use (Duley, 2007). The U.S. Preventive Services Task Force (USPSTF) recommends the use of low-dose aspirin (81 mg/day) after 12 weeks of gestation in women at high risk of developing preeclampsia (LeFevre, 2014). The USPSTF defines high risk as previous pregnancy with preeclampsia, multifetal gestation, chronic hypertension; type 1 or 2 diabetes mellitus; kidney disease; or autoimmune disease (antiphospholipid syndrome, systemic lupus erythematosus). Most pregnant patients followed in renal clinic will have chronic hypertension or CKD at baseline and hence, are considered to be high risk for preeclampsia. Low-dose aspirin should be offered for primary prophylaxis in all such patients unless there is a definite contraindication.

Management of Hypertension During Pregnancy

There are few data to support any specific BP targets in pregnancy. There are conflicting data on the benefits of antihypertensive therapy for mild to moderate hypertension (≤160/110 mm Hg), either chronic or de novo. A Cochrane meta-analysis that included 49 trials concluded that there is insufficient evidence to determine the effects of antihypertensive treatment in mild to moderate hypertension during pregnancy (Abalos, 2014). The risk of developing severe hypertension was reduced by half with the use of antihypertensive drugs but no differences were noted in maternal or fetal outcomes. With the availability of many safe antihypertensive medications (Table 25.4), it seems prudent to treat mild hypertension with a goal BP of 140/90 mm Hg in pregnant hypertensive women with CKD or end organ damage.

Angiotensin-Converting Enzyme Inhibitors and Angiotensin Receptor Blockers. Two classes of antihypertensive medications—angiotensin-converting enzyme (ACE) inhibitors and angiotensin receptor blockers (ARBs)—are strongly contraindicated in pregnancy. Adverse fetal outcomes have been reported with their use during all stages of pregnancy, although the evidence for association with first-trimester exposure is weak and conflicting. Fetal exposure to ACE inhibitors has been associated with oligohydramnios, renal dysplasia, and pulmonary

TABLE 25.4	**Antihypertensive Medications in Pregnancy**		

Medication	Dose	Side Effects/Comments	Safety Label
α-Methyldopa	500–3,000 mg in divided doses	Drug of choice	Category B
Labetalol	200–1,200 mg in divided doses	Widely used, efficacy and safety similar to methyldopa	Category B
Other β-blockers	Variable	Reports of IUGR and fetal bradycardia	Category C/D
Calcium channel blockers	Variable	Considered to be relatively safe	Category C
Diuretics	Variable	May cause diminished volume expansion	Category B/C
Clonidine	0.1–0.8 mg in divided doses	Limited data	Category C
Hydralazine	30–200 mg in divided doses	Widely used, might not be effective as a single agent	Category C
Minoxidil	2.5–10 mg in divided doses	Limited data	Category C
Spironolactone	Variable	Feminization of male fetus in animal studies, limited data in humans	Category C
α-Blockers	Variable	Limited data	Category B/C
ACE inhibitors	Contraindicated	Renal dysplasia, hypoplastic lungs	Category D
Angiotensin receptor blockers	Contraindicated	Neonatal anuric renal failure	Category D

Category B, animal studies show no fetal risk but human data lacking; Category C, animal studies show fetal risk but human data lacking; Category D, positive evidence of human fetal risk but potential benefits may warrant use; Category X, positive evidence of human fetal risk, the risks involved in use of the drug in pregnant women clearly outweigh potential benefits; IUGR, intrauterine growth retardation.

hypoplasia. Similar problems have been noted with exposure to ARBs in the second and third trimesters, with chronic renal insufficiency affecting surviving infants. Because multiple safe alternative antihypertensive medications are available, ACE inhibitors and ARBs should be avoided both during pregnancy and in women trying to conceive. However, exposure to ACE inhibitors in early first trimester should not prompt termination of pregnancy, as absolute risk of fetal malformations is relatively low with first-trimester exposure, and fertility rates are dismal in CKD patients.

Diuretics. There has been a strong aversion to the use of diuretics in pregnancy as they aggravate the decreased intravascular volume seen with preeclampsia; however, in a meta-analysis of nine randomized trials involving more than 7,000 normotensive pregnant patients receiving diuretics, there was a decrease in the tendency of treated women to develop edema, hypertension, or both, and there was no increase in adverse fetal outcomes (Collins, 1985). In pregnant women with CKD, in whom hypertension is related to volume expansion unrelated to pregnancy, diuretics are frequently needed for BP control. In such patients, diuretics can be safely used with appropriate caution.

α-Methyldopa. Methyldopa has been used in pregnant women since 1960. It minimally affects uteroplacental blood flow and fetal hemodynamics. The major reported side effect is somnolence as it acts centrally by decreasing sympathetic tone. Long-term follow-up studies done in children exposed to α-methyldopa in utero found no ill effects. It is not a potent BP-lowering medication and may need to be combined with a second agent for adequate BP control.

Calcium Channel Blockers. Once reserved for refractory hypertension, calcium channel blockers are now widely used as first-line drugs for the treatment of hypertensive pregnant women. Nifedipine is the most widely used in this. No increased risk of congenital anomalies has been reported. Concerns for neuromuscular blockade and severe hypotension with the simultaneous use of nifedipine and magnesium sulfate were not substantiated in a large retrospective review, but careful monitoring is advised.

β-Adrenergic Blockers and Labetalol. Labetalol combines α- and β-blockade and is the most widely used adrenergic blocker for hypertension in pregnancy as it has been associated with little adrenergic blockade in the newborn. Atenolol has been shown to decrease placental blood flow and affect fetal growth in a few small studies.

Hydralazine. Hydralazine has been widely used in pregnancy and is considered safe in pregnancy. Oral hydralazine is ineffective as a single agent. Neonatal thrombocytopenia and lupus have been reported.

Treatment of Severe Hypertension in Pregnancy
Acute-onset severe hypertension (SBP >160 or DBP >110 mm Hg or both) can occur in pregnancy or the early postpartum period. If severe hypertension is persistent for more than 15 minutes, it needs to be considered a hypertensive emergency (Committee on Obstetric Practice, 2015). Intravenous labetalol and hydralazine are considered first-line agents for the treatment of severe hypertension in pregnancy (Table 25.5).

PROTEINURIA IN PREGNANCY

Protein excretion of more than 300 mg in a day is considered abnormal in pregnancy and if noted for the first time after the 20th week of gestation, preeclampsia is a major concern. The most common cause of nephrotic syndrome in pregnancy is preeclampsia. Only a small fraction of patients with preeclampsia will develop heavy proteinuria,

TABLE 25.5	Medications for Treatment of Severe Hypertension in Pregnancy
Drug	**Dose**
Hydralazine	5–10-mg intravenous bolus every 20–30 minutes for a maximum of 20 mg, then infusion at 5–10 mg/h (Category C)
Labetalol	20-mg intravenous loading dose followed by 20–30 mg every 20–30 minutes to maximum of 300 mg or at a drip of 1–2 mg/min (Category B)
Nifedipine SR (sustained release)	20 mg oral; need to be cautious with simultaneous intravenous magnesium infusions (Category C)

but because preeclampsia is so common, the subset of preeclamptic patients who have nephrotic-range proteinuria make up the largest group of pregnant women with new-onset nephrotic syndrome. Increase in GFR and RPF along with anatomical changes induced by pregnancy can lead to an increase in protein excretion, which generally reverses postpartum. In a study that included 202 pregnant women with no baseline proteinuria, significant proteinuria defined as ≥1+ protein on urine dipstick was detected in 4%, 11%, and 11% in first, second, and third trimesters, respectively. Proteinuria disappeared in all patients postpartum and none had deterioration in renal function (Osman, 2011).

Studies in women with known CKD have shown that severe proteinuria early in pregnancy is a major risk factor for adverse neonatal outcomes irrespective of BP control. Proteinuria can be noted for the first time during pregnancy either because pre-existing renal disease is detected or because of new-onset renal disease. Definitive diagnosis can be delayed until after pregnancy, unless there is unexplained acute renal failure or serologic evidence of lupus or glomerulonephritis or in patients with profound hypoalbuminemia with severe complications of nephrotic syndrome. While spot protein/creatinine ratio can be used, 24-hour urine protein measurement remains the gold standard for evaluation of abnormal proteinuria in pregnancy.

Salt restriction is theoretically helpful and is useful if implemented before the development of edema. Low-dose diuretics are safe in pregnancy, but high doses are often required for effective diuresis in nephrotic syndrome; and in pregnancy, the safety of high-dose diuretics is not established.

URINARY TRACT INFECTIONS

Prevalence of asymptomatic bacteriuria is estimated to be around 5% to 7% in both pregnant and nonpregnant patients, but the risk of developing acute pyelonephritis is 40% higher in pregnancy (Cunningham and Lucas, 1994). Pregnancy is one of the indications for treating asymptomatic bacteriuria. If a first-trimester screening urine culture is negative in normal pregnancy, the development of asymptomatic bacteriuria later in pregnancy is unusual. However, in women with underlying CKD, particularly renal transplant recipients, bacteriuria can develop even after an initial negative screening culture.

Pyelonephritis is a serious medical condition when it occurs in a pregnant woman and is associated with both maternal and fetal morbidity. Adverse pregnancy complications associated with pyelonephritis include acute renal failure, septic shock leading to acute respiratory distress syndrome, low birth weight, premature labor, and premature rupture of membranes. Cephalosporins and penicillins, including combinations with clavulanic acid, generally are safe and effective. Treatment should be intravenous until the patient is afebrile and then continued for 14 days. Aminoglycosides can be used in the case of drug allergy or resistant bacteria, although they carry a theoretical risk of fetal ototoxicity. Tetracycline and quinolones should be avoided because of teratogenicity. Relapse occurs in 20% of treated cases of pyelonephritis; therefore, suppressive therapy, with nitrofurantoin in women with normal renal function or with a cephalosporin in women with abnormal renal function, is recommended (Jolley and Wing, 2010).

Hyperlipidemia

Plasma lipids undergo both qualitative and quantitative changes in pregnancy with significant increases noted in triglyceride and total cholesterol levels (Potter and Nestel, 1979). These alterations are thought to be due to changes in the hormonal milieu. This process can further be exacerbated in nephrotic syndrome. Hyperlipidemia generally is not treated until after pregnancy, as statins are classified as Category X (see Table 25.4). Various congenital malformations, ranging from vertebral to limb deformities, have been reported with statin use in the first trimester. Women of reproductive age who are taking statins need to be counseled to stop these agents when pregnancy is contemplated. In pregnant patients with severe hyperlipidemia or familial hypercholesterolemia, immunoadsorption to achieve cholesterol removal via lipoprotein apheresis can be considered.

Venous Thrombosis

There are no established guidelines for prevention of thromboembolic disease. Low-dose aspirin can be used safely in pregnant CKD patients. Heparin does not cross the placenta, and low-dose subcutaneous heparin use in a woman with profound hypoalbuminemia is reasonable, particularly if she has been prescribed bed rest or has membranous nephropathy. Women with documented thromboembolic disease should be fully anticoagulated, and this can be achieved by using high-dose subcutaneous heparin. Increased doses of heparin may be needed for clinical effectiveness because of gestational increases in heparin clearance. Low–molecular-weight heparins are considered to be safe in pregnancy but should be avoided in women with CKD because of increased bleeding risk from prolonged half-life.

Warfarin is teratogenic in the first trimester, and it crosses the placenta, putting the fetus at risk for bleeding later in pregnancy.

PROBLEMS SPECIFIC TO CHRONIC KIDNEY DISEASE PATIENTS

Rapid Decline in Renal Function

In most of the available literature on pregnancy in kidney disease, CKD was arbitrarily classified into three categories based on serum creatinine: mild (serum creatinine ≤1.4 mg/dL [125 mcmol/L]), moderate (1.4 to 2.7 mg/dL [125 to 240 mcmol/L]), and severe (≥2.8 mg/dL [≥250 mcmol/L]) renal dysfunction (Webster, 2017). While women with mild CKD are at increased risk of preeclampsia, hypertension, and worsening proteinuria, renal function is generally preserved. In pregnant women with CKD, renal impairment can progress rapidly, particularly if the initial serum creatinine is ≥1.4 mg/dL (125 mcmol/L) (Jones and Hayslett, 1996). A prospective study compared the rate of loss of renal function before and after conception in women with stages 3 to 5 CKD. The rate of GFR decline was not significantly different from conception to after delivery, but in subgroup analyses, women who had GFR <40 mL/min per 1.73 m^2 and 24-hour proteinuria >1 g had an increased risk of accelerated rate of GFR loss (Imbasciati, 2007). In a recently published report that compared outcomes in 504 pregnancies in women with CKD stages 1 to 5, to 836 pregnancies in women without CKD, there was an increasing trend of shift to a worse CKD stage. Only 47 of the 504 pregnancies were in women with stages 3 to 5 CKD, probably contributing to the statistically insignificant result (Piccoli, 2015).

There are several potential explanations for an adverse effect of pregnancy on the progression of renal disease, but none are entirely satisfactory. Increased intraglomerular pressure is generally blamed for the progressive decline in renal function in pregnant women with CKD. Normal pregnancy is accompanied by an increased GFR, but the increase is brought about by increased renal blood flow without any increase in intraglomerular pressure. Also, in women with more severe degrees of CKD, the normal pregnancy-associated increase in GFR is not frequently observed (Cunningham, 1990). Pregnancy in CKD is frequently accompanied by hypertension, but an accelerated decline in renal function has been described in some women during pregnancy despite having an unequivocally normal BP (90 to 100/60 mm Hg) throughout gestation (Jungers, 1997). Proteinuria usually is increased during pregnancy. Because proteinuria per se is thought to have a detrimental effect on renal function, one can speculate that a period of several months of increased proteinuria might have an adverse effect on renal function, but data to support this hypothesis are lacking. Imbasciati (2007) reported that proteinuria of >1 g/24 h was detrimental to renal function only when GFR was <40 mL/min per 1.73 m^2, and proteinuria had no significant independent adverse effect.

Whatever the mechanisms, pregnancy exerts adverse effects primarily in patients who have lost a critical amount of renal function prior to pregnancy. Once a pregnancy-related decline in renal function occurs, it cannot be predictably reversed even by terminating the pregnancy. Women who start dialysis for rapidly progressive renal insufficiency during pregnancy usually will require continued dialysis postpartum (Okundaye, 1998).

Anemia

A drop in hemoglobin is noted in normal pregnancy, because the red cell mass increases by only 18% to 30%, whereas the plasma volume expands by 40% to 50%. In women with CKD, this drop is further exacerbated by decreased erythropoietin generation. Also, pregnancy is an unusual cause of erythropoietin resistance. A sharp drop in hemoglobin generally is noted as early as the first few weeks of conception. Currently available forms of erythropoietin-stimulating agents (ESAs) are labeled as Category C drugs in pregnancy. ESAs are being used in pregnant dialysis patients with few untoward effects reported so far. In pregnancy in women with advanced CKD, doubling of the pre-existing erythropoietin dose is often required to reverse the drop in hemoglobin. Typically, in normal pregnancy, 700 to 1,000 mg of iron is required to support the increased demand, and one would expect the same amount of iron to be needed in nondialysis CKD patients. Iron stores should be repleted to allow adequate action of erythropoietin.

Bone Disease

Guidelines for management of bone disease in pregnant patients with CKD are lacking. Scant human data are available on the use of phosphate binders and vitamin D analogs in pregnancy, and few untoward effects have been reported so far. Among phosphate binders, calcium acetate, sevelamer, and lanthanum carbonate are all Category C drugs. Calcium acetate or sevelamer might be better to use than lanthanum, as lanthanum has been associated with some degree of lanthanum accumulation in animal studies. Of the active vitamin D compounds, calcitriol and paricalcitol are Category C, whereas doxercalciferol is Category B; thus the latter might be preferred. No untoward effects have been reported with cinacalcet use in pregnancy. Cinacalcet is a Category C drug, but given limited experience, it is not routinely recommended.

Low-Protein Diet

Pregnant patients are generally counseled to have high protein intake even though the ideal protein intake in normal pregnancy has yet to be determined. Low-protein diets are considered an important tool in management of CKD patients and are considered to slow CKD progression in selected patients. The different maternofetal requirements are at conflict in a pregnant CKD patient, and little is known about the risk/benefits of a low-protein diet in pregnant CKD patients. One report on 12 pregnancies in 11 patients did show that a vegetarian-supplemented low-protein diet was a safe option for pregnant CKD patients, with good maternal and fetal outcomes. The median week of delivery was 32 weeks, only one patient had doubling of serum creatinine, and none required dialysis (Piccoli, 2011). Use of a low-protein diet probably should be limited to the group of women with a high risk of accelerated progression of CKD.

LUPUS NEPHRITIS IN PREGNANCY

Lupus nephritis is among the most variable and most dangerous renal diseases affecting pregnant women (Moroni and Ponticelli, 2018). Despite significant improvements in fetal outcomes (a decrease in fetal loss from 40% to 17%), maternal mortality is still unacceptably high. A 20-fold increased risk in maternal mortality was found in lupus patients compared with their nonlupus counterparts (Clowse, 2008). The rule of renal failure not progressing when serum creatinine is <1.4 mg/dL (125 mcmol/L) does not apply to lupus. Increased risk of a lupus flare during pregnancy is reported in multiple studies where each patient's own nonpregnant course is used for comparison. In the multiethnic prospective study of pregnant patients with lupus, prior kidney disease (complete or partial remission) and low C4 at baseline were independently associated with higher risk of developing active nephritis during pregnancy (Buyon, 2017).

Lupus patients with **antiphospholipid syndrome** face a further increase in risk of thromboembolic events during pregnancy. A 54% reduction in pregnancy loss is reported with combination therapy of low-dose aspirin and heparin compared to aspirin alone in women with antiphospholipid syndrome (Empson, 2002). Aspirin is generally prescribed when conception is attempted and prophylactic dose of heparin (low–molecular-weight heparin is a safe alternative) at confirmation of intrauterine pregnancy. Use of intravenous immunoglobulin G has been associated with successful pregnancy outcomes in uncontrolled trials. Women with anti-SSA antibodies have an increased risk of having a baby with congenital heart block.

New-onset lupus or lupus flare is an indication for biopsy during pregnancy if the use of **cyclophosphamide** is being considered. Cyclophosphamide is teratogenic in the first trimester. There are case reports of cancer in children exposed to cyclophosphamide in utero. Evidence of teratogenic effects of **mycophenolate mofetil** continues to increase, and side effects on the fetus include bone marrow suppression, hypoplastic nails, cleft lip/palate hypertelorism, and abnormalities of the external ear. Mycophenolate mofetil should not be used during pregnancy. Cyclosporine, azathioprine, and prednisone are considered safe in pregnancy, with cyclosporine probably being the most effective in lupus nephritis. Rituximab has been used in a handful of pregnant women. It crosses the placenta and has been associated with neonatal infections including those due to cytomegalovirus. Fertility in women with lupus nephritis is similar to that of the general population if renal function is normal, unless they were treated with large doses of cyclophosphamide. Fertility is generally preserved if the total exposure to cyclophosphamide is less than 10 g.

For women with pre-existing lupus nephritis, pregnancy is safest if the disease has been in remission on <10 mg daily of prednisone for 6 months, serum creatinine is <1.5 mg/dL (130 mcmol/L), and blood pressure is well controlled.

CKD DIAGNOSED DURING PREGNANCY

Not uncommonly, CKD is diagnosed for the first time during pregnancy. Serum creatinine values of 1.0 mg/dL (90 mcmol/L), considered normal for nonpregnant conditions, are of concern in pregnancy, and such patients should be monitored closely. Kidney biopsy usually is avoided in pregnancy because of fear of bleeding from the biopsy site, but whether an increased bleeding risk truly exists is not clear.

If a condition causing either severe impairment of renal function or proteinuria is encountered where the likelihood of steroid responsiveness is high, then an empirical trial of corticosteroids can be tried, delaying biopsy until after pregnancy. However, a kidney biopsy is generally indicated when a treatable renal disorder is suspected, especially early in pregnancy or when there is rapid deterioration in renal function. Percutaneous ultrasound-guided biopsy can be done when needed in the usual prone position or with the patient lying on the right side.

For a woman with renal insufficiency who conceives, that pregnancy might be the last opportunity for childbearing. Whenever possible, pregnancy in women with CKD should be planned, and a team of high-risk obstetricians, nephrologists, and neonatologists should be involved in the patient's care.

References and Suggested Readings

Abalos E, Duley L, Steyn DW. Antihypertensive drug therapy for mild to moderate hypertension during pregnancy (Review). *Cochrane Database Syst Rev*. 2014;2: CD002252.

American College of Obstetricians and Gynecologists; Task Force on Hypertension in Pregnancy. Hypertension in pregnancy. Report of the American College of Obstetricians and Gynecologists' Task Force on Hypertension in Pregnancy. *Obstet Gynecol*. 2013;122:1122–1131.

Buyon JP, Kim MY, Guerra MM, et al. Kidney outcomes and risk factors for nephritis (flare/de novo) in a multiethnic cohort of pregnant patients with lupus. *Clin J Am Soc Nephrol*. 2017;12:940–946.

Chaiworapongsa T, Chaemsaithong P, Korzeniewski SJ, et al. Pre-eclampsia part 2: prediction, prevention and management. *Nat Rev Nephrol*. 2014;10:531–540.

Clowse ME, Jamison M, Myers E, et al. A national study of the complications of lupus in pregnancy. *Am J Obstet Gynecol*. 2008;199:127.e1–e6.

Collins R, Yusuf S, Peto R. Overview of randomized trials of diuretics in pregnancy. *Br Med J*. 1985;290:17–23.

Committee on Obstetric Practice. Committee Opinion No. 623: emergent therapy for acute-onset, severe hypertension during pregnancy and the postpartum period. *Obstet Gynecol*. 2015;125:521–525.

Cunningham FG, Cox SM, Harstad TW, et al. Chronic renal disease and pregnancy outcome. *Am J Obstet Gynecol*. 1990;163:453–459.

Cunningham FG, Lucas MJ. Urinary tract infections complicating pregnancy. *Bailleres Clin Obstet Gynaecol*. 1994;8:353–373.

Davison JM. The kidney in pregnancy: a review. *J R Soc Med*. 1983;76:485–501.

Duley L, Henderson-Smart DJ, Meher S, et al. Antiplatelet agents for preventing preeclampsia and its complications. *Cochrane Database Syst Rev*. 2007;CD004659.

Empson M, Lassere M, Craig JC, et al. Recurrent pregnancy loss with antiphospholipid antibody: a systematic review of therapeutic trials. *Obstet Gynecol.* 2002;99: 135–144.

Imbasciati E, Gregorini G, Cabiddu G, et al. Pregnancy in CKD stages 3 to 5: fetal and maternal outcomes. *Am J Kidney Dis.* 2007;49:753–762.

Jolley JA, Wing DA. Pyelonephritis in pregnancy: an update on treatment options for optimal outcomes. *Drugs.* 2010;70:1643–1655.

Jones DC, Hayslett JP. Outcome of pregnancy in women with moderate or severe renal insufficiency. *N Engl J Med.* 1996;335:226–232.

Jungers P, Chauveau D, Choukroun G, et al. Pregnancy in women with impaired renal function. *Clin Nephrol.* 1997;47:281–288.

LeFevre ML; U.S. Preventive Services Task Force. Low-dose aspirin use for the prevention of morbidity and mortality from preeclampsia: U.S. Preventive Services Task Force recommendation statement. *Ann Intern Med.* 2014;161:819–826.

Levine RJ, Lam C, Qian C, et al. Soluble endoglin and other circulating antiangiogenic factors in preeclampsia. *N Engl J Med.* 2006;355:992–1005.

Masuyama H, Nobumoto E, Okimoto N, et al. Superimposed preeclampsia in women with chronic kidney disease. *Gynecol Obstet Invest.* 2012;74:274–281.

Maynard SE, Karumanchi SA. Angiogenic factors and preeclampsia. *Semin Nephrol.* 2011;31:33–46.

Moroni G, Ponticelli C. Important considerations in pregnant patients with lupus nephritis. *Expert Rev Clin Immunol.* 2018;24:1–10.

Okundaye I, Abrinko P, Hou S. Registry for pregnancy in dialysis patients. *Am J Kidney Dis.* 1998;31:766–773.

Osman O, Bakare AO, Elamin S. The prevalence of proteinuria among pregnant women as detected by semi-quantitative method: a single center experience. *Arab J Nephrol Transplant.* 2011;4:77–82.

Piccoli GB, Attini R, Vasario E, et al. Vegetarian supplemented low-protein diets. A safe option for pregnant CKD patients: report of 12 pregnancies in 11 patients. *Nephrol Dial Transplant.* 2011;26:196–205.

Piccoli GB, Cabiddu G, Attini R, et al. Risk of adverse pregnancy outcomes in women with CKD. *J Am Soc Nephrol.* 2015;26:2011–2022.

Potter JM, Nestel PJ. The hyperlipidemia of pregnancy in normal and complicated pregnancies. *Am J Obstet Gynecol.* 1979;133:165–170.

Saxena AR, Ananth Karumanchi S, Fan SL, et al. Correlation of cystatin-C with glomerular filtration rate by inulin clearance in pregnancy. *Hypertens Pregnancy.* 2012;31:22–30.

Thadhani R, Hagmann H, Schaarschmidt W, et al. Removal of soluble Fms-like tyrosine kinase-1 by dextran sulfate apheresis in preeclampsia. *J Am Soc Nephrol.* 2016;27:903–913.

Tsatsaris V, Goffin F, Manaut C, et al. Overexpression of the soluble vascular growth factor receptor in preeclamptic patients: pathophysiological consequences. *J Clin Endocrinol Metab.* 2003;88:5555–5563.

Webster P, Lightstone L, McKay DB, et al. Pregnancy in chronic kidney disease and kidney transplantation. *Kidney Int.* 2017;91:1047–1056.

Wiles KS, Nelson-Piercy C, Bramham K. Reproductive health and pregnancy in women with chronic kidney disease. *Nat Rev Nephrol.* 2018;14:165–184.

Winkler K, Contini C, König B, et al. Treatment of very preterm preeclampsia via heparin-mediated extracorporeal LDL-precipitation (H.E.L.P.) apheresis: the Freiburg preeclampsia H.E.L.P.-apheresis study. *Pregnancy Hypertens.* 2018;12:136–143.

Woudstra DM, Chandra S, Hofmeyr GJ, et al. Corticosteroids for HELLP (hemolysis, elevated liver enzymes, low platelets) syndrome in pregnancy. *Cochrane Database Syst Rev.* 2010:CD008148.

Zerner J, Doil KL, Drewry J, et al. Intrauterine contraceptive device failures in renal transplant patients. *J Reprod Med.* 1981;26:99–102.

26

Management of Chronic Kidney Disease in Older Adults

Ann M. O'Hare and Brenda R. Hemmelgarn

Contemporary guidelines for the management of chronic kidney disease (CKD) are intended to apply to patients of all ages. Guidelines specific to older adults with CKD do not exist. Most nephrologists would agree that caring for older patients with CKD presents some unique challenges.

HOW DOES GLOMERULAR FILTRATION RATE CHANGE WITH AGE?

We know that mean glomerular filtration rate (GFR) is lower in older compared with younger persons (Fig. 26.1). It is unclear to what extent this phenomenon reflects "normal" aging versus an increased prevalence of conditions associated with CKD at older ages (e.g., hypertension, diabetes). Relatively little is known about how renal function changes with normal aging. What we do know comes almost entirely from early reports among a small number of participants in the Baltimore Longitudinal Study of Aging who underwent serial 24-hour urine creatinine clearance measurements over time. Among the subgroup of participants who did not have known renal disease or hypertension, creatinine clearance declined on average by 0.75 mL/min per year (Lindeman, 1985). Interestingly, a small number of people experienced an increase in creatinine clearance over time, suggesting, perhaps, that an age-related decline in renal function is not inevitable. In interpreting these results, it is important to note that this study population included only male subjects who were predominantly white and middle class, and few were older than 75.

WHAT IS THE PREVALENCE OF A LOW-ESTIMATED GLOMERULAR FILTRATION RATE IN OLDER ADULTS?

In the general population, approximately one in three adults older than 70 has an estimated glomerular filtration rate (eGFR) <60 mL/min per 1.73 m^2 (Coresh, 2007). The prevalence of CKD when defined as an eGFR below this level appears to be even higher in older populations receiving care. For example, in a national sample of Canadian nursing home residents ≥65 years, the prevalence of an eGFR <60 mL/min per 1.73 m^2 was almost 40%, and 50% among those older than 95 (Garg, 2004). Furthermore, older adults account for a substantial proportion of all cases of CKD. In the general population, those older than 70 are estimated to account for more than 50% of all cases of stage 3 or 4 CKD (Coresh, 2007). In a national cohort of veterans with stage 3 or 4 CKD, more than half were older than 75 (O'Hare, 2007b).

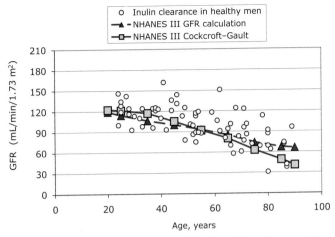

FIGURE 26.1 Mean level of estimated glomerular filtration rate by age in a community cohort. (Adapted from Coresh J, Astor BC, Greene T, et al. Prevalence of chronic kidney disease and decreased kidney function in the adult US population: Third National Health and Nutrition Examination Survey. *Am J Kidney Dis.* 2003;41:1–12.)

WHAT IS THE CLINICAL SIGNIFICANCE OF A LOW-ESTIMATED GLOMERULAR FILTRATION RATE IN OLDER ADULTS?

Contemporary guidelines define CKD largely based on fixed thresh-old levels of eGFR and albuminuria and thus implicitly do not account for the possibility that some decline in renal function may be expected to occur as part of normal aging. Indeed, there contin-ues to be disagreement within the nephrology community about whether modest reductions in eGFR (e.g., 45 to 59 mL/min per 1.73 m^2) in the older adult should always be considered to consti-tute "disease" (Glassock and Winearls, 2008). This debate—which is somewhat philosophical in nature—has been difficult to settle, not least because reasonable people may differ on the question of what constitutes disease, particularly in the absence of tissue diagnoses. Further adding to the confusion, among a biopsy series of healthy kidney donors, the presence of nephrosclerosis was strongly asso-ciated with advancing age, independent of level of renal function (Rule, 2010).

Regardless of the underlying explanation as to why mean eGFR decreases with age, it is clear that the prognostic significance of eGFR for both death and progression to end-stage renal disease (ESRD) varies systematically with age. Firstly, although mortality risk increases with declining eGFR among patients of all ages, the eGFR threshold below which absolute mortality rates rise above those for the referent category with an eGFR ≥60 mL/min per 1.73 m^2 is lower for older than younger persons. For example, among a large, predominantly male veteran cohort, those older than 65 with an

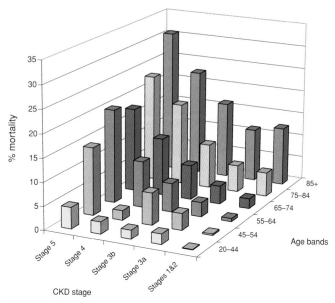

FIGURE 26.2 Mortality rates by age and estimated glomerular filtration rate. (From Raymond NT, Zehnder D, Smith SC, et al. Elevated relative mortality risk with mild-to-moderate chronic kidney disease decreases with age. *Nephrol Dial Transplant.* 2007; 22:3214–3220, with permission.)

eGFR that ranged from 50 to 59 had similar mortality rates to their age peers with an eGFR ≥60. Only at eGFR levels below 50 mL/min per 1.73 m^2 did mortality risk exceed that for the referent category (O'Hare, 2006). A similar phenomenon was observed among a community cohort in Coventry, England (Fig. 26.2) (Raymond, 2007). The precise eGFR threshold below which mortality risk increases relative to the referent category among older patients seems to vary across different populations and according to the referent category selected (Hallan, 2012).

The possibility that there are age differences in the relative and absolute risk of death among patients with similar levels of eGFR has important clinical and public health implications. Those older than 65 with very moderate reductions in eGFR (e.g., 45 to 60 mL/min per 1.73 m^2)—in whom mortality risk may be no higher than those with levels of eGFR ≥60 who do not meet criteria for CKD—account for the majority of older persons who meet these criteria. Thus, small changes in the eGFR threshold used to define CKD can make large differences in the size of the older population defined as having this condition.

Second, although eGFR is an excellent predictor of who will progress to ESRD, there are large differences in absolute risk of ESRD among patients of different ages with similar levels of eGFR: older patients are generally much less likely than their younger counterparts to progress to ESRD (O'Hare, 2007b). This phenomenon probably reflects a variety of different factors, including a higher competing risk of death, slower decline in eGFR among older persons with CKD, and age differences in rates of dialysis initiation among patients with similar levels of eGFR. In a national cohort of veterans, those aged 18 to 44 were more likely to progress to ESRD than to die when their eGFR was <45 mL/min per 1.73 m^2, whereas for those aged 75 to 84 years, risk of ESRD did not exceed risk of death until the eGFR was below 15. Among those older than 85, death was a more likely outcome than ESRD even at eGFR levels <15 (O'Hare, 2007b).

HOW DOES URINARY ALBUMIN EXCRETION CHANGE WITH AGE?

The prevalence of both microalbuminuria and proteinuria (or macroalbuminuria) increases with age (Coresh, 2007). This effect is amplified among those with diabetes or hypertension, both of which occur more frequently at older ages. Nevertheless, even among people without either of these conditions, there is an age-related increase in the prevalence of albuminuria (Coresh, 2007). Although the prevalence of albuminuria increases with age, this increase is outpaced by the rising prevalence of low eGFR. Thus, the majority of older persons who screen positive for CKD (McCullough, 2008) have a low eGFR (CKD stages 3 to 5). On the other hand, isolated albuminuria with preserved eGFR (CKD stages 1 and 2) is the most common presentation for CKD in younger persons. Thus, a relatively greater proportion of older adults with CKD will be identified by measurement of serum creatinine alone whereas many cases of CKD in younger adults would be missed without concurrent measurement of urinary albumin.

WHAT IS THE PROGNOSTIC VALUE OF ALBUMINURIA IN OLDER ADULTS?

The presence of micro- and macroalbuminuria has been shown to be associated with mortality in a variety of different populations, including patients with and without diabetes (Hallan, 2012; Hemmelgarn, 2010). Urinary albumin levels also appear to have prognostic value in older adults and may be helpful in identifying the subset with very moderate reductions in eGFR (e.g., stage 3a or 45 to 60 mL/min per 1.73 m^2) who are at greatest risk for mortality (Hallan, 2006; O'Hare, 2010). Proteinuria also appears to be associated with progression to ESRD in older adults, although limited data are available from older populations (Conway, 2009; Hemmelgarn, 2010).

TO WHAT EXTENT IS CHRONIC KIDNEY DISEASE ASSOCIATED WITH OTHER COMORBID CONDITIONS IN OLDER ADULTS?

The burden of comorbidity among patients with CKD tends to increase with age and is quite high in older populations with this condition (O'Hare, 2007b; Roderick, 2009). For example, among U.S. veterans with an eGFR <60 mL/min per 1.73 m^2, 85% or more of those older than 65 had at least one of the following comorbid conditions: coronary artery disease, congestive heart failure, peripheral arterial disease, hypertension, or stroke. The proportion of patients with CKD and diabetes peaked among those aged 55 to 75 and decreased thereafter. Indeed, the vast majority of older people with CKD do not have diabetes (O'Hare, 2009). In addition to cardiovascular disease, CKD is associated with a variety of different functional impairments and adverse outcomes, including disability, cognitive insufficiency, poor lower-extremity function, and frailty (Roderick, 2009; Shlipak, 2004). Many of the conditions that are prevalent in older adults with kidney disease are not closely tied to their underlying kidney disease but are nevertheless associated with adverse outcomes (Bowling, 2014). Multimorbidity is also extremely common in older adults with kidney disease. A recent qualitative study among veterans with moderate to severe CKD found that multimorbidity was a significant challenge to kidney disease self-management, highlighting the potential challenges and limitations of a disease-oriented approach to care in complex older adults with kidney disease (Bowling, 2017).

SHOULD OLDER ADULTS BE SCREENED FOR CHRONIC KIDNEY DISEASE?

Whether to screen older adults for CKD is recognized as an area of uncertainty in most clinical practice guidelines. Hallan (2006) modeled the accuracy of a variety of different screening strategies and found that the greatest sensitivity and specificity was achieved by screening those with diabetes, hypertension, or age >55 years. However, while inclusion of age as a screening criterion greatly improved capture of cases of CKD, the vast majority of participants older than 70 identified by screening did not go on to develop ESRD. Guidelines for hypertension and diabetes also recommend screening for CKD, thus the question of whether it makes sense to screen for CKD based on age is most relevant to those without either of these conditions.

HOW SHOULD RENAL FUNCTION BE MEASURED IN OLDER ADULTS?

Because of variation in serum creatinine with age, race, and sex, current KDIGO guidelines recommend that the Chronic Kidney Disease Epidemiology (CKD-EPI) equation be used to estimate GFR (see Chapter 1). This equation appears to provide more accurate estimates than the MDRD equation at GFR levels of 60 mL/min per 1.73 m^2 and higher in both older and younger adults. However, for older adults the GFR estimates from this equation appear to be no more accurate than the MDRD equation at eGFR levels <60 mL/min per 1.73 m^2. Several equations have been developed in older populations but these are not commonly used in clinical practice.

WHAT IS AN APPROPRIATE TARGET BLOOD PRESSURE IN OLDER PATIENTS WITH CHRONIC KIDNEY DISEASE?

Blood pressure is an important potential target for intervention to reduce cardiovascular risk and slow progression of kidney disease in older as in younger adults with this condition, and practice in this area tends to be strongly driven by the results of randomized controlled clinical trials. However, older adults with kidney disease often have multiple competing priorities, a high burden of other comorbid conditions, and limited life expectancy. Thus, an important consideration in generalizing the results of randomized controlled trials to the care of individual patients should involve assessing the the relevance of trial results to that person. In weighing the relevance of trial results to individual patients, consideration should be given to the questions addressed by the trial, the population studied the outcomes selected in relation to the specifics of that patient's situation and what is most important to them (American Geriatrics Society Expert Panel on the Care of Older Adults, 2012; O'Hare, 2016).

There has been much controversy in recent years about optimal blood pressure targets in both the general population and among those with CKD. The recent report from the committee members elected to JNC 8 recommends that blood pressure in patients with CKD be targeted to <140/90 mm Hg. The most recent KDIGO guideline however recommends use of a lower blood pressure target of <130/80 mm Hg for diabetic and nondiabetic patients with micro- or macroalbuminuria. For older adults with kidney disease, the guideline recommends tailoring blood pressure with careful consideration of "age, comorbidities and other therapies, with gradual escalation of treatment and close attention to adverse events related to BP treatment, including electrolyte disorders, acute deterioration in kidney function, orthostatic hypotension and drug side effects."

In general, the rationale for treating blood pressure in patients with CKD as for the general population is to reduce mortality and cardiovascular events. No randomized trials have provided convincing evidence that treatment to such a target slows progression of CKD or reduces other clinically significant outcomes in patients with CKD (Lewis, 2010). Most trials examining the effect of blood pressure lowering on other clinical outcomes in older adults have tended to use targets that are substantially higher than 130 systolic.

The recent SPRINT trial has led to renewed interest in more aggressive blood pressure targets in both the general population and those with CKD. This trial randomized high-risk, middle-aged, and older adults to a lower than usual blood pressure target of <120 mm Hg versus 140 mm Hg and found that among high risk patients without diabetes rates of fatal and nonfatal major cardiovascular events and death from any cause were lower in the intensive treatment group, although these patients did experience higher rates of adverse events, specifically hypotension, syncope, electrolyte abnormalities, and acute kidney injury (SPRINT Research Group, 2015). The results of SPRINT have been difficult to reconcile with the results of other major trials such as the Action to Control Cardiovascular Risk in Diabetes (ACCORD, 2010) which demonstrated that among patients with type 2 diabetes at high risk for cardiovascular events, targeting a systolic blood pressure of <120 mm Hg, as compared with <140 mm Hg, was not associated with a lower risk of fatal and nonfatal major cardiovascular events. There was also an increased risk for serious adverse events attributed to antihypertensive treatment, as well as higher rates of hypokalemia and elevations in serum creatinine level in the intensive therapy group.

One concern in extrapolating the results of SPRINT to individual older adults with kidney disease in the clinical setting is differences in the relatively low burden of comorbidity, baseline blood pressure, and number of hypertensive medications at baseline among older SPRINT participants compared with older adults with CKD in the clinical setting. Another concern is that methods for measuring blood pressure in SPRINT are not in routine use in clinical practice (Kovesdy, 2017).

WHAT AGENTS SHOULD BE PRESCRIBED TO SLOW PROGRESSION OF CHRONIC KIDNEY DISEASE IN OLDER ADULTS?

Angiotensin-converting enzyme inhibitors (ACEIs) or angiotensin receptor blockers (ARBs) are considered first-line agents for slowing progression of CKD because they both reduce proteinuria and lower blood pressure. KDIGO recommends these agents for patients with diabetic and nondiabetic proteinuric CKD, regardless of whether patients have hypertension. Based on recommendations from KDOQI, the 2014 Evidence-Based Guideline for the Management of High Blood Pressure in Adults from the JNC 8 panel recommend use of ACEIs or ARBs as either initial or add-on therapy in all patients with hypertension and CKD (James, 2014). In applying these guidelines to the management of older patients with CKD, it is important to note that many of the key studies supporting these recommendations did not enroll any participants older than 70 years of age (O'Hare, 2009) and that few data are available on the safety and efficacy of these agents in older adults. Furthermore, most guideline trials included only participants with micro- or macroalbuminuria.

The largest trial to date with the highest mean age (the Antihypertensive and Lipid Lowering to Prevent Heart Attack) failed to show a beneficial effect for ACEIs on renal outcomes (ALLHAT Officers and Coordinators for the ALLHAT Collaborative Research Group, 2002). Participants in this trial with an eGFR <60 mL/min per 1.73 m^2 had a similar risk of ESRD regardless of whether they received an ACEI, thiazide diuretic, or calcium channel blocker. However, the trial did not even require a threshold level of urinary protein (or even ascertain level of proteinuria) and likely included large numbers of older adults without proteinuria. In a secondary analysis among participants in the RENAAL trial (Reduction of Endpoints in Non-Insulin Dependent Diabetes Mellitus with the Angiotensin II Antagonist Losartan), those older than 65 derived a similar benefit from losartan as younger participants in terms of progression to ESRD (Winkelmayer, 2006).

Consistent with guidelines from the American Diabetes Association, we would recommend treatment with an ACEI or ARB in older patients with diabetes and micro- or macroalbuminuria, regardless of the presence of hypertension and if congruent with other treatment goals. Consistent with KDIGO guidelines, we would also recommend the use of these agents for patients with proteinuric nondiabetic CKD (e.g., protein excretion ≥200 mg/day), regardless of the presence of hypertension and if consistent with the patient's treatment goals. However, based on the results of ALLHAT, we suggest that for patients who have hypertension but do not have either proteinuria (if they are nondiabetic) or micro- or macroalbuminuria (if they are diabetic), other antihypertensive agents may be just as effective as ACEIs or ARBs in slowing progression of CKD.

For all older adults with CKD, we would recommend a patient-centered approach whereby choice of antihypertensive agent is guided by what is most important to the patient. These might include factors such as ease of administration, complexity of the overall treatment regimen, convenience of follow-up, and clinically relevant treatment targets, including, but not limited to, progression of kidney disease. For example, a repeat visit to test serum creatinine and potassium as recommended after initiation of an ACEI or a change in ACEI dose may be excessively burdensome for some older patients, perhaps favoring the use of an antihypertensive agent that does not require blood monitoring. Simpler treatment regimens (e.g., daily vs. twice or thrice daily dosing, minimizing the total number of agents) may be particularly helpful for patients who are cognitively impaired or who already have a heavy pill burden.

ARE THERE ADVERSE ASPECTS TO PROTEIN AND/OR CALORIE RESTRICTION IN OLDER ADULTS?

Mild protein restriction has long been considered as an effective way to reduce proteinuria and slow progression of CKD, although the largest trial addressing the effect of a low-protein diet on progression of CKD (MDRD) failed to show a benefit (see Chapter 7 for a complete discussion of this topic). Nevertheless, on the basis of the totality of evidence, most guidelines do recommend restricting protein intake to 0.8 g/kg per day in CKD patients. However, protein restriction should be approached with great care in older adults, in whom such restriction may be associated with sarcopenia. Protein restriction may be most relevant to the care of patients with advanced CKD close to needing dialysis. The results of a small randomized prospective study suggest that reduction of protein intake may be an effective way of delaying the need for dialysis (Brunori, 2007).

Although obesity is linked to increased morbidity and mortality risk in both the general population and in patients with diabetes, an inverse association between body mass index (BMI) and mortality risk has been demonstrated in older adults (Oreopoulos, 2009). In the general population, BMI has been shown to be associated with an increased risk of developing CKD or ESRD in some (Hsu, 2006), but not all (Foster, 2008) studies. Among older Medicare beneficiaries who had experienced an acute myocardial infarction, risk of both death and ESRD were generally lower for obese compared with patients with normal weight. However, data in more representative populations of older adults are currently lacking (Lea, 2009).

WHICH OLDER PATIENTS WITH CHRONIC KIDNEY DISEASE SHOULD BE REFERRED TO A NEPHROLOGIST?

Referral to a nephrologist serves multiple purposes, including diagnosis of the underlying etiology of CKD, management of the complications of CKD, and shared decision making around treatment options for advanced kidney disease. Current recommendations suggest that patients should at the very least be referred to a nephrologist when their eGFR falls below 30 mL/min per 1.73 m^2. This recommendation is based on the higher incidence of complications related to CKD and the greater risk of progression to ESRD in this group. The importance of nephrology referral has been suggested by studies among dialysis patients documenting that late referral to nephrology is associated with poorer quality of pre-ESRD care and increased mortality after dialysis initiation. Age and increased comorbidity have consistently been shown to be factors associated with late referral. However, as for all other decisions, whether to refer patients for nephrology care should hinge on the patient's goals and values and whether specialist care from a nephrologist would further these goals (Campbell, 2010).

In addition to the care of a nephrologist, older patients with CKD may benefit from **multidisciplinary care**, which includes specialized care by nurses, dieticians, and social workers who work together as a team in providing comprehensive management. Multidisciplinary care clinics have been shown based on randomized trials to result in improved morbidity and mortality among patients with chronic conditions such as diabetes and heart failure. Indeed, observational studies do suggest a survival advantage for older adults with CKD who received multidisciplinary care delivered by an interdisciplinary team (Hemmelgarn, 2007), although this remains to be confirmed in a randomized controlled trial.

WHAT PREPARATION IS NEEDED FOR HEMODIALYSIS?

Among patients who decide to initiate chronic hemodialysis and are ready to prepare for this, access to the bloodstream is essential, and a permanent form of vascular access, ideally a fistula rather than a graft or central venous catheter, is generally preferred, although several studies suggest that an AV graft may be a reasonable option in older adults with limited life expectancy. There is no consensus among clinical practice guidelines regarding the optimal time for referral for vascular access creation. In the clinical setting, expected time to initiation of dialysis usually is difficult to predict. Because of systematic age differences in the competing risk of death and in rates of loss of GFR, age can be an important consideration in deciding whether and when to refer a patient for vascular access creation.

We modeled the number of unnecessary procedures that would occur by age and level of eGFR using different threshold levels of eGFR for referral for vascular access among a large national cohort of U.S. Department of Veterans Affairs (VA) patients with an eGFR <25 mL/min per 1.73 m^2 (O'Hare, 2007b). Needless to say, the number of unnecessary procedures increased with age. In fact, among patients aged 85 to 100 years, placement of an access at an eGFR <25 mL/min per 1.73 m^2 would have turned out to be necessary in only one in six patients (O'Hare, 2007a). Often, a more targeted approach relying on additional factors that predict progression to ESRD (e.g., proteinuria or eGFR trajectory) may be required to identify older patients with a low eGFR who are most likely to benefit from preparation for ESRD.

WHAT ARE KEY CONSIDERATIONS IN FACILITATING INFORMED DECISION MAKING AMONG OLDER ADULTS WITH ADVANCED CHRONIC KIDNEY DISEASE?

When considering treatment options for advanced kidney disease, it is important that patients have a good understanding of what to expect with different treatment options and a realistic understanding of what these treatments can offer. For example, median survival after dialysis initiation ranges from a median of 2 years for those aged 65 to 79 years to just 8 months for those aged 90 and older (Table 26.1) (Kurella, 2007). Number of comorbid conditions (and presence of peripheral vascular disease in particular), increasing age, and poor functional status have been associated with increased mortality after dialysis initiation among older adults (Lamping, 2000). Among U.S. nursing home patients, survival after initiation of chronic dialysis was <1 year, and most surviving patients experienced a decline in functional status after dialysis initiation (Kurella Tamura, 2009). Several small studies outside the United States suggest that in very elderly patients with a high burden of comorbidity, dialysis may not be associated with a survival benefit compared with conservative therapy (Murtagh, 2007). Other studies suggest that dialysis may be associated with a survival benefit even in older adults with advanced CKD, but that these patients spend a much greater proportion of their remaining lifetime in a health care setting.

These findings combined with ethnographic work among outpatients with kidney disease suggesting that U.S. patients may feel

TABLE 26.1	Median Survival After Dialysis Initiation Among Older Adults in the United States	
Age at Dialysis Initiation (years)	**Median Survival (IQR^a), months**
65–79	24.9 (8.3–51.8)
80–84	15.6 (4.8–35.5)
85–89	11.6 (3.7–28.5)
≥90	8.4 (2.8–21.3)

^{a}IQR, interquartile range, the range enclosing the middle two quartiles of mid-50%.
Source: Adapted from Kurella M, Covinsky K, Collins A, et al. Octogenarians and nonagenarians starting dialysis in the United States. *Ann Intern Med.* 2007;146:177–183.

they have little option but to initiate dialysis (Kaufman, 2006) has led to a growing interest in conservative care in recent years, especially for patients not expected to do well with dialysis. Relatively little is known about dialysis initiation practices in the United States. In a large veteran cohort with stage 5 CKD followed for up to 10 years, more than two-thirds went on to initiate dialysis during follow-up (Wong, 2016a). There was an explicit or implicit decision not to pursue dialysis in less than 15% of patients. As reported previously for a large Canadian cohort (Hemmelgarn, 2012), patterns of dialysis initiation were heavily age dependent. Nevertheless, regardless of age, most patients received or were preparing to receive dialysis at the end of follow-up even in the oldest age group, with percentages ranging from 96.2% (95% confidence interval, 94.4% to 97.4%) for those <45 years old to 53.3% (95% confidence interval, 50.7% to 55.9%) for those aged ≥85 years. Results were similar after stratification by tertile of comorbidity score.

In addition to supporting the wishes of those patients who are certain they do not wish to start dialysis, there is also a need for a more patient-centered approach to dialysis initiation. Many patients would want dialysis if this was needed but wish to defer initiation as long as possible until they feel ready to start. Others are not sure if they would want dialysis and are not able to make this decision until they are faced with it. Available trial data suggest that dialysis can be safely deferred for significant periods of time in patients followed closely by a nephrologist (Cooper, 2010). Trial data also support the use of a low-protein diet as a way for delaying the need for dialysis in patients with advanced CKD (Brunori, 2007). In the absence of public support for robust alternatives to dialysis for patients with advanced kidney disease in the United States, dialysis can often be the default treatment for these patients (Wong, 2016b). Supporting patients who do not wish to initiate dialysis, who wish to defer this decision as long as possible, and who are unable to make a decision about dialysis until they become very sick will likely require public, political, and financial support for alternative multidisciplinary care models to meet the needs of these patients (Wong and O'Hare, 2017).

Given the often complex and challenging nature of decisions about dialysis initiation, it is well accepted that these decisions should in most instances be made through an iterative and ongoing process of shared decision making involving the physician, the patient, and the patient's family. Because it can be almost impossible for patients to know what the experience of being on dialysis will be like for them, a time-limited trial of dialysis may allow patients to gain a more personal understanding of what the benefits and harms are for them. Framing dialysis explicitly as a trial and following-up iteratively with the patient to learn about their experience and whether their thinking about dialysis has changed based on this experience may be particularly helpful for patients who are uncertain whether they want to receive chronic dialysis. The Renal Physicians Association (RPA) and American Society of Nephrology developed a clinical practice guideline on shared decision making in the appropriate initiation and withdrawal of dialysis (RPA, 2000). An update of this guideline was released by the RPA in 2010 (available at www.renalmd.org). This guideline serves as a valuable resource to guide shared decisions around dialysis initiation.

References and Suggested Readings

ACCORD Study Group; Cushman WC, Evans GW, Byington RP, et al. Effects of intensive blood-pressure control in type 2 diabetes mellitus. *N Engl J Med.* 2010;362: 1575–1585.

ALLHAT Officers and Coordinators for the ALLHAT Collaborative Research Group. Major outcomes in high-risk hypertensive patients randomized to angiotensin-converting enzyme inhibitor or calcium channel blocker vs diuretic: the Antihypertensive and Lipid-Lowering Treatment to Prevent Heart Attack Trial (ALLHAT). *JAMA.* 2002;288:2981–2997.

American Geriatrics Society Expert Panel on the Care of Older Adults With Multimorbidity. Guiding principles for the care of older adults with multimorbidity: an approach for clinicians. *J Am Geriatr Soc.* 2012;60:E1–E25.

Bowling CB, Booth JN 3rd, Gutierrez OM, et al. Nondisease-specific problems and all-cause mortality among older adults with CKD: the REGARDS Study. *Clin J Am Soc Nephrol.* 2014;9:1737–1745.

Bowling CB, Vandenberg AE, Phillips LS, et al. Older patients' perspectives on managing complexity in CKD self-management. *Clin J Am Soc Nephrol.* 2017;12:635–643.

Brunori G, Viola BF, Parrinello G, et al. Efficacy and safety of a very-low-protein diet when postponing dialysis in the elderly: a prospective randomized multicenter controlled study. *Am J Kidney Dis.* 2007;49:569–580.

Campbell KH, Sachs GA, Hemmerich JA, et al. Physician referral decisions for older chronic kidney disease patients: a pilot study of geriatricians, internists, and nephrologists. *J Am Geriatr Soc.* 2010;58:392–395.

Conway B, Webster A, Ramsay G, et al. Predicting mortality and uptake of renal replacement therapy in patients with stage 4 chronic kidney disease. *Nephrol Dial Transplant.* 2009;24:1930–1937.

Cooper BA, Branley P, Bulfone L, et al; IDEAL Study. A randomized, controlled trial of early versus late initiation of dialysis. *N Engl J Med.* 2010;363:609–619.

Coresh J, Selvin E, Stevens LA, et al. Prevalence of chronic kidney disease in the United States. *JAMA.* 2007;298:2038–2047.

Davison S, Torgunrud C. The creation of an advance care planning process for patients with ESRD. *Am J Kidney Dis.* 2007;49:27–36.

Foster MC, Hwang SJ, Larson MG, et al. Overweight, obesity, and the development of stage 3 CKD: the Framingham Heart Study. *Am J Kidney Dis.* 2008;52:39–48.

Garg AX, Papaioannou A, Ferko N, et al. Estimating the prevalence of renal insufficiency in seniors requiring long-term care. *Kidney Int.* 2004;65:649–653.

Gill J, Malyuk R, Djurdjev O, et al. Use of GFR equations to adjust drug doses in an elderly multi-ethnic group—a cautionary tale. *Nephrol Dial Transplant.* 2007;22: 2894–2899.

Glassock RJ, Winearls C. An epidemic of chronic kidney disease: fact or fiction? *Nephrol Dial Transplant.* 2008;23:1117–1121.

Hallan SI, Dahl K, Oien CM, et al. Screening strategies for chronic kidney disease in the general population: follow-up of cross sectional health survey. *BMJ.* 2006; 333:1047.

Hallan SI, Matsushita K, Sang Y, et al; Chronic Kidney Disease Prognosis Consortium. Age and association of kidney measures with mortality and end-stage renal disease. *JAMA.* 2012;308:2349–2360.

Hemmelgarn BR, James MT, Manns BJ, et al; Alberta Kidney Disease Network. Rates of treated and untreated kidney failure in older vs younger adults. *JAMA.* 2012;307:2507–2515.

Hemmelgarn BR, Manns BJ, Lloyd A, et al; Alberta Kidney Disease Network. Relation between kidney function, proteinuria, and adverse outcomes. *JAMA*. 2010;303:423–429.

Hemmelgarn BR, Manns BJ, Zhang J, et al. Association between multidisciplinary care and survival for elderly patients with chronic kidney disease. *J Am Soc Nephrol*. 2007;18:993–999.

Hsu CY, McCulloch CE, Iribarren C, et al. Body mass index and risk for end-stage renal disease. *Ann Intern Med*. 2006;144:21–28.

James PA, Oparil S, Carter BL, et al. 2014 evidence-based guideline for the management of high blood pressure in adults: report from the panel members appointed to the Eighth Joint National Committee (JNC 8). *JAMA*. 2014;311:507–520.

Kaufman SR, Shim JK, Russ AJ. Old age, life extension, and the character of medical choice. *J Gerontol B Psychol Sci Soc Sci*. 2006;61:S175–S184.

Kovesdy CP. The ideal blood pressure target for patients with chronic kidney disease-searching for the sweet spot. *JAMA Intern Med*. 2017;177:1506–1507.

Kurella Tamura M, Covinsky KE, Chertow GM, et al. Functional status of elderly adults before and after initiation of dialysis. *N Engl J Med*. 2009;361:1539–1547.

Kurella M, Covinsky KE, Collins AJ, et al. Octogenarians and nonagenarians starting dialysis in the United States. *Ann Intern Med*. 2007;146:177–183.

Lamping DL, Constantinovici N, Roderick P, et al. Clinical outcomes, quality of life, and costs in the North Thames Dialysis Study of elderly people on dialysis: a prospective cohort study. *Lancet*. 2000;356:1543–1550.

Lea JP, Crenshaw DO, Onufrak SJ, et al. Obesity, end-stage renal disease, and survival in an elderly cohort with cardiovascular disease. *Obesity (Silver Spring)*. 2009;17:2216–2222.

Lewis JB. Blood pressure control in chronic kidney disease: is less really more? *J Am Soc Nephrol*. 2010;21:1086–1092.

Lindeman RD, Tobin J, Shock NW. Longitudinal studies on the rate of decline in renal function with age. *J Am Geriatr Soc*. 1985;33:278–285.

McCullough PA, Li S, Jurkovitz CT, et al; Kidney Early Evaluation Program Investigators. CKD and cardiovascular disease in screened high-risk volunteer and general populations: the Kidney Early Evaluation Program (KEEP) and National Health and Nutrition Examination Survey (NHANES) 1999–2004. *Am J Kidney Dis*. 2008;51:S38–S45.

Murtagh F, Marsh JE, Donohoe P, et al. Dialysis or not? A comparative survival study of patients over 75 years with chronic kidney disease stage 5. *Nephrol Dial Transplant*. 2007;22:1955–1962.

O'Hare AM, Bertenthal D, Covinsky KE, et al. Mortality risk stratification in chronic kidney disease: one size for all ages? *J Am Soc Nephrol*. 2006;17:846–853.

O'Hare AM, Bertenthal D, Walter LC, et al. When to refer patients with chronic kidney disease for vascular access surgery: should age be a consideration? *Kidney Int*. 2007a;71:555–561.

O'Hare AM, Choi AI, Bertenthal D, et al. Age affects outcomes in chronic kidney disease. *J Am Soc Nephrol*. 2007b;18:2758–2765.

O'Hare AM, Hailpern SM, Pavkov ME, et al. Prognostic implications of the urinary albumin to creatinine ratio in veterans of different ages with diabetes. *Arch Intern Med*. 2010;170:930–936.

O'Hare AM, Kaufman JS, Covinsky KE, et al. Current guidelines for using angiotensin-converting enzyme inhibitors and angiotensin II-receptor antagonists in chronic kidney disease: is the evidence base relevant to older adults? *Ann Intern Med*. 2009;150:717–724.

O'Hare AM, Rodriguez RA, Bowling CB. Caring for patients with kidney disease: shifting the paradigm from evidence-based medicine to patient-centered care. *Nephrol Dial Transplant*. 2016;31:368–375.

Oreopoulos A, Kalantar-Zadeh K, Sharma AM, et al. The obesity paradox in the elderly: potential mechanisms and clinical implications. *Clin Geriatr Med*. 2009;25:643–659, VIII.

Raymond NT, Zehnder D, Smith SC, et al. Elevated relative mortality risk with mild-to-moderate chronic kidney disease decreases with age. *Nephrol Dial Transplant*. 2007;22:3214–3220.

Renal Physicians Association. RPA position on quality care at the end of life. *Clin Nephrol*. 2000;53:493–494.

Roderick PJ, Atkins RJ, Smeeth L, et al. CKD and mortality risk in older people: a community-based population study in the United Kingdom. *Am J Kidney Dis*. 2009;53:950–960.

Rule AD, Amer H, Cornell LD, et al. The association between age and nephrosclerosis on renal biopsy among healthy adults. *Ann Intern Med*. 2010;152:561–567.

Shlipak MG, Stehman-Breen C, Fried LF, et al. The presence of frailty in elderly persons with chronic renal insufficiency. *Am J Kidney Dis*. 2004;43:861–867.

SPRINT Research Group; Wright JT Jr, Williamson JD, Whelton PK, et al. A randomized trial of intensive versus standard blood-pressure control. *N Engl J Med*. 2015; 373:2103–2116.

Stevens LA, Coresh J, Feldman HI, et al. Evaluation of the modification of diet in renal disease study equation in a large diverse population. *J Am Soc Nephrol*. 2007;18:2749–2757.

Winkelmayer WC, Zhang Z, Shahinfar S, et al. Efficacy and safety of angiotensin II receptor blockade in elderly patients with diabetes. *Diabetes Care*. 2006;29:2210–2217.

Wong SP, Hebert PL, Laundry RJ, et al. Decisions about renal replacement therapy in patients with advanced kidney disease in the US Department of Veterans Affairs, 2000–2011. *Clin J Am Soc Nephrol*. 2016a;11:1825–1833.

Wong SPY, O'Hare AM. Making sense of prognostic information about maintenance dialysis versus conservative care for treatment of advanced kidney disease. *Nephron*. 2017;137:169–171.

Wong SP, Vig EK, Taylor JS, et al. Timing of initiation of maintenance dialysis: A qualitative analysis of the electronic medical records of a National Cohort of Patients From the Department of Veterans Affairs. *JAMA Intern Med*. 2016b;176:228–235.

27 | Chronic Kidney Disease in Asia

Philip Kam-Tao Li and Kai Ming Chow

The global epidemic of chronic kidney disease (CKD) is a major public health problem, not only in high-income countries but also in Asia. Practicing clinicians might benefit from recognizing several unique aspects of Asian patients with CKD that are highlighted in this chapter (Table 27.1).

ADJUSTMENT OF EQUATIONS FOR ESTIMATING GLOMERULAR FILTRATION RATES IN ASIANS

An accurate estimation of the glomerular filtration rate (GFR) is central to the classification, detection, and management of CKD. GFR estimation using prediction equations based on serum creatinine has been increasingly emphasized in clinical practice. The Asian population was underrepresented during the development of the two most commonly used equations, the Modification of Diet in Renal Disease (MDRD) study equation and the Chronic Kidney Disease-Epidemiology Collaboration (CKD-EPI) equation. These two equations only include a two-level variable for race: Black or non-Black. There is reason to believe that GFR estimation equations need modification and validation in Asian patients, as they have lower body muscle mass and creatinine production rate compared with Caucasians. Creatinine is generated from skeletal muscle catabolism and, to a lesser extent, from dietary protein (particularly cooked meat). Also, lower dietary meat intake in Indo-Asians when compared with Caucasians, could lead to lower creatinine excretion and hence different prediction coefficients in these estimating equations.

In fact, the MDRD equation or CKD-EPI equations have been modified for use in the Japanese, Korean, and Chinese populations with new correction coefficients. A four-level race equation (Black, Asian, Native American and Hispanic, and White (Caucasian) and other) was proposed to improve bias, for example, in Chinese subjects (Stevens, 2011). This equation is more accurate than the original two-level race CKD-EPI in some, but not all, populations. To overcome the need for an ethnicity coefficient, the use of cystatin C in combination with serum creatinine has been proposed in the estimation equations (Teo, 2018).

LOWER GLOMERULAR FILTRATION RATE/1.73 M² IN ASIANS

Apart from differences in creatinine-estimated GFR, actual measured GFR/1.73 m² in Asians appears to be lower than that found in Western populations. Data from healthy subjects, using ^{99m}Tc-diethylenetriamine penta-acetic acid (DTPA) plasma clearance, showed

Aspect	Implications
Lower creatinine appearance rate (possibly from both muscle and diet)	eGFR equations based on creatinine may need to be adjusted downward by about 20%
Lower GFR/1.73 m^2	Conventional staging of CKD may not apply because of a lower "healthy" range of GFR
High rates of hypertension, salt intake, smoking	Potential improvements that are due to education, dietary salt restriction, smoking cessation programs
High rates of glomerulonephritis	Possible improvement because of better sanitation and improvement of infections associated with glomerulonephritis
High rate of diabetes	Attention to diet and exercise; better detection of diabetes and treatments needed
Lower threshold of BMI for kidney damage	
Low nephron number at birth because of suboptimal maternal prenatal nutrition	Social and economic programs to focus on maternal health care
Lower level of kidney health awareness	Additional importance of screening and education
More rapid progression of CKD	Cause unknown
Better survival once CKD established	Cause unknown
Nephrotoxicity from herbal medicines	Better control and regulation and quality control of herbal medicines to avoid contaminants and adulterants
Environmental nephrotoxins	Community education and initiatives
Consumption of traditional foods with nephrotoxic potential or toxicity in CKD patients (djenkol, star fruit, fish gallbladder)	Patient education to avoid such foods

eGFR, estimated glomerular filtration rate; GFR, glomerular filtration rate; CKD, chronic kidney disease; BMI, body mass index.

that mean GFR values of young healthy Chinese (Ma, 2010) and Indians (Barai, 2005) were 104 to 110 mL/min per 1.73 m^2 and 81, respectively, both significantly lower than the reported value of 109 to 125 for Western populations. If confirmed, these data suggest that GFR thresholds used to define CKD in Western subjects might need to be modified for Asian populations.

ETIOLOGY OF KIDNEY DISEASE IN ASIAN COUNTRIES

Hypertension

Hypertension is a leading modifiable cause of CKD. The disease burden of hypertension in Asian countries remains enormous, especially in low- and middle-income countries. High blood pressure has been estimated to account for more than one-third of deaths and almost one-fifth of disability-adjusted life years in central Asia. There are several reasons. The prevalence of hypertension is high and increasing.

Awareness, treatment, and control of high blood pressure is exceedingly low, partly related to a low level of literacy and education, but also to a low level of access to medical care in South Asian countries. Data from national surveys suggest a low level of disease awareness and adequate treatment. For example, in a survey involving 142,000 Chinese adults, only 24% were aware of their hypertension (Wu, 2008). Percentage of hypertension awareness in most Asian countries has been <50%.

Several hypotheses have been suggested to explain the high prevalence of hypertension in developing Asian countries. Lifestyle changes associated with urbanization often are associated with adoption of a diet rich in salt and saturated fat and low-quality carbohydrates; such an explanation is supported by a higher prevalence of hypertension in the urban versus rural population in Asia. Widespread tobacco use (estimated to be 50% to 60% of adult men in many Asian countries) and increased salt consumption in Asia also contribute to the elevated hypertension rates. The role of poverty and intrauterine origin of CKD also could be part of the jigsaw puzzle. Epidemiologic evidence strongly supports a relationship between occurrence of adult hypertension and low birth weight resulting from either intrauterine growth restriction or preterm birth. Low birth weight is a common problem in low-income countries.

Insulin Resistance and Obesity

The downstream adverse consequences for any given severity of CKD risk factors may be worse in Asian populations. It has been suggested that ethnic susceptibility to insulin resistance renders the normal cutoff values of body mass index (BMI) derived in the Western population misleading when used for the Chinese, South Asian, and aboriginal populations. Asian people have a higher predisposition to insulin resistance at a lesser degree of obesity than people of European descent. For Chinese, the cutoff for central obesity is considered to be a waist circumference >90 cm in men and >80 cm in women (Li, 2008). This is compared with 94 cm and 80 cm, respectively, for Europids (white people of European origin, regardless of where they live in the world) as defined by the European Group for the Study of Insulin Resistance.

The impact of BMI on the kidney also appears to be different, such that one proposed definition of obesity in Asians has been not ≥30, but rather ≥25 kg/m^2 (Li, 2008). Deleterious effects of elevated BMI values, which generally are found in subjects with severe obesity, occur at lower BMI levels in the Chinese population. In a large multiethnic population screening study, each BMI category above 25 kg/m^2 was associated with a progressively higher odds ratio for the presence of proteinuria for the Chinese, whereas the relationship between BMI and proteinuria was only significant at BMI levels ≥30 kg/m^2 among the Malays (Ramirez, 2002). In the Chinese population, an increased risk of end-stage renal disease (ESRD) at the BMI threshold of 25 kg/m^2 also was shown in a large population-based cohort study (Reynolds, 2007). The impact of so-called metabolically healthy obesity on increased odds of CKD has also been confirmed in an Asian population (Jung, 2015).

Asian or Chinese people may be more likely to have **salt-sensitive hypertension**, in particular those with metabolic syndrome. If so, a public health strategy to reduce dietary salt intake could have considerable impact on the prevalence of hypertension and CKD in Asian countries.

Diabetes

Another connection between CKD burden and Asia is the diabetes epidemic. Given the population growth and rate of urbanization in Asia, it has been estimated that India and China will be the two countries with the highest numbers of people with diabetes by 2030. A dataset of 35 million patients in China from 2010 through 2015 confirmed that the percentage of patients with CKD related to diabetes surpassed that related to glomerulonephritis among both urban and rural residents (Zhang, 2016). Four other Asian countries are among the top 10 populations of diabetic patients around the world: Indonesia, Pakistan, Bangladesh, and the Philippines. Ethnic origin differences in the prevalence of diabetic nephropathy have been a focal point of interest in research. For example, in the United Kingdom Asian Diabetes Study (Dixon, 2006), researchers showed that among type 2 diabetes patients with normal, untreated blood pressure, the proportion who had microalbuminuria was three times higher among South Asian patients residing in the United Kingdom compared with the white European group. Most data from observational studies as well as clinical trials show that Asian patients with diabetes are more likely to develop ESRD than their Caucasian counterparts. Challenges for diabetes in India, China, and many other Asian countries include the need for education of the population and health care workers to manage diabetes more effectively.

Nephritis and Toxins

Other important causes of CKD in Asian countries include the high prevalence of chronic glomerulonephritis and interstitial nephritis, reflecting the presence of bacterial, viral, and parasitic infections that affect the kidneys. Environmental pollution (including soil pollution by organic compounds) and occupational exposure to chemicals such as lead and arsenic (Hsueh, 2009; Lin, 2003) also may play an important role.

Awareness of CKD and Education

Awareness of CKD is low in many low- and middle-income Asian regions. A recent survey from 12 countries including mostly Asian countries showed that only 6% of the general population (China, Mongolia, India, and Nepal) and 10% of a high-risk population (Bangladesh) were aware of their CKD status (Ene-Iordache, 2016). Local screening for CKD and its risk factors would thus be a public health priority, before education can be improved. We conducted a screening program named SHARE: Screening of Hong Kong Asymptomatic Renal Population and Evaluation (Li, 2005). Twelve hundred asymptomatic subjects with a mean age of 56 years were screened. The prevalence rates of proteinuria and microscopic hematuria in this cohort were 3% and 14%, respectively, and both increased with age. Ten percent of subjects aged 21 to 40 years, 24% of subjects aged 41 to 60 years, and 33% older than 60 years, all of whom had considered themselves to be healthy, had either high blood pressure or asymptomatic urinary abnormalities, the latter including proteinuria, microscopic hematuria, and/or glycosuria (Li, 2005). Our recent study on screening first-degree relatives of subjects with all stages of CKD found that such relatives are at risk of developing CKD. Parents, elderly, obese and male relatives were more likely to develop markers of kidney damage (Li, 2017). In 1st degree relatives of all stages of CKD patients, it is also found that proteinuria is more likely to occur in relatives of CKD patients secondary to Glomerulonephritis, high BMI increase their risk for hypertension and glycosuria and smoking increases their risk for lower eGFR and higher risk for proteinuria.

INCREASED RISK OF PROGRESSION

Disparities or excess risk of ESRD among Asians have been at least suggested from registry-level data. Although it is not easy to dissect socioeconomic effects from effects of ethnicity, socioeconomic conditions do not fully explain the increased risk for CKD progression in Asians. For example, the U.S. Renal Data System (USRDS) shows that U.S. Asians have a higher age- and sex-adjusted risk of ESRD compared with U.S. Caucasians. In a prospective multiethnic cohort of almost 300,000 adults who underwent a screening health checkup in northern California between 1964 and 1985, the age-adjusted rate of ESRD for Asians was more than twofold higher compared with Caucasian (Hall, 2005). Higher rates of progression of CKD in local Oriental Asian and South Asian CKD patients were recently confirmed in another cohort study done in Canada (Barbour, 2010). The reasons remain speculative. It is possible that metabolic abnormalities of CKD at any stage of CKD are differentially worse in Asian patients when compared with Caucasians. The same may be true for hypertension and proteinuria (Mathur, 2018).

INCREASED RATE OF SURVIVAL OF THOSE WITH CHRONIC KIDNEY DISEASE

Interestingly, despite a more rapid rate of renal decline for Asians (relative to Caucasians), Asians with CKD have better overall survival, whether measured before or after initiation of renal replacement therapy (Barbour, 2010; Li, 2003; Pei, 2000). Possible explanations include race-specific differences in diet, genetic factors, and the smaller body size of Asians.

DIETARY ASPECTS AND MEDICATION USE IN ASIA

In Asian patients, the need exists to look into medication use, and a detailed dietary history should always be taken because acute toxic nephropathy is rather common. One prospective study including more than 460,000 subjects from Taiwan found that regular users of herbal medicines had a 25% increased risk of developing CKD compared to nonusers (Wen, 2008). The results also showed an increasing proportion of herbal medicine users among those with more severe CKD. Another cross-sectional study in Taiwan confirmed that herbal therapy was associated independently with CKD (Guh, 2007). The association of folk medicine or herb-related kidney disease with CKD can be explained by direct herb nephrotoxicity, drug–herb interactions, herb contamination (such as nephrotoxic heavy metals) or adulteration (classically acetaminophen, indomethacin), and improper herb processing and preparation.

Toxic Herbs

Uncontrolled use and incorrect identification (inappropriate nomenclature and imprecise labeling) of medicinal herbs has been strongly suspected of being the underlying cause of aristolochic acid nephropathy (previously known as Chinese-herb nephropathy), a disease characterized by progressive renal interstitial fibrosis and frequently associated with urothelial malignancy. In a population-based case-control study, use of herbal products containing significant amounts of aristolochic acid (including Mu Tong and fangchi) was associated with an increased risk of ESRD (Lai, 2010). Suspicion of an herbal etiology for CKD of unknown cause has been raised in many parts of Asia, including Thailand, India, and Sri Lanka, especially among the rural population. Thus, better regulation and enforcement of quality assurance for herbal medicines are needed.

Toxic Foods and Food Supplements

Nephrotoxicity from other environmental sources and food products has been reported in Asian countries. In China, melamine toxicity (including risk of nephrolithiasis and acute kidney injury) from consumption of tainted powdered infant milk formula had been a cause of concern, and this problem should not reappear given proper food product surveillance and testing (Hau, 2009). Another source of food nephrotoxicity is related to consumption of **fish gallbladders**, classically from grass carp or *Ctenopharyngodon idellus*. Fish gallbladders are consumed in some Asian countries as a traditional medicine to improve symptoms of rheumatism, decreased visual acuity, and impotence. Ingestion of the raw gallbladders can induce acute tubular necrosis in addition to hepatotoxicity, presumably because of a cyprinol sulfate toxin.

Djenkol Bean or Jering

Djenkol bean or jering (*Pithecellobium jiringa*) is another traditional local delicacy consumed in tropical Asian countries, such as Malaysia and Indonesia, that has been reported to cause renal failure. The beans, usually eaten between September and February, contain djenkolic acid, which is a sulfur-containing amino acid. The exact pathogenesis of kidney injury is unknown but appears to be precipitation of djenkolic acids in the renal tubules as well in the ureters, causing irritation and obstruction of the urinary tract.

Star Fruit

Another food of concern is star fruit (*Averrhoa carambola*), a tropical fruit originating in Asia and grown in tropical countries such as Taiwan, India, and Thailand. This usually is consumed as a fresh fruit (yellowish-green in color with five lobes of fruit flesh) or as fruit juice. A wide range of neurotoxicity (including intractable hiccups, vomiting, altered level of consciousness, and seizures), sometimes fatal, has been reported. Patients with CKD should be warned to never eat star fruit or products containing it.

References and Suggested Readings

Barai S, Bandopadhayaya GP, Patel CD, et al. Do healthy potential kidney donors in India have an average glomerular filtration rate of 81.4 ml/min? *Nephron Physiol.* 2005;101:21–26.

Barbour SJ, Er L, Djurdjev O, et al. Differences in progression of CKD and mortality amongst Caucasian, Oriental Asian and South Asian CKD patients. *Nephrol Dial Transplant.* 2010;25:3663–3672.

Dixon AN, Raymond NT, Mughal S, et al. Prevalence of microalbuminuria and hypertension in South Asians and white Europeans with type 2 diabetes: a report from the United Kingdom Asian Diabetes Study (UKADS). *Diab Vasc Dis Res.* 2006;3:22–25.

Ene-Iordache B, Perico N, Bikbov B, et al. Chronic kidney disease and cardiovascular risk in six regions of the world (ISN-KDDC): a cross-sectional study. *Lancet Glob Health.* 2016;4:e307–e319.

Guh JY, Chen HC, Tsai JF, et al. Herbal therapy is associated with the risk of CKD in adults not using analgesics in Taiwan. *Am J Kidney Dis.* 2007;49:626–633.

Hall YN, Hsu CY, Iribarren C, et al. The conundrum of increased burden of end-stage renal disease in Asians. *Kidney Int.* 2005;68:2310–2316.

Hau AK, Kwan TH, Li PK. Melamine toxicity and the kidney. *J Am Soc Nephrol.* 2009; 20:245–250.

Hsueh YM, Chung CJ, Shiue HS, et al. Urinary arsenic species and CKD in a Taiwanese population: a case-control study. *Am J Kidney Dis.* 2009;54:859–870.

Jung CH, Lee MJ, Kang YM, et al. The risk of chronic kidney disease in a metabolically healthy obese population. *Kidney Int.* 2015;88:843–850.

Lai MN, Lai JN, Chen PC, et al. Risk of kidney failure associated with consumption of herbal products containing Mu Tong or Fangchi: a population-based case-control study. *Am J Kidney Dis.* 2010;55:507–518.

Leung TK, Luk AO, So WY, et al. Development and validation of equations estimating glomerular filtration rates in Chinese patients with type 2 diabetes. *Kidney Int.* 2010;77:729–735.

Li PK, Chow KM, Szeto CC. Is there a survival advantage in Asian peritoneal dialysis patients? *Int J Artif Organs.* 2003;26:363–372.

Li PK, Kwan BC, Leung CB, et al; Hong Kong Society of Nephrology. Prevalence of silent kidney disease in Hong Kong: The Screening for Hong Kong Asymptomatic Renal Population and Evaluation (SHARE) program. *Kidney Int.* 2005;64:S36–S40.

Li PK, Kwan BC, Szeto CC, et al. Metabolic syndrome in peritoneal dialysis patients. *NDT Plus.* 2008;1:206–214.

Li PK, Ng JK, Cheng YL, et al; Hong Kong Society of Nephrology. Relatives in silent kidney disease screening (RISKS) study: a Chinese cohort study. *Nephrology (Carlton).* 2017;22:35–42.

Lin JL, Lin-Tan DT, Hsu KH, et al. Environmental lead exposure and progression of chronic renal diseases in patients without diabetes. *N Engl J Med.* 2003;348:277–286.

Ma YC, Zuo L, Chen L, et al. Distribution of measured GFR in apparently healthy Chinese adults. *Am J Kidney Dis.* 2010;56:420–421.

Mathur R, Dreyer G, Yaqoob MM, et al. Ethnic differences in the progression of chronic kidney disease and risk of death in a UK diabetic population: an observational cohort study. *BMJ Open.* 2018;8:e020145.

Pei YP, Greenwood CM, Chery AL, et al. Racial differences in survival of patients on dialysis. *Kidney Int.* 2000;58:1293–1299.

Ramirez SP, McClellan W, Port FK, et al. Risk factors for proteinuria in a large, multiracial, Southeast Asian population. *J Am Soc Nephrol.* 2002;13:1907–1917.

Reynolds K, Gu D, Muntner P, et al. Body mass index and risk of ESRD in China. *Am J Kidney Dis.* 2007;50:754–764.

Stevens LA, Claybon MA, Schmid CH, et al. Evaluation of the Chronic Kidney Disease Epidemiology Collaboration equation for estimating the glomerular filtration rate in multiple ethnicities. *Kidney Int.* 2011;79:555–562.

Teo BW, Zhang L, Guh JY, et al. Glomerular filtration rates in Asians. *Adv Chronic Kidney Dis.* 2018;25:41–48.

Wen CP, Cheng TY, Tsai MK, et al. All-cause mortality attributable to chronic kidney disease: a prospective cohort based on 462 293 adults in Taiwan. *Lancet.* 2008;371:2173–2182.

Wu Y, Huxley R, Li L, et al; China NNHS Steering Committee; China NNHS Working Group. Prevalence, awareness, treatment, and control of hypertension in China: data from the China National Nutrition and Health Survey 2002. *Circulation.* 2008;118:2679–2686.

Zhang L, Long J, Jiang W, et al. Trends in chronic kidney disease in China. *N Engl J Med.* 2016;375:905–906.

28

Preemptive Kidney Transplantation

Warren L. Kupin

WHAT RENAL REPLACEMENT OPTIONS ARE AVAILABLE TO PATIENTS WITH CHRONIC KIDNEY DISEASE?

The Kidney Disease Outcomes Quality Initiative (KDOQI) guidelines recommend that all patients at stage 4 chronic kidney disease (CKD) (glomerular filtration rate [GFR] 15 to 29 mL/min) be referred to a nephrologist (Inker, 2014). At this level of GFR, nephrology consultation can assist in the management of the medical complications of CKD including optimizing acid–base balance, bone and mineral metabolism, anemia management, and most importantly start the education process regarding the different options of renal replacement therapy.

There are four main choices for patients to consider as they approach end-stage kidney failure (ESRD): hemodialysis, peritoneal dialysis, renal transplantation, or conservative management. Since the majority of patients will not start dialysis until the GFR is <10 mL/min, referral at stage 4 CKD allows time for the patient to assimilate the gravity of the situation and make an informed, non-urgent, and timely decision as to their wishes for renal replacement therapy. In spite of this recommendation by KDOQI, almost 50% of patients have never seen a nephrologist prior to the emergent need to start dialysis and are clinically unprepared without having a dialysis access (De Coster, 2010). Studies demonstrate that lack of nephrology care in the 12 months preceding the initiation of dialysis therapy leads to a significant increase in morbidity and mortality within the first year of starting dialysis and a decrease in the rate of early transplantation especially preemptive transplantation (Singhal, 2014).

Although this chapter will primarily focus on the renal replacement option of preemptive transplantation compared to either hemodialysis or peritoneal dialysis, the fourth option of conservative management has been an area that only recently is receiving more emphasis in nephrology and in primary care training programs (Cohen, 2006). Few patients are physically unable to receive long-term dialysis through either peritoneal or hemodialysis techniques, even in the presence of advanced congestive heart failure, malignancy, cirrhosis, or dementia. Even kidney transplantation can be performed as a successful technical procedure in the majority of dialysis patients. However, from a quality-of-life standpoint, nephrologists often are faced with the moral decision of not whether a patient *can* be dialyzed or undergo transplantation but rather whether the patient *should* be even offered either of these two options.

Patients permanently residing in long-term care facilities with minimal functional capacity, those with malignancy and expected survival times of <1 year, and patients with advanced cirrhosis who are not candidates for liver transplantation are examples of situations for which long-term dialysis or transplantation may not be advisable. Once the GFR is <20 mL/min, patients who decide to pursue only conservative care have an estimated survival of approximately 2 to 4 years and when the GFR declines to <10 mL/min the average survival is 6 months (Verberne, 2016). The role of the primary care physician in these cases is paramount to assist the nephrologist in the determination of whether an individual patient is a viable candidate for any form of renal replacement therapy because they have seen the patient and their family from a long-term social and medical perspective.

WHY IS TRANSPLANTATION A BETTER CHOICE THAN DIALYSIS FOR ESRD PATIENTS?

Any comparison between renal replacement options must be made with specifically defined end points in mind. The two primary end points used in transplantation are patient survival and quality of life. Once a patient develops ESRD, the expected life span of that individual begins to dramatically decrease because of a marked increase in cardiovascular disease, including myocardial infarction, stroke, congestive heart failure, and peripheral vascular disease. On average the life span of patients on either modality of dialysis is reduced to only 30% of the life span of an age-matched person in the general population (National Center for Health Statistics, 2016). As an example, a patient between the ages of 40 and 49 years in the general population would be expected to have 36 years of life remaining while the same patient on dialysis is expected to have only 10 years of additional survival (Table 28.1). If that same patient underwent kidney transplantation the expected survival would be 26 years, representing an additional life benefit of 16 years compared to remaining on dialysis. In spite of this survival benefit of transplantation, no patient with a kidney transplant is ever able to achieve a life span similar to the general population, and the number of years remaining in the lives of

TABLE 28.1 Remaining Years of Life by Renal Replacement Option

Age Group (years old)	General Population (years)	Dialysis (years)	Transplant (years)	Transplant Benefit Compared to Dialysis (years)
20–29	54.8	16.3	41.7	+25.4
30–39	45.3	12.8	33.8	+21
40–49	36	9.8	26.1	+16.3
50–59	27.3	7.7	19.1	+11.4
60–69	19.2	5.1	13.2	+8.1
70–79	12	3.6	9	+5.4

kidney transplant patients consistently track 20% to 30% lower than in the general population.

CKD and ESRD patients experience a magnified risk of cardiovascular disease, which is the result of not just the typical population risk factors of hypertension, diabetes, smoking, and hyperlipidemia, but also the numerous nontraditional factors unique to CKD, such as anemia, hyperuricemia, increased cytokine release, acidosis, proteinuria, and abnormalities of mineral–bone metabolism reflected by abnormally high levels of serum markers such as parathyroid hormone and fibroblast growth factor 23 (FGF23).

Prior to initiating dialysis the majority of patients with CKD die from cardiovascular disease rather than progress toward the need for dialysis. Most patients spend an average of 6 years within each stage of CKD, and during that time they are exposed to accelerated atherogenesis. Even at stage 4 CKD, only 20% of patients will eventually progress to dialysis, whereas 46% will die from cardiovascular disease (Levin, 2003). Once dialysis has been initiated, the average yearly mortality rate is approximately 20%, with 50% of the deaths resulting from cardiovascular disease. The mortality of dialysis patients is higher than the mortality in the general population from cancer, diabetes, congestive heart failure, cerebrovascular accident/transient ischemic attack, and acute myocardial infarction (National Center for Health Statistics, 2016).

In contrast, renal transplantation is associated with a 30% to 60% improvement in patient survival compared with dialysis, with a yearly mortality of only 3.5%. At any age up to 80 years, kidney transplant patients experience a significant survival advantage compared with those who remain on dialysis in spite of the perioperative risks and the need to be on lifelong immunosuppression. This finding holds true independent of race, cause of end-stage renal failure, and importantly, the presence or absence of diabetes. In fact, diabetic patients who undergo kidney transplantation experience an additional 6 years of benefit in survival compared to nondiabetic patients who receive a transplant (Pérez-Sáez and Pascual, 2015). This data supports the fact that diabetic patients who have the worst survival on long-term dialysis experience the greatest survival benefit from kidney transplantation.

The best group to compare transplant patients to is the 100,000 wait-listed dialysis patients (Wolfe, 2009). This unique group, which accounts for approximately 25% of the dialysis population, is composed of patients who have been accepted for transplantation but remain waiting for their allograft on dialysis for variable periods of time. Because they have been extensively screened for cardiovascular disease and malignancy, these patients have a markedly lower yearly mortality of only about 7% compared to the typical dialysis patient. However, transplant patients still maintain a survival advantage even compared with wait-listed patients (3.5%/yr vs. 7%/yr).

In summary, kidney transplantation significantly improves patient survival compared to continuing dialysis therapy in all patient groups regardless of age, race, gender, and cause of kidney failure (Davis, 2010).

WHAT IS "PREEMPTIVE" TRANSPLANTATION?

Preemptive transplantation refers specifically to the clinical scenario in which a patient receives a renal transplant before the initiation of any form of dialysis therapy. There has been a previous misconception among both patients and their primary care physicians that they must first undergo a period of dialysis before proceeding with transplantation. This concept may have had its roots based on two major concerns: posttransplant compliance and posttransplant recurrent disease in the allograft.

Approximately 25% of transplant patients demonstrate patterns of noncompliance with their immunosuppression, and this often leads to allograft rejection and graft loss (O'Grady, 2010). Demographic patterns identified a subgroup of patients who have a particular risk of noncompliance: young individuals, minority status, and <6 months of dialysis preceding transplantation. The impact of time on dialysis appeared to suggest that noncompliance in these younger patients was owing to the lack of mature understanding of the impact of ESRD on their mortality. It was once believed by many transplant physicians that perhaps 6 to 12 months of dialysis for a young patient at high risk of noncompliance would convince them to more reliably take their posttransplant medication. Although theoretically this concept may have some social validity, as will be discussed in this section, the survival benefits of preemptive transplantation clearly supersede any psychological benefit from intentionally placing a patient on dialysis even for a 6-month period of time (Pradel, 2008).

The second consideration of placing a patient on dialysis before transplantation focused on the risk of disease recurrence in the allograft. For patients with primary glomerular diseases such as focal segmental glomerulosclerosis (FSGS) or secondary renal diseases from systemic lupus erythematosus or vasculitis, this concept was formulated to allow the disease to "burn out" on dialysis and only afterward proceed to transplantation. Although it is true that patients with active autoimmune or vasculitic disease should not be transplanted until their disease is quiescent, the majority of patients with stage 5 CKD do not need any period of pretransplant dialysis and should proceed to transplantation (Menn-Josephy and Beck, 2015).

The United Network for Organ Sharing (UNOS), the independent, nonprofit organization responsible for the allocation of organs in the United States, does not have a prerequisite requirement for any period of dialysis before undergoing kidney transplantation and supports preemptive transplantation.

IS PREEMPTIVE TRANSPLANTATION BETTER THAN GETTING A TRANSPLANT AFTER THE INITIATION OF DIALYSIS?

The timing of renal transplantation significantly influences both short- and long-term outcome in adult and pediatric recipients. Patients who receive a preemptive transplant have higher success rates compared with patients who have already been started on dialysis even if dialysis therapy has been for <6 months. A preemptive transplant decreases the rate of allograft failure by 52% for recipients of a living donor kidney and by 25% for recipients of a cadaveric kidney. In addition, the risk of patient death was reduced by 31% for recipients of a living donor kidney and 16% for recipients of a cadaveric graft (Kallab, 2010). Pediatric recipients in particular benefit with improved graft survival after preemptive transplantation (Amaral, 2016).

The duration of time spent on dialysis before transplantation increases the risk of graft loss and patient death in a linear fashion. With 12 months on dialysis before transplantation, the risk of graft failure is 25% higher compared with preemptive transplantation; with 2 years on dialysis, the risk is 37% higher; and at 3 years of dialysis, the risk increases to 43% higher (Nishikawa and Terasaki, 2002). These results are independent of the dialysis modality: hemodialysis or peritoneal dialysis. A unique study looked at paired renal allografts from the same donor when one kidney went to a preemptive recipient and the other went to a patient on dialysis. Because the grafts came from the same donor, this removed from consideration all potential donor factors on the outcome. At 5- and 10-year follow-up, recipients of preemptive transplants had a significant survival advantage compared with the kidneys transplanted from the same donors into patients on long-term dialysis (78% vs. 63% at 5 years and 58% vs. 29% at 10 years). These data strongly support the singular detrimental effect of dialysis of any duration on the outcome of transplantation (Innocenti, 2007).

Even when the transplant is coming from a living donor, the usual survival advantages of living donation are adversely affected by the duration of time spent by the recipient on dialysis, especially as the time spent on dialysis approaches 2 years or more. If a living donor kidney is transplanted preemptively, the 3-year survival is 85% compared with 71% for the same living donor being used after the recipient has been on dialysis for >2 years. Thus, it appears far more advantageous for a living donor to step forward early and donate preemptively rather than to wait and see if the recipient can get a kidney from the cadaveric donor list first and only offer the option of donation if 1 to 2 years pass without a transplant being available. This "wait and see" option is not uncommon by living donors who may be hesitant to undergo the donation surgery and want to step in only if it appears that the wait for a cadaveric organ is going to be prolonged.

The mechanisms by which dialysis reduces the success of transplantation have not been defined. With hemodialysis, it is presumed that there is a constant inflammatory state that increases the risk of allograft loss through upregulation of the immune system. The uremic milieu in general may influence lymphocyte reactivity, response to immunosuppression, and risk of infectious and cardiovascular complications that together may reduce allograft function and decrease patient survival. Patients receiving a transplant after the start of dialysis have a 2.5 times higher risk of rejection, pointing to a biologic explanation for the outcome differences rather than patient selection.

An area not commonly discussed is the survival of patients who lose their allografts and return to dialysis. These patients do not simply go back to the previous mortality risks of standard dialysis patients of 20% per year. Patient mortality is 78% higher in patients with a failed allograft who return to dialysis—93% higher in diabetic patients and 69% higher in nondiabetic patients (Marcén and Teruel, 2008). This may be related to the lingering effects of long-term immunosuppression, the presence of the renal allograft leading to a chronic inflammatory state, and/or the persistence of posttransplant diabetes. Because preemptive transplantation has higher graft survival rates than transplantation after initiation of dialysis, fewer preemptively transplanted patients will need to return to dialysis and experience this marked increase in early mortality.

From a psychological perspective, preemptive transplantation leads to an improved sense of well-being and a perception of better health compared to transplant patients who had been on dialysis therapy. It appears that the depression of being on dialysis and the loss of a sense of health that diminishes with longer duration of dialysis carry over even after transplantation (Bzoma, 2016).

Cost

Although formal cost analyses have not been done, preemptive transplantation is considered to be more cost-effective than waiting to transplant until after the onset of dialysis. The economic break-even point for transplantation compared with dialysis is approximately 2.5 to 3 years. Although the initial year of transplantation has a threefold increased cost compared with dialysis, afterward the yearly maintenance expenses for immunosuppression are only 30% of the annual cost of dialysis. The frequency of yearly admissions decreases from 2 days/yr for dialysis patients to 0.8 days/yr for transplant patients (after the first year of transplantation). With the high yearly cost of dialysis and the expenses involved with vascular access complications, including hospitalizations, preemptive transplantation rapidly becomes cost advantageous to third-party payers.

HOW SOON CAN A PATIENT BE LISTED FOR PREEMPTIVE TRANSPLANTATION?

UNOS operates under a government contract and is responsible for developing transplant policies, facilitating organ distribution, and collecting and analyzing transplant data. All 244 U.S. renal transplant centers participate and follow UNOS guidelines. For renal transplantation, UNOS has established a GFR of <20 mL/min as the target value that a patient must have reached in order to be officially listed for transplantation. This GFR can be calculated from either a 24-hour urine sample or as an eGFR using the CKD-EPI formula.

The rationale for this target GFR level is based on the rate of decline of renal function and the anticipated time to wait for a cadaver organ. In general, with most renal diseases, GFR declines by an average of 1 to 4 mL/min per year depending on many variables, including blood pressure and blood sugar control and the use of renin–angiotensin–aldosterone system blocking drugs. Starting at a GFR of 20 mL/min, patients with that rate of decline in GFR will be able to be managed conservatively for 4 to 7 years before the GFR decreases to <10 mL/min, a level that would place them at imminent need of dialysis.

Currently, the average waiting time for a cadaveric renal transplant in the United States is approximately 3.5 years, and it is getting longer every year. Therefore, listing a patient with a GFR of 20 mL/min should allow sufficient leeway for a preemptive transplant. However, it is apparent that waiting for a cadaveric kidney transplant is an unpredictable situation, and as the GFR approaches 10 mL/min, a vascular access may need to be placed in anticipation of dialysis, even with the patient on the waiting list. In addition, patients who are sensitized as a result of prior blood transfusions or pregnancies often will have an even longer wait for transplantation and are unlikely to receive a preemptive transplant.

For those patients with one or more potential living donors, referral to a transplant center at a GFR <20 mL/min will allow ample time for all candidate donors to be screened and tested. The transplant surgery date can then be electively scheduled as the GFR approaches 15 mL/min.

HOW MANY PATIENTS ACTUALLY RECEIVE A PREEMPTIVE RENAL TRANSPLANT?

In spite of the established benefit of preemptive transplantation on graft survival, only 17% of all transplants performed in the United States are preemptive. This percentage has not changed appreciably over the past 10 years. Of all cadaveric transplants performed in the United States, only 11% are preemptive, whereas with living donor transplants, the rate of preemptive transplantation increases to 31%. As a result, 61% of all preemptive transplants are from living donors (Jay, 2016). In absolute terms the number of preemptive transplants in the United States has actually gone down over the past decade since there has been a 15% decrease in the number of total living donors and although the number of cadaveric transplants has increased, this does not offset the total loss of living donors and their greater contribution to preemptive transplantation.

Given the superior outcomes of preemptive transplantation, it is disappointing how few patients have the opportunity to take advantage of this option. Underlying reasons include delayed referral for nephrology consultation, lack of organ availability, and a prolonged delay in the evaluation and listing of patients (Sakhuja, 2016). In Europe, the same general situation exists with only 10% to 15% of all transplants being preemptive and the majority of those coming from living donors (ERA-EDTA Registry, 2015).

For every 3 months that a patient is followed by a nephrologist as opposed to their primary care physician before transplantation, the possibility of getting a preemptive transplant increases by 4%. In addition, when the patient first learns about dialysis and transplantation from a nephrologist as compared with their primary physician, they are four times more likely to get a preemptive transplant.

In addition to the problem of late referrals, there is a significant lack of cadaveric organs, resulting in unpredictable waiting times for most patients. The growth of the transplant waiting list continues to exceed the rate of transplantation and the waiting times have therefore progressively increased. One contribution to this lack of availability of cadaveric organs may have to do with the current national organ donation policy.

The United States has a "Required Request" Law for organ donation that requires all physicians to ask the families at the time of irreversible brain injury whether they would consent to organ donation. This allows families to OPT IN if they so desire for organ donation. This policy captures about two-thirds of all potential organ donations but a significant proportion of transplantable organs are not used due to family refusal. In contrast many European countries such as Spain have a "presumed consent" policy which requires patient families to OPT OUT of organ donation (Bendorf, 2013). In these countries it is already presumed that consent is given for organ donation and unless the families specifically intercede, every potential cadaveric donor is used. The donation rates in countries with "presumed consent" exceed the rate of donation in the United States. In the absence of a suitable supply of cadaveric and living donors, the rate of preemptive transplantation cannot be improved.

A number of socioeconomic issues may play a role as to whether a patient receives a preemptive transplant (Tong, 2014). Detailed analysis of the UNOS database indicates that Caucasian patients, patients with private insurance, patients who are employed, and those with a college education are more likely to receive a preemptive transplant. There are two major explanations as to how these patient demographics influence when a patient receives a transplant. First, these characteristics appear to influence the ability of the patient to complete the transplant workup in a timely fashion. Patients with a higher education and economic means appear to be able to move more quickly through the workup process and be listed at a much earlier time. Extra attention has to be paid to minority patients and those of limited educational status to assist them in finishing their pretransplant testing in an expeditious manner.

The second explanation as to why there may be racial differences in preemptive transplantation has to do with the availability of suitable living donors. The majority of preemptive transplants come from living donors, and fewer of these may be available to minority recipients due to medical reasons; for example, hypertension and type 2 diabetes, the two most common causes of renal failure in the United States, may affect the majority of siblings, offspring, and/or parents of a Black race or Hispanic patient, limiting the number of potential living donors.

More recently the major discovery of the negative impact of being a homozygous carrier for the apolipoprotein L1 gene mutations on the donor GFR and the outcome of transplantation in the recipient will also further limit living organ donation in patients of Black race. If a living donor is a carrier of this mutation, data have shown that they will experience a greater risk of CKD and even ESRD (Newell, 2017). Therefore although it is not yet a standard UNOS policy, many centers are disqualifying living donors who are homozygous for apolipoprotein L1 mutations since the long-term safety for the donor's renal function is not yet fully defined.

Overall cadaveric organ donation rates in minority groups also lag behind their representation on the waiting list. Currently Black patients represent 35% of the transplant waiting list, Hispanic patients 17%, and Asian patients 7%, whereas the organ donation percentage from these same groups is 14% for Black donors, 14% for Hispanic donors, and 3% for Asian donors. Because cadaveric transplants are distributed based on genetic matching criteria that often segregate by ethnicity, unless the minority donor pool is increased, minority patients will continue to wait longer than Caucasians for a good match and will be less likely to receive a preemptive transplant.

DOES THE NEW UNOS CADAVERIC ALLOCATION SYSTEM FAVOR PREEMPTIVE RENAL TRANSPLANTATION?

There has been a significant change in the methodology used to allocate cadaveric kidney transplants in the United States starting in December 2014 (Stegall, 2017). Previously the waiting list was treated as a relatively static hierarchy of patients based on how long they have been signed up by an individual transplant center after they completed their workup and were approved by each center's transplant committee. Patients "at the top of the list" were those who had been waiting the longest and they were generally assured with only a few exceptions of getting the next cadaveric graft available. This policy however adversely affected patients who were not promptly referred to a transplant center and may have been on dialysis for years before they were officially accepted for transplantation by a center. In addition, this policy did not account for maximizing the potential success for each organ transplanted since there was no formal assessment of the characteristics of the donor kidney.

The new allocation system is predicated on an effort to produce *longevity matching* for each cadaveric kidney transplanted. By assigning a unique calculated score to both the donor kidney and the recipient, this new system is an effort to transplant the best quality kidney into a recipient who is expected to get the best patient and

TABLE 28.2	Variables Comprising the KDPI and EPTS

EPTS (Expected Post Transplant Survival)	KDPI (Kidney Donor Profile Index)
Diabetes: yes or no	Age
Dialysis: yes or no, duration of dialysis	Height
Age	Weight
Previous transplant: yes or no	Ethnicity
	Stroke as a cause of death: yes or no
	Hypertension: yes or no
	Diabetes: yes or no
	Hepatitis C: yes or no
	Serum creatinine
	Donation after cardiac death

graft survival from that specific allograft. Each cadaveric kidney is now described by a Kidney Donor Profile Index (KDPI) that is a mathematical value based on the interaction of 10 different donor variables that have been determined to significantly influence the outcome of transplantation. Each potential recipient on the UNOS cadaver list also has a profile called the Expected Post Transplant Survival (EPTS) that is a mathematical score based on 4 recipient variables that influence the success of transplantation (Table 28.2). The values of the KDPI and EPTS are percentages of quality in an inverse scale so that a donor kidney with a KDPI of 15% would be a kidney whose qualities put it in the top 15% of grafts with expected prolonged survival and a recipient with a similar EPTS of 15% would be an individual who is expected to have an outcome of graft and patient survival in the top 15%. By mandate all kidneys with a KDPI of <20% should go to recipients with an EPTS of <20%.

One of the most important variables of the EPTS is "time spent on dialysis." As discussed, the longer a patient is on dialysis the lower the graft and patient survival, so preemptive patients have a significant opportunity to have an EPTS close to or below 20%.

However, the time a patient is on the waiting list is still a major factor in determining the ranking of patients. In this new system waiting time is now determined by the day they started dialysis and not the day the transplant center accepted them. For potential preemptive recipients the waiting time is still the day the transplant center accepted the patient or if it is available, the day the GFR went to <20 mL/min. What this means in practical terms is that starting in 2014 a major proportion of the patients on the list automatically gained many extra years of waiting time credited to them accounting for all the years they were on dialysis even before they were referred for transplantation, and all new patients being seen are now credited with waiting times back to the day they started dialysis.

Due to late referrals, potential preemptive patients do not have this opportunity to have prolonged waiting times and are often not listed until the GFRs are <15 mL/min. They rarely will be on the list for 3 to 5 years before they need to start dialysis which is the average waiting time that would make them competitive with regular dialysis patients to get a cadaveric graft. Although it is still too early to tell, theoretically, this policy will likely adversely affect the opportunity for a preemptive transplant from the cadaveric pool.

DOES PREEMPTIVE TRANSPLANTATION ALSO BENEFIT PATIENTS RECEIVING A COMBINED KIDNEY–PANCREAS TRANSPLANT?

Patients with CKD from diabetes may benefit from a combined kidney–pancreas transplant. This option is restricted primarily to patients with type 1 diabetes because of the absence of insulin production, which would be reversed by a pancreas transplant. Patients with type 2 diabetes have insulin resistance and high baseline insulin levels leading to the metabolic syndrome, and a pancreas transplant would not overcome this resistance; the newly transplanted pancreas would simply autoregulate downward its own insulin production, leading to minimal overall change in the patient's insulin levels. In the United States, diabetes is present in 35% to 40% of patients with ESRD, but of this group, only 10% have type 1 diabetes. Therefore, the vast majority of patients requiring dialysis who have diabetes do not qualify for a kidney/pancreas transplant.

Type 1 diabetic patients cannot be distinguished clearly from those with type 2 diabetes by clinical characteristics such as age at onset, family history, race, history of ketosis, or end-organ complications. The most sensitive method is the measurement of endogenous C-peptide production. Type 1 diabetic patients will have an absent/undetectable C-peptide production, whereas the C-peptide levels of type 2 diabetic patients will be very high, even in the presence of hyperglycemia.

Diabetic recipients, as mentioned, have a significant survival benefit with kidney transplantation compared with dialysis. Those who receive a combined kidney–pancreas transplant have an even better long-term survival compared with type 1 diabetic patients who receive a kidney transplant only (67% vs. 46%). The benefit of preemptive transplantation also holds true for combined kidney–pancreas transplant recipients; preemptively transplanted patients experience a 17% lower rate of graft loss and a 50% lower mortality compared with combined kidney–pancreas transplant recipients who were already receiving dialysis therapy (Morath, 2009).

CAN PREEMPTIVE TRANSPLANTATION BE DONE FOR A SECOND KIDNEY TRANSPLANT?

Preemptive transplantation is just as important before a second transplant as it is for a first transplant in regard to graft and patient survival. Repeat transplant recipients represent an important model for study because it removes any influence of delayed referral since these patients are already under the care of a transplant nephrologist. Only 8% of repeat transplants are done preemptively and living donors make up only 10% of this group which is in contrast to the prevalence of 31% for living donors with primary transplants. The benefit in graft outcome of preemptive transplantation with second transplants appears to be related to specific recipient immunologic issues that improved their ability to get transplanted at an earlier time, that is, degree of HLA sensitization. Patients who received a preemptive transplant had a much lower degree of sensitization compared to those that did not (panel reactive antibody titer of 28% vs. 70%) and this leads to a lower rate of rejection and improved survival. Consequently, every effort should be made to consider preemptive transplantation for recipients with failing primary transplants (Girerd, 2016).

WHAT ABOUT THE USE OF HEPATITIS C+ OR HIV+ PATIENTS TO EXPAND THE DONOR POOL?

In an effort to alleviate the organ shortage and reduce the waiting time for transplantation, specific populations of patients that were not previously approved for organ donation are now being considered. As previously discussed, preemptive transplantation is rarely possible from cadaver donors and therefore the majority of patients without living donors must wait on dialysis for years before a cadaveric organ becomes available. The use of hepatitis C+ donors (HCV+) and HIV+ donors has now been approved by UNOS in order to increase the donor pool and reduce the waiting time for transplantation.

Before the development of direct-acting antivirals (DAAs) for HCV, the implantation of HCV+ cadaveric kidneys into HCV– recipients was associated with increased mortality, higher risk of liver disease, increased risk of infection, and shorter graft survival compared to recipients of HCV– kidneys (Abbott, 2004). Consequently for many years, the use of HCV+ kidneys was not considered a viable option as a source of organs for kidney transplantation. However, the recent success of the new DAA class of therapy has led to a reconsideration of the use of HCV+ organs as a means of expanding the donor pool (Scalea, 2015).

In the case of recipients who are HCV+ who are activating replicating, the use of HCV+ organ donors is now an option in the United States (Levitsky, 2017). Approximately 2% to 3% of all adult donors are HCV+ which means that a considerable number of cadaveric organs that previously were discarded can now be used for select patients. Patients receiving these organs are initiated on DAA therapy at various time points early after the surgery to achieve a viral remission. Before the development of the newer DAA classes, HCV could not be effectively treated posttransplant using interferon-based regimens because of a significant risk of humoral-mediated rejection that resulted from this therapy. The new DAA classes are interferon-free regimens, and many combinations can now be used safely even in the setting of moderate reductions in GFR. Overall short- and long-term survival of HCV+ patients receiving an HCV+ donor kidney is significantly better than those remaining on the waiting list. Importantly, for this strategy to work, academic and community hepatologists need to be aware that they should not aggressively use DAA therapy for patients on the waiting list and eliminate their viremia because then this will not allow them to get an HCV+ donor and will actually prolong their waiting times (Reese, 2015).

Taking this concept a step further, the option was raised on using HCV+ organs for HCV− recipients. This would mean directly infecting a recipient with HCV from the donor organ which occurs in 100% of cases but then rescuing them by initiating DAA therapy right after the transplant. Patients potentially eligible for this strategy would be those with particularly prolonged waiting periods for transplantation or individuals at ages >70 years old, where waiting 4 to 5 years for an organ transplant may not be feasible. The THINKER trial (Transplanting Hepatitis C Kidneys into Negative Kidney Recipients) demonstrated the safety and efficacy of this protocol in patients with HCV genotype 1 as this genotype is especially sensitive to DAA therapy (Goldberg, 2017). In a recent survey, approximately 30% of HCV− patients on the waiting list agreed to accept an HCV+ donor kidney (McCauley, 2018). This unique approach to transplantation awaits further guidelines on which patients would be appropriate candidates (Durand, 2018).

Transplantation of HIV+ ESRD patients has now been widely accepted as a viable option. However HIV+ donor organs have previously not been utilized and have been discarded. In 2013, the HIV Organ Policy Equity (HOPE) Act was passed that allows for the use of HIV+ organs of both cadaveric and living donor origin specifically for HIV+ recipients (Haidar and Singh, 2017). HIV+ kidneys have been used successfully for HIV+ recipients in South Africa with outcomes comparable to the non-HIV+ population. All recipients were able to achieve viral suppression after transplantation with antiretroviral therapy (Muller and Barday, 2018).

Based on this success, even HIV+ living donors are now being considered for HIV+ recipients. Although the risk of CKD/ESRD is higher in these donors compared to the general living donor population, it was determined that (1) the risk is still extremely low and (2) with proper informed consent, HIV+ living donation is an option (Muzaale, 2017).

In summary, expanding the donor pool by using HCV+ donors and HIV+ donors is a novel, innovative, and important option in order to achieve preemptive transplantation for specific cohorts of patients.

WHAT TOOLS CAN BE USED TO HELP INCREASE THE RATES OF PREEMPTIVE TRANSPLANTATION?

A number of tools are available to both help increase the rate of preemptive transplant, as well as of transplantation in general. A group in Ohio (Sullivan, 2012) identified eight sequential steps that need to be followed to proceed to a kidney transplant: medical suitability, interest in transplant, referral to a transplant center, first visit to center, transplant workup, successful candidate, waiting list or identification of a living donor, and receipt of a transplant. They studied whether use of a "navigator," namely, a person to assist them in navigating through these steps, would result in an increase in the rate at which these steps would be completed. Their "navigators" were patients who themselves had received a kidney transplant. The transplant navigators would meet monthly with the patients (who were already on dialysis). Ninety-two patients were assigned navigators and 75 others were treated with usual care. Those assigned a navigator wound up completing twice as many steps toward a transplant than controls.

The Explore Transplant program, put together by Dr. Amy Waterman at the University of California, Los Angeles (UCLA) (www.explore-transplant.org), "is a family of educational programs that ensure that transplant patients and living donors make informed treatment choices. ET's educational resources include print brochures, videos, animated web applications, online web resources, and video story-telling applications in English and Spanish." The program has been adapted in many regions, including Ontario and Canada. A home-based educational program may be more effective than clinic-based programs (Rodrigue, 2008). A Live Donor Champion program (Garonzik-Wang, 2012) was launched at Johns Hopkins Medical Center, and would train a live donor champion, who might be a friend, family member, or community member willing to advocate for the transplant candidate in an advocacy role. The efficacy of this program has not yet been formally evaluated. Finally, a "mobile clinical decision aid," named the iChoose Kidney tool, that calculates the relative survival benefit of being treated with dialysis versus transplantation, has been developed and its efficacy is being tested in a clinical trial (Patzer, 2016).

WHAT IS TRANSPLANT TOURISM AND HOW DOES IT AFFECT PREEMPTIVE TRANSPLANTATION?

With the current prolonged waiting time for organ transplants coupled with the complications of long-term dialysis, many patients seek kidney transplants outside of the United States. The process by which a citizen of one country goes to another country to commercially acquire a renal transplant is called *transplant tourism* or *transplant trafficking*. The World Health Organization in 2004 issued a position statement that outlawed the sale of organs for transplantation. This is based not only on moral and ethical grounds but on potential medical complications that would occur from an unregulated black market for organ transplants. In addition, the Declaration of Istanbul on Organ Trafficking and Transplant Tourism signed by 78 countries in May 2008—and including the Transplantation Society, the International Society of Nephrology, and the World Health Organization—condemns the sale of organs and calls for all countries to establish monitoring organizations and prosecute any medical professional participating in this practice (International Summit on Transplant

Tourism and Organ Trafficking, 2008). Despite these constraints, commercially acquired transplants continue to be available in many countries. Usually, living donors are recruited from the local community and paid to donate a kidney to foreigners. Amnesty International has accused some countries of using prisoners and executed criminals as sources of these organs.

The quality of the donor organs, adequacy of surgical expertise, and perioperative care of such transplants are not monitored nor held to any standard of care. There is no oversight or data collection on these procedures, and the care of the donor or recipient cannot be guaranteed by any third party. Published reports show inferior short- and long-term graft survival for commercially acquired organs (Jafar, 2009). Inadvertent exposure to potentially serious infectious agents, such as tuberculosis, hepatitis B, hepatitis C, and HIV, has been reported anecdotally.

Transplant tourism is especially appealing to U.S. patients without living donors and who are not yet on dialysis, and are then told that the waiting time for a cadaveric transplant may take 3 to 5 years. This prolonged waiting time will more than likely mean that they will need to start dialysis before a transplant will be available. The fear of initiating dialysis is a major stimulus for patients who have the economic means to look elsewhere for a preemptive transplant.

All health care officials should be absolutely clear on the illegality of transplant tourism and the potential life-threatening risks that a patient will incur by attempting to proceed with this option.

CONCLUSIONS

- Kidney transplantation offers superior patient survival rates compared with either hemodialysis or peritoneal dialysis independent of multiple comorbid conditions.
- Preemptive transplants are associated with significantly higher patient and graft survival rates compared with patients receiving a transplant after any duration of dialysis.
- In spite of the benefits of preemptive transplantation, it is an underutilized option, accounting for only 17% of all transplants with the majority coming from living donors.
- The primary care provider can assist in improving the number of preemptive transplants by ensuring early timely referral for nephrology consultation, and nephrologists need to ensure that patients with GFR <20 mL/min are referred to a transplant center.
- Primary care providers can also encourage their patients and healthy family members to participate in organ donation which could increase the rate of preemptive transplantation.

References and Suggested Readings

Abbott KC, Lentine KL, Bucci JR, et al. The impact of transplantation with deceased donor hepatitis c-positive kidneys on survival in wait-listed long-term dialysis patients. *Am J Transplant*. 2004;4:2032–2037.

Amaral S, Sayed BA, Kutner N, et al. Preemptive kidney transplantation is associated with survival benefits among pediatric patients with end-stage renal disease. *Kidney Int*. 2016;90:1100–1108.

Bendorf A, Pussell BA, Kelly PJ, et al. Socioeconomic, demographic and policy comparisons of living and deceased kidney transplantation rates across 53 countries. *Nephrology (Carlton)*. 2013;18:633–640.

Bzoma B, Walerzak A, Dębska-Slizien A, et al. Psychological well-being in patients after preemptive kidney transplantation. *Transplant Proc*. 2016;48:1515–1518.

Cohen LM, Moss AH, Weisbord SD, et al. Renal palliative care. *J Palliat Med*. 2006; 9:977–992.

Davis CL. Preemptive transplantation and the transplant first initiative. *Curr Opinion Nephrol Hypertens*. 2010;19:592–597.

De Coster C, McLaughlin K, Noseworthy TW. Criteria for referring patients with renal disease for nephrology consultation: a review of the literature. *J Nephrol*. 2010;23:399–407.

Durand CM, Bowring MG, Brown DM, et al. Direct-acting antiviral prophylaxis in kidney transplantation from hepatitis C virus-infected donors to noninfected recipients: an open-label nonrandomized trial. *Ann Intern Med*. 2018;168:533–540.

ERA-EDTA Registry. ERA-EDTA Registry Annual Report 2013. Amsterdam, The Netherlands: Academic Medical Center, Department of Medical Informatics; 2015.

Garonzik-Wang JM, Berger JC, Ros RL, et al. Live donor champion: finding live kidney donors by separating the advocate from the patient. *Transplantation*. 2012; 93:1147–1150.

Girerd S, Girerd N, Aarnink A, et al. Temporal trend and time-varying effect of preemptive second kidney transplantation on graft survival: A 30-year single-center cohort study. *Transplant Proc*. 2016;48:2663–2668.

Goldberg DS, Abt PL, Blumberg EA, et al. Trial of transplantation of HCV-infected kidneys into uninfected recipients. *N Engl J Med*. 2017;376:2394–2395.

Haidar G, Singh N. The Times, They are a-Changing: HOPE for HIV-to-HIV organ transplantation. *Transplantation*. 2017;101:1987–1995.

Helmick RA, Jay CL, Price BA, et al. Identifying barriers to preemptive kidney transplantation in a living donor transplant cohort. *Transplant Direct*. 2018;4:e356.

Inker LA, Astor BC, Fox CH, et al. KDOQI US commentary on the 2012 KDIGO clinical practice guideline for the evaluation and management of CKD. *Am J Kidney Dis*. 2014;63:713–735.

Innocenti GR, Wadei HM, Prieto M, et al. Preemptive living donor kidney transplantation: do the benefits extend to all recipients? *Transplantation*. 2007;83:144–149.

International Summit on Transplant Tourism and Organ Trafficking. The declaration of Istanbul on organ trafficking and transplant tourism. *Clin J Am Soc Nephrol*. 2008;3:1227–1231.

Jafar TH. Organ trafficking: global solutions for a global problem. *Am J Kidney Dis*. 2009;54:1145–1157.

Jay CL, Dean PG, Helmick RA, et al. Reassessing preemptive kidney transplantation in the United States: Are we making progress? *Transplantation*. 2016;100: 1120–1127.

Kallab S, Bassil N, Esposito L, et al. Indications for and barriers to preemptive kidney transplantation: a review. *Transplant Proc*. 2010;42:782–784.

Kidney Disease: Improving Global Outcomes (KDIGO). KDIGO clinical practice guidelines for the prevention, diagnosis, evaluation, and treatment of hepatitis C in chronic kidney disease. *Kidney Int Suppl*. 2008:S1–S99.

Levin A. Clinical epidemiology of cardiovascular disease in chronic kidney disease prior to dialysis. *Semin Dial*. 2003;16:101–105.

Levitsky J, Formica RN, Bloom RD, et al. The American Society of Transplantation Consensus Conference on the use of hepatitis C viremic donors in solid organ transplantation. *Am J Transplant*. 2017;17:2790–2802.

Marcén R, Teruel JL. Patient outcomes after kidney allograft loss. *Transplant Rev (Orlando)*. 2008;22:62–72.

McCauley M, Mussell A, Goldberg D, et al. Race, risk, and willingness of end-stage renal disease patients without hepatitis C (HCV) to accept an HCV-infected kidney transplant. *Transplantation*. 2018;102:e163–e170.

Menn-Josephy H, Beck LH Jr. Recurrent glomerular disease in the kidney allograft. *Front Biosci (Elite Ed)*. 2015;7:135–148.

Morath C, Schmied BM, Mehrabi A, et al. Simultaneous kidney-pancreas transplant in type 1 diabetes. *Clin Transplant*. 2009;23:115–120.

Muller E, Barday Z. HIV-positive kidney donor selection for HIV-positive transplant recipients. *J Am Soc Nephrol*. 2018;29:1090–1095.

Muzaale AD, Althoff KN, Sperati CJ, et al. Risk of end-stage renal disease in HIV-positive potential live kidney donors. *Am J Transplant*. 2017;17:1823–1832.

National Center for Health Statistics. Table 7. Life expectancy at selected ages, by race, Hispanic origin, race for non-Hispanic population, and sex: United States, 2013. *National Vital Statistics Reports*. 2016;64:30.

Newell KA, Formica RN, Gill JS, et al. Integrating APOL1 gene variants into renal transplantation: considerations arising from the American Society of Transplantation Expert Conference. *Am J Transplant*. 2017;17:901–911.

Nishikawa K, Terasaki PI. Outcome of preemptive transplantation versus waiting time on dialysis. *Clin Transpl*. 2002:367–377.

O'Grady JG, Asderakis A, Bradley R, et al. Multidisciplinary insights into optimizing adherence after solid organ transplantation. *Transplantation*. 2010;89:627–632.

Patzer RE, Basu M, Mohan S, et al. A randomized controlled trial of a mobile clinical decision aid to improve access to kidney transplantation: iChoose Kidney. *Kidney Int Rep*. 2016;1:34–42.

Pérez-Sáez MJ, Pascual J. Kidney transplantation in the diabetic patient. *J Clin Med*. 2015;4:1269–1280.

Pradel FG, Jain R, Mullins CD, et al. A survey on nephrologists' views on preemptive transplantation. *Clin J Am Soc Nephrol*. 2008;3:1837–1845.

Reese PP, Abt PL, Blumberg EA, et al. Transplanting hepatitis C–positive kidneys. *N Engl J Med*. 2015;373:303–305.

Rodrigue JR, Cornell DL, Kaplan B, et al. A randomized trial of a home-based educational approach to increase live donor kidney transplantation: effects in blacks and whites. *Am J Kidney Dis*. 2008;51:663–670.

Sakhuja A, Naik A, Amer H, et al. Underutilization of timely kidney transplants in those with living donors. *Am J Transplant*. 2016;16:1007–1014.

Scalea JR, Barth RN, Munivenkatappa R, et al. Shorter waitlist times and improved graft survivals are observed in patients who accept hepatitis C virus+ renal allografts. *Transplantation*. 2015;99:1192–1196.

Singhal R, Hux JE, Alibhai SM, et al. Inadequate predialysis care and mortality after initiation of renal replacement therapy. *Kidney Int*. 2014;86:399–406.

Stegall MD, Stock P, Andreoni K, et al. Why do we have the kidney allocation system we have today? A history of the 2014 kidney allocation system. *Hum Immunol*. 2017;78:4–8.

Sullivan C, Leon JB, Sayre SS, et al. Impact of navigators on completion of steps in the kidney transplant process: a randomized, controlled trial. *Clin J Am Soc Nephrol*. 2012;7:1639–1645.

Tong A, Hanson CS, Chapman JR, et al. The preferences and perspectives of nephrologists on patients' access to kidney transplantation: a systematic review. *Transplantation*. 2014;98:682–691.

Verberne WR, Geers AB, Jellema WT, et al. Comparative survival among older adults with advanced kidney disease managed conservatively versus with dialysis. *Clin J Am Soc Nephrol*. 2016;11:633–640.

Wolfe RA, McCullough KP, Leichtman AB. Predictability of survival models for waiting list and transplant patients: calculating LYFT. *Am J Transplant*. 2009;9:1523–1527.

29

Preparing for Dialysis

**James E. Tattersall and
John T. Daugirdas**

OBJECTIVES IN LATER STAGES OF CHRONIC KIDNEY DISEASE

The overall set of actions required in advanced chronic kidney disease (CKD) is summarized in Table 29.1. The first aim is to prevent or at least delay progression. Although "delaying tactics" are best started at an early stage of CKD, they become even more important at later stages. Patients may be more likely to cooperate with treatment during these late stages when they may have experienced symptoms and when dialysis is being considered. Delaying or preventing CKD requires adequate diagnosis and treatment of the cause of CKD and management of contributing factors such as infection, inflammation, hypertension, and hyperglycemia. These measures should have been started long before the patient reaches CKD stages 4 to 5 but, in practice, many patients do not take or are not provided with this treatment until then (Sprangers, 2006). The most common underlying conditions requiring long-term dialysis (kidney disease due to hypertension, diabetes, and/or vascular disease) are potentially preventable. Our aim should be for no patient to ever require dialysis for a condition which is preventable.

The second aim of treatment is to manage the complications of CKD. This takes the form of nondialysis treatment of CKD and will address fluid overload, hypertension, acid/base abnormalities, anemia, bone metabolism, and nutrition. The third aim is to prevent or reduce associated comorbidity. This includes measures aimed at reducing cardiovascular risk. The fourth aim is to prepare for the possibility that the CKD will progress to the point that kidney function will no longer be able to support symptom-free life, even with all appropriate nondialysis treatment. At this point, palliative care, dialysis, or preemptive transplant would be required. This plan B is required in case our efforts to prevent progression are unsuccessful. The planning would include choosing the most appropriate strategy for the patient as kidney function dwindles. Effective planning requires knowledge of the rate of progression of CKD after all the delaying tactics have been implemented.

WHAT THE PATIENT CAN EXPECT FROM DIALYSIS

Dialysis is normally started when uremic symptoms can no longer be controlled by other means and there is no realistic prospect of improving renal function. In this case, the patient could expect dialysis to improve their uremic symptoms. This improvement may be

TABLE 29.1	Actions Required in Advanced Chronic Kidney Disease
Action	**Intended Outcome**
Educate patients on dialysis options.	Patient has made an informed choice on the type of dialysis at least 6 months before estimated dialysis start date. Patient starts dialysis with preferred dialysis type. Patient listed for transplant before dialysis starts when appropriate.
Control blood pressure and fluid overload. This may require high doses of loop diuretic. Suspect fluid overload when blood pressure does not respond to antihypertensive medication.	Blood pressure below 135/80 (130/80 if proteinuric). Avoid signs or symptoms of fluid overload or hypotension.
Seek and treat treatable causes of CKD or contributing factors. Renal biopsy may be required to establish diagnosis.	Delay or reverse deterioration in renal function by treating the underlying cause.
Control anemia. Provide intravenous iron and erythropoiesis agents if appropriate.	Maintain hemoglobin >10 g/dL. Avoid symptoms of anemia.
Provide dietary advice and monitor nutrition.	Maintain adequate nutrition state, especially for protein. Maintain serum potassium at safe level.
Prescribe ACEI/ARB if appropriate and assess its impact.	Especially if proteinuric or if renal function declining rapidly (>5 mL/min per year). May be counterproductive in advanced CKD.
Prescribe sodium bicarbonate if appropriate.	Maintain serum bicarbonate within normal range. May postpone need for dialysis.
Avoid cannulating arm veins.	Preserve arm veins for use as an AV fistula.
Avoid nephrotoxic drugs or contrast agents.	Preserve kidney function.
Plan and create dialysis access if appropriate. It may take several months to prepare a functioning fistula.	Adequate and appropriate dialysis access is established before dialysis is required. For hemodialysis, access should be a fistula wherever possible.
Control bone and mineral metabolism, especially serum phosphate.	Serum calcium within normal range, parathyroid hormone <10 times the upper normal limit, serum phosphate <1.5 mmol/L (4.64 mg/dL).
Control serum potassium by dietary restriction and medication if required.	Keep serum potassium within safe limits.
Monitor progression of CKD, estimate date required to start dialysis, and start dialysis at the appropriate time.	Start dialysis while patient is still relatively free of symptoms or significant CKD-associated morbidity. Prevent death or urgent admission caused by uremia. Prevent unplanned start to dialysis.

CKD, chronic kidney disease; ACEI, angiotensin-converting enzyme inhibitor; ARB, angiotensin receptor blocker; AV, arteriovenous.

marginal initially and, from the patient's point of view, hardly compensating for the burden of the dialysis treatment. Occasionally, an asymptomatic patient may start dialysis to avoid life-threatening metabolic abnormalities such as hyperkalemia or acidosis. In these cases, the patient is opting for dialysis for long-term benefit and risk reduction, rather than any immediate health benefit.

Dialysis may not prevent the development or progression of symptoms caused by diseases other than CKD or associated comorbidity. Dialysis patients are at an increased risk of certain health problems (e.g., infection, cardiovascular disease) (Sarnak and Levey, 1999). Patients treated by dialysis generally still need to continue nondialysis CKD treatment, including dietary restrictions. Even while treated by dialysis, residual kidney function helps to preserve health and improves outcome (Lee, 2017). Therefore, patients will continue with treatments aimed at preserving kidney function or delaying CKD progression after starting dialysis.

Dialysis treatments normally do not cause pain or other distressing symptoms. Patients treated by hemodialysis may experience symptoms of hypotension toward the end of treatment and may feel lethargic for several hours after dialysis. When they are present, symptoms caused by dialysis generally are mild and manageable. Younger and fitter patients are more likely to consider themselves disadvantaged by the practical limitations imposed by diet and dialysis rather than symptoms. A young person treated by dialysis, without significant comorbidity, may remain in a fully functioning state of health and employment for some decades. For the younger employed person, dialysis is likely to represent considerable practical challenges. Ideally the patient would be treated by a transplant, either preemptively (as discussed in Chapter 28) or as soon as possible after starting dialysis and before acquiring significant associated comorbidity. Elderly patients with poor physical function are more likely to be disadvantaged by the symptoms of dialysis. The practical limitations imposed by dialysis may be better tolerated by a retired person than by one who is employed.

OBJECTIVES FOR PATIENT EDUCATION

From the patient's point of view, the difficulties of starting dialysis can be limited by advance preparation. This preparation includes the timely provision of information, access to individuals who are knowledgeable about dialysis, and access to appropriate practical help. This provision of information is often delivered as a formal process involving home visits, provision of relevant literature, audiovisual presentations, lectures, and workshops. This preparation is generally provided by the facility or organization that will be providing the dialysis. The patient-education phase of the preparation requires substantial time, usually ranging from a few weeks to several months (Ravani, 2003).

Patients are likely to become symptomatic as renal function deteriorates close to the point where dialysis is being considered.

Patients are more likely to retain and consider information effectively at an earlier stage of their kidney disease, while still asymptomatic. On the other hand, there is little point in providing detailed information on treatment which may or may not become necessary in the distant future. The optimal time to provide the patient information will be informed by the patient's stage of life and expected rate of progression of the kidney disease.

Younger patients with CKD and few comorbidities are likely to find it more difficult to come to terms with chronic disease. They are more likely to enter a state of denial that could interfere with adequate treatment to delay or prevent CKD progression. In general, the psychological impact of impending adverse events is lessened by increasing the period of advance warning and by providing as much information about the adverse event as possible. For these reasons, older patients with multiple comorbidities need to start their dialysis preparation when they have reached stage 4 (glomerular filtration rate [GFR] <30) and long before they reach stage 5. Younger patients without comorbidity should be given general information on dialysis and all necessary psychological support as soon as they receive a diagnosis of CKD to help educate them about the benefits of complying with measures that may slow progression.

Elderly patients with advanced CKD may have cognitive impairment (approximately 20% of patients in one sample) (Murray, 2008). It is important that this be recognized early in the preparation process as it may have a reversible cause. Cognitive impairment could limit applicability of self-care treatments or the patient's competence to choose an appropriate strategy when renal function decreases to minimal levels.

CHOICES

The choices to be made by the patient include preemptive transplantation, dialysis, or end-of-life care (Table 29.2). If dialysis is chosen, there are still selections to be made: self-care or professionally provided care, treatment at home or in an outpatient dialysis unit. Self-care at home can be used to provide either hemodialysis (3 to 6 days or nights per week) or peritoneal dialysis (usually automated peritoneal dialysis done nightly). Dialysis in an outpatient unit generally is provided as hemodialysis either three times per week during the day, or if available, three nights per week or every other night.

Dialysis provided by health care professionals has the advantage that professionals take responsibility for delivering and monitoring the treatment and removing some of this burden from the patient. On the other hand, this professional care is likely to be relatively inflexible and less adaptable to the patient's individual needs. The patient will need to be available to receive the treatment at fixed times and at a defined location, dependent on the professional's schedule. There is generally a shortage of professionals who can provide this care. Professional care is expensive and may not be available for home treatments.

	TABLE 29.2	Some Common Renal Replacement Therapy Choices	
Modality	Description	Advantages	Disadvantages
Preemptive transplantation	Live or cadaver donor transplant before ever needing dialysis	See Chapter 28.	See Chapter 28.
Home hemodialysis	3–6 ×/wk, either during the day or at night. Usually assisted by a relative or caregiver; uncommonly, by a paid health care professional	When given more than 3 ×/wk, or when given as 8–10-hour treatments, 3–3.5 nights per week, evidence suggests better quality of life and better control of phosphate, blood pressure, and anemia; may also reduce left ventricular hypertrophy.	Home is changed into a hospital; partner burnout; with some home therapies, modification to home water systems is required; waste disposal; expense.
Home peritoneal dialysis	Automated cycler, with most of exchanges done during the night	Independence, relative simplicity.	Need for delivery of large volumes of peritoneal dialysis fluid; exposure to high amounts of glucose.
In-center nocturnal hemodialysis	Three 8–10-hour nocturnal treatments per week (or uncommonly, every other night) given in center (either staff assisted or self-care)	Marked increase in weekly dialysis time with better control of phosphate, blood pressure, and anemia. Home does not need to be converted into a clinic. Dialysis time spent sleeping.	Leaving home unattended on dialysis nights; travel to unit; relatively inflexible schedule.
In-center conventional hemodialysis	Either staff assisted (the norm) or self-care	Short amount of time spent on dialysis. Staff does all the work.	Travel to unit; relatively inflexible schedule. May be inadequate amount of dialysis.
Postponing dialysis	Very-low-protein diet plus ketoanalogs, careful fluid management	May work to postpone dialysis for about 1 year in elderly patients with few comorbidities (no heart failure, diabetes).	Expense of ketoanalogs.
Palliative care	Conservative management without dialysis	Good for those patients for whom dialysis is not expected to prolong life to a significant extent, or in whom overwhelming comorbidities are present.	Potentially reduced life expectancy.

Self-care dialysis typically is delivered and monitored by the patient or their family. With self-care dialysis, the patient attends the nephrology clinic at relatively infrequent intervals (1 to 6 months) but is supported by a community care team (comprising specialist clinical and technical staff) (Suri, 2006) that can provide telephone advice or visits as required (Lindley, 2006). The location and timing of self-care dialysis can be more flexible than professionally provided care. Self-care dialysis is more likely to result in full rehabilitation of the patient and is more compatible with full-time employment. With self-care dialysis, the treatment can be optimized for the patient's individual needs and may result in better quality of life and outcome (Loos-Ayav, 2008). Dialysis may be more reliably, safely, and effectively provided by the patient than by a professional who has to care for many patients simultaneously. Self-care is particularly suitable for dialysis provided at home.

Home dialysis (Marshall and Chan, 2016) generally is much more convenient for the patient, as it is delivered in a friendly, familiar environment and may allow the patient to participate in family activities during the treatment. Automated peritoneal dialysis usually is given by self-care in the home. The most effective schedules of hemodialysis are much easier to deliver at home and are rarely offered in an outpatient dialysis unit. Although home dialysis usually is delivered as a self-care treatment, frail patients, perhaps with cognitive impairment, may still have home dialysis assisted by a professional who comes to the patient's home for this purpose on a regular schedule (Oliver, 2007). Hemodialysis treatments given more frequently than three times per week have been associated with improved survival and reduced morbidity (Suri, 2006). Also, 3.5/week (every other night) long-session-length nocturnal dialysis also has been reported to have superior outcomes (Tang, 2011).

Choosing which form of dialysis a patient would prefer requires the patient to have a considerable amount of knowledge on the various types of treatments available. Whatever strategy is chosen, there will need to be some planning and preparation to ensure that each stage of the strategy can be implemented effectively at the appropriate time. In the case of an elderly patient with CKD and multiple other medical conditions, physical function and life expectancy may be limited by other medical conditions and not improved by dialysis (Kurella Tamura, 2009). These patients are less likely to cope with self-care dialysis and more likely to experience adverse symptoms of dialysis. An end-of-life care pathway not involving dialysis may be appropriate for some of these individuals.

Adequate preparation is likely to ameliorate the practical and psychological impact of starting dialysis or choosing an end-of-life pathway (Berzoff, 2008). Adequate preparation for dialysis is associated with better long-term outcome (Devins, 2005). When provided with adequate preparation and all strategy options, higher-functioning patients are relatively more likely to choose self-care dialysis (Goovaerts, 2005; Manns, 2005), whereas patients with extensive comorbidities are more likely to choose an end-of-life pathway not involving dialysis (Murtagh, 2007b). The proportion of patients choosing these options could be considered as a measure of the adequacy of preparation. The decision on the best dialysis or end-of-life strategy for the patient is very difficult. There is a lack of strong evidence to guide this decision. The decision should be informed by the patient's individual medical prognosis, social circumstances, and priorities. For these reasons, it is preferable or essential that the decisions are made by the patients themselves and that they are fully informed. When the patient has cognitive impairment or otherwise is incapable of deciding on strategy, input from family or others with a close relationship to the patient is required. There may be considerable ethical pitfalls when decisions are made on behalf of the patient (Davison and Holley, 2008).

THE DIALYSIS ACCESS: NEED FOR TIMELY PREPARATION

Hemodialysis requires access to an artery or a major vein. The best way to achieve this is by surgical creation of an arteriovenous (AV) fistula at the wrist or elbow. This causes the connected vein to become distended and its walls hypertrophied (arterialized). Needles are inserted into the arterialized vein to allow the hemodialysis equipment to access the blood. Fistula creation requires planning by radiologic mapping of the arm vessels. After the fistula has been formed, it may take up to 2 months for the arterialization to complete before the fistula can be used. In general, the process from planning to having a usable fistula may take a number of months, and the process may take longer when multiple attempts or corrective surgery is needed because of coexistence of vascular disease.

If a patient has to start hemodialysis without a functioning fistula, it will be necessary to create an alternative form of access that does not involve the time-consuming vein arterialization process. The alternatives here are a tunneled central venous catheter or an AV graft. Outcome for patients treated by hemodialysis is significantly better when a fistula is used for access rather than a central venous catheter or AV graft (Ethier, 2008). Therefore, a measurable objective for dialysis preparation is to aim to have all patients who plan for hemodialysis start with a functioning fistula. If a patient has opted for hemodialysis, the process of creating a fistula should be started 6 to 12 months before dialysis is likely to be required. Peritoneal dialysis (Saxena and West, 2006) requires access to the peritoneal cavity in the form of a tunneled catheter. This catheter is more likely to function correctly if it is inserted at least 1 week before it is first used. This time allows the tunnel track to seal, preventing leaks or infection.

Problems with dialysis access are a main cause of symptoms and poor health directly related to dialysis. A poorly functioning access may prevent adequate dialysis, allowing symptoms and complications of CKD to develop or progress. Access infections cause significant morbidity and mortality and may be difficult to treat. An infection in an AV graft or venous catheter used for hemodialysis access often results in septicemia and may be complicated by endocarditis. Infection of the catheter used for peritoneal dialysis may result in peritonitis. When the access involves artificial material, as in the case with grafts and catheters, usually it is necessary to remove the access to control infection. Many access infections are introduced during insertion. Infection is more likely if the access is created under urgent conditions or if the patient is uremic.

Avoiding Damage to Arm Veins

As explained above, a patient with severe CKD is likely to require AV access for hemodialysis. Even if a patient has chosen conservative care or peritoneal dialysis, it is possible that a period of hemodialysis may become necessary at some point. Successful creation of the fistula requires intact arm veins, and these should be preserved at all cost. For this reason, cannulation of the arm veins should be avoided. When arm vein cannulation is unavoidable, the small veins on the back of the hand may be used. As a last resort, the large cephalic vein in the antecubital fossa can be used.

Futility Versus Incomplete Preparation

When preparing stage 4 patients for dialysis by having them undergo a structured predialysis education program as well as insertion of an AV fistula, one is confronted with a need for balance. If a large number of patients undergo this education and training as well as AV fistula creation, but CKD does not progress, or if such patients die of other causes before needing dialysis, one might term this particular outcome *futility*. On the other hand, delaying training and AV fistula insertion until need for dialysis is more certain has the risk of a dialysis start with an incompletely prepared patient. Demoulin (2011) studied this issue in 386 patients with stage 4 CKD (mean eGFR approximately 23 ml/min) who were being treated in a single large Belgian clinic. The decision of when to create an AV fistula was left up to the treating nephrologists depending on their best judgment of rate of progression to dialysis. They found that approximately 6% of fistula insertions were futile because those patients never progressed to dialysis, mostly because of death from other causes, and another 6% were not yet on dialysis at the conclusion of the follow-up period. However, AV fistulas had been inserted in only half of the patients whose CKD progressed to the point of requiring hemodialysis. They concluded that perhaps earlier creation of AV fistulas may be preferred, but then a higher percentage would have been created in patients who may never need dialysis.

A further consideration in the planning for dialysis in elderly patients is the difficulty in creating a functioning fistula. Multiple vascular procedures may be required, especially when there is significant vascular disease. The increased operative risk for these patients and the increased chance of dying of nonrenal causes before requiring dialysis should be taken into account. Assisted peritoneal dialysis may be more appropriate in many of these patients.

END-OF-LIFE CARE WITHOUT DIALYSIS

For a CKD patient with poor physical function and life expectancy <1 year, dialysis may result in only a few months of extra life expectancy but will result in poorer quality of life (Germain and Cohen, 2008). In this case, a patient may consider that dialysis is not worthwhile. The patient may continue the nondialysis treatments and receive additional end-of-life or palliative care. Patients receiving end-of-life care without dialysis are much more likely to die at home (Smith, 2003), which is considered an advantage by some patients (Ratner, 2001).

   End-of-life care in CKD aims to control symptoms, maximize quality of life, and provide practical and psychological support (Burns and Carson, 2007). During the final months of life, specific support from community-based end-of-life care teams is likely to be required. Where no CKD-specific end-of-life care teams exist, cancer palliative care procedures may be adapted. Compared with cancer, CKD has similar practical and psychological effects. The terminal CKD patient will be anorexic and lethargic and have symptoms of pruritus and shortness of breath. Compared with cancer, CKD is much less likely to cause pain (Murtagh, 2007a).

Palliative Care Tool Kit From the Renal Physicians Association

In 2002, the American Society of Nephrology (ASN) and the Renal Physicians Association (RPA) issued a shared decision making guideline for the appropriate initiation and withdrawal from dialysis (RPA, 2000, 2010). The recommendations focused on nine areas: shared decision making, informed consent or refusal, estimation of prognosis, conflict resolution, advance directives, withholding/withdrawing dialysis, patients with special conditions, time-limited trial of dialysis, and foregoing dialysis and instituting palliative care. A second edition that substantially updated these guidelines was published in October of 2010. This position paper is available from the RPA (www.renalmd.org).

AVOIDING NEPHROTOXIC CONTRAST AGENTS

Patients preparing for dialysis often are elderly and with significant vascular disease. During the preparation for dialysis, it may be necessary to investigate the arterial supply for potential transplant or hemodialysis access. These investigations should minimize the use of nephrotoxic contrast agents wherever possible, as the failing kidney is unusually sensitive to toxic or hemodynamic insult. Planning for hemodialysis access usually can be achieved using ultrasound alone. Alternatively, for vascular mapping, very small amounts of contrast dye can successfully be used (Won, 2010) or CO_2 venography can be attempted (Heye, 2010).

THE USE OF ANGIOTENSIN-CONVERTING ENZYME INHIBITORS OR ANGIOTENSIN RECEPTOR BLOCKERS

Angiotensin-converting enzyme inhibitors (ACEIs) or angiotensin receptor blockers (ARBs) are generally beneficial in CKD patients. In general, good blood pressure control using ACEI/ARBs has the potential to reduce substantially the rate of deterioration of renal function. However, ACEI/ARB use may result in acute lowering of the GFR through hemodynamic mechanisms, typically by up to 20%, and hyperkalemia is more likely.

In the patient who is close to requiring dialysis, this fall in GFR caused by ACEI/ARB treatment may be counterproductive. A typical patient whose eGFR is declining at a rate of 4 mL/min per year and whose eGFR is 24 mL/min would be predicted to need dialysis in 4 years (when eGFR will be 8 mL/min). With treatment by ACEI/ARB, there may be an immediate fall in eGFR to 20 mL/min, but thereafter the deterioration would be expected to proceed at a slower rate, say 2 mL/min per year. In such a case, dialysis would not be required for 6 years, and treatment with an ACEI/ARB will have postponed the need for dialysis by 2 years.

If, on the other hand, ACEI/ARB is started when eGFR is 10 mL/min, a 20% deterioration in GFR caused by the ACEI/ARB would place the patient very close to a level of GFR at which dialysis would normally be required. Thus, a typical threshold of eGFR, below which starting ACEI/ARB may be counterproductive, might be about 12 mL/min. It also has been suggested that there may be a benefit to stopping ACEI/ARBs in advanced CKD. The resulting acute improvement in GFR could, in certain circumstances, buy valuable time for dialysis preparation if the cardiovascular problems and hypertension can be controlled by alternative agents. A progressive improvement in GFR has been described in a selected group of patients whose ACEI/ARB was stopped (Onuigbo, 2009).

Fluid Management

Abnormalities in salt and water homeostasis are part of the uremic syndrome in advanced CKD. Fluid overload contributes to hypertension, cardiovascular disease, and, potentially, deteriorating renal function, even when asymptomatic (Hung, 2015). When there is associated heart failure, peripheral and, especially, pulmonary edema, result in distressing symptoms and admissions. Patients with heart failure may need to be maintained in a relatively dehydrated state to avoid pulmonary edema. On the other hand, dehydration may cause symptoms and contribute to the decline in renal function (Khan, 2016). For these reasons, careful management of fluid status is required, usually controlled by dietary modification and varying diuretic doses. This is informed by regular clinical assessment of fluid status. These assessments may be enhanced by objective measurements such as bioimpedance.

Hyperkalemia

Patients with CKD stages 4 to 5 are at risk of hyperkalemia. This risk is increased by the use of potassium-sparing diuretics, ACEIs, angiotensin II antagonists, and aldosterone antagonists. These drugs are likely to be prescribed (and are generally beneficial) in CKD as they are used to treat cardiovascular disease and hypertension, and to delay the deterioration in kidney function. Use of nonsteroidal anti-inflammatory drugs or trimethoprim can worsen hyperkalemia, and alternative drugs should be used in CKD patients with potassium problems. Insulin-requiring diabetic patients are particularly at risk of hyperkalemia if adequate insulin is not provided at any time. As reviewed in Chapters 5 and 11, serum potassium levels >5.5 mmol/L are associated with markedly increased short-term risk of mortality.

The kidney's ability to excrete potassium is reduced in advanced CKD, but any tendency to increases in serum potassium can generally be managed or, ideally, prevented by a low-potassium diet and/or reducing or withdrawing drugs likely to increase serum potassium. A chronically increased serum potassium (>5.5 mmol/L), despite appropriate dietary and pharmacologic intervention, would be an indication for starting dialysis. Serum potassium tends to rise inexorably late in the course of CKD, especially when there is metabolic acidosis and malnutrition. Dialysis would normally be started before these events.

Acute rises of potassium (or when potassium is >6.5 mmol/L) can cause paralysis with respiratory muscle weakness, cardiac arrhythmias, and death, and constitutes a medical emergency. High serum potassium is considered to be particularly dangerous when there are electrocardiogram changes (e.g., tented T waves, depressed ST segments, arrhythmias). The cause is likely to be an acute deterioration in kidney function (the chronically failing kidney has little functional reserve and is more easily prone to acute kidney injury or drug side effect) or acutely excessive dietary potassium intake. Acute rises in serum potassium can also be caused by potassium leaking from the intracellular space when the potassium pumps at the cell surface run out of energy. This can occur in metabolic upsets such as diabetic ketoacidosis, hypoglycemia, or acidosis.

Acute rises in serum potassium are generally treated by dialysis. The serum potassium will fall significantly within several minutes of the start of a dialysis session. However, the hyperkalemic patient will be at significant risk of death during the time it takes to arrange dialysis (usually some hours, depending on the availability of equipment and staff). In this situation, other methods to reduce serum potassium are required (Table 29.3). Intravenous calcium protects against some of the acute effects of hyperkalemia without actually reducing potassium. It has a nearly immediate onset of action. It tends to be

TABLE 29.3	Treatments Used for Hyperkalemia		
Treatment	Onset	Duration	Mechanism
10 mL of 10% calcium gluconate solution IV over 10 minutes	1–3 minutes	30–60 minutes, can be repeated	Antagonizes potassium's effect on the myocardium Does not decrease serum potassium
Albuterol by nebulizer 10–20 mg in 4-mL saline over 10–20 minutes	Immediate	2–4 hours	Promotes potassium uptake into cells
Insulin 10 units + 50 mL of 50% dextrose IV over 20–30 minutes	15–60 minutes	4–6 hours	Promotes potassium uptake into cells
Sodium (or calcium) polystyrene sulfonate 30 g enema	2 hours	Several hours	Binds potassium in the colon, exchanges for sodium (or calcium)
Sodium (or calcium) polystyrene sulfonate 15 g 3–4 times daily, oral	4 hours	Ongoing	Binds potassium in the colon, exchanges for sodium (or calcium)

IV, intravenous.

used as the initial treatment for hyperkalemia with electrocardiographic changes. Treatment by inhalation or infusion of β-agonists and by intravenous glucose plus insulin, alone or in combination, can reduce serum potassium acutely by driving potassium into the cells. These treatments do not remove potassium from the body, and the effect lasts a few hours (Mahoney, 2005; Putcha and Allon, 2007).

Potassium-binding resin (e.g., sodium polystyrene sulfonate or calcium polystyrene sulfonate) exchanges potassium for sodium or calcium, effectively increasing potassium excretion in the colon. It can be administered orally or rectally. The rectal route has the fastest action, with onset within 2 hours. An oral dose will reduce serum potassium within 4 hours. In either case, potassium excretion can be maintained by repeated doses. The resins cause constipation and, rarely, colonic perforation. The relatively slow onset of action limits their usefulness in the acute situation, but they can be helpful when dialysis is not available or likely to be delayed, or when the rise in potassium is likely to be temporary (e.g., caused by dietary indiscretion) or can be reversed by other means. Potassium-binding resins tend to be used in combination with other treatments that have a more rapid and shorter action (Watson, 2010).

Patiromer is a novel, nonabsorbed polymer designed to bind and remove potassium, primarily in the colon, thereby decreasing serum potassium in patients with hyperkalemia (Li, 2016). In contrast to other available binding resins, patiromer does not release any other electrolyte in exchange for potassium. More experience with this drug is required to establish its role in CKD management. It has the potential to be an alternative or supplement to dialysis in the treatment of hyperkalemia. Patiromer currently is not approved for treatment of acute hyperkalemia in the United States because the time course of its action is moderately delayed. An alternative agent, sodium zirconium cyclosilicate, may have a more rapid onset of action (Meaney, 2017). Intravenous furosemide can reduce serum potassium rapidly, provided there is sufficient kidney function and the patient's hydration can be maintained. High doses (200 to 500 mg) may be required in CKD. If the patient is volume depleted, intravenous fluid (e.g., 0.9% saline) should be provided rapidly to dilute the serum potassium and, it is hoped, to restore some kidney function. Intravenous fluid must be delivered under careful supervision to avoid fluid overload. Any metabolic cause of the high serum potassium should be corrected. Intravenous sodium bicarbonate can be given to reverse acidosis.

Metabolic Acidosis

As discussed in Chapter 11, patients with CKD stages 4 to 5 are at risk of metabolic acidosis. A serum bicarbonate level below the lower end of the normal range has been shown to contribute to the malnutrition in the uremic state and may augment the dangers of hyperkalemia. The low bicarbonate can be corrected easily and cheaply by oral sodium bicarbonate, 2 to 4 g/day. This has been shown to improve nutrition and slow the deterioration in renal function. Although persistent acidosis, despite oral bicarbonate, often is given as an indication for starting dialysis, this is a rare reason to tip the scale in favor of abandoning conservative therapy. Usually such patients have marked problems with fluid overload, and the latter is the real reason that conservative treatment is abandoned.

Uremic Pericarditis, Bleeding, and Neuropathy/Encephalopathy

These are unusual but very important reasons for starting a CKD patient on dialysis. Uremic pericarditis is a serositis because of the accumulation of uremic toxins. The presentation can be quite subtle, and patients presenting with symptoms of acute heart failure and heart enlargement on x-ray should always undergo echocardiography to rule out presence of pericardial effusion. Sudden death can result if large effusions are not attended to. The pericarditis normally will resolve over a few weeks or days after starting adequate dialysis. Occasionally, a large pericardial effusion will require drainage to prevent or treat tamponade (Gunukula and Spodick, 2001). Uremia increases bleeding time, probably due to an inhibition of platelet function. In patients with unexplained bleeding and bleeding time prolongation, dialysis treatment often can resolve the problem. Anemia with Hb <10 g/dL may also be contributory. Uremia can cause an acute peripheral neuropathy, usually manifesting as a polyneuropathy with paresthesias and increased pain sensation and weakness in the limbs. Also, uremia can cause an encephalopathy, which in its most severe form can present as seizures and chronically may be manifested as cognitive deficit, muscle cramps, tremor, and asterixis. Uremic encephalopathy is a diagnosis of exclusion, and other causes must always be ruled out, especially stroke and intracerebral bleeding, which occur with increasing frequency in CKD.

EARLIER VERSUS LATER START OF DIALYSIS

Is it better to begin dialysis earlier or later in the course of CKD? Some observational studies have suggested that so-called early start of dialysis results in improved survival, although recent large observational analyses suggested the opposite (Klausner, 2009; Wright, 2010). Confounding by indication (putting sicker patients on dialysis sooner) and lead-time bias (starting the outcome time clock at time of dialysis for patients with both early and late start) are unsolvable problems when attempting to answer this question by observational studies alone. This question now has been partially answered by the randomized IDEAL trial (Initiation of Dialysis Early and Late) (Cooper, 2010). Here, patients with eGFR of 10 to 14 mL/min were randomly assigned to begin hemodialysis right away or to delay dialysis until either eGFR/1.73 m^2 decreased to <7 mL/min or uremic symptoms developed. Mortality was very similar in the early- and late-start groups, suggesting no benefit of an earlier start. Most patients in the late-start group started dialysis because of symptoms while eGFR/1.73 m^2 was still >7 mL/min. The separation in eGFR/1.73 m^2 between the two groups was only 2.2 mL/min, but the group assigned to later start did, on average, begin dialysis 6 months later than their early-start counterparts (Cooper, 2010). The results of this study suggest that it may be safe to delay starting dialysis until the patient develops symptoms as long as there is adequate clinical supervision and preparation, and highlight the fact that uremic-type symptoms generally occur while eGFR is >7 mL/min.

Deciding to Start Dialysis

Recent study has shown that a significant proportion of patients treated by long-term hemodialysis have sufficient renal function to stop dialysis, though it is not clear whether this is due to subsequent recovery of renal function or by starting dialysis unnecessarily (Fernandez-Lucas, 2012; Letachowicz, 2016). Hemodialysis with fluid removal by ultrafiltration is often used to control blood pressure and can reduce urine output, potentially masking renal function which could otherwise control uremia. Unnecessary dialysis may be avoided by delaying dialysis to the point where all efforts to preserve renal function have proven futile and the patient is already starting to experience symptoms.

The decision on when (or if) dialysis should be started is made jointly between patient and clinicians, based on estimation of risks, benefits, and disadvantages of dialysis from the patient's point of view. The cause, history, and family history of the patient's kidney disease are important here as it informs the likelihood of further progression. If continuing deterioration in renal function is inevitable, there is little advantage in delaying dialysis beyond the point where symptoms first appear.

TABLE 29.4	Indications for Starting Dialysis

- Anorexia, nausea, vomiting, especially if there is weight loss
- Inability to control fluid overload, despite high dose of loop diuretic and sodium restriction
- Serum potassium >6.5 mmol/L, especially if there are ECG T-wave changes
- Inability to control blood pressure
- Inability to maintain serum bicarbonate within normal range, despite oral bicarbonate
- eGFR <7 mL/min
- Emergency indications:
  Uremic pericarditis
  Uremic bleeding
  Uremic encephalopathy

ECG, electrocardiogram; eGFR, estimated glomerular filtration rate.

There are numerous advantages in patients' involvement in their treatment (self-care), ideally at home (Morfín, 2018). The patient is more likely to self-care and will cope better with the lifestyle changes required by dialysis if they are not also coping with significant symptoms.

Clinical indications for starting dialysis include otherwise unexplained symptoms of uremia (fatigue, anorexia, and weight loss). Indications for dialysis are given in Table 29.4. Most commonly, the patient will notice a change in energy level, although the presence of anemia to account for this always must be excluded. The best objective evidence for anorexia is an otherwise unexplained loss of weight. In patients with heart failure, resistant to diuretics, dialysis may be useful to control fluid overload, especially to avoid admissions due to pulmonary edema, even while serum creatinine is relatively low.

Incremental Start

In most cases, kidney function is not completely lost when dialysis starts. This residual kidney function can be taken into account, allowing a patient to start with a relatively low dose of dialysis, gradually increasing as or when kidney function falls. This incremental dialysis may include less frequent or shorter hemodialysis when there is adequate residual kidney function (Nolph, 1998). In this way the dialysis is initially required to top-up the kidney function. This low-dose dialysis may be better tolerated by the patient and allows more time for the patient to adjust to the treatment.

Based on urea measurements, standard dialysis is equivalent to a renal urea clearance (KrU) of 5 mL/min per 1.17 m². An incremental approach, maintaining adequate overall clearance by starting with once-weekly hemodialysis, increasing to twice weekly when KrU falls to 4 mL/min per 1.73 m² and thrice weekly when KrU is below 2 mL/min per 1.73 m² has been proposed (Casino and Basile, 2017).

A recent observational study compared 351 patients undergoing incremental twice-weekly hemodialysis in the United States with

8,000 matched patients undergoing conventional thrice-weekly dialysis. Residual renal function was better preserved in the incremental group. The incremental group had similar mortality rate to the conventional group except in those with lowest residual renal function (Obi, 2016). Incremental dialysis is commonly used in peritoneal dialysis (Ankawi, 2016).

Potential disadvantages of incremental dialysis include practical difficulties in measuring kidney function and a concern that patients may become acclimated to shorter dialysis times and then be less prone to agree to increased amounts of dialysis when residual renal function decreases.

Delaying Dialysis in the Elderly by Conservative Management Including a Very–Low-Protein Diet

Conservative treatment need not be synonymous with palliative care but can be thought of as a means to delay onset of dialysis. Brunori (2007) randomly assigned patients >70 years of age with GFR/1.73 m^2 (24-hour collection; average of urea and creatinine clearances) between 5 and 7 mL/min to either dialysis or to a very–low-protein diet (Brunori, 2007). There were a number of important exclusion criteria in this pilot study: patients with a cardiac ejection fraction <30%, patients with proteinuria >3 g/day, all diabetic patients, patients with previous history of heart failure, and patients with uremic symptoms. The diet contained 0.3 g/kg per day protein supplemented with ketoanalogs. Survival was actually a bit higher in the conservatively treated patients, and the hospitalization rate was markedly reduced compared with the dialyzed patients. Most (but not all) of the conservatively treated patients ultimately did require dialysis during the follow-up period. The median gain in time off dialysis was about 1 year.

CASE STUDY 29.1 — AN ELDERLY PATIENT WITH MULTIPLE COMORBIDITIES REFERRED LATE

The patient, age 78, lived alone and had diabetes, hypertension, and ischemic heart disease diagnosed many years ago. Despite this, the patient remained reasonably well, self-caring, and independent until 1 year ago. At this time, the patient reported shortness of breath on exertion and ankle swelling. Investigations revealed high blood pressure, CKD stage 3, moderate anemia (Hb 10 g/dL), and a hypertrophied, dysfunctional left ventricle. Heart failure was diagnosed, and the patient was treated by a loop diuretic and an ARB. He was admitted to a nursing home. Over the following few months, his serum creatinine increased and his blood pressure reduced. The ankle swelling persisted, despite the diuretics. His symptoms were attributed to heart failure, and the worsening CKD attributed to his diuretic and ARB. His diuretic dose was reduced, and the ARB was stopped. When the CKD was discussed with the patient, he stated that he did not want dialysis.

Recently his condition deteriorated. He is no longer able to walk unaided because of shortness of breath and weakness. He is at CKD stage 5. The anemia has worsened (Hb 8.5 g/dL). He was transferred from the nursing home to a nephrology service at a nearby hospital. On admission to the nephrology service, he was confused and unable to answer questions regarding his symptoms or past medical history. He was short of breath at rest. There was marked bilateral leg edema, evidence of pulmonary edema. Serum bicarbonate was low; phosphate and parathyroid hormone were high. After consulting with the family, a central venous catheter was inserted and dialysis started the same day.

Practice Points for Case 29.1

By first seeing the patient when he is already at CKD stage 5, the nephrology service is placed in a difficult position. It is possible that nondialysis treatments would be able to correct the fluid overload, anemia, acidosis, and other metabolic abnormalities, but there is insufficient time to implement these. The only options at this late stage are dialysis or death. The patient had stated that he did not want dialysis but it is not clear whether the decision had been adequately informed.

It is possible that, from the outset, the patient's CKD may have been contributing to his symptoms and poor physical function. Cardiovascular disease is strongly associated with CKD. Institution of appropriate nondialysis treatments for CKD at an earlier stage in the disease (i.e., 1 year ago) may have reversed his symptoms, improved cardiovascular function, and restored his independence. The patient's CKD was not severe 1 year previously. With appropriate treatment aimed at slowing the progression of CKD, the deterioration of CKD and the possible need for dialysis may have been avoided altogether.

CASE STUDY

AN ELDERLY PATIENT WITH CHRONIC KIDNEY DISEASE AND MULTIPLE COMORBIDITIES, OPTIMAL TREATMENT

The patient, age 78, has ischemic heart disease, arthritis, diabetes, and CKD stage 3. He reports shortness of breath and lack of energy. He has moderate bilateral ankle edema. Blood pressure is 182/93 mm Hg. He has moderate anemia (Hb 10 g/dL). He is started on an ARB and a loop diuretic. After increasing the diuretic dose, the eGFR/1.73 m^2 falls from 50 to 35, blood pressure falls to 132/80, and the edema disappears. The anemia persists and is treated by iron and an erythropoiesis-stimulating agent.

After 3 months the Hb has risen to 12 g/dL, eGFR/1.73 m^2 is 30 mL/min, and blood pressure and fluid overload remain well controlled. His treatment is considered optimal by medical staff with expertise in diabetes, kidney, and heart disease. The patient's mobility remains poor because of weakness and joint pain.

After a further 3 months with no change to treatment, the patient's symptoms are unchanged, but eGFR/1.73 m^2 has fallen to 25 mL/min. At the patient's current level of kidney function, the patient's symptoms are unlikely to be directly related to CKD and would not be improved by dialysis. Assuming that the CKD continues to progress at the same rate, it is estimated that the CKD would become symptomatic in 6 to 12 months unless dialysis was started before then. The patient starts discussions with a multidisciplinary nephrology team regarding his options, including dialysis.

Practice Points for Case 29.2

CKD stage 3 is common in elderly persons with cardiovascular disease and diabetes. The priority here is to start treatment aimed at delaying the progression of CKD and treating its effects, especially anemia, fluid overload, and hypertension. These treatments for CKD do not conflict with the treatment for diabetes or heart disease. With optimal treatment, CKD stages 3 to 4 should be asymptomatic, and there is a reasonable prospect that the CKD will not progress or at least progress so slowly that the need for dialysis can be postponed significantly. In elderly patients with multiple other conditions, any need for dialysis may be postponed beyond their expected duration of life. After several months of optimal treatment, if the CKD has progressed, it becomes possible to predict the requirement for dialysis, and dialysis preparation can begin. At this stage, the patient is still stable and has time to consider all the options.

CASE STUDY   **A YOUNG PERSON WITH CHRONIC KIDNEY DISEASE**

29.3   The patient, age 28, is diagnosed as having polycystic kidney disease during investigations for painless hematuria. Blood pressure averages 139/88 mm Hg, serum creatinine is normal. He has no abnormal symptoms and signs apart from the hematuria and palpable kidneys.

Practice Points for Case 29.3

The younger, asymptomatic patient will have difficulties accepting the diagnosis of chronic disease. He is not likely to take medication reliably. Health benefits in the distant future are unlikely to be a priority for the younger person. A poor prognosis is likely to result in denial. In the case of early CKD, there is the prospect of an excellent prognosis with appropriate treatment. The patient should be given all information, including information about dialysis, but offered the prospect of avoiding dialysis or postponing it by regular treatment. The patient should be offered psychological support and close follow-up. In this case, blood pressure, in particular, needs to be treated and monitored closely.

References and Suggested Readings

Ankawi GA, Woodcock NI, Jain AK, et al. The use of incremental peritoneal dialysis in a large contemporary peritoneal dialysis program. *Can J Kidney Health Dis*. 2016;3:2054358116679131.

Berzoff J, Swantkowski J, Cohen LM. Developing a renal supportive care team from the voices of patients, families, and palliative care staff. *Palliat Support Care*. 2008;6:133–139.

Brunori G, Viola BF, Parrinello G, et al. Efficacy and safety of a very–low-protein diet when postponing dialysis in the elderly: a prospective randomized multicenter controlled study. *Am J Kidney Dis*. 2007;49:569–580.

Burns A, Carson R. Maximum conservative management: a worthwhile treatment for elderly patients with renal failure who choose not to undergo dialysis. *J Palliat Med*. 2007;10:1245–1247.

Casino FG, Basile C. The variable target model: a paradigm shift in the incremental haemodialysis prescription. *Nephrol Dial Transplant*. 2017;32:182–190.

Cooper BA, Branley P, Bulfone L, et al; IDEAL Study. A randomized, controlled trial of early versus late initiation of dialysis. *N Engl J Med*. 2010;363:609–619.

Davison SN, Holley JL. Ethical issues in the care of vulnerable chronic kidney disease patients: the elderly, cognitively impaired, and those from different cultural backgrounds. *Adv Chronic Kidney Dis*. 2008;15:177–185.

Demoulin N, Beguin C, Labriola L, et al. Preparing renal replacement therapy in stage 4 CKD patients referred to nephrologists: a difficult balance between futility and insufficiency. A cohort study of 386 patients followed in Brussels. *Nephrol Dial Transplant*. 2011;26:220–226.

Devins GM, Mendelssohn DC, Barré PE, et al. Predialysis psychoeducational intervention extends survival in CKD: a 20-year follow-up. *Am J Kidney Dis*. 2005;46:1088–1098.

Ethier J, Mendelssohn DC, Elder SJ, et al. Vascular access use and outcomes: an international perspective from the dialysis outcomes and practice patterns study. *Nephrol Dial Transplant*. 2008;23:3219–3226.

Fernández-Lucas M, Teruel-Briones JL, Gomis A, et al. Recovery of renal function in patients receiving haemodialysis treatment. *Nefrologia*. 2012;32:166–171.

Germain MJ, Cohen LM. Maintaining quality of life at the end of life in the end-stage renal disease population. *Adv Chronic Kidney Dis*. 2008;15:133–139.

Goovaerts T, Jadoul M, Goffin E. Influence of a pre-dialysis education programme (PDEP) on the mode of renal replacement therapy. *Nephrol Dial Transplant*. 2005;20:1842–1847.

Gunukula SR, Spodick DH. Pericardial disease in renal patients. *Semin Nephrol*. 2001;21:52–56.

Heye S, Fourneau I, Maleux G, et al. Preoperative mapping for haemodialysis access surgery with CO(2) venography of the upper limb. *Eur J Vasc Endovasc Surg*. 2010;39:340–345.

Hung SC, Lai YS, Kuo KL, et al. Volume overload and adverse outcomes in chronic kidney disease: clinical observational and animal studies. *J Am Heart Assoc*. 2015;4:pii: e001918.

Khan YH, Sarriff A, Adnan AS, et al. Chronic kidney disease, fluid overload and diuretics: A complicated triangle. *PLoS One*. 2016;11:e0159335.

Klausner D, Wright S, Williams M, et al. Survivability of early and late start dialysis initiation. *J Am Soc Nephrol*. 2009;20:25A [abst].

Kurella Tamura M, Covinsky KE, Chertow GM, et al. Functional status of elderly adults before and after initiation of dialysis. *N Engl J Med*. 2009;361:1539–1547.

Lee MJ, Park JT, Park KS, et al. Prognostic value of residual urine volume, GFR by 24-hour urine collection, and eGFR in patients receiving dialysis. *Clin J Am Soc Nephrol*. 2017;12:426–434.

Letachowicz K, Madziarska K, Letachowicz W, et al. The possibility of renal function recovery in chronic hemodialysis patients should not be overlooked: single center experience. *Hemodial Int*. 2016;20:E12–E14.

Li L, Harrison SD, Cope MJ, et al. Mechanism of action and pharmacology of patiromer, a nonabsorbed cross-linked polymer that lowers serum potassium concentration in patients With hyperkalemia. *J Cardiovasc Pharmacol Ther*. 2016;21:456–465.

Lindley EJ, Thomas N, Hanna L, et al. Pre-dialysis education and patient choice. *J Ren Care*. 2006;32:214–220.

Loos-Ayav C, Frimat L, Kessler M, et al. Changes in health-related quality of life in patients of self-care vs. in-center dialysis during the first year. *Qual Life Res*. 2008;17:1–9.

Mahoney BA, Smith WA, Lo DS, et al. Emergency interventions for hyperkalaemia. *Cochrane Database Syst Rev*. 2005:CD003235.

Manns BJ, Taub K, Vanderstraeten C, et al. The impact of education on chronic kidney disease patients' plans to initiate dialysis with self-care dialysis: a randomized trial. *Kidney Int*. 2005;68:1777–1783.

Marshall MR, Chan CT, eds; on behalf of the Global Forum for Home Hemodialysis. *Implementing Hemodialysis in the Home. A Practical Manual*. Indianapolis, IN: International Society for Hemodialysis; 2016. Available from www.ishd.org

Meaney CJ, Beccari MV, Yang Y, et al. Systematic review and meta-analysis of patiromer and sodium zirconium cyclosilicate: A new armamentarium for the treatment of hyperkalemia. *Pharmacotherapy*. 2017;37:401–411.

Morfín JA, Yang A, Wang E, et al. Transitional dialysis care units: A new approach to increase home dialysis modality uptake and patient outcomes. *Semin Dial*. 2018;31:82–87.

Murray AM. Cognitive impairment in the aging dialysis and chronic kidney disease populations: an occult burden. *Adv Chronic Kidney Dis*. 2008;15:123–132.

Murtagh FE, Addington-Hall JM, Edmonds PM, et al. Symptoms in advanced renal disease: a cross-sectional survey of symptom prevalence in stage 5 chronic kidney disease managed without dialysis. *J Palliat Med*. 2007a;10:1266–1276.

Murtagh FE, Marsh JE, Donohoe P, et al. Dialysis or not? A comparative survival study of patients over 75 years with chronic kidney disease stage 5. *Nephrol Dial Transplant*. 2007b;22:1955–1962.

Nolph KD. Rationale for early incremental dialysis with continuous ambulatory peritoneal dialysis. *Nephrol Dial Transplant*. 1998;13:117–119.

Obi Y, Streja E, Rhee CM, et al. Incremental hemodialysis, residual kidney function, and mortality risk in incident dialysis patients: A cohort study. *Am J Kidney Dis*. 2016;68:256–265.

Oliver MJ, Quinn RR, Richardson EP, et al. Home care assistance and the utilization of peritoneal dialysis. *Kidney Int*. 2007;71:673–678.

Onuigbo MA. Does concurrent renin–angiotensin–aldosterone blockade in (older) chronic kidney disease patients play a role in the acute renal failure epidemic in US hospitalized patients?—Three cases of severe acute renal failure encountered in a northwestern Wisconsin nephrology practice. *Hemodial Int*. 2009;13: S24–S29.

Putcha N, Allon M. Management of hyperkalemia in dialysis patients. *Semin Dial*. 2007;20:431–439.

Ratner E, Norlander L, McSteen K. Death at home following a targeted advance-care planning process at home: the kitchen table discussion. *J Am Geriatr Soc*. 2001;49:778–781.

Ravani P, Marinangeli G, Tancredi M, et al. Multidisciplinary chronic kidney disease management improves survival on dialysis. *J Nephrol*. 2003;16:870–877.

Renal Physicians Association. RPA position on quality care at the end of life. *Clin Nephrol*. 2000;53:493–494.

Renal Physicians Association. *Shared Decision-Making in the Appropriate Initiation of and Withdrawal From Dialysis. Clinical Practice Guideline*. 2nd ed. Rockville, MD: RPA; 2010.

Sarnak MJ, Levey AS. "Epidemiology of cardiac disease" in dialysis patients: uremia-related risk factors. *Semin Dial*. 1999;12:69–76.

Saxena R, West C. Peritoneal dialysis: a primary care perspective. *J Am Board Fam Med*. 2006;19:380–389.

Smith C, Da Silva-Gane M, Chandna S, et al. Choosing not to dialyse: evaluation of planned non-dialytic management in a cohort of patients with end-stage renal failure. *Nephron Clin Pract*. 2003;95:c40–c46.

Sprangers B, Evenepoel P, Vanrenterghem Y. Late referral of patients with chronic kidney disease: no time to waste. *Mayo Clin Proc*. 2006;81:1487–1494.

Suri RS, Nesrallah GE, Mainra R, et al. Daily hemodialysis: a systematic review. *Clin J Am Soc Nephrol*. 2006;1:33–42.

Tang HL, Wong JH, Poon CK, et al. One year experience of nocturnal home haemodialysis with an alternate night schedule in Hong Kong. *Nephrology (Carlton)*. 2011;16:57–62.

Watson M, Abbott KC, Yuan CM. Damned if you do, damned if you don't: potassium binding resins in hyperkalemia. *Clin J Am Soc Nephrol*. 2010;5:1723–1726.

Won YD, Lee JY, Shin YS, et al. Small dose contrast venography as venous mapping in predialysis patients. *J Vasc Access*. 2010;11:122–127.

Wright S, Klausner D, Baird B, et al. Timing of dialysis initiation and survival in ESRD. *Clin J Am Soc Nephrol*. 2010;5:1828–1835.

Tool Kits and Web-Based Resources

Timothy T. Yau, Sandeep S. Soman, and Jerry Yee

INTRODUCTION

The detection and treatment of chronic kidney disease (CKD) requires implementation of a clinical action plan and/or clinical interventions based on CKD stage and comorbidities to improve outcomes. To optimize CKD stage-specific therapies, resources that assist in implementation of such an approach can be helpful. These have been compiled and organized as CKD tool kits in multiple websites and smartphone "apps" devoted to CKD care. Similar resources exist for practicing nephrology providers in both academic and nonacademic practice settings, or for the motivated patient, to help stay current with clinical updates regarding both CKD and related (non–CKD) disease-specific conditions.

CHRONIC KIDNEY DISEASE TOOL KITS

These generally are evidence-based distillations of national and/or international CKD-specific clinical practice guidelines (CPGs). They are briefly compared in Table 30.1.

Renal Physicians Association's Advanced Chronic Kidney Disease Patient Management Tool Kit

This resource www.renalmd.org/page/CKDToolkit, targeted to managing CKD stages 4 to 5, was compiled by the U.S.-based Renal Physicians Association (RPA). The tool kit incorporates the RPA's CKD CPGs, and is available either as a printed, binder-encased document, digitally as a CD-ROM, or as digital portable document format (PDF) files. The tool kit underwent field testing from 2004 to 2005 and was refined with the technical assistance of Duke University's Center for Clinical Health Policy Research. The evidence-based CPGs are complemented by peer-reviewed implementation tools and provider-based educational material as a slide presentation that outlines optimal management of CKD patients at an educational level appropriate for nephrologists and interested primary care physicians.

The tool kit is divided into five major sections: "Introduction," "Guide to Tool Selection," "Assessment Tools," "Implementation of Physician and Patient Tools," and "Evaluation Tools." In the "Guide to Tool Selection" section, certain tools recommended for nephrologists are different from those recommended for non-nephrologist physicians. However, practice assessment and evaluation methods do not

Tool Kit	Focus	Format	Web Availability	CD-ROM	Office Management Tools	Cost
Renal Physicians Association (RPA): Advanced Chronic Kidney Disease (CKD) Patient Management (Toolkit)	Nephrologists	Ring binder	Yes	Yes	Extensive	Free to RPA members
Kidney Health Australia: Chronic Kidney Disease (CKD) Management in General Practice, v. 3	General practitioners	56-page booklet	Yes	No	No	Free
Michigan Quality Improvement Consortium (MQIC) CKD Guidelines	General practitioners	1 page	Yes	No	No	Free
British Columbia Guidelines and Protocols: Identification, Evaluation and Management of Patients With CKD	Nephrologists	19 pages	Yes	No	Limited	Free
Henry Ford: CKD—Clinical Practice Recommendations for Primary Care Physicians & Healthcare Providers—A Collaborative Approach (Pocketbook)	Internists Family medicine physicians Physician assistants Nurse practitioners Nephrologists	76 pages	Yes	No	No	Free (Web)

TABLE 30.1 Comparison of Chronic Kidney Disease Educational and Practice Management Tool Kits

differ among the target user groups. The section on physician tools provides physician education material such as a CKD identification action plan card and wall poster, GFR slide rule, CKD chart flags/stickers, and sample referral and post-consult letter templates. The section also contains templates and algorithms for data collection and treatment. The latter differ modestly from those provided by the National Kidney Foundation Kidney Disease Outcomes Quality Initiative (NKF KDOQI)™ CPGs in scope and design.

An integral component of the patient tools section is a CKD patient diary that empowers the individual to achieve his or her care goals. In the diary, a convenient medication list section is presented alongside kidney diagrams that educate patients about their illness, including the need to preserve future vascular access sites. A "Vascular Access Passport" template that can easily be reproduced is also included for documentation of the historical record of vascular access anatomy, construction, and revision. Another section outlines a general approach to developing and/or enhancing CKD clinics. The unique "Evaluation Tools" section includes patient identification and management subsections. These facilitate the performance of continuous quality initiatives which may help the user to prepare efficient chart abstractions using the enclosed printed templates or preformatted Microsoft Excel spreadsheets.

The U.S. National Kidney Foundation's CKDinform Toolbox

The National Kidney Foundation (NKF) of the United States is dedicated to promotion of awareness, prevention and treatment of kidney disease for health care professionals, patients and their families, and for at-risk individuals (www.kidney.org). The NKF has put together the *CKDinform* (www.kidney.org/CKDinform) program, which is a collection of evidence-based resources for primary care practitioners (*PCPs*). This diverse "toolbox" has been created with the goal to enable PCPs to recognize *chronic kidney disease* (CKD) at an early stage and develop treatment protocols to slow progression.

The NKF also hosts a number of "apps" which can be downloaded from www.kidney.org/apps. These apps can assist with calculating eGFR, assessing relative risk for kidney disease, monitoring and referral in patients with CKD, care after transplant, and nutritional management.

Kidney Health Australia Handbook

This well-organized, 56-page booklet (kidney.org.au/health-professionals/prevent/chronic-kidney-disease-management-handbook) focuses its recommendations for diagnosing and managing CKD on general practitioners. The booklet provides the salient evidence and society-based recommendations for CKD detection and management. It includes detailed recommendations for CKD screening, proteinuria and hematuria evaluation, indications for nephrology referral, action plans for each stage of CKD, strategies for use of angiotensin-converting enzyme inhibitors (ACEIs) and angiotensin receptor blockers

(ARBs), and a discussion of how to manage patients in an interdisciplinary clinic. The booklet was last updated in 2015, and remains online for print-on-demand. CKD Go! is a free web-based app that allows one to view a personalized CKD Clinical Action Plan based on an individual's eGFR and urine albumin to creatinine ratio. Smartphone compatible, the app can be viewed and downloaded at http://kidney.org.au/health-professionals/detect/calculator-andtools/ckd-go.

The Michigan Quality Improvement Consortium Set of Clinical Action Plans

This group has standardized its various clinical action plans including that for CKD into handy one-page documents. The CKD guideline, last updated in November 2016, highlights the salient principles of screening for CKD and the recommendations for referral and management of CKD stages 1 to 5 (www.mqic.org/pdf/mqic_diagnosis_and_management_of_adults_with_chronic_kidney_disease_cpg.pdf).

The British Columbia Guidelines and Protocols Advisory Committee

This group has published a document that serves many of the functions of a tool kit. It is written as a series of clinical recommendations with accompanying algorithms and patient management tools. All guidelines are clear and supported by clinical evidence (www2.gov.bc.ca/gov/content/health/practitioner-professional-resources/bc-guidelines/chronic-kidney-disease).

Henry Ford Healthcare System Booklet

This 73-page booklet provides a resource for PCPs, nurses, and advanced practice providers. *Chronic Kidney Disease (CKD): Clinical Practice Recommendations for Primary Care Physicians & Healthcare Providers—A Collaborative Approach* is accessible from within the system's electronic health record and also downloadable as a digital PDF. The booklet is a mini-manual for nephrologists-in-training and internal medicine and family practice house staff. No patient educational material is included in this text.

The pocket-sized booklet is divided into sections pertaining to CKD recognition, staging and progression, and referral to the nephrologist. CKD is considered as a disease domain complex, with sections allocated to diabetic kidney disease, complications of CKD, and information regarding nutritional and immunization interventions. Each section is arranged by a statement of the problem, the rationale for targeted and specific therapy, and step-by-step methods that permit achievement of targeted outcomes. Sections include a summary of key points, tables, and algorithms that originate from Kidney Disease Outcomes Quality Initiative (KDOQI)/Kidney Disease Improving Global Outcomes (KDIGO) CPGs and recommendations. The tables and algorithms may be used quickly to provide answers to CKD-related issues, and background contextual matter can be reviewed later. Also featured are a comprehensive action plan, a CKD medication–related problem section, and a detailed, categorized, and itemized checklist of parameters that should be monitored in affected individuals. A small section details the utilization of medications that are familiar to the nephrologist but not necessarily to the primary care provider, for example, paricalcitol, renal-formulated vitamins, erythropoiesis-stimulating agents, and intravenous hematinics. The booklet is accompanied by a foldout that has evaluation and management information stratified by CKD stage. Lists of literature references provide a pathway for users who desire more detailed information (ghsrenal.com/ckd/HFHS_CKD_GUIDELINES_V7.0.pdf).

Updates to Tool Kits and Web Resources
Although most of these available tool kits are periodically modified, the rate at which they are modified may not maintain pace with new medical knowledge. In patients with CKD, the optimal hemoglobin and blood pressure levels, utility of statins in patients with near-normal cholesterol levels, and the risk/benefit ratio of using renin–angiotensin–aldosterone system dual blockade therapy (ACEI plus ARB or other combinations) to slow progression or CKD or reduce proteinuria are relatively rapidly evolving fields. The development of any patient's clinical action plan requires stringent comparisons of supplied algorithms and pathways to the current evidence base of medical literature.

EDUCATIONAL RESOURCES FOR THE NEPHROLOGY PROVIDER

Several web-based resources that target the practicing nephrology providers are freely available. Staying up-to-date with textbooks and journal publications is time consuming and involves effort. Although they are not replacements for journal publications or continuing medical education courses, these websites are tailored to provide access to high-yield information and promote peer-to-peer discussion.

UKidney
UKidney (ukidney.com) is a provider of educational tools for the study and practice of nephrology, hypertension management, and kidney transplantation. UKidney provides many resources that encompass general nephrology, hypertension, kidney transplant, toxicology, and nephropathology on its website. This site features essential educational contributions from major opinion leaders in nephrology and is continually updated and maintained by Dr. Jordan Weinstein. Registration is free but is required to access some of the educational content. Resources include the following, each of which is separately accessible:

- Slide presentations of multiple nephrology topics, arranged by category.
- Multimedia links to general nephrology, kidney transplant, dialytic technologies, and renal pathology videos.

■ An archive of key high-impact articles in nephrology, chosen by various contributors as recommended reading for nephrology trainees and practitioners. Articles are arranged by category, and include a PubMed link, Journal link, Visual Abstract, and Commentary section.

■ Toxicology primer written in collaboration with Extracorporeal Treatments in Poisoning Workgroup (EXTRIP).

■ Links to KDIGO guidelines, eGFR calculators, and many more external resources.

NephJC

NephJC (www.nephjc.com) is an online nephrology journal club that uses Twitter to discuss the trials, basic science research, clinical guidelines, and editorials that are driving nephrology. Website access is free. Participation in the discussion only requires a Twitter account to participate, at #nephJC. Meetings are held online twice monthly and moderated by one of the NephJC founders. High-impact articles are chosen by a selection committee. One week prior to the chat, a summary of the article is published on the website. These summaries act as home pages for the chats. Content experts or authors of the paper are invited to participate. The chat is synchronous, and allows real-time to-and-fro conversation akin to a face-to-face meeting. After chat completion, a summary highlighting the discussion is posted and the paper archived for future reference. For those that are unable to tune in to the online chat, the trials that have been discussed are archived for future reference and review.

American Society of Nephrology Communities

As a member benefit, the American Society of Nephrology (ASN) created the ASN Communities online platform (community.asn-online.org/home) where its membership can network, collaborate, and discuss important issues with peers and colleagues. Chats are organized by thread (e.g., acute kidney injury, glomerulonephritis, etc.) and moderated by internationally recognized experts in the field. Clinical or science questions may be posted, and members can view and reply to the questions in real-time, or via daily digest emails. Replies can be published publicly to an entire thread's participants or privately to an individual.

GENERAL PATIENT INFORMATION SITES REGARDING CARDIOVASCULAR DISEASE, DIABETES, AND HYPERTENSION

In the early stages of CKD, the problems faced by patients include general issues regarding maintenance of optimum weight, following a healthy diet, controlling blood glucose if diabetic, and controlling blood pressure if hypertensive. In this context, patients will not necessarily be limited to information available via CKD-focused sites.

Heart Hub for Patients

The American Heart Association sponsors this site, which includes valuable information on cholesterol, diabetes, high blood pressure, and diet (www.hearthub.org).

American Diabetes Association
The ADA has several patient resources and publications available on its home page (www.diabetes.org), including an ADA community forum.

National Institutes of Health-Related Resources
The National Heart, Lung, and Blood Institute (NHLBI) has prepared a set of patient-related educational materials and tutorials (www .nhlbi.nih.gov/health-topics/education-and-awareness). This includes National Diabetes Education Program (NDEP) resources, National High Blood Pressure Education Program (JNC8), and patient-specific information as well.

OTHER INFORMATIVE WEB SITES

National Institutes of Health Related
The National Kidney Disease Education Program (NKDEP) (nkdep.nih. gov) offerings for patients focus on CKD and include specific information about screening and nutrition. Many of the National Institutes of Health (NIH)-sponsored sites include resources in Spanish as well.

National Kidney Foundation
The material offered by the NKF (www.kidney.org) for patients includes a series of brochures describing many common problems faced by CKD patients. Nearly all brochures are free of charge. Of value are those that overview organ and tissue donation, donor family support, and children and adolescents' care. Other brochures outline Medicare patient education reimbursement for CKD4 patients under the Medicare Improvements for Patients and Providers Act (MIPPA).

American Association of Kidney Patients
The AAKP (www.aakp.org) has an active patient outreach program, including magazines and newsletters, an index by state of patient support groups, and periodic educational meetings that are held throughout the United States.

Medical Education Institute (homedialysis.org)
This website was created by the not-for-profit Medical Education Institute for the purposes of promoting home-dialysis therapies. Among the available resources is a list of centers in any given geographic area of the United States that offer home dialysis. It also can be a resource for outlining the different types of equipment and supplies necessary to arrange home therapies.

International Society for Hemodialysis
Under the aegis of the International Society for Hemodialysis (www. ishd.org/home-hd-toolkit), this useful website like homedialysis.org has resources for patients and practitioners invested in home-hemodialysis therapy. A modular tool kit is available as a comprehensive, peer-reviewed 282-page manual, *Implementing Hemodialysis in the*

Home: a Practical Manual, available for immediate downloading as a PDF manual. The modules include not only content directed toward patient care but also toward infrastructural and psychosocial issues. Membership in the International Society for Hemodialysis is not a requirement to access this material.

Sites for High-Information Patients

One problem for highly educated patients with kidney disease seeking information is that most material they find on the medical society and government websites has been prepared to reach the greatest possible audience and thus is available at a relatively general level. Patients seeking more advanced information may be misled when searching databases such as Medline for more detailed information about their particular condition(s). Although the "searching" patient may be well educated, it may prove difficult for him or her to properly evaluate multiple research articles directly, especially in areas where clear-cut consensus is lacking.

UpToDate for Patients

One potentially valuable site for such high-information patients is a website (www.uptodate.com/contents/table-of-contents/patient-education/kidneys-and-urinary-system) now owned by Wolters Kluwer that breaks down kidney disease (the site was created by a nephrologist) as well as other medical specialty areas into commonly encountered problem areas. The advantage of the site is that information regarding each problem area is updated every 3 to 6 months by an expert in the field. The free material directed toward patients is quite basic. More detailed information is available in the topic review pages developed for physicians, but also accessible to patients. Here, a paid subscription is required; patients can purchase a "7-day all-access pass" for $19.95 and a 1-month pass for $44.95.

Miscellaneous Physician and Nurse-Focused Internet Sites
KDOQI (www.kdoqi.org)

Open access provided via the website and also via the NKF's *American Journal of Kidney Diseases* with open access (ajkd.org/content/kdoqiguidelines).

KDIGO (www.kdigo.org)

Open access to the KDIGO guidelines, including those regarding CKD and treatment of high blood pressure and diabetes in kidney patients, is available via their website.

Nephrology Self-Assessment Program (NephSAP, www.asn-online.org/education/nephsap)

ASN self-assessment structured in clinical questions or vignettes. Free for ASN members.

*Kidney Self-Assessment Program (KSAP, www.asn-online.org/
education/ksap)*
Online self-assessment for ASN members that offers Continuing
Medical Education and maintenance of certification (MOC). Useful
resource for fellows preparing for board certification, or for practicing
physicians looking to recertify or renew. Four modules are available,
each costing $75 for ASN members.

American Nephrology Nurses Association (ANNA, www.annanurse.org)
Offers access to recorded sessions from its annual meeting, and man-
uscripts in the *Nephrology Nursing Journal.*

*European Dialysis and Transplant Nurses Association
(EDTNA/ERCA, www.edtnaerca.org)*
EDTNA has assembled a pocket guide, "Managing Stages 4 &
5 CKD—A Guide to Clinical Practice," published in 2008 and available
in seven languages.

References and Suggested Readings

Graham-Brown MPM, Oates T. Social media in medicine: a game changer? *Nephrol
    Dial Transplant.* 2017;32:1806–1808.
Miller EA, West DM. Characteristics associated with use of public and private Web
    sites as sources of health care information: results from a national survey. *Med
    Care.* 2007;45:245–251.
Patwardhan MB, Matchar DB, Samsa GP, et al. Utility of the advanced chronic kidney
    disease patient management tools: case studies. *Am J Med Qual.* 2008;23:105–114.
Sparks MA, Topf JM. NephMadness after 5 years: a recap and game plan for the future.
    Am J Kidney Dis. 2018;71:299–301. doi: https://doi.org/10.1053/j.ajkd.2017.12.001.
Watson AJ, Bell AG, Kvedar JC, et al. Reevaluating the digital divide: current lack of
    Internet use is not a barrier to adoption of novel health information technology.
    Diabetes Care. 2008;31:433–435.
Wilkinson I. Effects of a chronic kidney disease domain in the Quality and Outcomes
    Framework. *Br J Renal Med.* 2007;12:22–23. Available from http://www.bjrm.co.uk/
    journal_search_results.aspx?JournalID=2&sw=0&yrFrom=2007&yrTo=2007&sa=
    wilkinson&ef=False&notw=0&alw=True.
Woods M, Rosenberg ME. Educational tools: thinking outside the box. *Clin J Am Soc
    Nephrol.* 2016;11:518–526.
Yee J. Chronic kidney disease—a disease domain complex. *Geriatrics.* 2008;63:30–37.
Yee J, Krol GD. *Chronic Kidney Disease (CKD): Clinical Practice Recommendations
    for Primary Care Physicians & Healthcare Providers—A Collaborative Approach.* 7th
    ed. Detroit, MI: Henry Ford Health System; 2016. Available from http://ghsrenal.
    com/ckd/HFHS_CKD_GUIDELINES_V7.0.pdf.

31 International Guidelines for Chronic Kidney Disease, Cardiovascular Disease, and Diabetes

Jonathan C. Craig and Allison Tong

Clinical practice guidelines on the detection and management of early-stage chronic kidney disease (CKD) broadly cover identifying patients at risk for CKD, methods of diagnosis, referral to specialist care, and management to prevent disease progression. Guidelines with a primary focus on cardiovascular disease, diabetes, and hypertension may also provide recommendations relating to the primary and secondary prevention of CKD. This chapter reviews the main organizations issuing guidelines regarding CKD, cardiovascular disease, diabetes, and hypertension. For CKD guidelines published from 2010, we summarize the characteristics of the guideline organization, guideline development methods, and guideline recommendations for what we considered to be key areas for the generalist (Table 31.1). For guidelines primarily related to cardiovascular disease, diabetes, and hypertension, we summarize recommendations relating to CKD stages 1 to 4 (Table 31.2). The care of patients on dialysis or patients who have received a kidney transplant is not covered in this chapter.

The recommendations provided in Tables 31.1 and 31.2 are summarized from the original guideline. Readers are provided with website links (accessed June 2018) and journal sources of the original guidelines to access the complete guideline documents. Readers should be aware that existing guidelines are almost always updated periodically. These tables include selected internationally recognized guideline organizations (and not all guidelines worldwide). Guideline recommendations can help to inform clinical decision making, but health professionals should consider the context in which they practice and the patient's individual circumstances, preferences, and goals.

MAIN ORGANIZATIONS DEVELOPING GUIDELINES ON DETECTING AND MANAGING CHRONIC KIDNEY DISEASE

The major organizations that have published guidelines focused on CKD include both general guideline groups or kidney-specific groups: Canadian Society of Nephrology (CSN), European Renal Best Practice (ERBP), Kidney Health Australia—Caring for Australasians with Renal Impairment (KHA-CARI), Kidney Disease Improving Global Outcomes (KDIGO), National Institute for Health and Care

Excellence (NICE), National Kidney Foundation—Kidney Disease Outcomes Quality Initiative (NKF KDOQI), Scottish Intercollegiate Guidelines Network (SIGN), and the United Kingdom Renal Association (Table 31.1).

Canadian Society of Nephrology (CSN)

The CSN is a society of physicians and scientists specializing in the care of people with kidney disease and in research related to the kidney and kidney disease. They have published guidelines on CKD, peritoneal dialysis, hemodialysis, anemia, and kidney transplantation, which may be accessed using the following link: www.csnscn. ca/committees/clinical-practice-guidelines/library. In 2010, the CSN published a commentary on the 2009 KDIGO clinical practice guideline for the diagnosis, evaluation, and treatment of CKD—mineral and bone disorders (Manns, 2010).

Website: www.csnscn.ca

European Renal Best Practice (ERBP)

The European Renal Association—European Dialysis and Transplant Association (ERA-EDTA) is a professional organization based in the United Kingdom/Europe to advance medical science and clinical work in nephrology, dialysis, kidney transplantation, hypertension, and other related topics. The ERBP is a body of the ERA-EDTA responsible for producing guidelines. The ERBP guidelines cover clinical nephrology (including CKD, diabetes, anemia) and recently published guidelines on the management of older patients with CKD, and the management of patients with diabetes and CKD. The ERBP has also endorsed the 2009 KDIGO clinical practice guideline for the diagnosis, evaluation, and treatment of CKD—mineral and bone disorders and published a commentary (Goldsmith, 2010).

Website: www.european-renal-best-practice.org

Kidney Health Australia—Caring for Australasians With Renal Impairment (KHA-CARI)

The KHA-CARI commenced in 1999 to develop, publish, and implement evidence-based clinical practice guidelines to improve health care and outcome in children and adults with kidney disease. The guidelines cover CKD, dialysis (hemodialysis and peritoneal dialysis), and kidney transplantation. The most recent KHA-CARI guidelines on early CKD were published in 2013 and comprise 18 subtopics including diagnosis, classification and staging of CKD, education, disease progression, cardiovascular disease, diabetes, lifestyle and nutrition, and multidisciplinary care. Patients and family members were involved in the development of the guidelines (Tong, 2012), which helped to ensure that the guidelines addressed their priorities and preferences. KHA-CARI has also published commentaries on KDIGO guidelines on lipid management, blood pressure, and anemia in CKD.

Website: www.cari.org.au

TABLE 31.1 Guidelines Developed by General and Kidney Guideline Organizations (Published From 2010 Onward)

Guideline Organization Characteristics	European Renal Best Practice (ERBP)	Kidney Health Australia—Caring for Australasians with Renal Impairment (KHA-CARI)	Kidney Disease Improving Global Outcomes (KDIGO)	National Institute for Health and Care Excellence (NICE)	National Kidney Foundation—Kidney Disease Outcomes Quality Initiative (NKF KDOQI)	U.K. Renal Association
Name of guideline/s (CKD) and year of publication	Management of older patients with CKD stage 3b or higher. Management of patients with diabetes and CKD stage 3b or higher (2015).	Early CKD (2013)	Evaluation and management of CKD (2012) Management of blood pressure in CKD (2012) Anemia in CKD (2012) Lipids in CKD (2013)	CKD in adults: assessment and management (published 2014, updated 2015). Management of hyperphosphatemia (2013). Managing anemia (2015) CVD: risk assessment and reduction (published 2014, updated 2016).	Diabetes (2012) Nutrition in CKD (2010)	CKD-mineral and bone disorders (2015). Planning, initiating and withdrawal of renal replacement therapy (2014).
Organization/ governance	European Renal Association—European Dialysis and Transplant Association (ERA-EDTA).	Kidney Health Australia	Independent	Department of Health	National Kidney Foundation	U.K. Renal Association

Region	Europe	Australia, New Zealand	International	England	United States	United Kingdom
Target users	Health professionals	Health professionals, patients	Health professionals	Health professionals in primary and secondary care, patients and carers, commissioning organizations, service providers.	Health professionals	Health and social care professionals.
Guideline Development Process						
Work group members	Multidisciplinary	Multidisciplinary, patients/caregivers	Multidisciplinary	Multidisciplinary	Multidisciplinary	Multidisciplinary, patients/caregivers
Methods support	Methods support team	Editorial team	Evidence review team	Evidence review team (information specialist, systematic reviewer, economist).	Evidence review team	NS
Evidence base	Systematic literature review	Systematic literature review	Systematic literature review	Systematic literature review	Systematic literature review	Systematic literature review
Level of evidence	GRADE	GRADE	GRADE		GRADE	GRADE
Grade of recommendation	GRADE	GRADE	GRADE	NS	GRADE	GRADE
Guideline review	NS	Expert review, public consultation	Expert review, public consultation	Public, stakeholder consultation		Public review

(continued)

555

TABLE 31.1 Guidelines Developed by General and Kidney Guideline Organizations (Published From 2010 Onward) (Continued)

Guideline Organization	European Renal Best Practice (ERBP)	Kidney Health Australia—Caring for Australasians with Renal Impairment (KHA-CARI)	Kidney Disease Improving Global Outcomes (KDIGO)	National Institute for Health and Care Excellence (NICE)	National Kidney Foundation—Kidney Disease Outcomes Quality Initiative (NKF KDOQI)	U.K. Renal Association
Summary of Recommendations						
Detection						
Who to test	NS	Diabetes Hypertension CVD Obesity Lifestyle risk factors (smoking) Aboriginal and Torres Strait Islander peoples Family history	NS	Diabetes Hypertension CVD Acute kidney injury Structural renal tract disease, renal calculi, prostatic hypertrophy Multisystem diseases with potential kidney involvement Family history Opportunistic detection of hematuria or proteinuria	NS	NS

Proteinuria/PCR; Albuminuria/ACR; hematuria	NS	UACR in first void (or spot urine specimen); positive UACR to be repeated 1–2 times over 3 months.	In order of preference (early sample preferred): ACR, PCR, reagent strip urinalysis for total protein with automated reading, reagent strip urinalysis for total protein with manual reading.	ACR preferred to PCR ACR 3–70 mg/mmol should be confirmed by subsequent early morning sample. For hematuria, use reagent strips rather than urine microscopy (evaluate if 1+ or more).	NS	NS
Kidney function— evaluation of GFR	Use eGFR that corrects for differences in creatinine generation (older adults). Formal measurement recommended if a more accurate and precise estimate is required. CKD-EPI Cr-Cys may be an acceptable alternative (older adults).	eGFR	GFR and serum creatinine (initial). Use Cystatin C or clearance for confirmation.	eGFR (CKD-EPI), Cystatin C–based estimate of GFR at initial diagnosis to confirm/rule out CKD in people with eGFR creatinine 45–59 mL/min per 1.73 m^2 for 90 days, no proteinuria.	NS	NS

(continued)

TABLE 31.1 Guidelines Developed by General and Kidney Guideline Organizations (Published From 2010 Onward) (*Continued*)

Guideline Organization	European Renal Best Practice (ERBP)	Kidney Health Australia—Caring for Australasians with Renal Impairment (KHA-CARI)	Kidney Disease Improving Global Outcomes (KDIGO)	National Institute for Health and Care Excellence (NICE)	National Kidney Foundation—Kidney Disease Outcomes Quality Initiative (NKF KDOQI)	U.K. Renal Association
Classification	NS	Kidney function stages 1–5 and kidney damage stage based on GFR and kidney damage irrespective of the underlying diagnosis.	Based on cause, GFR (G1–G5), and albuminuria (A1–A3).	Refer to KDIGO (use of GFR and ACR categories). Increased ACR and decreased GFR in combination multiply the risk of adverse outcomes.	CKD stages 1–5	NS
Management						
Blood pressure—target	Suggest against applying lower blood pressure targets in patients with diabetes and CKD stage 3b or higher (eGFR <45 mL/min per 1.73 m^2) than in the general population.	≤140/90 ≤130/80 in people with micro- or macroalbuminuria (UACR). >3.5 mg/mmol in women; UACR >2.5 mg/mmol in men. ≤30/80 in all people with diabetes.	140/90 UAE <30 mg; 130/80 UAE ≥30 mg.	140/90 mm Hg In people with an ACR ≥70 mg/mmol, aim below 130/80.	NS	NS

| Hypertension—first-line therapy (ACEIs, ARBs) | In patients with diabetes and CKD stage 3b or higher (eGFR <45 mL/min per 1.73 m²) but without proteinuria, all blood pressure–lowering drugs can be used equally to lower blood pressure. CKD stage 3b or higher (eGFR <45 mL/min per 1.73 m² or on dialysis) with diabetes who have a cardiovascular indication (heart failure, ischemic heart disease)—treated with an ACEI at maximally tolerated dose. Insufficient evidence to justify the start of an ARB in adults with CKD stage 3b or higher and diabetes who have a cardiovascular indication (heart failure, ischemic heart disease) but intolerance for ACEI. Combination therapy is not recommended | Nondiabetic kidney disease—ACEI or ARB (first line)—combination should be avoided. Diabetic kidney disease—ACEI or ARB as first line, avoid combination therapy. | ARB or ACEI (diabetics w/ UAE 30–300 mg/24 h) ARB or ACEI (UAE >300 mg/24 h) | ACEI or ARB for people with CKD and: diabetes and ACR ≥3 mg/mmol, hypertension and ACR ≥30 mg/mmol, ACR ≥70 mg/mmol—avoid combination. Refer to NICE hypertension guidelines. | Do not recommend using an ACEI/ARB for the primary prevention of diabetic kidney disease in normotensive–normoalbuminuric patients with diabetes. Use an ACEI or an ARB in normotensive patients with diabetes and albuminuria levels >30 mg/g who are at high risk of diabetic kidney disease or its progression. | NS |

(continued)

TABLE 31.1

Guidelines Developed by General and Kidney Guideline Organizations (Published From 2010 Onward) *(Continued)*

Guideline Organization	European Renal Best Practice (ERBP)	Kidney Health Australia—Caring for Australasians with Renal Impairment (KHA-CARI)	Kidney Disease Improving Global Outcomes (KDIGO)	National Institute for Health and Care Excellence (NICE)	National Kidney Foundation—Kidney Disease Outcomes Quality Initiative (NKF KDOQI)	U.K. Renal Association
Hypertension—second-line therapy (e.g., calcium channel blockers, diuretics, β blockers).	Start a selective β-blocking agent as primary prevention in patients with diabetes and CKD stage 3b or higher and then continue it when tolerated. Prescribe lipophilic rather than hydrophilic β-blocking agents in patients with diabetes and CKD stage 3b or higher (eGFR <45 mL/min).	Diabetic kidney disease—β blockers, calcium channel blockers, and thiazide diuretics appropriate.	NS	NS	NS	NS

| Dyslipidemia—statins | Start a statin in patients with diabetes and CKD stages 3b and 4. Fibrates can replace statins in patients with CKD stage 3b who do not tolerate statins. | Statin therapy (with or without ezetimibe) to reduce the risk of atherosclerotic events. | ≥50 years with eGFR<60 mL/min per 1.73 m² treat with statin or statin/ezetimibe combination. ≥50 years with CKD and eGFR 60 mL/min per 1.73 m² treat with statin. 18–49 years use statin in patients with one or more of the following: coronary disease, diabetes, prior ischemic stroke, estimated 10-year incidence of coronary death or nonfatal MI. | Offer atorvastatin 20 mg for the primary or secondary prevention of CVD. Increase the dose if >40% reduction in non-HDL cholesterol is not achieved and eGFR is 30 mL/min per 1.73 m² or more. Agree the use of higher doses with a nephrologist. | Use LDL-C lowering medicines, such as statins or statin/ezetimibe combination, to reduce risk of major atherosclerotic events in patients with diabetes and CKD. | NS |

(continued)

TABLE 31.1 Guidelines Developed by General and Kidney Guideline Organizations (Published From 2010 Onward) (*Continued*)

Guideline Organization	European Renal Best Practice (ERBP)	Kidney Health Australia—Caring for Australasians with Renal Impairment (KHA-CARI)	Kidney Disease Improving Global Outcomes (KDIGO)	National Institute for Health and Care Excellence (NICE)	National Kidney Foundation—Kidney Disease Outcomes Quality Initiative (NKF KDOQI)	U.K. Renal Association
Antiplatelet therapy—aspirin	Do not add glycoprotein IIb/IIIa inhibitors to standard care to reduce death, myocardial infarction, or need for coronary revascularization in patients with diabetes and CKD stage 3b or higher and acute coronary syndromes (ACSs) or high-risk coronary artery intervention. Start aspirin as secondary prevention, unless there is a contraindication, side effect, or intolerance. Start aspirin as primary prevention only in patients without additional risk factors for major bleeding.	Not routinely recommended as the risk/benefit for primary prevention of CVD in patients with early CKD is uncertain.	Offer treatment with antiplatelet agents to patients at risk for atherosclerotic events.	Offer antiplatelet medications for secondary prevention of CVD.	NS	NS

Diet and nutrition—salt reduction, protein restriction, potassium, phosphate.	Supervision by a dietitian	Individualized diet intervention with qualified dietitian. Normal protein diet 0.75–1 g/kg per day with adequate energy. Low-protein diet (≤0.6 g/kg per day) is not recommended. Restrict sodium intake to 100 mmol/day. No restriction on dietary phosphate. Patients with persistent hyperkalemia may restrict dietary potassium intake with support from a dietitian. Polyphenol-enriched diets may slow progression of diabetic nephropathy. Mediterranean style and high-fibre diet recommended.	Protein restriction (0.8 g/kg per day) for GFR <30 mL/min per 1.73 m². Avoid high-protein intake (>1.3 g/kg per day) in adults with CKD at risk of progression. Lower salt intake to <90 mmol Expert dietary advice and information (salt, phosphate, potassium, protein).	Offer dietary advice about potassium, phosphate, calorie, and salt intake. Do not offer low-protein diets (dietary protein intake <0.6–0.8 g/kg per day) to people with CKD.	Medical nutrition therapy provided by a registered dietitian. Without diabetes, not on dialysis, with an eGFR <50 mL/min per 1.73 m² protein-controlled diet providing 0.6–0.8 g/kg per day. Very-low-protein intake 0.3–0.5 g/kg per day for eGFR <20 mL/min per 1.73 m². Diabetic nephropathy 0.8–0.9 g/kg per day. CKD stages 3–5, 10–12 mg phosphorus per gram of protein. Sodium intake <2.4 g. Potassium intake <2.4 g.	NS

(continued)

					National Kidney Foundation—Kidney Disease Outcomes Quality Initiative (NKF KDOQI)	
Guideline Organization	European Renal Best Practice (ERBP)	Kidney Health Australia—Caring for Australasians with Renal Impairment (KHA-CARI)	Kidney Disease Improving Global Outcomes (KDIGO)	National Institute for Health and Care Excellence (NICE)		U.K. Renal Association
Diabetes—glucose control	Recommend against tighter glycemic control if this results in severe hypoglycemic episodes. Tighten glycemic control with the intention to lower HbA_{1c} when values are >8.5% (69 mmol/mol). Use HbA_{1c} as a routine reference to assess longer-term glycemic control in patients with CKD stage 3b or higher (eGFR <45 mL/min per 1.73 m²).	Patients with diabetes mellitus aim to achieve an HbA_{1c} <7.0%	Target HbA_{1c} <7%	NS	Target hemoglobin A1c (HbA_{1c}) 7.0% Do not treat to an HbA_{1c} target of <7.0% in patients at risk of hypoglycemia. Target HbA_{1c} be extended above 7.0% in individuals with comorbidities or limited life expectancy and risk of hypoglycemia.	NS

TABLE 31.1 Guidelines Developed by General and Kidney Guideline Organizations (Published From 2010 Onward) (Continued)

| Anemia—iron, ESA, red cell transfusion | NS | Refer to KDIGO | Diagnose anemia when the Hb concentration is <13.0 g/dL (males) and <12.0 g/dL (females). Iron: patients on ESA therapy who are not receiving iron supplementation—trial of IV iron. ESA: Hb concentration <10.0 g/dL—initiation of ESA is individualized based on the rate of fall of Hb concentration, prior response to iron therapy, risk of needing a transfusion, symptoms. ESAs not to be used to maintain Hb concentration >11.5 g/dL. | Offer ESA to people with anemia of CKD who are likely to benefit in terms of quality of life and physical function. Correction to normal levels of Hb with ESAs is not usually recommended in people with anemia of CKD. Offer iron therapy to people with anemia of CKD who are iron deficient and who are not receiving ESA therapy, before discussing ESA therapy. Offer iron therapy to people with anemia of CKD who are iron deficient and who are receiving ESA therapy. | Oral or IV iron administration if serum ferritin <100 ng/mL and TSAT <20%. | NS |

(continued)

565

TABLE 31.1 Guidelines Developed by General and Kidney Guideline Organizations (Published From 2010 Onward) (*Continued*)

Guideline Organization	European Renal Best Practice (ERBP)	Kidney Health Australia—Caring for Australasians with Renal Impairment (KHA-CARI)	Kidney Disease Improving Global Outcomes (KDIGO)	National Institute for Health and Care Excellence (NICE)	National Kidney Foundation—Kidney Disease Outcomes Quality Initiative (NKF KDOQI)	U.K. Renal Association
Bone disease	NS	Vitamin D deficiency and insufficiency can be corrected using strategies recommended for the general population.	Vitamin D and bisphosphonates not routinely prescribed unless clinically indicated.	Offer bisphosphonates if indicated for prevention and treatment of osteoporosis in people with GFR ≥30 mL/min per 1.73 m². Vitamin D not to be routinely offered. Offer cholecalciferol or ergocalciferol to treat vitamin D deficiency in people with CKD and vitamin D deficiency.	Vitamin D supplementation to maintain adequate levels of vitamin D if the serum level of 25-hydroxyvitamin D <30 ng/mL. Following initiation of vitamin D therapy, the use of cholecalciferol or ergocalciferol therapy should be coordinated with the serum calcium and phosphorus levels.	Serum calcium, adjusted for albumin concentration, should be maintained within the normal reference range (2.2 and 2.5 mmol/L). Serum phosphate in patients with CKD stages 3b–5 should be maintained between 0.9 and 1.5 mmol/L.

Metabolic acidosis	NS	Oral bicarbonate supplementation for serum bicarbonate concentrations <22 mmol/L treatment unless contraindicated.	If vitamin D deficiency has been corrected and symptoms of CKD—mineral and bone disorders persist, offer alfacalcidol or calcitriol to people with a GFR of <30 mL/min per 1.73 m². Consider oral sodium bicarbonate supplementation GFR <30 mL/min per 1.73 m² with serum bicarbonate concentration <20 mmol/L.	NS
Psychosocial support—information, education, lifestyle advice		Comprehensive and structured CKD education on risk factors and psychological impact.	Patients with progressive CKD to have access to counseling, education, psychosocial care. Provide information and education tailored to severity of CKD, complications, and risk of progression. Facilitate informed decision making about treatment. Offer access to psychosocial support as needed.	Education and counseling regarding self-management.

(continued)

TABLE 31.1	Guidelines Developed by General and Kidney Guideline Organizations (Published From 2010 Onward) (Continued)					
Guideline Organization	European Renal Best Practice (ERBP)	Kidney Health Australia—Caring for Australasians with Renal Impairment (KHA-CARI)	Kidney Disease Improving Global Outcomes (KDIGO)	National Institute for Health and Care Excellence (NICE)	National Kidney Foundation—Kidney Disease Outcomes Quality Initiative (NKF KDOQI)	U.K. Renal Association
Lifestyle modification— smoking, weight management, exercise	Additional physical exercise for patients with diabetes and CKD stage 3b or higher (eGFR <45 mL/min). Exercise training to be offered in a structured and individualized manner to avoid adverse events (older adults).	Regular physical exercise Smoking cessation Minimize carbonated beverages Drink fluids in moderation Maintain a healthy weight	Physical activity compatible with CV health and tolerance, weight management (BMI 20–25).	Exercise Achieve a healthy weight Smoking cessation	Increase frequency or duration of physical activity as tolerated.	NS

Referral					
NS	CKD stages 4–5 GFR <30 mL/min per 1.73 m² Persistent significant albuminuria Consistent decline in eGFR from baseline of <60 mL/min per 1.73 m². Glomerular hematuria with macroalbuminuria; CKD and hypertension that cannot be treated to target with at least three agents.	CKD stages 4–5 GFR <30 mL/min per 1.73 m² Consistent significant albuminuria (ACR ≥300 mg/g or AER ≥300 mg/24 h Urinary red cell casts CKD and hypertension refractory to treatment with four or more antihypertensive agents. Persistent abnormalities of serum potassium Recurrent or extensive nephrolithiasis Hereditary kidney disease	CKD stages 4–5 GFR <30 mL/min per 1.73 m² ACR ≥70 mg/mmol unless known to be caused by diabetes and already appropriately treated. ACR ≥30 mg/mmol or more with hematuria Sustained decrease in GFR of 25% or more, and a change in GFR category or sustained. Decrease in GFR of ≥15 mL/min per 1.73 m² within 12 months. Uncontrolled hypertension despite the use of at least four antihypertensive drugs. Known or suspected rare or genetic causes of CKD. Suspected renal artery stenosis.	NS	CKD stages 4–5 GFR <30 mL/min per 1.73 m² At least 1 year prior to anticipated renal replacement therapy.

ACEI, angiotensin-converting enzyme inhibitor; ACR, albumin–creatinine ratio; ARB, angiotensin receptor blocker; C, cholesterol; CKD, chronic kidney disease; Cr-Cys, creatinine-cystatin; CVD, cardiovascular disease; eGFR, estimated glomerular filtration rate; ESA, erythropoietin-stimulating agent; Hb, hemoglobin; IV, intravenous; LDL, low-density lipoprotein; MI, myocardial infarction; NS, no suggestions/recommendation on this topic; PCR, protein–creatinine ratio; UACR, urinary albumin-to-creatinine ratio; UAE, urinary albumin excretion; U.K., United Kingdom.

TABLE 31.2 Related Guidelines on Cardiovascular Disease, Hypertension, and Diabetes

Guideline Organization	Guideline and Year of Publication	Country/ Region	Source	CKD Related Recommendations and Suggestions (CKD Stages 1–4)
Cardiovascular Disease and Hypertension				
American College of Physicians and American Academy of Family Physicians	Pharmacologic treatment of hypertension in adults aged 60 years or older to higher versus lower blood pressure targets.	United States	*Ann Intern Med.* 2017;166:430–437.	An SBP target of less than 140 mm Hg is a reasonable goal for some patients with increased cardiovascular risk (including CKD).
Eighth Joint National Committee (JNC 8)	Evidence-based guideline for the management of high blood pressure in adults (2014).	United States	*JAMA.* 2014;311:507–520.	For patients aged 18 years or over with CKD, initiate pharmacologic treatment to lower BP at SBP ≥40 mm Hg or DBP ≥90 mm Hg and treat to goal SBP <140 mm Hg and goal DBP <90 mm Hg. In the population aged 18 years or older with CKD, initial (or add-on) antihypertensive treatment should include an ACEI or ARB to improve kidney outcomes. This applies to all CKD patients with hypertension regardless of race or diabetes status.
European Society of Cardiology in collaboration with the European Association for the Study of Diabetes	European guidelines on cardiovascular disease prevention in clinical practice (2016).	Europe	*Eur Heart J.* 2016; 37:2315–2381.	No consensus on which measure of renal function (i.e., which formula, and creatinine or cystatin C–based) best predicts CVD. Statin therapy has a beneficial effect on CVD outcomes in CKD and in some studies slows the rate of loss of kidney function. ACEIs and ARBs are particularly effective in reducing LVH, reducing microalbuminuria and proteinuria, preserving renal function and delaying ESKD.

Organization	Title	Country	Reference	Recommendations
Hypertension Canada	Diagnosis, risk assessment, prevention, and treatment of hypertension in adults (2017)	Canada	*Can J Cardiol.* 2017;33:557–576.	For patients with nondiabetic CKD, target BP is <140/90 mm Hg. For patients with hypertension and proteinuric CKD (urinary protein >500 mg/24 h or albumin/creatinine ratio >30 mg/mmol), initial therapy should be an ACEI or an ARB if there is intolerance to ACEIs. For patients with hypertension and proteinuric CKD (urinary protein >500 mg/24 h or albumin/creatinine ratio >30 mg/mmol), initial therapy should be an ACEI or an ARB if there is intolerance to ACEIs. The combination of an ACEI and ARB is not recommended for patients with nonproteinuric CKD.
Joint British Societies[a]	Consensus recommendations for the prevention of cardiovascular disease (2014)	United Kingdom	*JBS3 Heart.* 2014; 100:ii1–ii67.	In adults with stages 3–5 CKD, with or without diabetes, BP should be treated to maintain systolic <140 mm Hg and diastolic <90 mm Hg. In adults with CKD, with or without diabetes, in whom urinary albumin excretion exceeds 30 mg/day (equivalent to an ACR of 3 mg/mmol), these targets should be reduced to systolic <130 mm Hg and diastolic <80 mm Hg. All antihypertensive agents are effective in adults with stages 3–5 CKD. ACEIs or ARBs should be included in the antihypertensive regimen, particularly in people with albuminuria >30 mg/day (equivalent to an ACR of 3 mg/mmol). In adults with stages 3–5 CKD, lipid-lowering therapy with statins should be considered in all patients. Routine use of aspirin is not recommended for primary prevention in CKD.

(continued)

TABLE 31.2 Related Guidelines on Cardiovascular Disease, Hypertension, and Diabetes (*Continued*)

Guideline Organization	Guideline and Year of Publication	Country/ Region	Source	CKD Related Recommendations and Suggestions (CKD Stages 1–4)
National Heart Foundation of Australia	Guideline for the diagnosis and management of hypertension in adults (2016)	Australia	www. heartfoundation. org.au/images/ uploads/ publications/ PRO-167_ Hypertension-guideline-2016_ WEB.pdf	Any first-line antihypertensive agent to reduce blood pressure is recommended for patients with hypertension and CKD. In the presence of micro- or macro albuminuria, an ARB or ACEI should be considered as first-line therapy. In patients with CKD, antihypertensive therapy should be started in those with SBP consistently >140/90 mm Hg and treated to a target of <140/90 mm Hg. Dual renin–angiotensin system blockade is not recommended in patients with CKD. Aiming toward SBP <120 mm Hg has shown benefit, where well tolerated. Close follow-up of patients is recommended in patients treated to <120 mm Hg systolic to identify treatment-related adverse effects including hypotension, syncope, electrolyte abnormalities, and acute kidney injury. Aldosterone antagonists should be used with caution.
Singapore Ministry of Health	Screening for cardiovascular disease and risk factors	Singapore	www.moh.gov.sg	In patients at risk of CKD, screening for risk factors for CVD and for coronary artery disease is recommended at baseline and when patients become symptomatic of renal disease.

Diabetes

Organization	Title	Country	Source	Recommendations
American Association of Clinical Endocrinologists and American College of Endocrinology	Clinical practice guidelines for developing a diabetes mellitus comprehensive care plan (2015)	United States	*Endocr Pract.* 2015;21(Suppl 1): 1–87.	Annual assessment of serum creatinine to determine the eGFR and urine AER should be performed to identify, stage, and monitor progression of diabetic nephropathy.
American Diabetes Association	Standards of medical care in diabetes (2017)	United States	https://professional.diabetes.org/content/clinical-practice-recommendations	At least once a year, assess urinary albumin (e.g., spot urinary ACR) and eGFR in patients with type 1 diabetes with duration of ≥5 years, in all patients with type 2 diabetes, and in all patients with comorbid hypertension. Optimize glucose control to reduce the risk or slow the progression of diabetic kidney disease. Physical activity can acutely increase urinary albumin excretion. However, there is no evidence that vigorous-intensity exercise increases the rate of progression of diabetic kidney disease, and there appears to be no need for specific exercise restrictions for people with diabetic kidney disease.
Diabetes Canada	Clinical practice guidelines for the prevention and management of diabetes in Canada (2013)	Canada	*Can J Diabetes.* 2013;37:A3–A13.	In adults, screening for CKD in diabetes should be conducted using a random urine ACR and a serum creatinine converted into an eGFR. Screening should commence at diagnosis of diabetes in individuals with type 2 diabetes and 5 years after diagnosis in adults with type 1 diabetes and repeated yearly thereafter. A diagnosis of CKD should be made in patients with a random urine ACR ≥2.0 mg/mmol and/or an eGFR <60 mL/min on at least 2 of 3 samples over a 3-month period.

(continued)

TABLE 31.2 Related Guidelines on Cardiovascular Disease, Hypertension, and Diabetes (*Continued*)

Guideline Organization	Guideline and Year of Publication	Country/ Region	Source	CKD Related Recommendations and Suggestions (CKD Stages 1–4)
European Society of Cardiology in collaboration with the European Association for the Study of Diabetes	European guidelines on cardiovascular disease prevention in clinical practice (2016)	Europe	*Eur Heart J.* 2016; 37:2315–2381.	Metformin, acarbose, and most sulphonylureas should be avoided in stages 3–4 CKD, while insulin therapy and pioglitazone can be used in their place as required.
	ESC guidelines on diabetes, pre-diabetes, and cardiovascular diseases developed in collaboration with the EASD (2013)		*Eur Heart J.* 2013; 34:3035–3037.	
International Diabetes Federation	Global guideline for type 2 diabetes (2012)	International	www.idf. org/e-library/ guidelines/79-global-guideline-for-type-2-diabetes.html	Assess kidney function with urine test for albuminuria, measurement of serum creatinine, and calculation of eGFR. ACR an early morning void specimen is preferred (or random spot is acceptable). CKD is diagnosed on the basis of a raised urine albumin/protein or reduced eGFR (<60 mL/min per 1.73 m²) calculated from MDRD formula and using a standardized creatinine assay. Monitor renal function and use metformin with caution if eGFR <45 mL/min per 1.73 m².

Singapore Ministry of Health	Diabetes mellitus (2014)	Singapore	www.moh.gov.sg	Perform an annual test to assess urine albumin excretion starting at diagnosis.
				Measure serum creatinine at least annually in all adults with diabetes. The serum creatinine should be used to estimate GFR and stage the level of CKD, if present.
				Estimate renal function with the modification of diet in renal disease (MDRD) equation when eGFR is below 60 mL/min per 1.73 m^2.

[a]Joint British Societies: British Cardiovascular Society, Association of British Clinical Diabetologists, British Association for Cardiovascular Prevention & Rehabilitation, British Association for Nursing in Cardiovascular Care, British Heart Foundation, British Hypertension Society, British Renal Society, Diabetes UK, HEART UK, Renal Association, Stroke Association.
ACEI, angiotensin-converting enzyme inhibitor; AER, albumin excretion rate; ACR, albumin–creatinine ratio; ARB, angiotensin receptor blocker; BP, blood pressure; CKD, chronic kidney disease; CVD, cardiovascular disease; DBP, diastolic blood pressure; ESKD, end-stage kidney disease; LVF, left ventricular hypertrophy; SBP, systolic blood pressure.

Kidney Disease Improving Global Outcomes

The KDIGO is an international organization that develops and implements evidence-based clinical practice guidelines in kidney disease. It was originally established in 2003 by the U.S. National Kidney Foundation and in 2013 became an independently incorporated nonprofit foundation governed by an international Executive Committee. To date, KDIGO has published nine clinical practice guidelines. KDIGO also convened Controversies Conferences to bring together key opinion leaders to discuss and debate nephrology-related topics. KDIGO guidelines in CKD address topics including anemia, blood pressure, evaluation and management, mineral and bone disorder, hepatitis C, and lipids. In 2012, KDIGO released the clinical practice guideline for the evaluation and management of CKD. The guidelines are published in *Kidney International* as a supplement.

Website: www.kdigo.org

National Institute for Health and Care Excellence

The NICE provides national guidance and advice to improve health and social care in the United Kingdom. The guidelines are for general practitioners, local government, public health professionals, and members of the public. NICE has produced guidelines on CKD, specifically on management of hyperphosphatemia (CKD stage 4/5), assessment and management of CKD in adults, and management of anemia.

Website: www.nice.org.uk

National Kidney Foundation—Kidney Disease Outcomes Quality Initiative

The National Kidney Foundation produces guidelines through the NKF KDOQI for all stages of CKD and related complications, which cover topics including anemia, bone metabolism, cardiovascular disease, diabetes, classification of CKD, and nutrition. The 2002 KDOQI clinical practice guidelines for chronic kidney disease: evaluation, classification and stratification have been replaced by the KDIGO 2012 clinical practice guideline for the evaluation and management of chronic kidney disease. KDOQI has published various commentaries on KDIGO guidelines including evaluation and management of CKD (2012); blood pressure (2012); and anemia (2012). Currently, they are collaborating with the U.S. Academy of Nutrition and Dietetics to update the KDOQI clinical practice guideline on nutrition in CKD.

Website: www.kidney.org

Scottish Intercollegiate Guidelines Network

The SIGN was formed in 1993 to develop and disseminate national clinical practice guidelines based on current evidence. SIGN includes health professionals from all medical specialties. In 2008, SIGN issued a guideline on the diagnosis and management of CKD and contains recommendation on how to diagnose CKD, slow the progression of CKD, reduce the risk of cardiovascular disease, manage the complications of CKD, provide psychosocial support, and improve quality of life in patients with CKD.

Website: www.sign.ac.uk

U.K. Renal Association

The Renal Association is a professional body for nephrologists (renal physicians or kidney doctors) and renal scientists in the United Kingdom. The U.K. Renal Association established the Clinical Practice Guidelines Committee to prepare guidelines for the management of patients with kidney disease. The process for guideline development has been accredited by the U.K. NICE. Current accredited guidelines include CKD—mineral and bone disorders, planning, initiating and withdrawal of renal replacement therapy, post-operative care in the kidney transplant recipient, and vascular access for hemodialysis.

Website: www.renal.org

CARDIOVASCULAR, HYPERTENSION, AND DIABETES GUIDELINES ADDRESSING ISSUES RELATING TO CHRONIC KIDNEY DISEASE

Guidelines with a primary focus on cardiovascular disease, diabetes, and hypertension include recommendations relating to patients who are at risk for or have been diagnosed with CKD. Please refer to Table 31.2 for an overview of selected guidelines. With regard to CKD-related issues, the following broad principles almost always apply:

Cardiovascular Disease

Patients with CKD are identified to be at an increased risk for cardiovascular disease and cardiovascular mortality. Recommendations for screening patients with cardiovascular disease using estimated glomerular filtration (eGFR) rate and albumin–creatinine ratio are given.

Hypertension

Hypertension guidelines provide recommendations on the drug treatment threshold and blood pressure targets for people diagnosed with CKD. The threshold for treatment in patients with CKD ranges from systolic blood pressure of <125 to 140 mm Hg and diastolic blood pressure <75 to 90 mm Hg, depending on the level of proteinuria and other clinical circumstances.

Diabetes

Patients with diabetes should be screened for CKD by measuring albuminuria and calculating eGFR. Glucose control is recommended to reduce the risk or slow the progression of diabetic nephropathy. Angiotensin-converting enzyme inhibitors (ACEIs) or angiotensin receptor blockers (ARBs) are recommended to optimize blood pressure control.

References and Suggested Readings

Goldsmith DJ, Covic A, Fouque D, et al. Endorsement of the Kidney Disease Improving Global Outcomes (KDIGO) Chronic Kidney Disease-Mineral and Bone Disorder (CKD-MBD) Guidelines: a European Renal Best Practice (ERBP) commentary statement. *Nephrol Dial Transplant.* 2010;25:3823–3831.

Manns BJ, Hodsman A, Zimmerman DL, et al. Canadian Society of Nephrology commentary on the 2009 KDIGO clinical practice guideline for the diagnosis, evaluation, and treatment of CKD-mineral and bone disorder (CKD-MBD). *Am J Kidney Dis.* 2010;55:800–812.

Tong A, Lopez-Vargas P, Howell M, et al. Consumer involvement in topic and outcome selection in the development of clinical practice guidelines. *Health Expect.* 2012;15:410–423.

More Equations for Estimating Glomerular Filtration Rate and Expected Daily Creatinine Excretion Rate

John T. Daugirdas

CHRONIC KIDNEY DISEASE EPIDEMIOLOGY COLLABORATION (CKD-EPI) EQUATION SET FOR CALCULATING ESTIMATED GLOMERULAR FILTRATION RATE (EGFR)

Note: *Designed for use when serum creatinine (SCr) is entered as mg/dL. To convert SCr from mcmol/L to mg/dL, multiply by 0.0113.*

African-American Woman
If SCr ≤0.7

$$eGFR/1.73 \text{ m}^2 = 166 \times (SCr/0.7)^{-0.329} \times 0.993^{Age}$$

If SCr >0.7

$$eGFR/1.73 \text{ m}^2 = 166 \times (SCr/0.7)^{-1.209} \times 0.993^{Age}$$

African-American Man
If SCr ≤0.9

$$eGFR/1.73 \text{ m}^2 = 163 \times (SCr/0.9)^{-0.411} \times 0.993^{Age}$$

If SCr >0.9

$$eGFR/1.73 \text{ m}^2 = 163 \times (SCr/0.9)^{-1.209} \times 0.993^{Age}$$

White (or Other Race) Woman
If SCr ≤0.7

$$eGFR/1.73 \text{ m}^2 = 144 \times (SCr/0.7)^{-0.329} \times 0.993^{Age}$$

If SCr >0.7

$$eGFR/1.73 \text{ m}^2 = 144 \times (SCr/0.7)^{-1.209} \times 0.993^{Age}$$

White (or Other Race) Man
If SCr ≤0.9

$$eGFR/1.73 \text{ m}^2 = 141 \times (SCr/0.9)^{-0.411} \times 0.993^{Age}$$

If SCr >0.9

$$eGFR/1.73 \text{ m}^2 = 141 \times (SCr/0.9)^{-1.209} \times 0.993^{Age}$$

EXPECTED 24-HOUR CREATININE EXCRETION RATES

Figure A1.1 shows in graphic form the expected 24-hour creatinine excretion amounts for a man or a woman of different ages as a function of body weight. Whenever a 24-hour urine specimen is collected, the amount recovered can be compared to these values. The estimates were derived from an equation published by Ix and colleagues (2011).

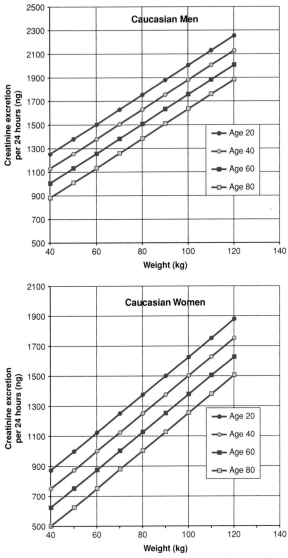

FIGURE A1.1 The expected 24-hour creatinine excretion rate in whites according to an equation by Ix and colleagues (2011).

SALAZAR–CORCORAN EQUATION

The Salazar–Corcoran equation can be used to estimate creatinine clearance (not indexed to body surface area) in obese persons. The equation is as follows:

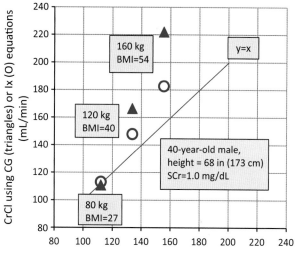

FIGURE A1.2 Differences in three creatinine clearance estimating equations in three 40-year-old male subjects, all having a serum creatinine of 1.0 mg/dL (88.4 mcmol/L) and all being of the same height, but weighing 80, 120, or 160 kg. Both the Cockcroft and Gault (CG) and Ix equations tend to overestimate creatinine clearance in markedly obese subjects.

Man:

$$\text{CrCl} = \frac{(137 - \text{age})\,[(0.285\,\text{Wt}) + (12.1\,\text{Ht}^2)]}{51\,\text{SCr}}$$

Woman:

$$\text{CrCl} = \frac{(146 - \text{age})\,[(0.287\,\text{Wt}) + (9.74\,\text{Ht}^2)]}{60\,\text{SCr}}$$

where Wt = actual body weight in kg and Ht = height in meters. SCr = serum creatinine in mg/dL.

As shown in Figure A1.2, as body mass index (BMI) increases, relative to clearance estimated by the Salazar–Corcoran equation, Cockcroft and Gault estimates (solid triangles) are unphysiologically high. This overestimation is partially, but not completely, corrected by using the Ix equation.

References and Suggested Readings

Cockcroft DW, Gault MH. Prediction of creatinine clearance from serum creatinine. *Nephron.* 1976;16:31–41.

Ix JH, Wassel CL, Stevens LA, et al. Equations to estimate creatinine excretion rate: the CKD Epidemiology Collaboration. *Clin J Am Soc Nephrol.* 2011;6:184–191.

Levey AS, Stevens LA, Schmid CH, et al; CKD-EPI (Chronic Kidney Disease Epidemiology Collaboration). A new equation to estimate glomerular filtration rate. *Ann Intern Med.* 2009;150:604–612.

Salazar DE, Corcoran GB. Predicting creatinine clearance and renal drug clearance in obese patients from estimated fat-free body mass. *Am J Med.* 1988;84:1053–1060.

Ideal, Lean, Median Standard, and Adjusted Body Weights

John T. Daugirdas

IDEAL BODY WEIGHT EQUATIONS (KG)

Method of Devine (1974)
Men: 50 + 2.3 kg for each inch over 5 feet
Women: 45.5 + 2.3 kg for each inch over 5 feet

Method of Robinson (1983)
Men: 52 + 1.9 kg for each inch over 5 feet
Women: 49 + 1.7 kg for each inch over 5 feet

ADJUSTED BODY WEIGHT (KG)

There are two methods of computing adjusted body weight in widespread use. The first, used for protein and calorie recommendations by Kidney Disease Outcomes Quality Initiative (KDOQI) is:

$$adjBW = edfreeBW + (stdBW - edfreeBW) \times 0.25$$

where edfreeBW is the edema-free actual body weight, and stdBW is the median standard weight. The median standard body weight

Table A2.1 Frame Size as Determined by Elbow Breadth (cm)

Age (years)	Frame Size		
	Small	Medium	Large
Men			
18–24	≤6.6	>6.6 and <7.7	≥7.7
25–34	≤6.7	>6.7 and <7.9	≥7.9
35–44	≤6.7	>6.7 and <8.0	≥8.0
45–54	≤6.7	>6.7 and <8.1	≥8.1
55–64	≤6.7	>6.7 and <8.1	≥8.1
65–74	≤6.7	>6.7 and <8.1	≥8.1
Women			
18–24	≤5.6	>5.6 and <6.5	≥6.5
25–34	≤5.7	>5.7 and <6.8	≥6.8
35–44	≤5.7	>5.7 and <7.1	≥7.1
45–54	≤5.7	>5.7 and <7.2	≥7.2
55–64	≤5.8	>5.8 and <7.2	≥7.2
65–74	≤5.8	>5.8 and <7.2	≥7.2

Derived from the U.S. population in the National Health and Nutrition Examination Surveys (NHANES) 1 and NHANES 2 data sets.
Source: Data from Frisancho AR. New standards of weight and body composition by frame size and height for assessment of nutritional status of adults and the elderly. *Am J Clin Nutr.* 1984;40:808–819.

Table A2.2 Median Standard Weights for Men and Women in the United States by Age, Height, and Frame Size (Used to Compute Adjusted Body Weight)

Height		Median Standard Weight (kg)						Compare: Ideal Body Weight (kg) (Robinson)
		Age 25–54			Age 55–74			
		Frame Size[a]						
inches	cm	S	M	L	S	M	L	
Men								
62	157	64	68	82	61	68	77	55.8
63	160	61	71	83	62	70	80	57.7
64	163	66	71	84	63	71	77	59.6
65	165	66	74	84	70	72	79	61.5
66	168	67	75	84	68	74	80	63.4
67	170	71	77	84	69	78	85	65.3
68	173	71	78	86	70	78	83	67.2
69	175	74	78	89	75	77	84	69.1
70	178	75	81	87	76	80	87	71
71	180	76	81	91	69	84	84	72.9
72	183	74	84	91	76	81	90	74.8
73	185	79	85	93	78	88	88	76.7
74	188	80	88	92	77	95	89	78.6
Women								
58	147	52	63	86	54	57	78	45.6
59	150	53	66	78	55	62	78	47.3
60	152	53	60	87	54	62	78	49
61	155	54	61	81	56	64	79	50.7
62	157	55	61	81	58	64	82	52.4
63	160	55	62	83	58	65	80	54.1
64	163	57	62	79	60	66	77	55.8
65	165	60	63	81	60	67	80	57.5
66	168	58	63	75	68	66	82	59.2
67	170	59	65	80	61	72	80	60.9
68	173	62	67	76	61	70	79	62.6
69	175	63	68	79	62	72	85	64.3
70	178	64	70	76	63	73	85	66

[a]Frame size as defined in Table A2.1. S, small; M, medium; L, large.
Data for median standard weight derived from the combined National Health and Nutrition Examination Surveys (NHANES) I and NHANES II data sets (Frisancho AR. New standards of weight and body composition by frame size and height for assessment of nutritional status of adults and the elderly. *Am J Clin Nutr.* 1984;40:808–819). Ideal body weight computed according to Robinson JD, Lupkiewicz SM, Palenik L, et al. Determination of ideal body weight for drug dosage calculations. *Am J Hosp Pharm.* 1983;40:1016–1019.

depends on the frame size, which in turn can be determined from the elbow breadth measured in cm (Table A2.1). Once the frame size has been categorized as small (S), medium (M), or large (L), Table A2.2 can be used to determine the median standard body weight. In the table, the ideal body weight calculated using the Robinson equation has been added for comparison.

Another version, commonly used in drug dosing, is:

$$\text{Adjusted body weight} = \text{IBW} + 0.4 \times (\text{edfreeBW} - \text{IBW})$$

where IBW = ideal body weight calculated according to Devine or Robinson as described above.

LEAN BODY WEIGHT EQUATIONS (KG)

Janmahasatian (2005):

Men: $9{,}270 \times wt(kg)/(6{,}680 + 216 \times$ body mass index [BMI])
Women: $9{,}270 \times wt(kg)/(8{,}780 + 244 \times BMI)$

References and Suggested Readings

Devine BJ. Gentamicin therapy. *Drug Intell Clin Pharm.* 1974;8:650–655.

Frisancho AR. New standards of weight and body composition by frame size and height for assessment of nutritional status of adults and the elderly. *Am J Clin Nutr.* 1984;40:808–819.

Hallynck TH, Soep HH, Thomis JA, et al. Should clearance be normalised to body surface or to lean body mass? *Br J Clin Pharmacol.* 1981;11:523–526.

Hume R. Prediction of lean body mass from height and weight. *J Clin Pathol.* 1966;19:389–391.

Janmahasatian S, Duffull SB, Ash S, et al. Quantification of lean bodyweight. *Clin Pharmacokinet.* 2005;44:1051–1065.

Mitchell SJ, Kirkpatrick CM, Le Couteur DG. Estimation of lean body mass in older community-dwelling men. *Br J Clin Pharmacol.* 2010;69:118–127.

Pai MP. Estimating the glomerular filtration rate in obese adult patients for drug dosing. *Adv Chronic Kidney Dis.* 2010;17:e53–e62.

Pai MP, Paloucek FP. The origin of the "ideal" body weight equations. *Ann Pharmacother.* 2000;34:1066–1069.

Robinson JD, Lupkiewicz SM, Palenik L, et al. Determination of ideal body weight for drug dosage calculations. *Am J Hosp Pharm.* 1983;40:1016–1019.

Note: Page locators followed by f and t indicate figures and tables respectively.